Occupational Therapy and Mental Health

For Churchill Livingstone:

Editorial Director (Health Professions): Mary Law
Project Development Manager: Dinah Thom
Project Manager: Derek Robertson

www.harcourt-international.com

Bringing you products from all Harcourt Health Sciences companies including Baillière Tindall, Churchill Livingstone, Mosby and W.B. Saunders

..., journals and

NHS Sta   St James's

This

▸ **Search for information** on over 20 000 published titles with full product information including tables of contents and sample chapters

▸ **Keep up to date** with our extensive publishing programme in your field by registering with **eAlert** or requesting postal updates

▸ **Secure online ordering** with prompt delivery, as well as full contact details to order by phone, fax or post

▸ **News** of special features and promotions

If you are based in the following countries, please visit the country-specific site to receive full details of product availability and local ordering information

USA: www.harcourthealth.com

Canada: www.harcourtcanada.com

Australia: www.harcourt.com.au

 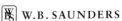
Baillière Tindall   CHURCHILL LIVINGSTONE   Mosby   W.B. SAUNDERS

Occupational Therapy and Mental Health

Edited by

Jennifer Creek DipCOT
Freelance Occupational Therapist,
North Yorkshire

THIRD EDITION

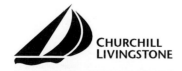
CHURCHILL
LIVINGSTONE

EDINBURGH LONDON NEW YORK PHILADELPHIA ST LOUIS SYDNEY TORONTO 2002

CHURCHILL LIVINGSTONE
An imprint of Harcourt Publishers Limited

© Longman Group UK Limited 1990
© Pearson Professional Limited 1997
© Harcourt Publishers Limited 2002

First published 1990
Second edition 1997
Third edition 2002

ISBN 0443 06447 4

British Library Cataloguing in Publication Data
A catalogue record for this book is available from the British
Library

Library of Congress Cataloging in Publication Data
A catalog record for this book is available from the Library
of Congress

Note
Medical knowledge is constantly changing. As new
information becomes available, changes in treatment,
procedures, equipment and the use of drugs become
necessary. The editor, contributors and the publishers have
taken care to ensure that the information given in this text is
accurate and up-to-date. However, readers are strongly
advised to confirm that the information, especially with
regard to drug usage, complies with the latest legislation
and standards of practice.

The
Publisher's
policy is to use
**paper manufactured
from sustainable forests**

Printed in China

Contents

Contributors

Lynne Barr MBA DipCOT SROT
Director of Occupational Therapy and Orthotics
Services, Occupational Therapy Department,
South Cleveland Hospital, Middlesbrough

Sheena E. E. Blair MEd DipCOT
Senior Lecturer/Course Leader, Department of
Occupational Therapy and Art Therapy, Queen
Margaret University College, Edinburgh

Mary Booth BSc(Hons) DipCOT
Head Occupational Therapist, Tees and North
East Yorkshire NHS Trust, Middlesbrough

Hazel Bracegirdle MSc BA DipCOT PGCE
Lecturer in Psychology, Ridge Danyers College,
Stockport

Sarah Burton DipCOT
Senior I/Head III Occupational Therapist,
Ridgeway Community Mental Healthcare Trust,
Tindal Centre, Aylesbury

John Chacksfield DipCOT PGCE
Head Occupational Therapist, Forensic Services,
John Howard Centre, Hackney, London

Sarah Cook MEd DipCOT
Lecturer/PhD student, University of Sheffield,
Sheffield

Jennifer Creek DipCOT
Freelance Occupational Therapist,
North Yorkshire

Sheila Dudley SRN RMN
Directorate Manager, Adult Mental Health,
Tameside General Hospital,
Ashton-under-Lyne

Linda Finlay PhD BA(Hons) DipCOT
Associate Lecturer, Open University,
Scarborough, North Yorkshire

Anne Fleming BSc DipCOT
Head II Occupational Therapist, Forth Valley
Primary Care NHS Trust, Larbert

Marjorie Gardner BSc(Hons) DipCOT MA
Freelance Occupational Therapist,
West Yorkshire

Saroj Gujral MBA DipOT DMS
Freelance Consultant, Surrey

Clephane A. Hume MTh BA DipCOT CertFE
Honorary Secretary, World Federation of
Occupational Therapists, Edinburgh

Lily I. H. Jeffrey FCOT SROT UCCAP
Occupational Therapy Manager,
West Lothian Healthcare NHS Trust,
St John's Hospital, Livingston

Valerie Johnstone BSc SROT
Senior I Occupational Therapist,
Northumberland Mental Health NHS Trust,
Occupational Therapy Department,
St George's Hospital, Morpeth

Anne Joice DipCOT
Divisional Head of Profession: Occupational
Therapy in Mental Health, Florence Street
Resource Centre, Glasgow

Jenny Lancaster DipCOT
Senior I Occupational Therapist, BKCW Mental
Health Trust, Substance Misuse Service, London

Penny Lewis MSc DipCOT
Quality Assurance Manager, Wonford House
Hospital, Exeter

Lesley Lougher BScSoc DipCOT
Community CAMHS Manager,
North West Anglia Healthcare NHS Trust

Mhairi McAughtrie DipCOT
Project Manager, Community Based Learning
Disability Services, Stirling Council

Jean J. Maclean MEd SROT CertFE
Fieldwork Coordinator, Department of
Occupational Therapy and Art Therapy, Queen
Margaret University College, Edinburgh

Lesley McNaughton BSc
formerly Senior Occupational Therapist,
Forth Valley Primary Care NHS Trust

Tom Miller
Senior Occupational Therapist,
Exmouth Community Mental Health Team,
North & East Devon Partnership NHS Trust,
Exmouth, Devon

Ruth Mitchell DipCOT
Senior I Occupational Therapist, Forth Valley
Primary Care NHS Trust, Larbert

The late **Gary Molden** BA(Hons) DipCOT
Senior Occupational Therapist, Tameside
General Hospital, Ashton-under-Lyne

Cathy Ormston
formerly Head of Occupational Therapy Services,
Northumberland Mental Health NHS Trust

Catherine F. Paterson MEd FCOT TDipCOT SROT
Director of Occupational Therapy,
Department of Occupational Therapy,
Robert Gordon University, Aberdeen

Jackie Pool DipCOT
Occupational Therapist, Dementia Concern,
Hampshire

Mary Roberts MSc DipCOT FETC
Assistant Team Manager, West Berkshire
Council Social Services, Theale

Alison Rogowski BPhil DipCOT SROT
Head Occupational Therapist, Forensic Services,
Frameside Clinic, Bristol

Kath Snowden DipCOT
Head III Occupational Therapist/Day Services
Manager, Tameside General Hospital,
Ashton-under-Lyne

Penny Spreadbury MBA DipCOT
Therapy Services Manager, Nottingham City
Hospital NHS Trust, Nottingham

Averil Stewart BA FCOT TDipCOT
Professor and Head of Department of
Occupational Therapy and Art Therapy,
Queen Margaret University College, Edinburgh

Ian E. Thompson BA(Hons) PhD
formerly Professor of Philosophy and Ethics,
University of Notre Dame Australia, Fremantle,
Western Australia

Tania Tulloch DipCOT SROT
Team Manager and Head Occupational
Therapist for Mental Health, Ripon

Jo Vaughan DipCOT
Senior I Community Occupational Therapist,
Tindal Centre, Aylesbury

Lynn Yarwood BSc DipCOT SROT
Head III Occupational Therapist,
Northumberland Mental Health NHS Trust,
Occupational Therapy Department, St George's
Hospital, Morpeth

Preface

During the past few years, the contexts in which occupational therapists practise have continued to change rapidly, but the profession has retained its capacity to evolve and fit into new systems and structures. Occupational therapy has always been a dynamic, flexible profession which appears to thrive on change and, even, adversity. The most exciting innovations can be seen in countries where occupational therapists are struggling to cope with underfunding, insecurity and overwhelming need.

Some of the contextual changes in the UK have been more comfortable than others for occupational therapists. For example, the National Service Framework for Mental Health provides guidelines which are mostly compatible with our professional philosophy, and the move, within social services, away from maintaining dependency towards an enabling culture allows us to use our skills to the full. On the other hand, the drive for practice to be based on sound evidence of effectiveness has, to some extent, caught us unprepared. Our research base is still inadequate and we struggle to demonstrate conclusively that our interventions do what we say they do.

Other recent influences on practice include the introduction of clinical governance, the move towards a primary care led health service, greater involvement of service users and carers in the planning and provision of services, a new focus on health improvement and pressure to work across professional and organisational boundaries in order to provide seamless care.

Occupational therapists have a concern with human function and a broad knowledge base that ensure we have a useful role in almost any health or social care context. The breadth of our domain of concern is one of our greatest strengths, but it is also a source of anxiety. We worry that other people – purchasers, service users and fellow professionals – do not fully understand the contribution we are able to make. As our field of practice has expanded, we have tried to articulate more clearly our core beliefs, values and skills, but there is still a need to strengthen our own awareness of what it is that makes occupational therapy unique.

During the past decade, we have moved beyond the need to define ourselves by models of practice and we are attempting to find theoretical frameworks which can encompass a more flexible, person-centred way of working. Occupational therapy is looking for a way to retain the art of practice alongside strengthening our scientific credibility. A development which supports this endeavour is the growth of occupational science. This is a new academic discipline which crosses disciplinary boundaries but will provide us with the theories of occupation that we need in order to understand the relationships between people, occupation and health and to develop the most effective interventions.

Preparing the third edition of *Occupational therapy and mental health* has been a challenging process. I have tried to retain what I see as the strengths of the previous two editions while incorporating new material to support students in developing the knowledge and skills they will require for practice in the modern world. This has led to an updating of all existing chapters and the inclusion of three new ones.

Section 1 covers aspects of occupational therapy philosophy and theory. Chapter 1, a short history of occupational therapy in mental health, sets the profession in its historical context, helping the reader to understand how it has evolved into the form that we see today. The chapter on health and wellness remains crucial in the light of the current concern with improving health rather than only treating disease. The chapter on the knowledge base of occupational therapy has been revised to incorporate recent developments in occupational therapy theory. The research chapter gives an overview of current issues in research rather than looking at specific methodologies.

Section 2 describes the occupational therapy process, from the frames of reference used through assessment and intervention to evaluation. Chapter 9 has been renamed 'Clinical governance' to reflect the updated content of the previous chapter on quality assurance and clinical audit.

Section 3 discusses the context of occupational therapy practice. Chapter 10, 'Roles and settings', has been completely rewritten, using more examples of occupational therapists at work so that the reader can see what influences the ways in which the therapist's role develops.

Section 4, 'Media and methods', gives a broad picture of how different media might be applied in practice. It is impossible to cover the full range of activities that the occupational therapist might use, but the chapters cover physical activity, cognitive approaches, groupwork, creative activities, skills training and the therapeutic use of play.

Section 5 includes chapters on working with 12 different client groups: acute, long-term, rehabilitation, older people, children and adolescents, people with learning disabilities, those in community care, primary care, people in a transcultural context, forensic, substance misusers and people suffering from loss and grief. It has been extensively revised to reflect the changes that have taken and are still taking place. Three new chapters have been added – primary care, substance misuse and loss and grief. Primary care is a very new area for mental health occupational therapy, so the chapter gives real examples of five different ways in which a mental health occupational therapy service has been introduced into a primary care setting.

Section 6 covers the organisation and management of occupational therapy services, including new chapters on management and budgeting. This section also incorporates a chapter on fieldwork education, since most therapists are likely to be involved in supervising students at some time in their career.

ACKNOWLEDGEMENTS

For this edition (and Chapter 25 in the second edition), Chapter 26 has been revised by Saroj Gujral. We are grateful to Clephane Hume for allowing some of her material from the first edition to be reused in these later editions.

Philosophy and theory base

1

A short history of occupational therapy in psychiatry

Catherine F. Paterson

INTRODUCTION

Although the concept of the therapeutic use of occupation dates back to antiquity, the term 'occupational therapy' was not coined until early in the 20th century, and the first training course in the UK was not started until 1930. The study of the history of occupational therapy helps to put into perspective both the achievements and the limitations of the profession, and provides a clearer understanding of its philosophy and potential. Occupational therapy has been developed in many different areas of practice, but only the history of occupational therapy in the field of mental health is reviewed here. However, it can only be considered in the wider context of the social and medical history of psychiatry, and the development of the profession as a whole.

This chapter briefly surveys some of the earliest references to occupation as treatment, explores the moral movement in psychiatry in the late 18th and early 19th centuries, discusses the contribution of psychiatrists Adolf Meyer, David Henderson and Elizabeth Casson to the founding of the profession of occupational therapy, and identifies some of the major developments in psychiatry and occupational therapy in the 20th century. Finally, there is a brief discussion of the professional organisations, training and state registration which are important to the professionalisation of occupational therapy.

PSYCHIATRY AND OCCUPATION BEFORE THE 19TH CENTURY

Throughout history, the social and medical care of the mentally ill has been dependent on public attitudes and medical opinion of the times. What constitutes 'normal' and 'abnormal' behaviour, and what is considered 'mad' or 'bad' has varied throughout the ages. Beliefs about the causes of mental illness have had a significant influence on the way sufferers have been treated. Prevailing ideas of causation have included possession by evil spirits, over-stimulation of the senses, brain disease, genetic inheritance, psychological trauma and faulty biochemistry. Finally, the national economy and society's willingness to pay have dictated limitations to the provision of services. Consequently the therapeutic use of occupation has fluctuated in relation to social, medical and economic factors.

From the very earliest surviving manuscripts and throughout the ages, both in Eastern and in Western culture, we find reference to the belief that occupation in the form of exercise, work, recreation and amusements can both influence and be used to improve mental and physical health and well-being. The Greek physician Hippocrates, in the 4th century BC, taught that the brain was the seat of the mind and described how mental health depended on a balance of four bodily humours, blood, choler, phlegm and bile (Digby 1985). Galen, the most influential of the Roman physicians, followed the methods of Hippocrates, especially when mental aberrations occurred in the course of somatic disease. Seigel (1973) outlined Galen's psychotherapeutic concepts, stating: 'Since he treated mostly well-to-do patients, he advised good nursing care; demanded kindness with the emotionally ill; employed as physical methods hydrotherapy, showers, sweating, local application of heat and sunbathing. . . . In milder cases he recommended travel, occupational therapy and, for the educated, an increasing participation in lectures, discussions, reading and in pastime creative activities.'

While the idea that madness was caused by evil spirits, witchcraft, sin or divine intervention dominated popular thinking throughout the Dark and Middle Ages, physicians in Europe continued to accept Hippocrates' and Galen's explanation of the humoral basis of madness well into the 18th century.

In Britain at that time, the rich person with a mental illness would likely be attended at home by a physician or placed in a private 'madhouse'. On the other hand, the 'mad' poor were most likely to be treated no differently from other social deviants, being classed with the destitute, vagrants and criminals. Some were incarcerated in prisons or workhouses, or in one of the few hospitals for pauper patients, such as Bethlem Hospital in London (Dickenson 1990). The conditions in which the mentally ill were kept, whether at home or in an institution, usually included the use of physical restraint, often by manacles and chains. There was usually no heat or lighting, little food, clothing, bedding or sanitation, no segregation of the violent from the quiet and withdrawn, and no meaningful occupation. There was even wrongful confinement, by their relatives, of people who were not in fact mentally ill. Traditional medical remedies were aimed at reestablishing humoral balance and included special diets, bleeding, purging, emetics and blistering, often on a seasonal basis (Jones 1972).

Eventually scandals, changes in public opinion and the example of a few asylums run on humanitarian principles led to a period of reform. Of particular significance was the Act of 1808 and the Select Committee of 1815–16. The Act, for 'the better Care and Maintenance of Lunatics, being Paupers or Criminals, in England', laid down detailed specifications for the construction and maintenance of county asylums, and the Select Committee investigated allegations of maltreatment in public institutions of the insane (Jones 1972). However, the transformation of the treatment of pauper lunatics made slow progress until the great expansion of the county asylum system in the 1840s (Walton 1981).

PSYCHIATRY AND OCCUPATION IN THE 19TH CENTURY

The moral movement

At the beginning of the 19th century, the two asylums most celebrated for introducing reforms were the Bicêtre in Paris, under Dr Philippe Pinel (1745–1826), and the York Retreat, founded by layman William Tuke (1732–1822). Pinel and Tuke became internationally acclaimed for their introduction of moral treatment for the mentally ill, that is, psychological rather than physical treatment.

Pinel was appointed to the medical staff of the Bicêtre in 1794, during the French Revolution, when the institution housed upwards of 200 male patients, who were regarded not only as incurable but also as extremely dangerous. Instead of blows and chains he introduced light and fresh air, cleanliness, workshops and areas for walking, but above all kindliness and understanding (Batchelor 1975). Pinel wrote in his 1806 treatise on insanity (Pinel 1962):

It is no longer a problem to be solved, . . . that in all public asylums as well as prisons and hospitals, the surest, and perhaps, the only method of securing health, good order, and good manners, is to carry into decided and habitual execution the natural law of bodily labour, so contributive and essential to human happiness. . . . I am convinced that no useful and durable establishments . . . can be founded excepting on the basis of interesting and laborious employment.

William Tuke and the Society of Friends founded the Retreat at York in 1796 on the Quaker principles of compassion and humanity. The central emphasis was on trying to help the patient gain enough self-discipline to master his illness. To this end it was thought important to create a comfortable, domestic environment in which the patient could experience normal civilised daily living conditions, which would help the process of self-control. Anne Digby (1985) summarised the regime as follows:

The need to balance the emotions and distract the patient from painful thoughts and associations led to the central feature of the moral therapy: the creation of varied employment and amusements. The key to moral treatment lay in the quality of personal relationships between staff and patients. This is what makes the term moral treatment so elusive, and also made the treatment so difficult to translate successfully from the Retreat to other institutions in the mid-nineteenth century.

By 1839 it was reported that patients at the Retreat were cultivating a 2-acre field with potatoes and turnips under the supervision of an attendant employed for the purpose. There were also attempts to occupy the patients along the lines of their former posts; a surveyor's assistant made a survey of the estate, while a watch repairer and a carpenter were employed in their customary tasks. By 1844 two carpenter's shops had been set up to provide a greater variety of occupation for men. There were also opportunities for convalescent patients to go shopping or attend meetings in York, or to take tea with local Quakers. Some patients looked after kittens and birds, while others found pleasure in the grounds. Outdoor amusements were also available, from helping in the hayfield, to archery or cricket. At Christmas, the carol singers visited the Retreat, and, on Plough Monday, the Morris dancers. Indeed, Digby reported that the Lunacy Commissioners commented in 1847 that 'every means of amusement and occupation appear to be provided for the patients' (Digby 1985).

Although Pinel and Tuke are most frequently credited with the introduction of moral treatment, there were other asylum superintendents at the beginning of the 19th century who were particularly interested in the therapeutic use of occupation as part of a humane regime of care. These included William Hallaran (1765–1825), the first physician of the Cork Asylum, Sir William C. Ellis (1780–1839), medical superintendent of the Hanwell Hospital, and William A. F. Brown (1805–1885), the first medical superintendent of the Crichton Institution at Dumfries.

Hallaran published a book in 1810 in which he laid stress 'On the Cure of Insanity', especially by suitable occupation for 'the convalescent maniac', combining 'corporeal action, with the regular employment of the mind'. He was the first physician to recognise the danger of institutional neurosis and gave the first account of the benefit derived from being allow to paint (Box 1.1). He concluded that this case proved the need to introduce a systematic arrangement of daily labour which could help convalescent patients to become once more useful members of society (Hunter & MacAlpine 1963).

Another of the early medical superintendents who championed the use of occupation was William Ellis. Ellis was appointed to the newly opened Wakefield Asylum in 1818, with his wife as matron. He later became medical superintendent at Hanwell (later St Bernard's Hospital, Southall), where he paved the way for his successor, John Conolly (1794–1866), renowned for the abolition of all physical restraint (Hunter & MacAlpine 1963). Samuel Tuke (1841), grandson of William Tuke, credited Ellis with:

the first extensive and successful experiment to introduce labour systematically into our public asylums. He carried it out . . . with a skill, vigour, and kindliness towards the patients which were alike

---

Box 1.1   From W. Hallaran, On the Cure of Insanity (1810)

A young man . . . came under my care in a state of acute mania, and continued so full three months without remission. The symptoms having at length given way, he was treated as a convalescent patient, and every means tried to encourage him to some light work, merely as a pastime, but all to no purpose. Though the maniacal appearances had totally subsided, he still betrayed an imbecility of mind and bordered closely on dementia, and it was found impossible to excite in him the smallest interest . . . when by accident he was discovered in the act of amusing himself, with some rude colouring, on the walls of his apartment. . . . He was questioned as to his knowledge of drawing, and he, having signified some acquaintance with that art, was immediately promised colours of a better description, if he would undertake to use them. This evidently gave immediate cheerfulness to his countenance, . . . he immediately commenced a systematic combination of colours, having completed his arrangements, he requested one of the attendants to sit for him. . . . The portrait was an exact representation of the person who sat before him, and in a few days there were several other proofs of his skill in this line, which bore testimony to his ability. He soon became elated with the approbation he had met with, and continued to employ himself in this manner for nearly two months after, with progressive improvement as to his mental faculties, when he was dismissed cured. (Hallaran 1810, reprinted in Hunter & MacAlpine 1963.)

---

creditable to his understanding and his heart. He proved, that there was less danger from putting the spade and the hoe into the hands of a large proportion of insane persons, than from shutting them up together in idleness, though under the guards of straps, strait-waistcoats, or chains. (Tuke, cited by Hunter & MacAlpine 1963)

While the men at Hanwell were encouraged either to follow their own trade or to learn a new one, Lady Ellis organised the female patients under a 'workwoman' to make 'useful and fancy articles' which were sold at bazaars and outside the asylum:

She borrowed of the treasurer twenty-three pounds eighteen shillings; this she laid out in the purchase of a few articles in the first instance as patterns, and in buying the requisite materials. These are made up and worked by the patients, and sold by the workwomen to visitors at the bazaar, or are sent off to order. The scheme has answered beyond the most sanguine expectations . . . It is hardly possible to conceive the benefit the patients derived from this employment. (Ellis 1838, reprinted in Hunter & MacAlpine 1963)

The foremost of the moral physicians in Scotland was W. A. F. Browne. His first position was as medical superintendent at the Montrose Asylum, where in 1837 he wrote an influential treatise entitled 'What asylums were, are and aught to be'. He wrote extensively on the prescription of occupation:

It is not enough to have the insane playing the part of busy automatons, or to wear out their muscular energies vicariously, in order to relieve the drooping heart of its load. There must be an active, and, if possible, intelligent and willing participation on the part of the labourer, and such portion of interest, amusement, and mental exertion associated with the labour, that neither lassitude not fatigue may follow. The more elevated, the more useful the description of the occupation provided then, the better. (Browne 1837)

Browne was able to put many of his ideas into practice in the establishment of the well-endowed Crichton Institution in Dumfries, where the use of occupations is well recorded in all the annual reports. He appointed a superintendent of outdoor recreations and a superintendent of the workroom, where they made not only the 'usual articles of bed and body clothing', but also 'articles of embroidery and fancy work'.

Growth of the asylums in the 19th century

The Victorian era in Britain was characterised by the building of large public asylums on the outskirts of every large town in response to the legislation of 1808 for the 'better care and maintenance of lunatics'. Many of these asylums became the mental hospitals which were later closed or contracted in response to the Care in the Community legislation of the 1990s. These institutions were, themselves, the product of social reforms, at a time when the urban industrialised working class in Britain lived in conditions of squalor and grinding poverty (Jones 1972).

However, the optimism that cures could be effected through treatment in an asylum could not be sustained. Patients became quieter and more manageable but most were still unable to return to their former situations. The success of the asylums led to the admission of more and more inmates, so that their very size – many containing 2000 or more patients – made them the antithesis of the domestic surroundings necessary for treatment on moral principles. Many asylums found it impossible to attract the number and calibre of attendants required to manage disturbed patients without resorting to measures of restraint. Thus, during the latter half of the 19th century, the individualised prescription of occupation gave way to the widespread use of the physically fit patients for work in the kitchens, laundry, farm and gardens of the asylums, as much for economic as for therapeutic reasons (Jones 1972).

DEVELOPMENTS IN THE 20TH CENTURY

Institutionalisation and deinstitutionalisation

At the turn of the last century, the most important influences on psychiatry were the theories of Sigmund Freud (1856–1939) and his associates Alfred Adler (1870–1937) and Carl Jung (1875–1961), who developed psychoanalysis and psychotherapy. Although these new disciplines had a significant influence on the way people thought about mental processes, and on consulting room practice, they had little effect on regimes within British asylums. Denis Martin (1968) described asylums as benignly authoritarian, in that the satisfactory running of the hospital depended on the submission of the patients to authority with the minimum of resistance. Methods of dealing with those who were unable to submit included locked doors, various forms of mechanical restraint, segregation of the sexes, heavy sedation, electroconvulsive therapy, prolonged sleep and prefrontal leucotomy, which were administered as treatment but which could be perceived or even used as punishment. However, the same authority was benevolent since the hospital provided security and met the patients' physical needs, so that the final result was 'institutionalisation' (Martin 1968). During the early part of the 20th century, conditions remained largely unchanged in the hospitals. However, the move beyond the asylum can be traced back to the changes in practice during the First World War, when the problem of shellshock required a new response to mental distress (Stone 1985). The Mental Treatment Act of 1930 provided a further impetus for the development of outpatient clinics and after-care services as well as admission of patients on a voluntary basis (Jones 1972). The 1950s saw the introduction of the first effective antipsychotic and antidepressant drugs and the beginnings of a sustained debate about the legitimacy of custodial care. The criticisms were led by psychiatrists Ronald Laing, David Cooper and Thomas Szasz – collectively dubbed 'antipsychiatrists' – and by Erving Goffman, whose seminal work *Asylums*, published in 1961, drew attention to the dangers of the 'total institution' (Pilgrim & Rogers 1993). The ideological and financial pressures on the psychiatric hospitals, together with the advent of effective medication, facilitated the deinstitutionalisation movement which began slowly in the 1960s and finally gained momentum with the Care in the Community legislation in the 1990s. The widespread reliance on drugs to control symptoms also reestablished the somatic basis of mental illness as the dominant view.

The beginning of the profession of occupational therapy in the USA

At the end of the 19th century, in the USA as in Britain, the asylums were suffering from overcrowding and economic pressures. However, there was a resurgence of interest in reform and in structuring the patient's day in a more productive manner. A major influence on psychiatry on both sides of the Atlantic was Dr Adolf Meyer (1866–1950), who emigrated from Switzerland to America in 1892. According to Rowe & Mink (1993), Meyer viewed mental illness as the outcome of a person's maladaptive interaction with the environment. His emphasis on objective observation of patient behaviour and on habit was compatible with the psychology of learning that was being developed by American psychologists, and his views anticipated the biopsychosocial model currently adopted by many psychiatrists (Rowe & Mink 1993).

As early as 1892 Meyer observed that 'the proper use of time in some helpful and gratifying activity appeared to me a fundamental issue in the treatment of any neuropsychiatric patient'. In 1895, Meyer's wife, a social worker, introduced a systematic type of activity into the wards of the state institution in Worcester, Massachusetts, so that: 'A pleasure in achievement, a real pleasure in the use and activity of one's hands and muscles and a happy appreciation of time began to be used as incentives in the management of our patients.' Meyer considered that:

The whole of human organization has its shape in a kind of rhythm. . . . night and day, of sleep and waking hours, of hunger and its gratification . . . work and play and rest and sleep, which our organism must be able to balance even under difficulty. The only way to attain balance in all this is actual doing, actual practice, a program of wholesome living as the basis of wholesome feeling and thinking and fancy and interests. (Meyer 1922, reprinted 1977)

Meyer is generally regarded as one of the founders of occupational therapy in the USA, along with other professionals who were developing the use of occupation quite independently. These were Susan E. Tracy, a nurse, Eleanor Clarke Slagle, a social worker, William Rush Dunton Jnr, another psychiatrist, and finally Thomas B. Kidner and George Barton, who both originally trained as architects. Barton became an advocate after his own illness, when he experienced the beneficial effects of directed occupation. He founded an institution in Clifton Springs, where people with chronic ill health could be retrained or adjusted to gainful living by means of occupation. It is Barton who is credited with introducing the term 'occupational therapy' at a meeting in 1914, and it was at Clifton Springs in 1917 that the National Society for the Promotion of Occupational Therapy was formed, with Barton as its first president. In 1923, the name was changed to the American Occupational Therapy Association (Licht 1967).

The beginning of the profession of occupational therapy in Scotland

Professor Sir David K. Henderson (1884–1965) (Fig. 1.1), a prominent Scottish psychiatrist during the first half of the 20th century, was much

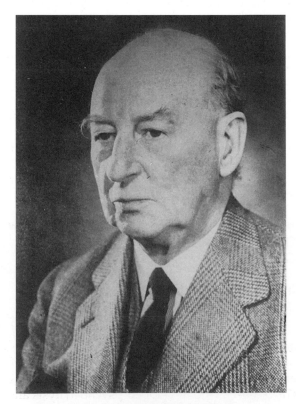

Figure 1.1   Professor Sir David K. Henderson.

influenced by Meyer, with whom he had worked in New York and Baltimore. On returning to Scotland, Henderson's first position was at the Gartnavel Royal Hospital in Glasgow (Figs 1.2, 1.3), where he employed, in 1922, Dorothea Robertson, the first instructress in occupational therapy in Britain (Henderson 1925). Miss Robertson, although a graduate of Cambridge University, did not have the benefit of any training in occupational therapy, but within months, she had made sufficient impact that the Commissioners of the General Board of Control for Scotland reported that:

For many years the advantages of farm and garden work for men and domestic work for women have been recognised from curative and ameliorative aspects and many patients have been so employed. There are, however, many patients not physically fitted for these strenuous labours or whose mental disorder such, for instance, as epilepsy, requires that they be under constant supervision. In all such cases the occupational therapy is being tried with excellent results. Patients were seen under a competent instructress making, baskets, toys, rugs, etc. So successful has the treatment been that it is proposed to erect a special building within the grounds of the establishment where manifold light occupations can be carried out. (General Board of Control for Scotland 1923)

Henderson considered that mental disorder, whatever its underlying reason, resulted in patients being unable to adapt. This made patients, for the time being, social failures, and that no matter how they attempted to compensate, their innermost reaction was one of hopelessness. In a lecture to the Scottish Division of the Medico-Psychological Association in 1924, Henderson emphasised that:

there is nothing which will sooner and more satisfactorily increase a person's self-esteem than his ability to accomplish something . . . It is therefore our duty to attempt to establish well co-ordinated, purposeful ways of doing things, instead of idleness, apathy, or inadequate reaction. We must plan and organise our patient's day, so that adequate time is provided for work and rest and play, so that interests are stimulated, and to borrow a word from Meyer – exteriorized. Even although the patient has been a failure in the world at large, we must attempt to make him a success in the hospital environment. (Henderson 1925)

Henderson was an influential figure in the development of occupational therapy in Scotland, particularly in his encouragement of the founding of the Scottish Association of Occupational Therapy in 1932, and in the

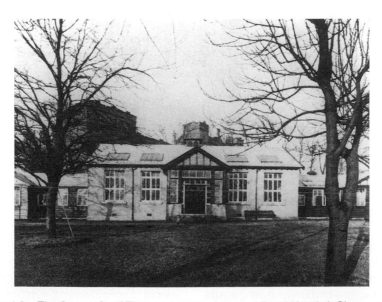

Figure 1.2   The Occupational Therapy Pavilion, Gartnavel Royal Hospital, Glasgow, 1923.

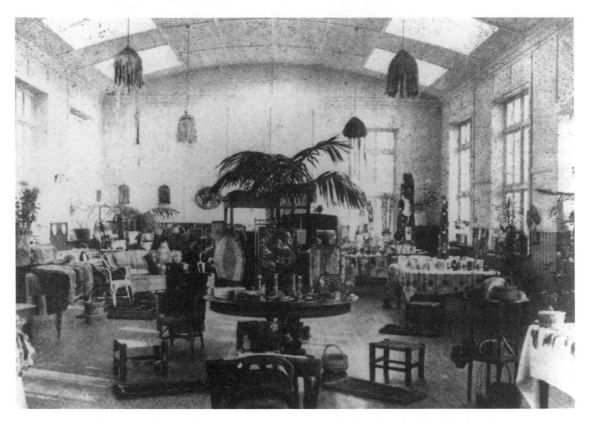

Figure 1.3 The interior of the Occupational Therapy Pavilion, Gartnavel Royal Hospital, Glasgow.

reconstitution of the Association after the war in 1946, when he became its president (Groundes Peace 1957).

The first qualified occupational therapist to work in Britain was Margaret Barr Fulton (1900–1989) (Fig. 1.4), who became interested in occupational therapy during a holiday in the USA and who trained in Philadelphia. At first, Miss Fulton found it difficult to find a position; however, she was eventually given an introduction to Henderson in Glasgow. Unable to employ her himself, Henderson referred her to a former colleague, Dr R. Dods Brown, medical superintendent of the Royal Aberdeen Mental Hospital, who secured her services immediately.

In 1929, Dods Brown published an article entitled 'Some observations on the treatment of mental diseases' in which he gave a description of occupational therapy, which was based in an army hut erected in the grounds of his hospital.

His paper was illustrated with case material, including the reports in Box 1.2.

Following the appointment of Miss Robertson and Miss Fulton, it appears that many Scottish mental hospitals followed suit in appointing instructresses in arts and crafts, most of whom held art college diplomas. By 1932, there were eleven such ladies who, under the direction of Miss Fulton, and with the encouragement of Dr Henderson, formed themselves into the Scottish Association of Occupational Therapy (SAOT) (Groundes Peace 1957).

Although Miss Fulton continued to work at the Royal Aberdeen Mental Hospital until her retirement in 1963, her influence was considerable both throughout Scotland and worldwide in her capacity as one of the founders in 1952 of the World Federation of Occupational Therapists and as its first president.

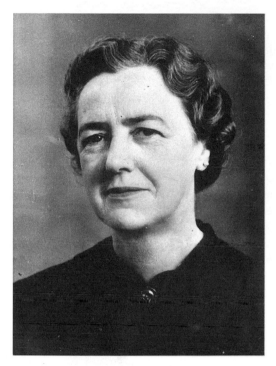

Figure 1.4   Miss Margaret Barr Fulton MBE.

The beginning of the profession of occupational therapy in England

Among the delegates at the conference where Henderson described the occupational therapy department at the Gartnavel Royal Hospital in 1924 was Dr Elizabeth Casson (1881–1954) (Fig. 1.5), who was also destined to play an important role in the development of occupational therapy in Britain. Casson qualified as one of the first women doctors at Bristol in 1919, and chose to specialise in psychological medicine. In 1926, while on holiday in America she visited an occupational therapy department at Bloomingdale Hospital, New York, and the Boston School of Occupational Therapy, where the idea of an English school on similar lines was implanted in her mind (Casson 1955).

At that time Casson was employed at the Holloway Sanatorium, where there was a tradition of many forms of occupation including games, entertainments, competitions and the annual sports. One of the instructresses, Alice Constance Tebbit (1906–1976), later Mrs Glyn Owens, obtained a scholarship at the

Box 1.2   From Dods Brown, Some Observations on the Treatment of Mental Diseases

A man, aged 69, had been in hospital for several months, during which time he did not improve. He spoke to no-one, and would not employ himself in any way. He seemed to be deteriorating rapidly, and to be passing into dementia. He was sent to 'The Hut' every day, but for more than a week he showed not the slightest interest in anything he saw nor what was said to him. Later he was induced to do a little sandpapering, which he did in an entirely mechanical way. After a time he was given a fret saw to use, and this seemed to arouse some interest in him. As the days passed it was apparent that his interest was growing more and more, not only in the work, but also in his personal appearance, because one day he objected to the sawdust getting on his clothes. As time went on he was given more difficult work to do, and in this he became thoroughly interested and indeed enthusiastic, and when his discharge was being discussed, he was reluctant to leave the institution. He made a thoroughly good recovery.

A woman who had been in a depressed, and somewhat agitated condition, and who had maintained almost complete silence for about two years, and who, on account of delusions of unworthiness, had refused her food, and had been tube-fed for several months, was put to the occupational therapy department. From that time she began to converse, and to take an interest in things outside herself. She improved steadily and rapidly, and was discharged recovered. (Dods Brown 1929.)

Philadelphia School of Occupational Therapy and qualified in 1929 (Casson 1955).

By this time, Casson had fulfilled her ambition of founding a residential clinic for women psychiatric patients at Dorset House in Bristol, to which was attached the first school of occupational therapy in the UK, which opened on 1 January 1930 with Miss Tebbit as its first principal. The school later moved to Dorset House in Oxford, where it is now part of the Oxford Brookes University. At the Bristol clinic, Dr Casson:

decided to establish a treatment centre where each patient's daily life would be so planned that it fitted the individual's need like a well tailored garment. She planned that each member of the household, whether patient or staff, should feel an integral part of the whole and each would contribute, according to capacity, to the welfare of the whole. There would be no sharp social or professional distinctions between members of staff and every patient would be made to eradicate any unnecessary dividing line between the

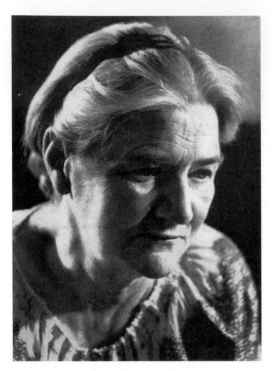

Figure 1.5 Dr Elizabeth Casson OBE.

patients and the staff. In this community everyone would be essential and therefore would feel valued and valuable. (Owens, 1955)

These last sentiments anticipated the concept of the therapeutic community developed after the Second World War by Maxwell Jones and Denis Martin. Early in the 1930s, there was a 6-month course at the Maudsley Hospital for state registered nurses for training in occupation work (Board of Control 1933), and schools of occupational therapy were opened in Edinburgh in 1937 and in Liverpool in 1946.

Dr Casson was a source of inspiration and encouragement to occupational therapists throughout her life, which is commemorated by the Casson Memorial Lecture delivered at the annual conference of the College of Occupational Therapists.

Associations of occupational therapy

While the Scottish Association of Occupational Therapy (SAOT) had been formed in 1932, the Association of Occupational Therapists (AOT), covering the rest of the UK, had its inaugural meeting in 1935, when Mrs Owens was elected chairman. In the few years leading up to the Second World War, the Association organised the first national examinations in occupational therapy and launched its *Journal* (Hume & Lock 1982). From 1939 to 1945 the Association was immersed in the war effort, including the organisation of shortened courses for occupational therapy auxiliaries for the military hospitals, and the development of a realistic form of treatment in the physical field. Evelyn Mary Macdonald (1905–1993), a recent graduate at the time and later principal of Dorset House recalled that:

While Occupational Therapy was receiving this impetus in the physical field, the work in mental hospitals was sadly curtailed. Departments were taken over for emergency beds, materials were difficult to obtain and priority of supplies went to hospitals dealing with physically disabled civilian and service cases. The Occupational Therapists doing psychological work struggled on bravely . . . It is interesting to note the trends in occupations at this time. In the physical field the choice was controlled largely by the materials made available through the special government priority system. These were mainly those for 'handicrafts' – in some cases almost too light and diversional in the eyes of keen therapists. A second controlling factor was that the occupations were deliberately limited by the government to 'crafts' and excursions in the realms of trade were not permitted. In the psychological field, however, the Occupational Therapists, without the materials required for much of the usual craft work, turned the patients' interests to other and what might be termed more realistic occupations. This was in fact a progressive step and these are proving useful and acceptable in the treatment in both fields to-day. (Macdonald 1957)

After the war, in 1948, the whole management of health care services was revolutionised by the formation of the National Health Service, when responsibility for all psychiatric services, except some small homes, became a national rather than a local authority responsibility, with services being free at the point of delivery. Most occupational therapists became employees of the NHS.

A commission was soon set up to consider the staffing and training requirements of the new service, and representatives of the AOT and SAOT became involved in protracted negotiations with the Ministry of Health and the British Medical Association (BMA) on how occupational therapy should be regulated. The BMA wanted to continue to control the 'auxiliary professions', including occupational therapy, while the professions themselves wanted autonomy. The outcome was a compromise. The Professions Supplementary to Medicine (CPSM) Act (1960) provided for boards for each of the eight professions, regulated by a council responsible to the Privy Council. The boards and council had strong medical representation, albeit not sufficient to outvote the professions (Mendez 1978).

The Act was significant in that it recognised the need for properly qualified and registered occupational therapists to work in the NHS ; and the Occupational Therapists Board recognised the diplomas of the two associations as qualifications for entry to the Register. The CPSM is being replaced by the Health Professions Council in April 2002.

In 1952, Mrs Owens, then Principal of the Liverpool School, hosted a meeting to form the World Federation of Occupational Therapists (WFOT). The constitution drawn up required that the AOT and SAOT should be jointly represented on the WFOT Council, which led to the Joint Council of the Associations of Occupational Therapy in the UK. Cooperation between the two associations inevitably led to amalgamation and to the formation of the British Association of Occupational Therapists in 1974 (Hume & Lock 1982).

One of the outcomes of this amalgamation was revision of occupational therapy training, particularly the phasing out of the national diploma examinations, a system which had become unwieldy with increasing numbers of students. The new system of validation of courses paved the way for the development of degree courses, the first being approved in Belfast and Edinburgh in 1986. By 1994 there were 30 pre-registration courses, mostly in universities, and the profession had achieved all-graduate entry.

SUMMARY

Historically, the use of occupation as an integral aspect of treatment has fluctuated in relation to prevailing ideas about the causes of mental illness and other social and political factors. Of particular importance was the moral treatment developed in small asylums in the early 19th century, where individualised programmes of work and leisure and good interpersonal relationships between staff and patients were paramount.

From the inspiration of three psychiatrists and a handful of remarkable pioneering occupational therapists, the profession in Britain has developed in the relatively short period of 70 years, with over 20 000 occupational therapists being registered in 2000. Having been involved in the treatment of the most intractable patients before the introduction of effective drugs in the 1950s and the gradual deinstitutionalisation of patients since then, the profession has an even greater challenge in the new millennium. Occupational therapists have demonstrated the contribution they can make to the independence of people with physical disabilities in the community: with the closure of the psychiatric hospitals they need to be proactive in the provision of effective services for people with mental health problems in the community. Occupational therapists should continue to be mindful of the humanistic ideals on which the profession was founded: the belief in the therapeutic value of occupation, and the need for satisfying interpersonal relationships and balance in the daily routines of work, self-care and leisure.

REFERENCES

Batchelor I R C 1975 Henderson and Gillespie's textbook of psychiatry. Oxford University Press, London

Board of Control 1933 Memorandum on occupation therapy for mental patients. HMSO, London

Browne W A F 1837 What asylums were, are and aught to be. Reprinted in: Scull A 1991 The asylum as Utopia: W A F Browne and the mid-nineteenth century consolidation of psychiatry. Tavistock/Routledge, London

Casson E 1955 How the Dorset House School of Occupational Therapy came into being. Occupational Therapy 18(3): 92–94

Dickenson E 1990 From madness to mental health: a brief history of psychiatric treatments in the UK from 1800 to the present. British Journal of Occupational Therapy 53(10): 419–424

Digby A 1985 Moral treatment at the Retreat, 1796–1846. In: Bynum W, Porter R, Shepherd M (eds) The anatomy of madness: essays on the history of psychiatry. Tavistock, London

Dods Brown R 1929 Some observations on the treatment of mental diseases. Edinburgh Medical Journal 36(11): 657–686

General Board of Control for Scotland 1923 Tenth Annual Report. HMSO, Edinburgh

Groundes Peace Z 1957 An outline of the development of occupational therapy in Scotland. Scottish Journal of Occupational Therapy 30: 16–43

Henderson D K 1925 Occupational therapy. Journal of Mental Science 71(292): 59–73

Hume C A, Lock S J 1982 The Golden Jubilee, 1932–1982: an historical survey. British Journal of Occupational Therapy 45(5): 151–153

Hunter R, MacAlpine I 1963 Three hundred years of psychiatry, 1535–1860. Oxford University Press, London

Jones K 1972 A history of the mental health services. Routledge and Kegan Paul, London

Licht S 1967 The founding and founders of the American Occupational Therapy Association. American Journal of Occupational Therapy 21(5): 269–277

Macdonald E M 1957 History of the Association Chapter IV, 1942–1945. Occupational Therapy June: 30–33

Martin D V 1968 Adventure in psychiatry. Bruno Cassirer, Oxford

Mendez M A 1978 Dr Elizabeth Casson Memorial Lecture. Processes of change: some speculations for the future. British Journal of Occupational Therapy 41(7): 225–228

Meyer A 1922 The philosophy of occupation therapy. Archives of Occupational Therapy. 1: 1–10. Reprinted in: American Journal of Occupational Therapy 1977 31(10): 639–642

Owens C 1955 Recollections, 1925–1933. Occupational Therapy 18(3): 95–97

Pilgrim D, Rogers A 1993 A sociology of mental health and illness. Open University Press, Buckingham

Pinel P 1962 A treatise on insanity, trans. D D Davis. Hafner, New York [first published 1806]

Rowe C J, Mink W D 1993 An outline of psychiatry. Brown and Benchmark, Madison

Seigel R E 1973 Galen on psychology, psychopathology, and function and diseases of the nervous system. S Karger, Basel

Walton J 1981 The treatment of pauper lunatics in Victorian England: the case of the Lancaster Asylum, 1816–1870. In: Scull A Madhouses, mad-doctors and madmen: the social history of psychiatry in the Victorian era. Athlone Press, London

2

Health, wellness and occupation

Sheena E. E. Blair
Clephane A. Hume

INTRODUCTION

It is fitting that a book which is concerned with occupational therapy and mental health acknowledges the contribution which the profession can make towards understanding and promoting a state of health and well-being. However, in the third edition of this book, and in revisiting this chapter, the need to amend the chapter title to include the word occupation seemed overdue. This perhaps reflects the natural progression of knowledge whereby tacit values, principles and theories become subject to systematic enquiry.

Interest in the promotion of mental health has a history of more than 100 years, dating back to the formation of the Finnish Association for Mental Health in 1897. The World Federation of Mental Health was founded in 1948 to promote better understanding of mental illness and to serve as a means of drawing attention to mental health. More recently, an initiative between the European Commission and the World Health Organization (WHO 1999d) acknowledged that issues surrounding mental health problems contribute to five of the ten leading causes of disability worldwide, and that while improvement can be detected concerning physical health, this is not the case in the area of mental health. Tudor (1998) has offered a comprehensive and critical analysis of the whole area of mental health promotion as distinct from the prevention of mental health disorder. His work has contributed significantly towards emphasising the concept of mental health as positive and distinctive.

There is little doubt that health is an important component of well-being and, according to Argyle (1987), it is one of the main sources of happiness. Equally, positive social relationships insulate people against the adverse effects of stress and are a major factor in the state of well-being. However, Downie et al (1993) noted the difficulties in qualifying a state of well-being and argued that subjective feelings of well-being cannot accurately be seen to equate with positive health. For example, the latter authors might take exception to the American definition of Johnson (1986), who described well-being as a 'state that transcends the limitations of body, space, time and circumstances and in which one is at peace with oneself and with others'. While this is a pleasing, gentle and ethereal explanation, it may not be as pragmatic as the specific goal-setting which health promotion espouses.

In this chapter we consider features of health, some influences upon it, and the relationship between occupational therapy and well-being across the life cycle.

Definition of terms

The key terms used in this chapter – health, wellness, well-being, health promotion and health education – are defined below.

Health

Defining health is a complex matter as the concept defies neat description. The World Health Organization (1946) gave the following definition: 'Health is a state of complete physical, mental and social well-being, and not merely the absence of disease or infirmity.' Webb (1994), however, noted that this definition is problematic in that it implies a static rather than a dynamic phenomenon. A pivotal interpretation of health potential was given by the philosopher Seedhouse (1986, p. 61); it recognises the dynamic nature of health and acknowledges individual differences:

A person's optimum state of health is equivalent to the state of the set of conditions which fulfil or enable a person to work to fulfil his or her realistic chosen and biological potentials. Some of these conditions are of the highest importance for all people. Others are variable dependent upon individual abilities and circumstances.

Likewise, a later World Health Organization (1986) publication, the Ottawa Charter for Health Promotion, stated: 'Health is therefore seen as a resource for everyday life, not the objective of living; it is a positive concept emphasising social and personal resources as well as physical capacities.'

Wellness

This state was defined by Johnson (1986) as proactive and as a 'context for living, a state of being, a place from which to come as individuals commit themselves to improve life for all of humanity'. According to this definition, a harmony is sought between mind, body and spirit and between the individual and society.

Well-being

As with the concept of health, the state of well-being is multifaceted; Downie et al (1993) considered that true well-being involves and reflects a quality of empowerment. They emphasised that a biomedical approach can involve a subjective sense of well-being through the prescription of a drug, but that the health promotion approach involves a sense of individual control.

Health promotion

Since the mid-1980s, a confusing array of terms has been used in the area of health promotion, including health education, health protection and wellness education. Downie et al (1993) offered the following definition: 'Health promotion comprises effort to enhance positive health and prevent ill-health, through the overlapping spheres of health education, prevention and health protection.'

Downie et al's definition contrasts with that offered by Ewles & Simnett (1993), who used the

World Health Organization definition of health promotion: 'Health promotion is the process of enabling people to increase control over and to improve their health.' This definition emphasises the element of empowerment.

It becomes clear when reading the literature that health education is now understood as an intrinsic component of health promotion which 'seeks to improve the health status of individuals and communities' (Webb 1994).

Health education All health care professionals have a responsibility in terms of health education; this has been described by Downie et al (1993) as seeking 'to enhance positive health and to prevent or diminish ill-health through influencing beliefs, attitudes and behaviour'. It can operate at a number of different levels. These were described most simply by Draper et al (1980) as follows:

- Type 1 health education is about the body and its maintenance.
- Type 2 health education involves information about access to and appropriate use of health services.
- Type 3 is health education in a wider context, including education about national, regional and local politics which have ramifications involving health.

Psychologists have been concerned with issues which relate to mental health since the early part of the 20th century. The accent on health inevitably moves psychology away from the study of mental processes towards human beings who are affected by dynamic forces in social contexts. The contribution of health psychology has allowed greater understanding of the attitudes, beliefs and consequent behaviour of human beings. The close relationship between psychology and education has produced research revealing factors which affect attitudes which in turn affect the wish to change. In addition, health psychology has enabled other health professionals to explore alternative models and approaches to managing stress, pain or crisis.

A key feature in the whole debate about health education and promotion has been the problem of evaluating how effective it is (Baric 1980).

Health psychologists have made a contribution in this area by offering methodologies which are relevant to the study of the process of health promotion as well as outcome measures.

FEATURES OF HEALTH

Traditional Western health care has been challenged in terms of its ideology, management and interventions many times over the last 50 years. Dissatisfaction with the medicalisation of health has promoted new philosophies which, since the mid-1980s, have placed health in the context of the community. Consequently, the challenge for all health-care professionals has become the quest for more proactive approaches which could promote and maintain sound physical and mental health. Inherent in the new philosophies of care for people in the community are ideas of individual responsibility, self-determination, empowerment and a more equitable partnership between client and health professional.

The mid-1980s seemed to be a crucial time for a number of interested groups to make formal declarations of their interest in health promotion. In 1986, the first international Conference on Health Promotion occurred in Ottawa, primarily to acknowledge the changing worldwide expectations for a new emphasis in the public movement (WHO 1986). A charter was presented 'for action to achieve Health for All by the year 2000 and beyond'. It endorsed the need to work towards healthy communities and a reorientation of health services which will include health research and changes in professional education. In the same year, the Division of Health Psychology of the British Psychological Society was established. Again, an accent on health rather than illness was the primary aim with a drive towards a 'psychology of prevention' rather than treatment (Niven 1989).

Health education also shifted in emphasis away from the traditional imparting of sensible information, which had attracted the criticism that it assumes the notion of rational human beings who are free to choose healthy lifestyles. It became part of a broader approach to promoting health which incorporates efforts to change political, social and economic conditions for individual groups and communities.

This implies cooperation between agencies, in both the statutory and the voluntary sector. In an even more comprehensive manner, in response to the worldwide prevalence of mental health problems, (10.5% of Disability Adjusted Life Years lost in 1990) (WHO 1999a) the World Health Organization, governments and local authorities have set targets for the promotion of health, such as, for example, the UK Health of the Nation health strategy (HMSO 1991).

Definitions of mental health

This has been defined from many theoretical perspectives: the current consensus among writers is that every attempt to define the concept has to recognise 'inherent cultural assumptions' (Chwedorowicz 1992). Originally, the World Health Organization (1951) characterised mental health as being:

- not merely absence of illness
- a state of well-being and feeling able to cope
- influenced by biological and social factors
- subject to variations and fluctuations of degree.

Within these factors, consideration must be given to:

- harmonious relationships with others
- participation in/contribution towards changes in social and physical environment, and
- internal homeostatis (i.e. balanced lifestyle and coping with stresses/conflicts).

More recently, the World Health Organization has defined mental health as 'a state of well-being in which the individual realises his or her own abilities, can cope with the normal stresses of life, can work productively and fruitfully and is able to make a contribution to his or her community' (WHO 1999d).

Mental health promotion (WHO 1999b) is an umbrella term that covers a variety of strategies, all concerned with exerting a positive effect upon mental health, the encouragement of individual resources and skills and making improvements in the socio-economic environment. Tudor (1996) avoided a definition, but considered the interrelationship between mental ill health prevention and mental health promotion by identifying target elements for practice:

- coping
- tension and stress management
- self-concept and identity
- self-esteem
- self-development
- autonomy
- change
- social support and involvement.

To this, occupational therapists would add another dimension, that of the occupational lives of individuals and the contribution this makes to mental health.

Factors contributing to health and ill health

A number of authors (e.g. Argyle 1987, Brugha 1991) have emphasised the importance of social contacts and social support as factors in well-being. Brown & Harris's (1978) seminal work on depression described clearly the vulnerability experienced by women who lack supportive relationships. Wood (1990) introduced the concept of being life-affirming and noted seven characteristics of people who have this quality: emotional stability, sociability, self-confidence, control of their lives, having a sense of purpose, optimism and having the capacity to enjoy life. Such people have confidence in their own self-worth and are happy about their lifestyle. Affective well-being leads to competence, autonomy, ability to set goals and to achieve them, so that the person is actively engaged in a purposeful life. Inherent in this is spiritual well-being.

Homeostasis, as described above, means being in balance. When this balance is disturbed, either by external or by internal factors, the relationship between stress and ability to cope with the demands of everyday life can be depicted in the form of a curve, in which performance increases while the individual is in a state of ever-heightening arousal. This arousal prevents attention to the warning signs of fatigue, culminating in physical or psychological ill health. Factors which affect the balance have been considered by many authors but, broadly speaking, they can be divided into three categories: biological, psychological and sociological/environmental. Some examples of each are given in Table 2.1.

A model of how interacting demands can contribute to illness is of value in understanding the concept of well-being, or the state of being in control and at peace with the pressures of life (Fig. 2.1). Everyone experiences a range of life transitions, such as leaving home, starting work, marriage or retirement. These transitions will be stressful but are regarded as normal stages in development. Individuals in general have considerable capacity to withstand the stresses both of transitions and of more traumatic events. Holmes & Rahe (1975) identified life events which are significant and rated these according to the degree of stress they provoke. Events relating to loss – such as bereavements, unemployment, ill health – are examples of crisis situations which are significant. Even more positive events such as marriage are not without stress!

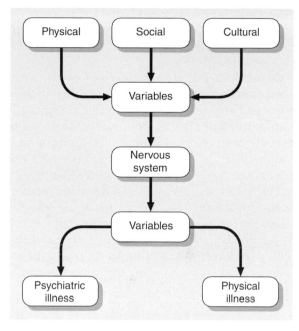

Figure 2.1   Interaction between stressors and health.

and satisfactory lifestyle. Consensus also exists between writers within the profession that, while health status may be a fluctuating phenomenon, there is a link between involvement in occupation and a sense of well-being.

OCCUPATIONAL THERAPY

A central tenet of occupational therapy, since its inception, has been the promotion of a balanced

Occupational therapy and wellness

Although the term wellness is philosophically consistent with British usage, it is American in

Table 2.1   Factors which may affect health

Biological	Psychological	Sociological/environmental
Biochemical	Stressful life events	Deprivation and poverty, including homelessness
Cerebrovascular accident	Learned behaviours	Low social status, marginalisation
Trauma (e.g. head injury)	Relationships	Unemployment
Genetic	expressed emotion	Gender
Toxins (e.g. alcohol)	double bind	Racism
Deafness	Loss	Vandalism
Physical ill health	Loneliness	Migration
	Mental health problems	Climate
	Stigma	Noise
		Nuclear threat/disasters
		Terrorism
		Pace of living

origin and Johnson (1986), who wrote a text on the subject, explained it as 'an emerging concept that reflects individual responsibility for health and well being'.

Brown (1987), also speaking from an American perspective, considered that occupational therapy was an 'unrecognised forerunner in the wellness movement'; however, it is important to note that the promotion of positive health must be a combined effort between all agencies who are committed to ideas of health and well-being.

The value of activity is central to the profession's philosophy and to its focus on occupational performance. The health-promoting value of purposeful participation in activity has been well documented in textbooks on occupational therapy and is inherent in the concept of self-actualisation. Through *doing*, people are confronted with the evidence of their ability to function competently and take control of their lives as far as they are able. Personal dignity and beliefs are enhanced and sense of worth is developed. Nothing succeeds like success and the occupational therapist is well able to facilitate this; Reed & Sanderson (1992), however, are keen to emphasise that there is 'no perfect or ideal model of health for occupational therapy to follow'.

Occupational therapy and health promotion

The recommendations in the Ottawa Charter for Health Promotion (WHO 1986) have been realised in the curriculum content of undergraduate programmes, where both health psychology and health promotion have a prominent place. Research is also increasingly targeted towards studying what keeps people healthy and responsible for their own health status.

While few occupational therapists in the UK work comprehensively with the well population, they have been involved for many years, in working with carers, offering support, advice and education. The shift towards helping individuals to recognise their own power and the contribution of occupational therapy in enabling individuals to make choices are not new (Stewart 1993). However, working in different venues and with different levels of health has required occupational therapists to adopt new approaches. Finn (1972) considered that for occupational therapists to work within prevention programmes required an expansion of the role from therapist to 'health agent'.

An interesting example of this comes from Stead (1994) who, as an occupational therapist,

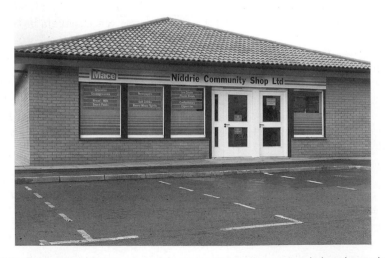

Figure 2.2   This community store is an important collaborative venture in learning and working.

was one of the members of a voluntary board of directors involved in setting up a community store in Edinburgh (Fig. 2.2). As a community business, the store provides not only a valuable service but also employment and training opportunities for members of the local community. This initiative represents an important collaborative venture of learning and working which contributes to the health and wellness of a community. It also endorses the view of Tudor (1996) and others that there needs to be attention to community mental health and that contributing to the community fulfils an altruistic purpose.

In other circumstances, occupational therapists may become involved in networking procedures within communities whereby an in-depth knowledge of the area and resources is used to develop social contacts. Community schools, voluntary organisations, church groups and the resources of certain industries can all be used as sites and venues to draw attention to the promotion of sound mental health. In this manner, occupational therapists, with other health professionals, can also keep attention to mental health on the political agenda at local level.

Occupational therapy and well-being

Factors which have been cited as having a detrimental effect on mental health are reflected in the occupational therapy process, as outlined by Reed & Sanderson (1992). This focuses on aspects of the person's life with respect to leisure, personal care and occupation, in relation to the physical, psychological, social, economic and spiritual aspects of life. External factors, sociological and environmental, are taken into account and there is an emphasis on building on abilities and enhancing the competence of the individual rather than highlighting areas of disability or malfunction. This philosophy, which is essentially holistic and focused towards recognising individual power, is compatible with health promotion and its concepts of personal responsibility and control. Any treatment programme should be devised in consultation with the individual and carers and should prioritise the expressed needs of the client. Some people will, of course, need advocacy support.

According to Johnson (1986), the wellness and holistic health movement in the USA emerged from 'the human potential and counterculture movements in the 1960s and 1970s'. It coincided with philosophies in occupational therapy which acknowledge the dynamic interaction of mind, body, spirit and social context. The focus on spiritual well-being encompasses the values of the individual and recognises the need for self-esteem and affirmation. The centrality of spirituality is recognised in the 1997 revision of the Canadian model of occupational performance (CAOT 1997). Without some awareness of the spiritual dimension of human beings there is a lack of meaning in life which can often be identified in loneliness, depression and feelings of powerlessness (Neuhaus 1997).

It can be seen that a client-centred focus will, in itself, help to combat problems. Many people lack experience of warm and supportive relationships and the therapist can provide these and, at the same time, facilitate the expansion of social networks to enhance feelings of well-being. A sense of well-being and feelings of confidence lead to an increase in motivation. Equally, 'challenges can be more valuable than tender loving care' and by involving clients in purposeful activity, their self-esteem can be developed (Clark 1984).

Some of the factors which promote a sense of well-being are listed below:

- **Contribution**. An old Indian proverb states that the smile you send out returns to you. This is a sense of being able to give to others.
- **Comfort/change/calm/content**. Self-regard and acceptance of one's lot lead to being at ease in one's surroundings. Parallel with this is the ability to change and adapt so that the individual does not sink into stagnation.
- **Contact/companionship**. The degree of support from others which the person perceives that he is receiving is a crucial factor in ability to cope. Involvement and social networks are essential for human survival. Empathy with others is an aspect of this.

- **Choice**. The degree to which the person feels in control, the sense of power and choice, is also significant.
- **Competence**. The ability to cope gives a self-concept which reinforces competence. Carrying out activities proficiently promotes self-esteem.
- **Commitment**. This includes a sense of purpose and belonging and a sense of direction in life.

Activity and health

A historical review of how occupational therapy in the USA has evolved to contribute to preventive health activities and wellness was offered by Reitz (1992). In terms of policy and practice, the review noted a strong commitment to directing energy towards helping society to understand not only the relationship between ill health and lifestyle, but also the relationship between involvement in occupation and health.

In discussing this from the perspective of leisure, Argyle (1987) considered that Scottish country dancing epitomises the totality of an enhancing activity in which there is social contact, skill, exercise and involvement in culture. Gardening can be understood in the same light. Although different in the pace of activity, it provides the participant with closeness to the seasons and the rhythm of life. It enhances the quality of life by the provision of colour, smell and actual experiences and the produce which results from careful tending (Fig. 2.3).

These ideas of the value of activities and links with well-being are central to many writers in occupational therapy. For example, Kielhofner (1992) explained that although human beings achieve meaning in a myriad of different ways, 'occupation is an important pathway for the creation of personal meaning'.

From an occupational therapy perspective then, mental health can be observed through the purpose and meaning inherent in the activities with which a person chooses to become involved. Choices, however, are dependent upon opportunity, resources and the confidence to make them. Working within a community, atten-

tion to factors that restrict choice, such as homelessness, unemployment and limited finances, seems to be part of the thinking of Wilcock (1993). She suggests that, in terms of the occupational therapist's contribution to prevention of ill health, research should be undertaken into the effect of occupational deprivation and occupational stress.

The contribution of occupational science

The discipline of occupational science is concerned with the form, the function and the meaning of occupation. While the relationship with the practice of occupational therapy is a robust one, it draws its knowledge base from diverse interdisciplinary sources. This provides a rich contribution in terms of analysis of how occupation affects mental health and subsequent well-being.

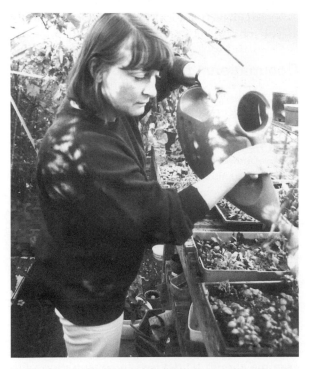

Figure 2.3 Gardening can enhance the quality of life and health.

Yerxa (1993) was an early proponent of this new science, believing that it offers a new way to comprehend the occupational nature of human beings and how this can enhance human potential and personal growth. A number of theorists, including Clark (1993), extended those ideas, building a knowledge base from doctoral programmes of study at the University of Southern California. Clark also offered a type of qualitative research methodology in the form of narrative analysis which revealed how engagement in meaningful occupation can transform the rehabilitative process. The idea that engagement in occupation and reflection upon it could be a transformative experience is also shown in the work of Townsend (1997). She extended the notion to include the potential for social change. All these theorists have adhered to an idea of interconnectedness between occupation, perceived quality of life and well-being. It is Wilcock (1998), however, who has offered the most comprehensive text to date on an occupational perspective on health. In her view, mental well-being can be enhanced by the significant social, spiritual, psychological and biological features which a balanced occupational life offers.

Occupational science is concerned with understanding people as occupational beings. It has exciting possibilities as a field of study alongside new public health initiatives which emphasise primary health care, prevention of ill-health and promotion of health.

HEALTH, WELLNESS AND THE LIFE CYCLE

A substantial body of knowledge exists which indicates that both unexpected life events and normal transitions, such as those shown in Table 2.2, have important implications for health and well-being. How individuals manage such events depends upon a complex mix of personal, social and economic factors. Research over the past two decades, particularly in the social sciences, has sought to link micro- and macro-type evidence about how social contexts shape human lives.

Occupational therapists are particularly concerned with the way in which 'various forms of occupation are recognised as existing in a dynamic relationship to each other through the life span' (Kielhofner 1992). This sense of continuity is an important element in understanding an individual's strengths and coping capacity when faced with transitions in life.

Kaplan & Sadock (1991), in a general text on psychiatry, included a section on 'phase of life problems'. The DSM111-R (American Psychiatric Association 1980) acknowledged that this category can be used when the key aspect of a presenting problem is problems related to stresses in the life cycle. Stress is a process in which perceived demands (internal or external) severely tax or exceed available coping resources (Fig. 2.4). This leads to a vicious circle of effects in which mood (depression) influences feelings ('I am useless') and tends to alter behaviour (not participating in activities) which increases the level of depression. When coping mechanisms fail, the results can be as shown in Table 2.3.

Table 2.2 Transitions and life events

Possible critical transition points	Unanticipated life events
Birth	Accidents
Adolescence	Life-threatening disorders
Marriage/partnership	Natural disasters
Pregnancy	Wars
Separation/divorce	Physical/mental illness
Unemployment/retirement	Loss of status/prestige
Death	

Table 2.3 Success and failure of coping mechanisms

Mental health	Mental illness
High self-esteem	Reality distorted
Stress opposing (experience of success)	Symptoms
	Relationships difficult
Intimate relationships	Behaviour dangerous to
Social support networks	self/others
Reasonable mood swings	Emotions uncontrolled
Balance between relaxation and stress	Problems overtake person's life
Coping	Not coping

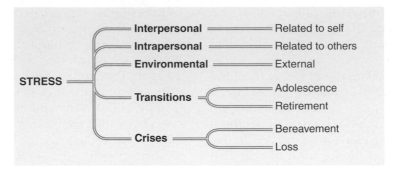

Figure 2.4 Types of stress.

The context in which life events occur is obviously of importance: the widower with young children who is made redundant will not experience the same problems as the older man with a grown-up family. The 'undefined and hidden' burden consequent on mental health problems was acknowledged in a recent statement by the World Health Organization (1999c) as contributing to stigma and to emotional and socioeconomic difficulties for patients and carers alike. It is an important shift from emphasis on pathology to an awareness of other factors which can cause difficulties in coping. The degree to which individuals adjust and adapt is a central concern of occupational therapists.

It is evident that external events are more likely to overwhelm someone's adaptive ability if:

- the events are unexpected
- the events are numerous
- the resulting stress is chronic and unremitting
- one loss triggers many other necessary adjustments.

Robustness of personality plus sound support systems usually enable people to negotiate transitions, but anxiety and depression can result from major life-cycle changes such as marriage, parenthood, unemployment, retirement or loss. Studies have shown that perceived support is one of the key factors in ability to cope when life events threaten a person's sense of well-being. However, one person's stress is another person's motivation to continue, and many people operate at high stress levels, producing excellent work.

The factors which seem to protect individuals are:

- a history of coping successfully with transitions
- strong family connections
- being in employment and having a reasonable income
- a pattern of regular leisure activities
- ability to manage daily routine
- personal strengths, such as flexibility and reliability
- an outlook which incorporates hope and purpose in life
- ability to set realistic goals
- mature defence mechanisms, such as a sense of humour.

Adams et al (1976) offered a succinct account of the process of transition plus a model which is helpful in analysing the potential phases which an individual may go through. It is therefore possible to identify potential target groups and mobilise appropriate agencies if necessary.

A number of psychological approaches in promoting coping skills have been described by Moos (1986) and by Danish & D'Augelli (1982) who designed a comprehensive system to teach life-skills. The role of the health professional is to help individuals set goals for themselves which are reasonable, manageable and can be developed into identifiable skills. This is familiar territory for the occupational therapist, who often has the role of facilitator or teacher.

Another form of brief therapy which lends itself well to community settings and preventive approaches is solution-orientated therapy, as described by O'Hanlon & Weiner-Davies (1989). This is an approach to problem solving which keeps control firmly in the hands of the client. An optimistic and collaborative ethos is created by engaging in a spirit of mutual investigation. No attempt is made to site the problem in some past circumstances; instead, this approach has an orientation towards the future. Occupational therapists can use this approach as a guiding principle in helping clients to approach change in a less fearful manner.

WELLNESS AND OLDER PEOPLE

Throughout this chapter, the connection has been made between health and engagement in activity. This aspect becomes more salient when considering older people. A number of interesting texts, for example, Macheath (1984) and Bernard (1985), have examined activities, health and fitness with a primary aim of weakening the notion that growing older is synonymous with illness (Fig. 2.5).

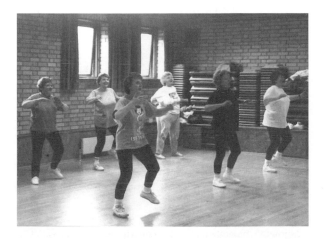

Figure 2.5   Growing older is not synonymous with illness.

More recently, Miller (1991), in trying to determine factors which promoted wellness in older people, found a complexity and scarcity of available information. Miller believed that ideas about healthy ageing should emerge from older people themselves, and designed a small ethnographic study to explore this. Interview results conveyed a healthy, vibrant attitude, in that the subjects remained interested in their community and world affairs. The idea of meta ageing which, according to Maslow (1970), was a form of self-actualisation was also evident in an integration of selfhood in later years. Valued activities and relationships were the main components of a state of wellness. This study is important for occupational therapists in helping to understand the values and attitudes which older people have concerning leisure, learning and social relationships.

Alford & Futrell (1992) suggested that there is a need for longitudinal studies of all facets of wellness and health promotion of people as they age. This is an attempt from nursing to make the relationship between theory and practice strong. However, it has implications for all workers in health care as attention turns from concentration on pathology towards an attempt to identify and sustain factors concerning a state of well-being.

Recently, Seymour (1999) identified occupational therapists working with the elderly as having mixed attitudes towards health promotion and proposed strategies for maximising the therapist's potential role in this area.

The case study in Box 2.1 describes a resilient person who can set goals which are manageable and can, if necessary, ask for help. She could take advantage of community facilities without professional encouragement. Nevertheless, support would be available from all voluntary groups associated with Alzheimer's-type dementia if Joan wished to be involved. Her general practitioner should be aware of her circumstances and of the network of possibilities in the community which could be used if necessary.

It is, therefore, vital to inform general practitioners about services which can be offered and to remind them and other professionals in

Box 2.1 A case history

Joan is 68 and, apart from slightly raised blood pressure, has no health problems. Her husband died 6 months ago, having had Alzheimer-type dementia for the last 5 years. She has three children, one of whom lives nearby, and four grandchildren. As the youngest member of her family she has one remaining brother and a sister-in-law.

During her husband's illness, much of Joan's time was devoted to caring for him, especially during the last few months. She did not want him to go into care but eventually he needed to be admitted to hospital, where he died after rapid worsening of his condition. This was a very stressful time for Joan but she was later glad that he did not have to go into a home, something he had not wanted.

Joan's family is supportive and she enjoys baby-sitting for her small granddaughters. She has a variety of interests and is beginning to become involved in some of these now that she has more time. Prior to the birth of her children she worked in an insurance office and later (before her husband became ill) she was actively involved in voluntary works, which gave her a wide range of social contacts. She has support from her church, visits and entertains friends, and is planning to extend these activities. She is a friendly person who can easily exchange conversation with people she meets when walking the dog. Two months ago, Joan and her unmarried son went to visit friends in Germany and she was pleased that she had completed part of the journey alone. She now plans to take up an invitation to go to America.

Joan readily admits that she has her ups and downs and regards this as part of the grief process. She feels pleased with herself that she is coping alone and has a range of goals for the future, which give her a sense of purpose. She is determined to work towards achieving these but, at the same time, she is ready to be patient with herself when things do not work well. She plans to develop her social networks, including contact with married friends.

In short, Joan has drive and determination, she is sociable and not lacking in self-esteem. She also has the ability to ask for support when she needs it without feeling that this is a sign of inadequacy. She knows that she is able to cope with change and she is not afraid to attempt new things.

primary care about the contribution of occupational therapy towards mental health.

SUMMARY

The profession of occupational therapy is not concerned with prescription of activities or the mystique of unusual techniques. Occupational therapists consider that significant change occurs within the context of day to day occupation.

The underlying philosophy of occupational therapy is consistent with models of health which focus on helping individuals to become aware of their own power by gaining life skills that give them a greater sense of personal control. It is concerned with the constellation of activities which give meaning to life by determining roles, values, habits and routines. Those aspects give shape and purpose to our lives and provide the vital ingredients which contribute to a sense of well-being.

REFERENCES

Adams J, Hayes J, Hopson B (eds) 1976 Transition: understanding and managing personal change. Martin Robertson, London
Alford D M, Futrell M 1992 Wellness and health promotion of the elderly. Nursing Outlook 50(5): 221–226
American Psychiatric Association 1980 Diagnostic and statistical manual of mental disorders, 3rd edn. APA, Washington DC
Argyle M 1987 The psychology of happiness. Methuen, London
Baric L 1980 Evaluation: obstacles and potentialities. International Journal of Health Education 23: 142–149

Bernard M 1985 Health education and activities for older people: a review of current practice. Health Education Council No. 2. Department of Adult Education, University of Keele, Keele
Brown G, Harris T 1978 Social origins of depression. Tavistock, London
Brown K M 1987 Wellness: past visions, future roles. In: Cromwell F (ed) Sociocultural implications in treatment planning in occupational therapy. Howarth Press, New York
Brugha T S 1991 Support and personal relationships. In: Bennet D, Freeman A L (eds) Community psychiatry. Churchill Livingstone, Edinburgh

CAOT 1997 Enabling occupation: an occupational therapy perspective. CAOT Publications, ACE, Ottawa

Chwedorowicz A (1992) Psychic hygiene in mental health promotion. In: Trent D P (ed) Promotion of mental health. Avebury, Aldershot, vol 1, pp 241–246

Clark D H 1984 The development of a psychiatric rehabilitation service. Lancet 2: 625–627

Clark F 1993 Occupation embedded in a real life: interweaving occupational science and occupational therapy. American Journal of Occupational Therapy 47 (17): 1067–1078

Danish S J, D'Augelli A R 1982 Helping skills II. Life development intervention. Human Sciences Press, New York

Downie R S, Fyfe C, Tannahill A 1993 Health promotion models and values. Oxford University Press, Oxford

Draper P, Griffiths J, Dennis J, Popjay J 1980 Three types of health education. British Medical Journal 280: 493–495

Ewles L, Simnett I 1993 Promoting health: a practical guide. Scutari Press, London

Finn G L 1972 The occupational therapist in prevention programmes. American Journal of Occupational Therapy 26(2): 59

HMSO 1991 The health of the nation: a consultative document for health in England. Cm 5523, HMSO, London

Holmes T H, Rahe R H 1975 The Social Readjustment Rating Scale. Journal of Psychosomatic Research 11: 213–218

Johnson J A 1986 Wellness: a context for living. Slack, New Jersey

Kaplan H, Sadock B J 1991 Synopsis of psychiatry. Williams and Wilkins, Baltimore

Kielhofner G 1992 Conceptual foundations of occupational therapy. F A Davis, Philadelphia

Macheath J A 1984 Activity, health and fitness in old age. Croom Helm, London

Maslow A 1970 Motivation and personality. Harper Rowe, New York

Miller M P 1991 Factors promoting wellness in the aged person: an ethnographic study. Advances in Nursing Science 13(4): 38–51

Moos R H 1986 Coping with life crisis: an integrated approach. Plenum, New York

Neuhaus B 1997 Including hope in occupational therapy practice: a pilot study. American Journal of Occupational Therapy 51(3): 228–234

Niven N 1989 Health psychology. Churchill Livingstone, Edinburgh

O'Hanlon W H, Weiner-Davis M 1989 In search of solutions: a new direction in psychotherapy. W W Norton, New York

Reed K L, Sanderson S N 1992 Concepts of occupational therapy, 2nd edn. Williams and Wilkins, Baltimore

Reitz M S 1992 A historical review of occupational therapy's role in preventive health and wellness. American Journal of Occupational Therapy 46(1): 50–55

Seedhouse D 1986 Health: the foundations for achievement. Wiley

Seymour S 1999 Occupational therapy and health promotion: a focus on elderly people. British Journal of Occupational Therapy 62(7): 313–317

Stead J 1994 The newsletter (summer). Community Enterprise Lothian, Edinburgh

Stewart A 1993 Empowerment and enablement: occupational therapy 2001. Inaugural Lecture, 1 December 1993. Queen Margaret College, Edinburgh

Townsend E 1997 Occupation: potential for personal and social transformation. 4 (1)

Tudor K 1996 Mental health promotion. Routledge, London

Webb P (ed) 1994 Health promotion and patient education. Chapman and Hall, London

Wilcock A A 1993 Keynote paper: biological and sociocultural aspects of occupation health and health promotion. British Journal of Occupational Therapy 30(6): 203

Wilcock A 1998 An occupational perspective of health. Slack, New Jersey

Wood C 1990 Say yes to life. Dent, Edinburgh

World Health Organization 1946 Constitution. WHO, Geneva

World Health Organization 1951 Committee on Mental Health. WHO, Geneva

World Health Organization 1986 Ottawa Charter for Health Promotion. WHO, Geneva

World Health Organization 1999a Fact sheet no. 217. WHO, Geneva

World Health Organization 1999b Press release WHO/21 March. WHO, Geneva

World Health Organization 1999c Fact sheet no. 218, April. WHO, Geneva

World Health Organization 1999d Fact sheet 220. WHO, Geneva

Yerxa E 1993 Occupational science: a new source of power for participants in occupational therapy. Occupational Science 1(1)

Zemke R, Clark F 1996 Occupational science: the evolving discipline. F A Davis, Philadelphia

3

The knowledge base of occupational therapy

Jennifer Creek

INTRODUCTION

In the first chapter we looked at the development of occupational therapy into a modern-day profession. Using this information as a background, we can now look more closely at the current philosophical and theoretical base of occupational therapy. We will do this by analysing the following:

- the development of professional philosophy in the modern age
- the philosophical assumptions that underpin practice today
- the main areas of knowledge from which occupational therapy derives its theoretical base
- the relationship of the theoretical base to the practice of occupational therapy.

THE PHILOSOPHICAL DEVELOPMENT OF THE MODERN PROFESSION

As described in Chapter 1, the profession of occupational therapy as we know it today dates from about 1917. Since that time the profession has undergone, and is still undergoing, changes in its outlook and philosophy. Professional philosophy is the system of shared beliefs and values held by members of a profession – for those whose profession is occupational therapy, this includes beliefs about the nature of human beings, society, health and ill health, the nature and purpose of occupational therapy and the relationships between these various elements.

The early years

When the profession of occupational therapy began, it operated with a pragmatic and humanistic view of human beings and their relationship with occupation. Some of the main proponents of this philosophy of pragmatism, such as John Dewey and George Herbert Mead, worked in Chicago, where the first occupational therapy course was started in 1908. Pragmatism 'recognizes the inextricable influences on each other of the mental and physical aspects of human beings, their artifacts, their environments, and the societies and times in which they live' (Breines 1995, p. 16). This philosophy permeated early writings on occupational therapy, for example, Adolph Meyer (1917, cited by Young & Quinn 1992, p. 118) argued that mental disorders can be understood only 'in the context of the total personality, and in the light of the many interacting factors that conspire to bring them about'.

Humanism views people as 'growing, developing, creating being(s), with the ability to take full self-responsibility' (Cracknell 1984). This includes taking responsibility for maintaining their own health and for making choices that determine what they become.

These beliefs in the mind–body–environment–time interrelationship and in the capacity of human beings to achieve health through what they do led occupational therapists to use broad and balanced programmes of occupation to treat mental health problems.

In 1922, Meyer wrote about the value of occupation in the management of psychiatric patients. Although he did not attempt to define occupational therapy, Meyer was aware that 'the proper use of time in some helpful and gratifying activity appeared to be a fundamental issue in the treatment of the neuropsychiatric patient'. He also outlined his philosophy as a recognition of:

the need of adaptation and the value of work as a sovereign help in the problems of adaptation . . . our conception of man is that of an organism that

maintains and balances itself in the world of reality and actuality by being in active life and active use . . .

. . . Our role (as occupational therapists) consists in giving opportunities rather than prescriptions . . . Man learns to organise time and he does it in terms of doing things. (Meyer 1922)

Key concepts from the foundation of the profession which still inform practice today include taking a temporal perspective of the client and being concerned with the balance of activities in an individual's life over time, not just with single activities. Occupational therapists are concerned not only with the person as he is now, at the moment of intervention, but also with how he functions at different times and in different environments. We are interested in the person's past, how he functioned previously, and in his future, what he expects to do after the intervention is finished and for the rest of his life.

The whole-person approach is still considered to be a crucial aspect of occupational therapy intervention. Mattingly & Fleming (1994) described this as a concern with 'the patient's relationship with the disease . . . with disability as a meaningful experience, especially inasmuch as it has affected the patient's capacity to move through the world, and to take up the occupations that have shaped his or her life and given it significance.'

The influence of reductionism

Throughout the 1950s and 1960s, occupational therapy gradually changed its philosophy under the influence of the reductionist model of science which was then being adopted by all the life sciences in an attempt to become scientifically respectable. Reductionism is based on the belief that the structure and function of the whole can best be understood from a detailed study of the parts by observation and experiment (Smith 1983). Reilly (1962) said that each person's need to be occupied should not be inferred from global generalisations but was being rigorously investigated under laboratory conditions. This comment sat uncomfortably within a talk which emphasised a view of human beings as complex organisms developing and functioning within their own environments, and demonstrates some of the confusion of identity that occupational therapists were experiencing at that time.

Shannon (1977, p. 231) claimed that occupational therapists at this period not only lost sight of the beliefs of the founders of the profession, but also adopted the medical model with 'its focus on pathology . . . and on the minute and measurable'. Medicine is concerned with acute illness or with the acute phase of illness, whereas occupational therapy is traditionally and most usefully concerned with the needs of people with chronic health problems. Therapy began to focus on pathology and on the therapeutic techniques used rather than on the person, and became concerned with reducing symptoms and working with people who could be cured rather than those with complex, long-term needs.

With the increasing complexity of treatment and accompanying need for specialisation, the focus moved from health to illness and the responsibility for wellness moved from the individual to the medical profession. Occupational therapy, in accepting this change, lost its humanistic perspective and began to prescribe activities for patients rather than giving them opportunities to influence their own health through occupation.

By adopting the reductionist model, occupational therapists were able to develop a great depth of expertise in various fields of practice – for example, many therapists became highly skilled in the use of projective media in analytic group psychotherapy – but the profession as a whole suffered from role diffusion and loss of identity (Kielhofner & Burke 1977).

Reassessing our beliefs

The 1970s and 1980s saw a conscious effort on the part of occupational therapists to reassess the original philosophy of the profession, which had become obscured during the 1950s and 1960s.

West (1984) suggested that society was moving from a mechanistic view of man and health to a systems view which is congruent with the pragmatic and humanistic perspective of occupational therapy: 'Health care of the future will consist of restoring and maintaining the dynamic balance of individuals, families and social groups, and it will mean people taking care of their own health individually, as a society, and with the help of therapists.'

The profession attempted to reassert the validity of occupational therapy traditions and values without losing the very real advances in theory and practice made during the reductionist era. The areas of belief which were examined and agreed to be still relevant to occupational therapy practice in mental health can be summarised as follows:

- a concern with the person as a physical, thinking, emotional, spiritual and social being, who has a past, present and future, and who functions within physical and social environments
- a belief in intrinsic motivation – an innate predisposition to explore and act on the environment and to use one's capacities
- a recognition of each person's need for a balance of occupations in his life in order to: facilitate development, give meaning to life, satisfy inherent needs, realise personal and biological potentials, adapt to changing circumstances and maintain health
- an acceptance of the social nature of people and of the importance of social interaction in shaping what we become
- a recognition of the importance of what we do in determining what we become – the primacy of function over structure
- a view of health as a subjective experience of well-being, resulting from being able to achieve and maintain a sense of meaning and balance in life
- a belief in the responsibility and capability of people to find healthy ways of adapting to changing circumstances by what they do
- an acceptance of the role of occupational therapists in serving the occupational needs of people in order to help them restore meaning and balance to their lives
- a belief in occupation as the central organising concept of the profession and in the use of activity as the main treatment medium.

The continuing search for a clearer understanding of occupational therapy is not an academic exercise but a response to major changes both in society and within the profession. The remainder of this chapter is a brief review of three aspects of occupational therapy:

- the philosophical assumptions underpinning current practice
- the theoretical base of the profession
- the ways in which theory is linked to practice.

PHILOSOPHICAL ASSUMPTIONS

A professional philosophy is a system of shared beliefs and values held by members of a profession. Philosophical assumptions are the basic beliefs which make up this system and which show how members of a particular profession view people and the profession's goals and function (Mosey 1986). In occupational therapy, we accept as true certain beliefs about the nature of people, for example that 'All people experience the need to engage in occupational behaviour because of their species common combination of anatomical features and physiological mechanisms. Such engagement in occupation is an integral part of complex health maintenance systems' (Wilcock 1995, p. 69). Without this belief we would not be convinced of the value of occupation as therapy. This sharing of fundamental beliefs contributes to our sense of identity as a profession.

The three areas of belief central to occupational therapy are beliefs about:

- the nature of human beings
- the nature of health and illness
- the nature and purpose of occupational therapy.

View of human beings

Occupational therapy is essentially person-centred. The individual is seen 'not as an object or thing to be manipulated, controlled or made to conform but as a unique individual whose very humanness entitles him to choices in determin-

ing his own destiny' (Yerxa 1967). This belief in the right of the individual to be himself is made up of three separate beliefs:

- a concern with the whole person within his environment
- a belief in intrinsic motivation to be active
- an understanding of the social nature of people.

Concern with the whole person

Occupational therapists take a holistic view of human beings, that is, they see each person as a unique individual whose body, mind and spirit function together and cannot be seen or understood as separate entities. People also change, according to this view, if they are separated from the environmental influences that have shaped who they are. These influences include the physical environment, cultural environment, societal factors and social support (Christiansen 1997).

The holistic approach assumes that people can only be understood by seeing the relationships between body, mind, spirit and environment over time. Occupational therapists are concerned with the person as he is now, at this moment, and with how he functions at different times and in different environments. We are concerned with the balance of occupations in the individual's life over time, not just with single activities. Meyer wrote, in 1922, that 'the culminating feature of evolution is man's capacity of imagination and the use of time with foresight based on a corresponding appreciation of the past and the present.' Occupational therapists are interested in the person's past, how he functioned previously, and with his future, what he expects to do with the rest of his life.

People as initiators of action

Western medical science is founded on the principle that human life should be preserved if possible. Occupational therapy takes the principle that human function should be preserved or restored where possible. It is the basic premise of our profession that being in a state of function is a desirable condition (Reilly 1962).

Indeed, it can be argued that human life and human function are the same thing; for Sartre, 'human reality does not exist first in order to act later; but for human reality, to be is to act, and to cease to act is to cease to be' (Sartre 1966). People have an intrinsic motivation to act on the environment in order to discover their own potential and to develop their capacities. We do not wait for the environment to impinge on us and then respond; we are able to visualise the ends we wish to achieve and act to realise them. West (1984) summarised the writings on philosophy of several occupational therapists as follows:

activity is the essence of living and is significantly interrelated with high morale . . . to some degree life itself is seen as purposeful occupation – that is to say, as activity, as task, as challenge . . . it is the purposefulness of behaviour and activity that gives human life order . . . the basic philosophy of occupational therapy speaks to Man as an active being and to the use of purposeful activity as Man's interaction with and manipulation of his environment.

People as social animals

People do not act in isolation. We are essentially social animals who develop and live in the context of a group. Human interaction stimulates biological, psychological, emotional and social development, and people deprived of human company do not thrive. There is a long period of physical and emotional dependency in childhood, and it is both normal and healthy to retain some emotional dependence on others once physical maturity is reached.

Social groupings take different forms in different cultures, but within all cultures a small and stable social group is considered most desirable. We do not cope well with living in groups that are too large for us to know everyone else, and we have had to devise coping strategies, for example for living in cities.

View of health

Occupational therapists do not view health as merely the absence of disease, or disease as the absence of health. Health, as defined by occupational therapists, is the ability to function adequately in a balanced variety of roles, appropriate to the individual's culture, stage of

life and circumstances, and to achieve a sense of satisfaction from them. It is a dynamic balance, since each individual's needs, and the roles expected of him, change throughout the life cycle.

The individual is in a state of function when he has learned the skills necessary for successful participation in the range of roles he is expected to play throughout his life. These roles change throughout the life cycle and there may be times when existing skills lag behind new needs. Dysfunction occurs when the individual is unable to maintain himself within his environment because he does not have the skills necessary for coping with the current situation. Dysfunction is very individual. For a violinist, the loss of a finger could be a major disability; for a singer, the same injury may be only a minor inconvenience.

The World Health Organization (2000) described the relationship between disease and activity thus: 'an individual's functioning in a specific domain is an interaction or complex relationship between the health condition and the contextual factors (i.e. environmental and personal factors)' (Fig. 3.1).

Not only do we believe that health can be defined by what we are able to do, we also believe that what we do makes us healthy or

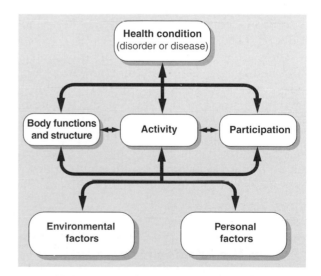

Figure 3.1 World Health Organization classification of functioning, disability and health

unhealthy. Occupational therapists believe that occupation is the highest level of human function, that it develops and integrates the individual's potentials of body, mind and will through the process of doing. What people do creates functional demands that drive neuroplastic changes and organisation, therefore occupations shape what we become: physically, mentally, socially and spiritually.

Why dysfunction occurs

Causes of dysfunction fall into four main groups:

- failure to develop and mature normally due to physical abnormality or environmental deprivation, for example Down's syndrome or emotional abuse
- environmental or personal changes that the individual cannot cope with, such as bereavement or redundancy
- new physiological or psychological needs, such as maternity, which cannot be met using existing skills
- pathology or trauma causing loss of skills, for example head injury or schizophrenia.

When the individual encounters a new situation, he uses his existing skills to try to master it. If these fail, he will try to learn effective new skills. Eventually, if the situation still remains outside his control, he will experience disequilibrium or crisis.

The pace at which change occurs is important for maintaining equilibrium; too fast a pace means that new skills are not learned quickly enough, adaptation is disturbed and a state of dysfunction may occur (Clark 1979, Mosey 1968). The degree and pace of change that a person can manage without losing equilibrium is dependent on both internal factors (e.g. the ability to learn new skills quickly) and external factors (e.g. the amount of support available in the social environment).

View of the profession

The uniqueness of the occupational therapy approach to psychosocial dysfunction lies in the philosophy of human beings having the ability to influence their own health through what they do. Occupational therapy is concerned with the consequences of disease or injury as they affect a person's ability to function, rather than with the primary pathology. For example, the occupational therapist will try to slow down the process of dementia by involving the client in a balanced programme of activities to maintain physical and cognitive functioning, rather than by tackling the disease itself.

The aim of intervention is to develop each person's potentials to their highest possible level, to enhance his quality of life and sense of wellbeing and to increase his satisfaction in daily living. The core of occupational therapy practice is activity analysis, synthesis and application. The outcome of intervention should be that the client is able to enact a balanced range of occupations which will enable him to maintain physical and mental health.

THE THEORETICAL FOUNDATIONS OF OCCUPATIONAL THERAPY

The theoretical foundation of a profession is made up of selected theories from various disciplines and fields of inquiry (Mosey 1981). The main areas of study from which occupational therapy draws its knowledge base are:

- theories of occupation
- biological sciences
- developmental theory
- physical medicine
- psychiatry
- psychology
- sociology.

The wide-ranging nature of this list presents a problem in itself, as no one can be fully informed on all of these subjects, especially with the recent explosion of knowledge in all fields. It is important, therefore, to appreciate how these very varied subjects are of relevance to occupational therapy.

The following sections deal with each of the above areas of knowledge, concentrating on the aspects that are particularly relevant to the practice of psychosocial occupational therapy.

Although occupational therapy was founded on a set of beliefs about the occupational nature of people, it is only in recent years that the profession has begun to formulate its own theories about occupation. Occupational science is a new academic discipline 'focusing on the study of the human as an occupational being' (Yerxa 2000). It brings together knowledge from different disciplines with the intention of providing a knowledge base in human occupation for the practice of occupational therapy.

Some theories of occupation are described below. However, since occupational therapy is primarily a practical profession rather than an academic discipline, it is likely that we will continue to develop our theoretical base by drawing on the work of other disciplines. Occupational therapists need to be skilled in selecting, adapting and applying new knowledge, from whatever source, as it becomes available.

Theories of occupation

The profession of occupational therapy was founded on the belief that people can influence their own health by being proficient in occupations which allow them to explore and interact with their environment in an adaptive way.

In order to understand this interaction and its effects, it is necessary to develop a theory of occupation, including:

- the nature of human occupation
- the function of human occupation
- classification of occupations
- occupational genesis
- occupational role
- occupational performance
- occupational behaviour and occupational choice
- the relationship between occupation and health.

What is human occupation?

The words 'activity' and 'occupation' are often used synonymously, even by occupational thera-

pists, but it is important to clarify the difference. Reilly (1962) suggested that the very existence of occupational therapy depends on our knowledge of the difference between the two terms and our capacity to act on that knowledge. Christiansen & Baum (1991, p. 847) offered a teleological definition of activity, as 'productive action required for development, maturation, and use of sensory, motor, social psychological, and cognitive functions'. Hagedorn (1997, p. 143) defined activity descriptively as 'an integrated sequence of tasks which takes place on a specific occasion, during a finite period, for a particular purpose.' This definition makes it easier to differentiate activity from occupation, which has been variously defined as:

- 'a form of human endeavour which provides longitudinal organisation of time or effort in a person's life' (Hagedorn 1997)
- 'a cluster of activities that can be grouped under a name and form part of a social role' (Breines 1998, unpublished lecture)
- 'a general term that refers to engagement in activities, tasks and roles for the purpose of meeting the requirements of living' (Levine & Brayley 1991)
- 'chunks of culturally and personally meaningful activity in which humans engage that can be named in the lexicon of our culture' (Clark et al 1991)
- 'that which occupies us between birth and death, and can be classified into occupations relating to play, leisure, work and self-care. Occupations have meaning and value for the individual' (Pretorius 1997).

Occupations, then, can be named – for example child care, teaching, carpentry, painting and decorating. If a set of activities does not have a name, then it does not constitute an occupation. A second feature of occupations is that they take place over time and help to organise how time is spent. Thirdly, occupations are social in nature and always have a social context. Even the most private occupations, such as maintaining personal hygiene, are shaped by the society in which we live. In the 1950s it was common for people in the UK to take a bath once a week; now, many people bath or shower every day.

For occupational therapists, the key feature that differentiates occupation from activity is the social dimension of occupations: an occupation has meaning for the individual and forms a part of his personal and social identity. Activity is a narrower concept in that the activities we do are part of the occupations that make up our lives.

Activities have purpose and meaning for the person carrying them out, although the meaning will differ for different individuals and for the same person at different times. Purposeful activities have been defined as 'doing processes that require the use of thought and energy and are directed towards an intended or desired end result' (Mosey 1986).

The function of human occupation

People have a basic need to engage in activity which has meaning and value for them. Reilly (1962) claimed that 'man has a vital need for occupation and that his central nervous system demands the rich and varied stimuli that solving life problems provides him'. Occupations, and the activities by which they are enacted, can serve various functions in daily life:

- Human development is influenced by the physical and mental activity of the growing child.
- Activity is a tool for exploring and learning about our own potential, about others and about the environment (Finlay 1988).
- People relate to the human and non-human world, and test out their perceptions, through what they do.
- Occupations contribute to an individual's personal sense of identity.
- Occupations form an important part of each person's position in society and social status.
- People use activity as a means to satisfy many of their physical and psychological needs.
- Engaging in purposeful activity gives the individual a sense of control over his life and contributes to a sense of quality of life.
- The health of the individual is influenced by what he does.

Occupational therapists use the characteristics of meaningful activity to bring about change in their clients. For example, someone with chronic depression can be distracted from morbid preoccupation with thoughts of suicide by engagement in an interesting, pleasurable activity such as silk painting. This temporary distraction allows the individual to *experience* what it feels like not to be depressed, opening the way for the use of depression management techniques for long-term relief. The therapeutic goals of purposeful activity are summarised in Figure 3.2.

Classification of occupations

One of the most simple theories of occupation is the identification and classification of different types of occupation. Three categories are usually employed:

- self-care
- play/leisure
- productivity/work.

These are artificial differentiations, since an occupation can move from one category to

Enhancing consciousness
Providing opportunities
Providing extrinsic motivation
Accessing intrinsic motivation
Teaching skills
Increasing competence
Rehearsing future events
Improving self-awareness
Enhancing the development of autonomy
Assisting in the construction of meaning
Helping to clarify values and intentions
Helping to identify personal goals
Offering purpose
Assisting with the development of volition
Helping to create identity
Respecting choices
Improving temporal orientation
Enabling achievement
Assisting towards the attainment of personal goals
Enhancing self-image

Figure 3.2 The therapeutic goals of purposeful activity (from Creek 1998).

another or belong in more than one category at the same time. For example, cooking may be self-care if it is to satisfy an individual's hunger, it may be work if it is to feed a family, or it may be leisure if it is to give a dinner party to friends.

Self-care. Self-care is occupation that enables the individual to survive and that promotes and maintains health. It includes:

- Basic physical functions such as eating, sleeping, excreting, keeping clean and keeping warm.
- Survival functions such as cooking, dressing, shopping, maintaining one's living environment, and keeping fit. Many of these functions have become specialised and have been delegated to members of society who have special skills, such as builders and bakers, but some remain with the individual.

The standard of self-care varies from person to person, although society tries to set minimum standards for certain aspects such as housing, clothing and nutrition.

Play/leisure. Man is a very adaptable species. This adaptability has been achieved by developing flexible behaviour rather than specialised behaviour (Kielhofner 1980). Play is the medium through which the child is able to learn and rehearse a wide range of skills that will enable him to respond appropriately and adaptively in different situations. Even in adult life, new skills are learned more thoroughly and integrated more successfully into the pattern of daily life if the individual approaches learning in a playful and explorative manner.

Play also allows children to practise participating in their culture and to learn its norms and values through the games and folk literature which are specific to that culture. For example, competitive games teach a child both society's rules and expectations about competition and his own position in the pecking order of a competitive society (Kielhofner 1980).

In adult life, play is usually called 'leisure' and is often used to satisfy individual needs that are not met by either self-care or work occupations. For example, amateur dramatics can improve the physical well-being of a person who has an otherwise sedentary lifestyle, provide intellectual stimulation for a full-time mother of small children, create social contacts for an unemployed person or enhance the self-esteem of someone who has a low-level position at work.

Productivity/work. Work is any productive activity, whether paid or unpaid, that contributes to the maintenance or advancement of society as well as to the individual's own survival or development. Work may help to maintain society (e.g. refuse collection), or contribute to its advance (e.g. theoretical physics).

The work in which a person spends most of his time usually becomes an important part of his personal identity and a major social role, giving him his position in society and a sense of his own value as a contributing member. Different jobs are given different social values so that people in certain jobs are considered to be more important than others, irrespective of how necessary their work is to the continuation of society. For example, a doctor is more highly valued in Western society than a housewife.

Work serves many functions for the individual:

- It gives the person a major role in society and a social position.
- It usually provides the person with a means of livelihood.
- It gives a structure to time around which other activities can be planned.
- It can give a sense of purpose and value to life.
- It can be an important part of an individual's personal identity and a source of self-esteem.
- It can be a forum for meeting people and building different types of relationships.
- It can be an important interest and a source of satisfaction.

Anyone who is unable to work misses all these benefits and is, in addition, usually seen as a negative factor in society.

Balance of occupations

Each person takes on many occupations in the course of his life. These fit together in what

Bateson (1997, p. 7) called 'the framework of a life'. Self-care, play and work exist in a balance which is not static but changes at different stages of the life cycle and varies from individual to individual. People are not pre-programmed to follow a daily routine of activities; they continually make choices about what to do with their time and how to structure their daily routine. 'The net effect is engagement in a daily blend of occupations, each of which may be experienced as work, rest, play, leisure or self-care and which shape, in part, one's perception of the quality of life' (Yerxa et al 1989).

The healthy individual has his daily life activities organised into a satisfying pattern which meets his needs and which is socially acceptable. The balance of occupations in a person's life is determined by personal interests and abilities, social expectations, age, environment and personal circumstances. For example, a professional woman with no children may find that she enjoys a variety of social and sporting activities which keep her fit, relieve the stress of working and enable her to meet people. A single mother with four children and a low-paid job, on the other hand, may not have the resources of time, energy or money to engage in a range of leisure activities.

Some patterns of activity can be seen to be unbalanced. For example, the 50-year-old man who works up to 12 hours a day, rarely sees his children, has no social life outside work and has no other important interests could not be said to have a balanced range of occupations. If he loses his job, he may develop serious health problems. For occupational therapists, the balanced use of time in daily living activities not only influences health but is an indicator of health.

The term 'temporal adaptation' is used to refer to the normal use of time in a purposeful daily routine of activities. Occupational therapists are not so much concerned with a person's ability to carry out specific tasks at particular points in time as with the way in which he uses and organises time in daily life. In order to achieve a balance, the individual must have an awareness of time and of himself within time. Using time adaptively requires remembering past experiences and acting on them, being aware of future consequences of actions, planning ahead, acting on those plans and monitoring the effects of actions.

Occupational genesis

It is the nature of human beings to be active, therefore activity has always been a part of human life. However, the activities which have purpose and meaning for people and which take up a large part of their time have changed over the ages, from the physical activities of hunter/gatherer societies to the more passive, sedentary lifestyle of modern Western people. Breines (1995) called this evolution of human activity 'occupational genesis': 'Occupational genesis describes the evolving adaptive process in which humans engage in purposeful activities that are meaningful to their lives as their world and their experiences change.'

Occupational genesis applies to societies, to the nature of human occupations that have predominated at different times in history. Breines (1995) described the activities and skills that have enabled people to survive and develop through the ages, from the very early people, 'searching their world for food, shelter, and understanding', to modern people solving the problems of their world with the tools and skills available to them. Occupational genesis also applies to the process of change in the nature and balance of occupations throughout an individual's lifespan. To some extent, the ontogenesis of the individual follows the pattern of phylogenesis of society, as the developing child learns about himself and his world through doing, just as the human race has survived and evolved through doing.

Breines (1995) described occupations taking place in three realms, each associated with one of the meanings of this complex term, as shown in Figure 3.3. The egocentric realm is oriented towards the self so that the world is seen in relation to the self, for example a child sees his mother's broken arm in terms of what mother can and cannot do for him. The exocentric realm is oriented towards the external world, for example an

Term	Meaning	Realm
To be occupied	Mind and body	Egocentric
To occupy	Time and space	Exocentric
Occupation	Work, play and self-care	Consensual

Figure 3.3 Dimensions of occupation (from Breines 1995).

employed man votes for the political party which will increase taxes to pay for better social security because he is concerned about the plight of homeless people. The consensual realm is where a world view is shared with others, for example members of a church share the same spiritual beliefs. Activities which have meaning for the individual integrate these three elements in a wholesome relationship.

Engagement in activities which are age- and culturally appropriate can ground the individual in his own community and lead to a sense of connectedness with others. Conversely, an inability to perform the activities that are considered normal in society, or that the individual would consider appropriate for himself, can lead to feelings of exclusion and worthlessness. The theory of occupational genesis assists the occupational therapist to understand which activities will enhance a sense of belonging and worth in the client.

Occupational roles

Each person fulfils a number of roles during his lifetime. At any one time the individual may adopt a variety of roles, and these roles will change at different stages of life. For example, a child may have the roles of: daughter, sibling, school pupil, friend, Brownie, niece, dog owner. A decade later, some of these roles will have been dropped and new ones taken up, so that she is now: daughter, sibling, student, friend, flatmate, lover, waitress, and so on.

An occupation and a social role may share the same name, for example 'mother' is both a role and an occupation. Occupation incorporates what a mother does for her children, which is influenced by social expectations and her sense of identity as a mother. The concept of occupation is mainly concerned with activity, the actions that a person takes to achieve his purposes, while the concept of role is mainly concerned with social expectations and the mechanisms by which society shapes the actions of individuals to achieve harmony.

Roles are social constructs which carry behavioural expectations and which contribute to a person's self-image and sense of identity. They are 'the sets of behaviours that individuals occupying specific positions within a group are expected to perform' (Baron & Byrne 1997, p. 437). Roles are allocated by society and adopted by the individual, that is, a role is both a social position and a set of tasks performed by the individual. Each person will interpret a role in a unique way. For example, the role of mother carries expectations about the care and nurturing of children. Women in the UK normally play a major part in bringing up their own children because that is the expectation in Western society. Different women will interpret the role in different ways, perhaps delegating some parts of the task of mothering to a relative or a paid childminder. If society feels that a woman is not fulfilling her role adequately, then it may be taken away from her and her children given into the care of others. Or a woman may choose not to accept the role of mother and may voluntarily give her children into full-time care.

The activities required for the fulfilment of one role may come into conflict with the activities required for the fulfilment of a different role. Blair (1998) suggested three ways in which this might occur:

- incompatible expectations, such as a proposal for team building initiatives after hours producing conflict between the roles of co-worker and family member
- overload arising from demands beyond the individual's capacity, such as the demands on a therapist for effective intervention with a large number of people and a large volume of paperwork
- ambiguity and uncertainty about what is expected of a worker or the standard of work expected.

Social role is linked to social status. 'Status' refers to the position of the individual within the social structure and 'role' is what the person does in that position. The status we achieve through our major social roles influences both the way that other people in our social group treat us and our expectations of how we will be treated. If we have a high social status, we are more likely to expect to be treated with respect and consideration.

Roles carry both rights within society and obligations to that society. For example, a university student has the obligation to attend a certain number of teaching sessions, to behave in an acceptable way during those sessions, to make an effort to learn the topics presented and to complete a prescribed number of assignments within a given timescale. In return, the student is given money, a position in society and the possibility of paid employment at the end of the programme of study.

Early occupational therapy theorists (Moorhead 1969, Matsutsuyu 1971) classified roles as: family roles, personal sexual roles and occupational roles, and considered that the main concern of the occupational therapist was with occupational roles. More recent writings (Kielhofner 1992, Reed & Sanderson 1992) suggest that the pattern of occupations we engage in is influenced by the roles that society gives us, although we have some control over the individual occupations we choose within that pattern.

Occupational performance

The word 'occupation' is used to refer to both the performance of an activity and the pre-existing format that guides or structures that performance (Nelson 1988). For example, there is an established format of rules, procedures, equipment and environment for playing football. This is the 'occupational form', which is socially constructed and exists independently of performance. Football has a physical environment which includes materials, location, human context and temporal context. It also has a sociocultural reality that depends on a social or cultural consensus and allows the occupational form to be interpreted differently in different social contexts, such as

the major differences between a game of football for schoolchildren and an FA cup championship match. The playing football, the doing, is 'occupational performance'. The way in which we perform within a given occupational form also depends on our level of competence and the meanings that we give to the occupation. For example, a professional goalkeeper may deliberately allow the ball into the net if he is trying to encourage a young child to learn the game, or he may do his best to keep it out to help his team to win an international match.

Christiansen & Baum (1997, p. 600) defined occupational performance as 'the unique term used by occupational therapy to express function as it reflects the individual's dynamic experience of engaging in daily occupations within the environment.'

Mosey (1986) classified occupational performance into five areas:

• family interactions
• activities of daily living
• school/work
• play/leisure/recreation
• temporal adaptation.

The first four categories are social roles, while the fifth, temporal adaptation, 'refers to the ability to organize one's time in order to fulfil adequately the responsibilities and enjoy the pleasures of one's required and/or desired social roles' (Mosey 1986, p. 8).

Occupational performance involves a sequence of skilled actions and depends on:

• a range of learned skills
• developmental maturation
• the ability to combine and apply skills appropriately at the right time and place (Reed & Sanderson 1992).

A skill is 'the ability to put skill components together in smoothly integrated and sequenced, competent performance' (Hagedorn 1995). Skill components are the structures and processes that underpin performance.

Competence 'To be competent means to be sufficient or adequate to meet the demands of a situation or task' (White 1971). Competence is a relative state, so that we can talk about someone being more competent at one task than another, or about one person being more competent than another at a particular task. Competence in occupational performance develops with practice, therefore it can be expected that a child or a novice will be competent in a narrower range of activities than an experienced adult, and will be less competent in the tasks he can perform.

People have an intrinsic drive to realise their potentials and to exert an influence on the environment. It is this drive which leads to the development of competence, as the individual tests his capacities on the outside world and gains confidence in his ability (White 1971).

Occupational behaviour and occupational choice

The term 'occupational behaviour' was coined to refer to active engagement in occupation. Occupational behaviour has been defined as 'the entire developmental continuum of play and work' (Reilly 1969). It includes:

- an act of the will
- an experience of engagement, and
- a planning and organising of resources (Yerxa et al 1989).

Occupational behaviour evolves throughout the life cycle. Children learn the rules for acceptable behaviour in society through play, and their play experiences lead on to choice of occupations in adult life. The major occupation of many adults is work, and the process of choosing a job or career is called 'occupational choice'.

Ginzberg and colleagues (1951) studied how people choose their main work occupation, finding that such an important decision is not made in one step but is the culmination of many smaller decisions made over many years. This long process of decision making allows the individual to accumulate knowledge of what he likes doing, what he does well and what activities he values. Ginzberg and his associates described occupational choice as a series of choices and the elimination of choices, as changes occur in the individual and the environment, which lead eventually to a narrowing of choice and to decisions being made. They identified four elements that influence the occupational choices made by individuals:

- awareness of one's own capacities
- interests
- personal goals and values
- time perspective of occupations.

In addition, the opportunity for making a particular choice must be present.

What people may choose to do in the short or long term is partly influenced by the nature of the choices available. The range of choices is determined by social factors, such as public disapproval, and by the physical environment, such as the location of sport and leisure facilities. In order to choose to do something, the individual also has to be aware of what his choices are. This awareness includes knowing what activities are available and knowing how to access them. It also implies having the capacity to see opportunities for action and having enough information on which to base choices.

The relationship between occupation and health

Occupational therapists claim that there is a link between occupation and health but there has been, until recently, no strong theory to explain that link. In the 1990s, an Australian occupational therapist, Wilcock, published a series of papers and a book outlining a theory of the relationship between occupation and health (Wilcock 1995, 1998a, 1998b).

Wilcock (1998a, p. 5) argued that humans are occupational beings with a central nervous system that has the capacity to 'analyse, organise, understand, produce, judge, plan, activate, formulate and execute complex occupation'. Occupations are, therefore, innate human behaviours that encompass all the things that people do, serving both a social and a biological function. Humans have evolved as occupational beings and it is through occupation that we adapt to, or insulate ourselves from, our physical, cultural and social environments.

Wilcock (1998a) further suggested that the two evolutionary functions of occupation are survival and health. It is through occupations that we meet our basic survival needs of safety, food, water, warmth and shelter. Health, which can be seen as the natural state for a person to be in, is also achieved through occupation, first by having all the basic survival needs met and then by 'having physical, mental and social capacities maintained, exercised and in balance' (p. 6).

Health can be a positive experience of well-being and not just the absence of disease or infirmity. Wilcock (1998b, p. 103) described mental well-being as a condition in which people can 'be creative and adventurous as they experience all human emotions, explore and adapt appropriately, and without undue disruption meet their life needs'.

The three occupational factors which can cause a breakdown of health are occupational imbalance, deprivation and alienation (Wilcock 1998b). Occupational imbalance is a lack of balance between work, rest and play causing a loss of harmony between internal bodily systems and between the person and the environment. Occupational deprivation arises when external circumstances prevent the individual from using his capacities to the full, leading to imbalance and failure to develop or maintain normal functioning. Occupational alienation occurs when a person engages in activity which is not in accordance with the occupational nature of the species or the individual. The results are frustration, boredom, unhappiness and stress.

Occupational therapy can intervene either at the level of the individual or at the level of society, as in health promotion or community development, in order to counteract the negative effects of occupational imbalance, deprivation and alienation. This theory suggests that the most appropriate arena for the work of the occupational therapist is not in secondary or tertiary health care systems but in public health.

Biological sciences

When working with people whose problem is emotional or behavioural, it is essential to have a grounding in the biological sciences, since physical structures and systems underpin development in all other areas, and there are many physical abnormalities associated with psychosocial disorders. It is not within the scope of this book to cover the biological sciences in any detail but to review their importance to the knowledge base of occupational therapy.

Anatomy is the study of physical structures and systems. Physiology is the study of body functions. The understanding of certain organic disorders, for example dementia, depends on knowledge of anatomy and physiology, especially neuroanatomy and neurophysiology.

Some illnesses and handicaps are caused by chromosomal abnormalities, such as trisomy 21 (Down's syndrome), or genetic abnormalities, such as inherited microcephaly. Handicaps may also result from damage to the central nervous system of the foetus or young child by infection, toxins, anoxia or trauma. Effective intervention with such major handicaps depends on understanding the normal functioning of the nervous system and knowing where the focus of damage is. Other psychosocial problems arising from central nervous system malfunction include epilepsy, organic brain disease and the side-effects of certain groups of drugs used in treatment.

Problems which may not have a physical cause but which have an important physical component in their presentation include eating disorders, addictions, anxiety neurosis, autism, catatonia, mania and depression.

Kinesiology is the study of the mechanics of movement, including range and coordination of movements and muscle strength. Movement and coordination are often affected in psychosocial disorders, for example stereotyped movements in autism or depressive stupor. Common features of learning disability are abnormal muscle tone, poor posture and unusual gait. Some methods of treatment can also affect the way a person looks and moves, for example certain groups of drugs affect the central nervous system to produce Parkinsonian rigidity and tremor.

Any abnormality of appearance immediately marks a person as different and can interfere with his acceptance by society, so effective treatment of movement patterns is essential in any resettlement programme.

The link between mind and body and the use of physical activity as treatment are covered in more detail in Chapter 12.

Developmental theory

In order to understand and treat people with functional deficits it is necessary for the occupational therapist to have a basic understanding of normal structures, functions and sequences of development.

Development is the gradual evolution of an organism through a series of predictable stages to full growth. In the case of human beings, this means the process of realising their genetic potential by passing through a series of stages of growth and maturation, in areas that are relatively independent of environmental influences. Psychological and social development are dependent on, but also influence, physical growth and maturation. Maturation is the process of coming to full growth and development, mentally, physically and socially.

Competent performance of age-appropriate skills depends on development and maturation occurring in the appropriate sequence and at an appropriate pace.

Conditions for development

Each person is born with genetic programming that determines his physical and psychological potential. However, in order to realise that potential, certain environmental factors must be present.

The growing child needs to have physiological needs met, such as food, sleep, warmth, touch and physical handling. He needs to be protected from trauma by disease or injury, to be given loving attention and opportunities to explore safely his own potential and the environment. He interacts with his environment and reaches his potential through occupation; without occupation, development will not proceed normally.

Finally, the child needs a sense of security and belonging if he is to develop the confidence to move away from a strong attachment to the mother figure towards greater independence and social adjustment (Smith 1993).

Physical development

Physical development follows a recognised sequence in which certain skills are always learned before others – for example all children stand before they walk. Many skills are learned at the same time, especially in the first years of life, but not at the same rate – for example some children are able to talk quite well before they can walk while others learn to walk first. Various stages are passed through in learning new skills but not all children pass through all stages – for example some children never crawl before they walk.

Cognitive development

Cognitive development is a function of the interaction between an individual and his environment. It is dependent on and influenced by both:

- the development of other adaptive skills, such as physical and social skills
- environmental stimuli and opportunities for exploration.

Each person's pace of development is unique, determined by these two factors, but there are patterns that are common to everyone. It is these patterns that are studied in cognitive developmental theory.

Cognition develops through a series of predictable stages that are qualitatively distinct from each other, as the nervous system matures and as the infant receives feedback on his actions from environmental stimuli. Each level of skills must be mastered before the child can move on to the next stage, and earlier skills must be integrated with new ones. Norms can be established for the age at which a child might be expected to reach each stage, depending on his cultural background. Although individual variations in the pattern might occur, no stage can be missed out if new learning is to be integrated with existing knowledge.

There are many ways of looking at how cognition develops and breaking it into stages, including theories of the development of self-awareness, of thinking, of language and of ethical reasoning.

Personality development

Each person is born with a genetic potential for personality, just as for physical characteristics. Individual differences are apparent from birth but personality is also shaped by experience. Some characteristics are influenced by the culture that the child grows up in, for example aggression and competition are highly valued in some cultures but actively discouraged in others.

Although many people share a culture and have experiences of it, each person has unique experiences throughout life which shape his personality and self-concept (Smith 1993). For example, the child of a soldier may be widely travelled and have been to many schools by the time he leaves home, while the child of a single, unemployed parent from the same town and same social background is more likely to have stayed in the same house and at the same school throughout his school career. These two people will have very different views of the world and different responses to events.

Psychosocial development

People are essentially social animals who develop and live in the context of groups. Human interaction stimulates biological, psychological, emotional and social development and people deprived of human contact do not thrive.

The type of contact the developing child needs changes from the intense relationship with the mother, through various levels of group interactions, to adult intimacy and progressive emotional interdependence. Erik Erikson (1965) proposed eight stages of psychosocial development from birth to old age (Table 3.1). He suggested that each stage involves a crisis that must be resolved if development is to continue normally.

Physical medicine

In medicine, disease is classified according to aetiology or symptomatology. Care is taken to establish an accurate diagnosis so that the most appropriate treatment can be given. This may be to:

- remove the cause of the disease (e.g. surgery to remove a tumour)
- correct the pathology of the disease (e.g. insulin injections for diabetes mellitus)
- give symptom relief (e.g. neuroleptic medication to control psychotic symptoms).

The occupational therapy student studies the classification, aetiology, presentation, treatment and prognosis of diseases affecting the vascular, locomotor, respiratory, digestive, urogenital and endocrine systems. Emphasis is placed on neurology, including diseases and injuries affecting the nervous system such as brain, spinal cord and peripheral nerve injuries, cerebral palsy, poliomyelitis, chorea, multiple sclerosis and cerebrovascular accidents.

A knowledge of basic medical theory and language is important to occupational therapists because we work within a system which has a strong bias towards the medical model. This model helps us to understand in depth some aspects of disease and illness but it can nevertheless be limiting, as it does not normally take account of the whole person functioning in his environment and in time (Lyons 1985).

Table 3.1 Erikson's stages of psychosocial development

Age	Psychosocial crisis	Key relationships
0–1	Trust vs. mistrust	Mother
2–3	Autonomy vs. shame and doubt	Parallel play
4–5	Initiative vs. guilt	Interactive play
6–puberty	Industry vs. inferiority	Idols
Adolescence	Identity vs. role confusion	Peer group
Early adulthood	Intimacy vs. isolation	Life partner
Middle adulthood	Generativity vs. self-absorption	Children
Late adulthood	Ego-integrity vs. despair	Self-sufficiency

Psychiatry

Psychiatry uses a medical model, seeing mental disorder in terms of predisposing and precipitating factors (aetiology), signs and symptoms, course, treatment and prognosis. Psychiatric diseases are usually classified by signs and symptoms. Treatment can be physical, for example electroconvulsive therapy (ECT), or psychological, for example cognitive behavioural therapy.

Most psychiatrists take into account a range of factors affecting the client, such as premorbid personality, family history and social circumstances, but these are added on the medical model.

Occupational therapy students study the aetiology, presentation, classification and treatment of the more common psychiatric disorders including psychoneuroses, psychoses, organic states, substance misuse, personality disorders, psychiatric problems of children and developmental delay (learning disability).

As in physical medicine, this model is useful in focusing on particular aspects of disease and for communicating with colleagues about those aspects, but it can be limiting with its emphasis on treatment techniques rather than on people and social systems.

Psychology

Psychology is an important area of study throughout the 3 or 4 years of occupational therapy education. As well as providing theories to explain many aspects of human beings, such as personality and motivation, it has produced certain assessment and treatment techniques which have been widely adopted by occupational therapists, for example some anxiety management techniques.

Areas of study include psychological development, which covers personality development, cognitive development and psychosocial development. Perception, consciousness, memory, motivation, language and thinking are basic areas of study. Learning theory and conditioning are considered to be important to the occupational therapist, although some of the behavioural methods derived from these theories do not fit with the humanistic, person-centred approach. Humanistic psychology and psychoanalytic theory are studied in some depth and both give alternative insights into basic drives and motivation. Intelligence, creativity and methods of measuring these are studied, although occupational therapists are not usually expected to do formal testing. Knowledge of the effects of stress and methods used to cope with it are of particular importance to the occupational therapist. Finally, counselling techniques are being given increasing emphasis.

Sociology

The body of knowledge in sociology has been expanding rapidly in recent years and has become increasingly important to occupational therapists. In the past, when occupational therapists were mostly based in hospitals, clients were often treated in isolation from their families and social networks. With the shift in emphasis from care in hospitals to care in the community, an understanding of how people function in society has become even more vital.

Topics studied include: social behaviour; the process of socialisation; social relationships; social stratification and social class; the social construction of age, gender, illness and disability; deviance, stigma and normalisation; social trends; family, community and kinship; the multicultural society; power and inequality; organisations; work and leisure; the social and cultural context of health and illness; and social policy.

Use of the knowledge base The breadth of occupational therapy practice requires that the profession has this extensive knowledge base but different fields of practice will draw on different areas of knowledge. The ways in which the knowledge base is organised for use are covered in the section below, 'therapy', and in Chapter 5.

OCCUPATIONAL THERAPY THEORY INTO PRACTICE

In order to understand the ways in which the knowledge base of occupational therapy is organised, it is necessary to have an understanding of various terms, which are defined below. They include: theory, frame of reference, approach, model and paradigm. The section then offers a framework for understanding the relationship of theory to practice in occupational therapy and finishes by describing the occupational therapy process.

Defining terms

Theory

Theories are conceptual systems or frameworks used to organise knowledge. A theory consists of a description of a set of phenomena, an explanation of how and under what circumstances they occur, and a demonstration of how they relate to each other. A theory is not reality and should not be confused with reality. A theory is a framework constructed to understand or shape reality in order to achieve some particular purpose, and a good theory will fulfil the purpose for which it was designed.

Occupational therapists use theories from a variety of disciplines, as shown above. The breadth of the theoretical base, and the complexity of some of the theories we use, could seem overwhelming. However, not all occupational therapists need to know all the theories that make up the total body of knowledge of the profession. We use different theories depending on the area in which we work, the kind of problems we are dealing with in that setting and our own knowledge, skill and preferences. Theories that work well together and that can be applied within a particular field of practice can be organised as frames of reference.

Frame of reference

A frame of reference is an individual's 'personal notion of reality, their cultural, social, and psychological biases, their values and beliefs, and how these factors influence the practice of occupational therapy' (Krefting 1985). So, in its widest sense, a frame of reference is the way a person sees the world.

Llorens (1984) offered a narrower definition for occupational therapists: 'Theoretical frames of reference organise what is known in a field and permit description or depiction of relationships and interrelationships among facts and concepts.' A frame of reference, therefore, is made up of selected theories that are compatible with each other and that can be applied within a particular field of practice. Bruce & Borg (1993) wrote that a frame of reference refers to the principles behind practice with particular client groups.

Within occupational therapy there are many frames of reference, some of which can be used in more than one field and some of which are for very specific purposes. The choice of a frame of reference is influenced by the presenting problems of the client, the ethos of the unit where the intervention takes place and the knowledge of the therapist (Hurff 1985).

Approach

The terms 'frame of reference' and 'approach' are often used synonymously. A simple definition of an approach is 'ways and means of putting theory into practice' (Creek et al 1993).

Model

For some decades there has been a growing body of literature on models in occupational therapy. A basic definition of a model is: 'A simplified representation of the structure and content of a phenomenon or system that describes or explains the complex relationships between concepts within the system and integrates elements of theory and practice' (Creek et al 1993). However, different writers use the term in different ways. Krefting (1985) suggested that there are generic models which encompass all aspects of the profession, as shown at the higher level in Figure 3.4. There are also models which have a narrower focus and are only relevant within a particular field of practice as shown at the lower level in Figure 3.4.

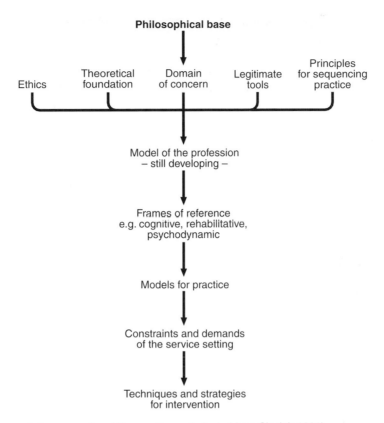

Figure 3.4   Basic framework for occupational therapy theory (adapted from Sinclair 1991).

Paradigm

Mosey (1986) used the term 'model' in the way that most other writers use the term 'paradigm', to refer to:

the particular way in which a profession perceives itself, its relationship to other professions, and its association with the society to which it is responsible. A model is the reservoir of the collected knowledge and beliefs of a profession. It is characterised by a description of the profession's philosophical assumptions, ethical code, body of knowledge, domain of concern, the nature of and principles for sequencing the various aspects of practice, and the profession's legitimate tools.

Creek & Feaver (1993) suggested that a paradigm is 'the profession's world view that encompasses philosophies, theories, frames of reference and models for practice'.

Framework for occupational therapy theory

Philosophies, theories, frames of reference and models for practice can be organised into a flexible framework which depicts the relationship between each of these components of occupational therapy and shows how they influence practice (Fig. 3.4).

As explained, occupational therapists share certain beliefs and values which make up the profession's philosophical base. This base gives rise to:

- the ethical values which direct practice and set standards for therapists
- the theories which are selected to support practice
- the domain of concern which delineates the legitimate goals of the profession and the

people with whom it is appropriate for occupational therapists to work

- the legitimate tools of the profession which are the methods and media occupational therapists can claim to have competence in using
- the principles for sequencing practice which inform the occupational therapy process.

These components of occupational therapy make up the model or paradigm of the profession. Occupational therapy is a dynamic profession in a rapidly changing world, therefore it does not have a fixed and universally agreed model.

Theories are organised into frames of reference that can be applied within particular fields of practice. Theories may also be used to create models for practice which give more specific guidelines for intervention in particular areas.

The ways in which intervention is carried out are influenced by the constraints and demands of the setting where the therapeutic encounter takes place, as well as by the nature and goals of occupational therapy.

Finally, occupational therapists carry out treatment using techniques and strategies which are designed or adopted from other disciplines to achieve therapeutic goals in the ways suggested by the frame of reference being used.

The philosophical base and theoretical foundation of occupational therapy have been described in this chapter. The other components of this framework are described in more detail in Chapter 5 (the occupational therapy process, frames of reference, models for practice), Chapters 6–8 (legitimate tools), Chapter 10 (domain of concern) and Chapter 11 (ethics).

SUMMARY

In this chapter, a concise overview was given of the knowledge base of occupational therapy. Specialist textbooks on the different subjects will provide more details.

There was first a discussion of the changes that have taken place in the beliefs and values espoused by members of the profession during the past 90 years. The philosophical assumptions underpinning present-day practice were briefly reviewed under the headings of beliefs about people, beliefs about health and beliefs about the nature and purpose of the occupational therapy profession.

The knowledge base of occupational therapy is drawn from a wide range of disciplines. The various theories of occupation that have been and are still being developed, many under the banner of occupational science, were described. Some of the other fields of knowledge were reviewed more briefly, including: biological sciences, developmental theories, physical medicine, psychiatry, psychology and sociology. It was emphasised that, although occupational therapists are now developing their own theories of the relationships between people, health and occupation, occupational therapy will continue to benefit from drawing on new theories from other disciplines, as it has always done.

In conclusion, a framework was offered for understanding how the various components of occupational therapy fit together and allow theory to be translated into practice.

The next chapter considers the importance of research in the development of occupational therapy and practice.

REFERENCES

Bateson M C 1997 Enfolded activity and the concept of occupation. In: Zemke R, Clark F (eds) Occupational science: the evolving discipline. F A Davis, Philadelphia

Breines E B 1995 Occupational therapy activities from clay to computers: theory and practice. F A Davis, Philadelphia

Christiansen C 1997 Person-environment occupational performance. In: Christiansen C, Baum (eds) C Enabling function and well-being. Slack, Thorofare

Christiansen C, Baum C (eds) 1991 Occupational therapy: overcoming human performance deficits. Slack, Thorofare

Clark P N 1979 Human development through occupation: a philosophy and conceptual model for practice, part 2. American Journal of Occupational Therapy 33(8): 577–585

Creek J 1998 Purposeful activity. In: Creek J (ed) Occupational therapy: new perspectives. Whurr, London

Creek J, Feaver S 1993 Models for practice in occupational therapy, part 1: defining terms. British Journal of Occupational Therapy 56(1): 4–6

Creek J, Hagedorn R, Foster and Turner 1993 Unpublished discussion.

Erikson E H 1965 Childhood and society. Triad Paladin, London

Finlay L 1988 Occupational therapy practice in psychiatry. Croom Helm, London

Ginzberg E, Ginsberg S W, Axelrad S, Herma J L 1951 Occupational choice: an approach to a general theory. Columbia University Press, New York

Hagedorn R 1995 Occupational therapy perspectives and processes. Churchill Livingstone, Edinburgh

Hagedorn R 1997 Foundations for practice in occupational therapy, 2nd edn. Churchill Livingstone, Edinburgh

Hurff J M 1985 Visualisation: a decision-making tool for assessment and treatment planning. Occupational Therapy in Health Care 1(2): 5–12

Kielhofner G 1980 A model of human occupation, part 2: ontogenesis from the perspective of temporal adaptation. American Journal of Occupational Therapy 34(10): 657–663

Kielhofner G 1992 Conceptual foundations of occupational therapy. F A Davis, Philadelphia

Kielhofner G, Burke J P 1977 Occupational therapy after 60 years: an account of changing identity and knowledge. American Journal of Occupational Therapy 31(10): 675–689

Krefting L H 1985 The use of conceptual models in clinical practice. Canadian Journal of Occupational Therapy 52(4): 173–178

Llorens L 1984 Theoretical conceptualisations of occupational therapy: 1960–1982. Occupational Therapy and Mental Health 4(2): 1–14

Lyons M 1985 Paradise lost! . . . Paradise regained? Putting the promise of occupational therapy into practice. Australian Occupational Therapy Journal 32(2): 45–53

Matsutsuyu J S 1971 Occupational behaviour – a perspective on work and play. American Journal of Occupational Therapy 25(6): 291–294

Mattingley C, Fleming M F 1994 Clinical reasoning: forms of inquiry in a therapeutic practice. F A Davis, Philadelphia

Meyer A 1922 The philosophy of occupation therapy. Archives of Occupational Therapy 1:1–10. Reprinted in: American Journal of Occupational Therapy 1977 31(10): 639–642

Moorhead L 1969 The occupational history. American Journal of Occupational Therapy 23(4): 329–334

Mosey A C 1968 Recapitulation of ontogenesis: a theory for the practice of occupational therapy. American Journal of Occupational Therapy 22(5): 426–438

Mosey A C 1981 Occupational therapy: configuration of a profession. Raven Press, New York

Mosey A C 1986 Psychological components of occupational therapy. Raven Press, New York

Nelson D L 1988 Occupation: form and performance. American Journal of Occupational Therapy 42(10): 633–641

Pretorius J 1997 A model of ontogenesis and the dynamics of occupational function and dysfunction. In: Crouch R B, Alers V M (eds) Occupational therapy in psychiatry and mental health. Maskew Miller, Cape Town

Reed K L, Sanderson S N 1992 Concepts of occupational therapy, 3rd edn. Williams and Wilkins, Baltimore

Reilly M 1962 Occupational therapy can be one of the great ideas of 20th century medicine. American Journal of Occupational Therapy 16(1): 1–9

Reilly M 1969 The educational process. American Journal of Occupational Therapy 23(4): 299–307

Sartre J P 1943 Being and nothingness, trans. H E Barnes 1966. Methuen, London

Shannon P D 1977 The derailment of occupational therapy. American Journal of Occupational Therapy 31(4): 229–234

Sinclair K A 1991 Basic framework for occupational therapy theory. Unpublished teaching material.

Smith A G 1983 Holistic philosophy and general systems theory: an overview for occupational therapy. Journal of the New Zealand Association of Occupational Therapists 34(1): 13–18

Smith R E 1993 Psychology. West Publishing Company, Minneapolis

West W L 1984 A reaffirmed philosophy and practice of occupational therapy for the 1980s. American Journal of Occupational Therapy 38(1): 15–23

White R W 1971 The urge towards competence. American Journal of Occupational Therapy 25(6): 271–274

Wilcock A A 1995 The occupational brain: a theory of human nature. Journal of Occupational Science: Australia 2(1): 68–73

Wilcock A A 1998a A theory of occupation and health. In: Creek J (ed) Occupational therapy: new perspectives. Whurr, London

Wilcock A A 1998b An occupational perspective of health. Slack, Thorofare

World Health Organization 2000 International classification of functioning, disability and health. WHO, Geneva

Yerxa E J 1967 Authentic occupational therapy. American Journal of Occupational Therapy 21(1): 1–9

Yerxa E J 2000 Confessions of an occupational therapist who became a detective. British Journal of Occupational Therapy 63(5): 192–199

Yerxa E J et al 1989 An introduction to occupational science, a foundation for occupational therapy in the 21st century. Occupational Therapy Health Care 6(4): 1–17

Young M E, Quinn E 1992 Theories and principles of occupational therapy. Churchill Livingstone, Edinburgh

4

Research and professional effectiveness

Averil Stewart

INTRODUCTION

Nullius in verba (Don't take anybody's word for it)

(Motto of the Royal Society of London for improving natural knowledge – founded 1660)

Since the second edition of this book was published, there have been a number of developments which have led to this chapter taking on board the importance of evidence based practice (EBP) leading to clinical effectiveness. The issues of clinical governance and clinical audit are dealt with in Chapter 9, but these are inevitably interwoven with the search for clinical, and hence professional, effectiveness. Standards and guidelines are being set by national, local and professional bodies, and the process audited in order to achieve improved quality of care.

The management of research and development is tied into national and local needs, working across disciplines and institutions, through partnerships and networks, and focusing on ethical concerns, accountability, effectiveness and quality. The desire to be as effective as possible must be at the heart of any professional practice. In order to use effective interventions, as well as the personal artistry involved in being a therapist, the occupational therapy practitioner has to be up-to-date, aware of relevant literature, and should maintain a questioning research-minded, approach, rather than a blind acceptance that something is so because it was always so!

An increasing number of organisations and support mechanisms are available in the UK to make this possible. At governmental level, a range of papers have brought about change; they include the White Paper 'A first class service' (DoH 1998), which has led to the establishment of the National Institute for Clinical Excellence (NICE). The institute will work closely with organisations to examine the evidence of best practice and disseminate guidelines for effective interventions. At professional level, the College of Occupational Therapists has produced position statements, for example on clinical governance; the college has also appointed a research and development officer, and helps fund research projects. Information technology has made access possible to an abundance of information through the internet, professional databases and the Cochrane Databases of Systematic Reviews (CDSR). This is a worldwide network of reviewers who are increasingly looking at interprofessional collaboration and the development of health care policy as the outcomes of systematic reviews of research data. Their teamwork and enthusiasm lead to rigour and accessibility of information for other professionals seeking to make their practice evidence based. There are, however, controversies and dilemmas for therapists in this strongly scientific approach (Clemence 1998). Whatever the barriers, including weaknesses in research and the attitudes of clinicians, there is an imperative for all practising therapists to be involved in lifelong learning, self-appraisal and continuing professional development.

This chapter seeks to contribute to that lifelong learning as well as to provide a base for the new student and would-be researcher. It aims to explore some of the debates associated with research methodologies, and the role of research in the development of individual therapists, in the development of the profession as a whole and, most important of all, in ensuring quality interventions for clients. It does not deal in any detail with the research process, about which there are many excellent recent texts. These include Reid (1993), French (1994), Hart & Bond (1995), Crombie & Davies (1996), Bailey (1997), Silverman (1997) and DePoy & Gitlin (1998).

RESEARCH VERSUS COMMON SENSE

From an early age children try to make sense of their environment and of the meaning of life. They ask questions of enormous importance – 'Why did granny die?', 'Where is heaven?' – questions which adults often find difficult, resulting in answers which may curtail future questioning or lead to resigned acceptance: 'That's the way it is.' Palliative rather than explanatory answers may be given in order to ease the uncertainty of the unknown. Some questions, however, do not need explicit or verbal answers; through conditioning, young Johnny knows big brother will hit him hard if he takes away his ball. Custom and habit, regular observations and routine behaviours lead to predictions about probable outcomes. It is common sense to expect to have a disturbed night if too much has been drunk before going to bed.

The Compact Oxford English Dictionary (1991) defines 'common sense' as 'normal or average understanding; good sound practical sense in dealing with everyday affairs of life; general sagacity'. While this is a relatively vague definition, Popper (1972) argues as to whether or not 'All science, and all philosophy, are enlightened common sense'. It may be contended that, over the years, practical, thinking occupational therapists have been applying good principles founded on common sense and backed up by observation and experience. However, this is no longer enough. Knowledge, validated by systematic data collection, is now required in order to place occupational therapy on a similar footing to other professions and to increase the evidence for theoretical underpinnings.

Definition and hierarchy of research

The definition of 'research' in the Compact Oxford English Dictionary (1991) is 'a search or investigation directed to the discovery of some fact by careful consideration or study of a subject; a course of critical or scientific enquiry'. In order to make sense of the world and to gain some control, children from an early age will sort by category, collect objects and attempt to classify on the basis of self-determined criteria, for example who has the biggest conker or biscuit. Adults, scientists and researchers also attempt to classify through rigorous observation and analysis. Hence the development of plant taxonomies, the classification of diseases and, currently, the establishment of uniform terminology and taxonomies in occupational therapy (Christiansen 1994). The emerging discipline of occupational science, as found in the journal of that name, is attempting to describe and analyse humans as occupational beings and subsequently to provide a systematic study of dysfunction in occupational performance which is the basis for occupational therapy. There are many difficulties associated with this commendable aim, not least the need to agree on a common worldwide language, but at least it is a start.

Comparison between natural, medical and social sciences

Establishing cause and effect is very complex, although it might appear easier in the field of natural sciences and medicine than in social sciences. This is not necessarily the case for, while influences on physical and biological processes under investigation can be controlled and manipulated more readily than psychological and social influences, there are similar problems affecting rigour. For example, there is growing acceptance that 'experimenter effects', first elucidated by psychologists in the 1950s and 1960s, can apply to physical, chemical and biological processes as well as to behaviour.

Another issue concerns observability. As with some internal psychological processes, not all physical processes are observable or subject to experimentation. Einstein himself conducted research through thought experiments because he could not directly observe the behaviour of the subject of his enquiry, the universe. Equally, a brain biochemist has to infer what is going on in neurochemical terms by manipulating input and observing output, in much the same way as a psychologist.

In its purest sense, scientific method involves controlled trials that should be repeatable, so that other researchers, undertaking similar observations of the same subject under the same conditions, would get the same result. The personal opinions of an expert, no matter how much his professionalism **may** be respected, are not in themselves scientifically sound. They have a subjectivity, albeit grown out of experience. Opinions need to be backed up by evidence, data and explanation. Put another way, the strength of evidence can be described on the basis of five different categories (Muir Gray 1997), as shown in Table 4.1. Such a hierarchy of evidence highlights the problems for health care professions where there can be a paucity of research, particularly of randomised controlled trials, or research is qualitative in nature. Others (Reid 1993, DePoy & Gitlin 1999) describe these strengths as a continuum, with scientific experimentation at one end and phenomenology at the other.

Occupational therapists, like many others, are more concerned about the subjective experience of individuals and conducting research which seeks to understand the many variables which can interact with therapy. It is widely accepted that, when dealing with people, there is a multiplicity of factors which may influence who does

Table 4.1   The five strengths of evidence (Muir Gray 1997)

Type	Strength of evidence
I	Strong evidence from at least one systematic review of multiple well-designed randomised controlled trials
II	Strong evidence from at least one properly designed randomised controlled trial of appropriate size
III	Evidence from well-designed trials without randomisation, single group pre-post, cohort, time series or matched case-control studies
IV	Evidence from well-designed non-experimental studies from more than one centre or research group
V	Opinions of respected authorities, based on clinical evidence, descriptive studies or reports of expert committees

or does not produce certain behaviours as a result of, for example, increasing stress. To take this theme further, studies by Gentry & Kobasa (1984) examined personality characteristics, such as hardiness, to help explain apparent resistance to stress and other health-related behaviours, thus demonstrating how human behaviour is governed by many different factors.

Research and professional life

Research, therefore, is about understanding our world and the specific contexts in which we work. It is also about identifying limits and looking for alternative theories or approaches. There is a challenge within this which requires time for reflection, to examine alternatives and change a course of action as necessary. Such challenges are not the sole prerogative of researchers but are part of the practical thinking person's repertoire. Complacency and blind acceptance are not the hallmarks of professional education and development. 'Habit is all the test of truth, it must be right, I've done it since my youth' (Crabbe 1810, quoted in Smith 1989) is no longer an acceptable attitude. Autonomous practice now requires critical awareness.

Research, clinical reasoning, reflective practice and, indeed, philosophy have much in common. They require detachment, standing back in order to avoid blinkered thinking and automatic behaviour. Seedhouse (1986), in discussing philosophy, suggests that 'personal, intellectual insecurity is a great strength if it is coupled with a stubborn energy and patience'. Like philosophy, research is a process which attempts to elucidate, to clarify and to explain events. It is a process which develops the person as well as producing knowledge and understanding. As such it should pervade professional practice. It is not a superior activity but is rather like being a detective seeking clues, asking questions and following up hunches in order to produce new information and possible explanations. With increasing emphasis now on evidence based practice, if this is to become inherent in the way of working, then therapists will have to be prepared to take on board the seeking of evidence through systematic reviews of available research, and to publish their own.

THE ART AND SCIENCE OF RESEARCH IN OCCUPATIONAL THERAPY

The art of research lies in asking the right questions and, as already suggested, a questioning attitude should be part of life for the problem-solving and imaginative therapist. If this is so, then research need not be something that is superimposed but is, by its nature, already part of the ethos of practice. Every record and routine statistic has the potential for contributing towards descriptive, explanatory study.

Of course, this type of data does have limitations. Simply collecting data on its own, without reason for doing so and without analysis and interpretation, is meaningless. Detailed description of everyday behaviour, with no attempt to explain relevance, has the potential for becoming a vice, or, as Popper (1972) indicates, in order to observe we must know what to observe and have definite questions or hypotheses in mind. However, it is often from analysis of accumulated records that the germ of an idea, or a hunch worth following up, emerges. Log and source books from student days, observational studies, first impressions, diaries and case studies can capture thoughts and ideas that on their own may appear insignificant but, once noted, may lead to more systematic study. Reflective diaries and, just as important, recorded discussions with colleagues help to keep the mind open to different perceptions, to promoting debate, prompting the search for evidence and developing a reflectiveness that is a critical component of practice. The use of reflexivity (Finlay 1998) and narratives (Ryan & McKay 1999) are increasingly showing the importance of intellectual reasoning and are gaining in respectability. Description of practice, with analysis of subjective experience, can enhance the validity of that research, but one needs to move from subjective confidence to consensus opinion and, where data is lacking, attempt to fill the gaps.

This idea leads neatly into the science of research. If the art is about asking the right questions, the science is choosing the best method, adopting appropriate protocols and planning the process, constantly checking that the question being asked is being addressed. There are many texts to elaborate on methods and define terminology. This next section considers some of the debates around methodology.

METHODOLOGICAL DEBATES

It might seem as though the more mature sciences, cosmology and chemistry for example, have traditions and structures which give them a kind of internal connectedness or holding-together, with greater stability and power to assimilate more information and develop predictive capability, yet even here, according to Popper's methodology, every recognition of a truth is preceded by an imaginative preconception of what that truth might be (Medawar 1984).

Medical science follows much of the traditional methodology but, in so doing, often has to reduce concepts to that which can be measured, and not all of medical intervention is based on scientifically validated procedures. Professional and ethical factors can be fundamental obstacles to research where, for example, there is resistance to evaluating procedures using placebo comparisons. In addition, and particularly in relation to the current concept of health, medical intervention is reduced to that which can be costed, bought and sold, indicating the political and economic influences on research. Indeed, it can be asked 'What is health?' and 'To what extent do medical interventions enhance health' (Box 4.1)?

This is the dilemma and controversy surrounding evidenced based practice, where randomised controlled trials are considered to be the highest order of evidence yet sit uncomfortably with many therapists. Debates abound concerning the scientific method and the acceptability or otherwise of unorthodox methods. Those using the latter have often been unfairly criticised and their findings rejected because their critics have neither scrutinised the methodology nor kept an open mind.

Box 4.1 Case for comment

What is health?
Health is more than the absence of disease.

Do you agree?

Illness and disease are the concerns of medical science.

Where does individual responsibility fit in?

A precise definition offered by Seedhouse (1986) is that 'A person's optimum state of health is equivalent to the state of the set of conditions which fulfil or enable a person to work to fulfil his or her realistic chosen and biological potentials. Some of these conditions are of the highest importance for all people. Others are variable dependent upon individual abilities and circumstances.'

Does this cover all possibilities and how can it be studied?

Seedhouse (1986) also says that 'All theories of health and all approaches designed to increase health are intended to advise against, to prevent the creation of, or to remove, obstacles to the achievement of human potential. These obstacles may be biological, environmental, societal, familial, or personal.'

Are occupational therapy interventions covered by this?

A belief that medical science has the solutions to one's ailments or more serious life-threatening conditions can inhibit taking personal responsibility for one's health, the development of personal strengths and potential to accept and adapt to situations. Potential solutions are complex and personal. For example, should obstetricians be seeking the use of eggs from aborted fetuses to help infertile women or should they (or counsellors, or therapists) be helping these women instead to come to terms with their disappointment and loss?

Inductive versus deductive approaches

There is general agreement on the notion of two different philosophical approaches to research, namely the inductive and deductive. Readers are recommended to study recent texts such as Reed & Proctor (1995), Bailey (1997) and DePoy & Gitlin (1998) for detailed discussion. The following, however, helps set the scene, introducing a number of overlapping terms. Their interrelatedness is explained as the chapter develops.

The inductive approach

The inductive approach aims to explain phenomena in the social world, to describe what is observed, interpret what is happening and so generate theories about human behaviour under certain circumstances. It moves from the complex but not abstract study of whole units, such as human experience within specific situations, to grounding theory in observations.

The inductive approach focuses on specific contexts and on selected subjects from whom qualitative data may be obtained. The knowledge acquired in naturalistic settings is based on the perceptions of the subjects and their understanding of the world within their own social contexts. Hence it is described as a holistic view, or holism. This deeper understanding does not necessarily lead to predictions but can help one anticipate what might happen elsewhere.

There is inevitably a problem in attempting to explain the circumstances experienced by one person, the subject, through the investigative methods and perceptions of another, the researcher. The authenticity of the descriptions and the dependability and credibility of the researcher become key features in inducing theoretical explanations of the subject's world. Indeed, the very presence of a researcher, such as an anthropologist, will distort the subject's normal world and hence the behaviour which the researcher wishes to study. The tensions which exist within inductive methods may require the researcher to 'go native' and abandon preconceived ideas and prejudices in order to be open to alternative explanations for behaviour.

In the same way, tensions can exist if occupational therapists are to carry out research into occupational therapy. Their value judgements and past professional experience could influence their interpretations, attributing features which were not intended by the subjects. Inductive research aims to understand but not to judge human behaviour.

The deductive approach

The deductive approach, on the other hand, aims to identify causes and so to predict future outcomes. It aims to test theories by identifying variables, setting up a hypothesis, and gaining quantitative data which will substantiate or refute the theory. The concept of objective meas-

urement and numerical calculation enables statistical analysis to be carried out. This may show the significance, or otherwise, of particular interventions for the sample population studied. From statistical significance, probabilities, as opposed to chance happenings, allow findings to be generalised to a wider similar population, thereby leading to future predictions.

In deductive research, the variables are predetermined by the researcher and the data are quantified, resulting in what is sometimes called the positivist notion of the experimental approach. In other words it moves from theory to indicating what can be expected, testing the relationship between two or more specific variables in the search for predictive laws or generalised statements. The hypothesis reduces the theory to more concrete and measurable components. There is, therefore, a logical process of moving from the abstract of the theory to that which is concrete and observable.

These two approaches, the inductive and the deductive, are complementary and not mutually exclusive. Indeed, it has been argued by several authors that both approaches are necessary. Thus, there is a cyclical nature to research which will be discussed more fully later in this chapter. At the same time, DePoy and Gitlin (1998) have proposed that qualitative and quantitative research designs can be spread along a continuum with naturalistic settings at one end and true experimental designs, in which control, manipulation and randomisation are all present, at the other end (Bailey 1997). The research design chosen will depend on what is being compared and the links in the research process.

Let us have a look at some of these terms.

Phenomena and phenomenology

One usually starts research with a particular phenomenon in mind that one wants to understand better. Phenomena are everyday experiences and include the whole complex gamut of human behaviour and interactions. Phenomenology is the study of these behaviours with meaning being attributed to them by the researcher's analytic inductive approach. Interpretation should gradually emerge from the data and its verification through triangulation processes. This means taking bearings through different research methods and checking out the credibility or convergent validity of the findings, in order to interpret the data with confidence. Phenomenological research is a form of naturalistic enquiry, sometimes called the interpretative method, and it follows an inductive approach.

Naturalistic research

According to DePoy & Gitlin (1998), this form of research is in direct contrast to experimental, scientific research and hence is associated with qualitative and inductive methods. It places the researcher in the natural environment of the subject, sometimes having to 'go native'.

Naturalistic research must be differentiated from the naturalism which Reid (1993) associates with positivism and the orthodox scientific approach. Such subtle differences in the use of words can lead to confusion, which emphasises the reader's and would-be researcher's need for constant vigilance and questioning. In other words: *Nullius in verba*, or, 'Don't take anybody's word for it'.

Positivism

Positivism is a methodological ideal which should be applied to all scientific research leading to causal explanations. The method is logical and rational, under the control of the researcher, following long established procedures of identifying variables and hypotheses which are sometimes referred to as the hypothetical-deductive method. It tends to focus on laboratory situations, such as randomised controlled trials (RCTs), which through the use of standard techniques reduce researcher bias and produce quantifiable and verifiable results.

Towards the end of the 19th century an antipositivist philosophy became prominent, with historians and social scientists looking for more diversified approaches which would help them understand the individual and unique features of their subjects. Until recently, orthodox scientific traditions have been considered the

ideal to be aimed for, with the softer methods of the social sciences lagging behind in terms of rigour and precision (Krefting 1991, Short-DeGraff & Fisher 1993, Gliner 1994). This shift to a post-modern climate has been growing over the past two decades, allowing for greater emphasis on interpretation and meaning based on qualitative, narrative and discursive study rather than deductive, logical and positivist rational scientific approaches (Reid 1993, DePoy & Gitlin 1998). The quantitative-deductive approach is seeking the truth through replication while the qualitative-inductive seeks to understand. Both should be complementary but, alas, this shift does not seem to be reflected in the EBP literature (Rogers & Perrin 1999). For many therapists, research through RCTs is unattainable, but this should not deter the gathering of evidence from well designed non-experimental studies from more than one centre, and the use of wider research databases.

The cyclical nature of research

Stewart (1990), Wallace (1985) and, more recently, Frankfort-Nachmias & Nachmias (1992) have suggested that the research process is cyclical, with theory being induced from practice and this in turn leading to formal testing in order to verify or refute the theory (Fig. 4.1). This simple

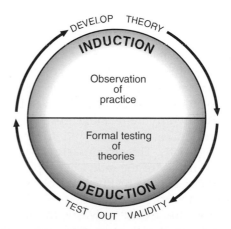

Figure 4.1 The cyclical nature of research showing the relationship between the development of theory as part of induction and formal testing within deduction.

model shows how relationships stemming from observations might be explained through induction on one hand, while on the other established theories enable predictions to be made (i.e. there is a deductive approach). It is timely to expand on this model, identifying differences and demonstrating how methods can be combined in order to give an eclectic, integrated approach to research. It should be noted that there is a simplicity in this analysis and that its emphasis is on the human condition.

As has been suggested, there are two philosophical traditions in research, naturalistic enquiry on the one hand and scientific on the other (Fig. 4.2).

Naturalistic enquiry is considered to have a more holistic perspective and is based on the following beliefs:

- that reality, and perhaps therefore truth for individuals, is determined by events and understood through each person's unique experience
- that multiple realities exist and that human experience is complex and cannot be understood from examining only its parts.

In this, the inductive and phenomenological perspective, it is the insider, the person being investigated, who is considered the knowledgeable one, the person being observed or sharing insights into experiences of disability or pain or whatever phenomenon is being studied (Fig. 4.3). The researcher abandons assumptions and preconceptions in favour of the perspectives of the subject being studied. As a result, the search for understanding and interrelation becomes a dynamic process. As concepts, such as that of pain, are abstracted and developed into constructs identifying relationships, so are theoretical principles generated and theory developed (Fig. 4.4). This theory stems from the subjective reality of the individual's perceptions or behaviour, not the reality of the observer.

Where subjects have limited powers of communication, the extent to which the researcher imposes his perceptions on the phenomena is debatable. For example, it was Piaget's detailed observations of his young children within the

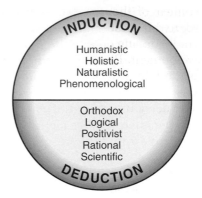

Figure 4.2 A comparison of some of the characteristics of induction with some of those of deduction.

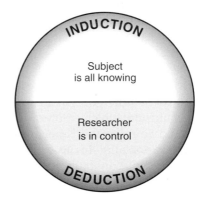

Figure 4.3 The difference between the subject's role in induction and the researcher's in deduction.

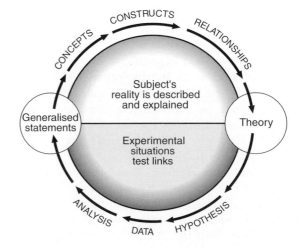

Figure 4.4 The transformation of information within the scientific process.

natural context of their home life in the 1920s which led to his description, explanation and subsequent theorising concerning children's cognitive development. Piaget's theories have since been subjected to extensive scientific scrutiny and criticism (e.g. Donaldson 1978, Box 4.2) and applied to education and health-related interventions.

What is theory?

The word theory has several definitions, from the popular ones which are of limited value to the more scientific, such as 'a summary statement of the principles or laws which make up a given explanation of a phenomenon' (Reed 1984). Theories may be offered to help understand relationships or to explain cause and effect, but this does not mean that they are true.

The many theories being put forward regarding occupational therapy are good examples of the different ways in which interactions between therapist, client, purposeful activity and the environment, and subsequent outcomes, can be explained (Hagedorn 1997). These, often competing, theories are offered as solutions to problems of understanding. They may offer solutions to some problems but not necessarily to all. Some are applicable to people with physical disabilities while others are appropriate for those with psychological difficulties.

According to sources quoted in Reid (1993), occupational therapy, physiotherapy and nursing have all been striving to find their own unique and unifying theory as though their futures depended on it. Such efforts are questionable if they exclude drawing on appropriate theories from other branches of the social and physical sciences. It is, therefore, important for thinking therapists to look for the best testable theory for their own area of practice and it is incumbent on therapists, as part of their professional development, to be actively seeking the theory or theories which best explain the process and give most information. At the same time it is important to refute and discard those theories which do not work (Popper 1972).

Qualitative versus quantitative methods

Distinctions between inductive/naturalistic and deductive/scientific approaches open up the debate about qualitative versus quantitative

---

Box 4.2 Challenging the long-held theories of Piaget

Piaget devoted many years to making detailed observations and devising tasks to enable him to analyse children's behaviour in terms of their cognitive and intellectual development. These observations were then generalised to all children and his theory established. His work is described as being unprecedented in its complexity. His findings were intricate and persuasive and for many years were upheld as being reliable. Claims about the development of children's cognitive processes were backed by much supporting evidence, leading to his theories being widely accepted and indeed influential in undergraduate education, with subsequent application to education and health-related interventions. The theories were induced from field observations and analysis. More recently they have been subjected to testing, with different results.

For example, Piaget claimed that children were highly egocentric up to the age of 6 or 7 years, and this view was central to his theories about children's capabilities. Donaldson, in her extremely important book Children's Minds (1978), challenges his assumptions with much concrete evidence from other sources and with alternative explanations. She suggests that failure to communicate effectively with children can account for their failure in tasks rather than an inherent inability to perform the tasks in the first place. In other words, when tasks are presented in familiar and understandable contexts, children can adopt another's perspective.

Donaldson claims that:

- gaps between children and adults are not so great as has been widely believed
- children are not so limited in their ability to reason deductively as Piaget and others have claimed
- children are probably first making sense of the situation and then using this kind of understanding to help make sense of what is being said.

If children can appreciate another's point of view and 'decentre' then this has far-reaching implications for the way in which they learn and how adults behave towards them.

methods (Fig. 4.5). It has been contended that qualitative methods should supplant the traditional reductionist quantitative approach to human problems (Short-DeGraff 1994) and that health professionals are not particularly enthusiastic about the low face validity of number-crunching approaches involved in quantitative methods (Reid 1993).

While qualitative methods may lead to the development of theory and quantitative approaches test out the validity of theory, there should be no dogmatic commitment to one or the other but rather a recognition that both are of value. Both offer different perspectives leading to different kinds of knowledge which can inform each other. The qualitative approach gives rich understanding while quantitative methods give hard data for subsequent verification of the theory. Each approach is also more or less appropriate at different stages of the research cycle.

The findings will be shaped by the design of the research and how information has been obtained.

Qualitative methods

Qualitative methods (as used in the study described in Box 4.3) draw on the experiences of the subjects. Case studies, or open-ended questions in surveys and interviews, or illuminative studies based on letters, documents, field notes and observations, are all typical of qualitative methods. Others, such as the Delphi technique, are well described in the many research methodology texts which are available (for example Reid 1993).

When using qualitative methods, the researcher may have little (if any) knowledge of the area but have a hunch or curiosity and enthusiasm to understand more about human experiences and to explore causal links between different factors. It is not easy, however, to establish criteria which will help define subjective concepts such as dignity or self-determination. The researcher's questions or detailed observations of phenomena gradually become more specific as the data lead to categorisation and potential identification of relationships.

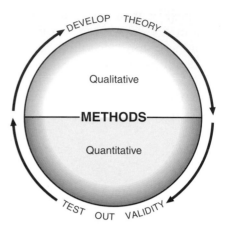

Figure 4.5   The relationship between qualitative methods for developing theory and quantitative methods for testing validity.

The methods followed offer a degree of structure which helps to focus on issues of interest. A vast amount of data can be accumulated and this can be very time-consuming to process, collate, categorise and analyse. The findings are based on the reality of the subjects under study and may not necessarily be open to generalisations. Transferability of knowledge may be limited although helpful in offering insights into subjective experiences and hence informing future practice with that group of people under similar conditions.

Box 4.3   A study of residents in a community home, part 1

A student researcher is interested in the level of independence, or interdependence, which is encouraged by staff in a group of residents in a community home for people with learning difficulties. An observer/participant role is developed with frequent visits being made at various times of the day and detailed notes made of the interactions and individual behaviours. The data accumulated are grounded in those attributes which are associated with independence and interdependent behaviour, and compared with those that reflect institutional behaviour. The many limitations and ambiguities of this method are identified. The credibility and potential transferability of the findings are checked out with staff in an open-ended but semistructured interview. (A similar study of deinstitutionalised adults was carried out by Kielhofner in 1981.)

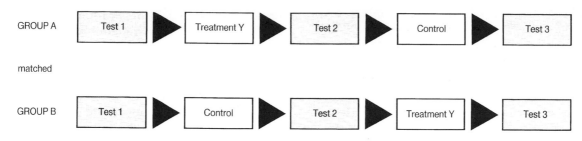

Figure 4.6   Two runs with experimental and control conditions reversed.

The credibility of the researcher, not necessarily having years of experience but having integrity and an imaginative yet systematic approach, makes the resulting theory, grounded in meticulously recorded data, more acceptable. According to Krefting (1991), credibility, transferability, dependability and confirmability are key concepts in strengthening the acceptability of qualitative research.

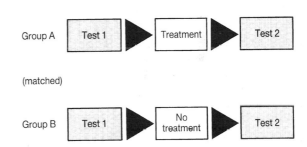

Figure 4.7   The pre- and post-test method.

Quantitative methods

The use of quantitative methods permits specific factors (e.g. the increase in heart rate during exercise) to be measured, surveyed and analysed, thereby leading to predictions about normal behaviour. Unambiguous results and data which can be subjected to statistical analysis have advantages and provide a gauge for the outcomes of future interventions. One tends to think of quantifiable methods as being evidence of the scientific approach, and that experimental designs involve random assignment of subjects, control and manipulation of the variables by the researcher and accumulation of data both before and after treatment (Fig. 4.6). Comparisons of results then confirm or refute the relationship between cause and effect.

However, methods described as quasi-experimental may be used when true experiments are impractical or unethical. The 'one group, pre-test, post-test' approach is an example of a quasi-experimental method (Fig. 4.7).

Quasi-experimental methods may be advocated by those concerned with health care and social sciences, but this view is challenged by Ernst (1993) who argues that 'randomised trials are

essential for evaluating the effectiveness of any therapy, complementary or not, and such studies are feasible, even for highly individualised therapies'. Ernst claims there is no better research protocol than the classic scientific method with randomised, placebo-controlled, double-blind trials, and that a substantial part of health care research should be into the placebo effect, or what some might describe as the natural healing effect of our bodies and the potential influence of therapeutic relationships with or without direct physical contact.

Research in occupational therapy often draws on quasi-experimental methods. External validity should mean that generalisations are possible, but it can never be completely guaranteed (Box 4.4).

Integrated research methods

There are obvious differences between the qualitative methods of the naturalistic approach and the quantitative methods of the more experimental, logical positivist approach. Put somewhat simplistically, these relate to the nature of the reality under study, the relationship between

Box 4.4 A study of residents in a community home, part 2

Let us consider the case of community residents (see Box 4.3) and the researcher's interest in finding out how independent they are. Using a deductive, quantitative approach, the hypothesis based on criteria associated with the concept of independence might be that 'residents cannot make decisions for themselves, and instead seek out staff guidance'. The research design might be based on a time sampling analysis with behaviours observed at regular predetermined intervals and recorded in a number of present and mutually exclusive categories of behaviour typical within the residence. Large quantities of data will be accumulated, multiplied by the number of time intervals per hour, the number of residents and the number of sessions during which recordings are undertaken. Statistical procedures and allowance for sampling errors give probability scores permitting the hypothesis to be tested.

Take this a step further and let us develop some action research, whereby the residents follow a programme designed to increase their independence in decision making, and are subsequently observed again using the same method of time sampling. If there is a significant increase in the number of decision-making situations, the conclusion might be drawn that the programme has had a beneficial effect. However, again the possibility of cause and effect has to be viewed with caution, for there might also have been a change of staff, or a shift in any number of variables, all of which, within quasi-experimental conditions, cannot be controlled. Nevertheless, this is a simple example of the pre- and post-test method with a substantial amount of data having been accumulated.

subject and researcher, and the possibility of developing or testing theory and of giving explanations or making causal links and subsequent generalisations.

Table 4.2 (influenced by Gliner 1994) shows the differences between naturalistic and positivist research methods with regard to seven different factors associated with qualitative and quantitative designs.

In order to increase the confidence with which results can be viewed, different research methods may be adopted in the same study. This is known as triangulation and helps to give additional insights into the same phenomena as well as enhancing the credibility of findings. The combination of different strategies can strengthen the research effort and further contribute to the understanding of the issues being studied.

It is, however, important to acknowledge the strengths and limitations of each method (Short-DeGraff & Fisher 1993). By employing several different methods it is possible to avoid overlapping weaknesses and therefore to exploit their complementary strengths.

The integration of different research designs is well established in the social sciences and is now gaining increasing respectability in health care and medical sciences. As Robertson (1994) says, 'it is simply not feasible to develop and evaluate a single therapeutic "package" for a given category of neuropsychological disorder, given that even superficially similar neuropsychological deficits can be caused by quite different patterns of underlying neuropsychological breakdown'. In other words, while single subject studies may prove fruitful in increasing understanding, other methods must be used to give evidence of how large numbers of people with cognitive defects can be rehabilitated cost-effectively. Later, we will return to this issue, in relation to patient profiling.

Table 4.2 Differences between research approaches

Factors	Naturalistic enquiry/qualitative	Positivistic/quantitative
Research strategy	Unstructured	Structured
Nature of reality	Described and explained, socially constructed by subject	Predicted and controlled by researcher
Nature of data	Rich, deep, soft, subjective	Hard, factual, reliable
Relationship of subject and researcher to situation	Subject is the knowing one Subject is close/insider	Researcher is in control Researcher is distant/outsider
Possibility of generalisation	Development of theory	Confirmation and verification or refuting of theory
Possibility of causal links	Attempt to explain	Tested
Evidence of rigour	Confirmability of data Credibility of researcher	Tests of reliability and validity

OCCUPATIONAL THERAPY RESEARCH IN RELATION TO MEDICAL AND SOCIAL SCIENCES

Moving from the general to the specific, it has to be asked how occupational therapy research fits into medical sciences. Since the profession is more concerned with the person who has the disease, rather than the disease which the person has, it crosses boundaries between medical science and the social sciences. Table 4.3, influenced by Seedhouse (1986), shows some distinctions between assumptions in the two fields but, like everything else, such distinctions must be treated with a degree of circumspection and be a topic of discussion with colleagues.

RESEARCH IN PRACTICE

WHY GET INVOLVED IN RESEARCH?

It is time now to ask where these debates on the nature of knowledge and on what constitutes research are leading us, and how they can be applied in practice. There are many reasons why practising therapists and students should get involved in research.

At the personal, subjective level there is the satisfaction – even if preceded by frustration – of the increase in knowledge and understanding. Quest and discovery stimulate the mind and counteract possibilities of passive acceptance of, and complacency with, the status quo. Involvement in research can be an excellent antidote to low morale, by focusing the mind on a process which opens up new ideas and possible approaches. Involvement at both undergraduate and postgraduate level helps to ensure one is a more effective consumer of others' research findings. The ability to sift out relevant material and its potential for application comes with practice and with appreciation of what the originator has gone through in terms of subjective experience and methodology. The ability to digest critically what has been written is very important and may well trigger action to follow up some of the references or check out findings with other sources of information. Consumers of research should not be passive recipients. Remember: *Nullius in verba*.

Whatever might be gained at a personal level has a knock-on effect at the professional level, for the two are intrinsically bound together. Indeed, to suggest a distinction is somewhat arbitrary. In terms of professional practice and the development of the profession, there are many reasons for involvement as consumer or researcher. These include:

- setting up, agreeing and using taxonomies
- understanding the theoretical bases and assumptions of the profession
- developing/testing assessment instruments
- establishing consumer perceptions and satisfaction with the service
- assessing treatment effectiveness and outcomes

Table 4.3 Social and medical sciences and occupational therapy

Social sciences	Medical sciences
Health is more than a target for medicine	Health occurs when disease is absent
People can influence their own health	Health is a commodity
Everyday activity can influence health	Drugs and technology are important
Psychosocial influences are studied in relation to health	Knowledge focuses on our bodies

If occupational therapy fits somewhere between the two, the following statements might be added:

Occupational therapy
Survival depends on a balance between health and occupation
People can adapt to ill health and disability and develop their potential
Meaningful activity is essential to health
Knowledge focuses on the individual's physical, psychological and socioeconomic circumstances
as well as on personal aspirations

- evaluating one's own practice against that of others; assessing what is the most appropriate
- identifying resources provided and their effectiveness in meeting needs
- investigating approaches to learning and implications for educational programmes.

This list is not exhaustive and could be written in other ways, emphasising how the research agenda can be influenced by the political context of health services, focusing, for example, on needs-based assessments, on the cost-effectiveness of service delivery, on the implications of ageing populations, on user involvement with empowerment, on quality of service, on evaluations and audits, and so on.

If the outcomes of research are to have relevance to the delivery of today's services, then researchers have to be sensitive to current legislation and the finite resources which are available to an ever growing and ever more demanding public. In other words, research should not be undertaken just for its own sake. Containment of costs is all the more reason for establishing the effectiveness of different therapies, the results of which must be communicated to others, including policy makers and managers.

Let us now look at the profession's theoretical base.

Understanding the theoretical base

One of the hallmarks of a profession is its supposedly unique body of knowledge and the systematic and continued pursuit of further knowledge by its members.

Occupational therapy has drawn much of its knowledge from the social sciences, from psychology and from sociology but until recently very little has been included about the nature of occupation and its significance to humans. Occupational science is beginning to redress this through articulating, qualifying and quantifying the effect of occupation on various parts of our lives. It involves psychosocial issues and is researched through a range of methods.

As stated in the *Journal of Occupational Science Australia* (Journal of Occupational Science Australia 1993):

Occupational science is the rigorous study of

- the human need to be occupied,
- the purpose of occupation in survival and health,
- the effects of occupation or occupation deprivation,
- why humans strive for occupational competence and mastery,
- what prevents or enhances occupational performance,
- how social, cultural and political structures affect occupation,
- how occupation provides for biological and sociocultural needs,
- how occupation is necessary in the development of human capacities.

The *Journal of Occupational Science* gives occupational therapists and others worldwide the opportunity to share attempts to understand the many different issues that impings on occupation in all its forms, for all categories of people, from able-bodied to disabled, employed to unemployed, male and female, young and old.

Another area for research grows from the many different models of practice (see e.g. Box 4.5) which are being developed. Currently, many different theories are being expounded in order to summarise the principles that help explain occupational therapy. These theories are being developed – and criticised – by practising clinicians and theorists (Mosey 1986, Kielhofner 1992, Hagedorn 1995, 1997). A surfeit of theories should not be seen as a problem but as a challenge to select out those which best suit the needs of a particular area and group of clients, or those which lend themselves to testing and explaining process and potential outcomes most effectively. Once there is a theory, no matter how imprecise, it gives a base for others to work from and encourages healthy debate about strengths and shortcomings. The aim should be to progress by successive approximations towards the truth.

The search for truth is complicated. For example, research may demonstrate the effectiveness of a particular therapeutic intervention, yet no satisfactory theoretical explanation may be available. Conversely, the most elegant of theories may be impotent in practice. Popper (1972) says there is an infinite number of possibly true theories. Pragmatic preferences may win the day

Box 4.5   A debate

The 'Stewart' model, which is used to explain the occupational therapy process (Stewart 1992), resembles the Scottish saltire (Fig. 4.8). The four components, namely client, therapist, activity (or occupation) and environment, are placed at the corners. Dynamic interactions, which are identified around the perimeter and as a diagonal cross, complete the diagram in order to give one person's attempt to get a 'good fit' and so explain the occupational therapy process.

However, if an occupational therapist makes an orthosis for a client – which means doing something to him rather than the client being active himself – does this fit the model? In other words, does the theory require all components to be interacting in a dynamic way simultaneously or is there another component, that of time, which needs to be added? Such an addition would legitimise the making of an orthosis as a function of preparation for activity by the client.

The question is then raised: does this addition to the theory enhance its explanatory properties, and how can it be subjected to rigorous investigation? What does it tell us about the nature of the relationship between the therapist and the client? Is it one of empowerment or of professional control?

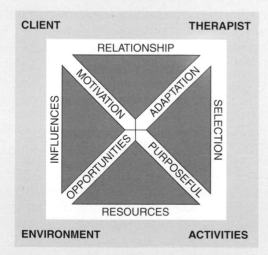

Figure 4.8   The 'Stewart' model for occupational therapy showing the relationship between client, therapist, activities and the environment.

but therapists must nevertheless be aware of the surrounding debates, as, for example, between the Bobath and Johnstone approaches to the treatment of people who have suffered strokes.

There is no guarantee that a better theory will be found but one should keep questioning and retain a degree of healthy scepticism. Indeed, this scepticism should be fundamental to the educational and professional development of students and be inherent in the life of the practising therapist. The search for a sound explanatory base may be justified in terms of helping to strengthen and validate the profession but it can only be sustained by empirical research (Reid 1993). Theorising is a scholarly activity but it should not become detached from the real world. Research in occupational therapy should be scholarly activity in pursuit of understanding, not only about the people with whom occupational therapists work, but also about the influences of occupation on all people and the meanings they derive from their occupations. The use of reflective diaries and case stories contributes to that understanding.

RESEARCH INTO PRACTICE

The development of a firm theoretical base for the profession is one reason for research activity. Others relate to effective use of the expertise of occupational therapists and hence improvements in the quality of service to clients. Therapists should be helping to fill gaps in the evidence not only by asking the appropriate questions but also by being active consumers of others' research. If a profession is to have greater autonomy and credibility then it must monitor its practices and define the characteristics and functions that make it unique; yet can occupational therapy claim occupation as its own, when it is so central to all human endeavour (Ilott 1999)?

For many therapists, their *raison d'être* is to work with clients, promoting their independence. Yet the change in emphasis within the profession, from group work and the therapeutic use of a wide range of activities to increasing focus on activities of daily living and returning clients to work and/or to live in the community, must raise many questions. Not least are the questions: 'Could others have done this work as effectively, or even more effectively than occupational therapists?' and 'What would have been the consequences of not having done the work?'

In these days of overlapping roles and increasing financial stringencies, there is an even greater need to monitor and evaluate existing services. Lest there is confusion, a distinction needs to be made between research and audit. They have much in common and may use similar methods, with research aiming to inform what is best practice and to ensure what is the right thing to do, while audit ensures the right thing is done right (Sealey 1999)!

Among an abundance of helpful literature is the position paper on research, education and practice in mental health from the College of Occupational Therapists (Craik et al 1998). It resulted from a survey which emphasised the central role of occupation in assessment, intervention and increasing well-being for people with mental health problems. Therapists are recommended to focus on the profession's core skills and on working as specialists in a multidisciplinary team, not as generalist mental health workers.

The following sections look at research which has been carried out into: the development and effectiveness of assessment tools, consumer perceptions and effectiveness of the service, aspects of management and, finally, community care and the empowerment of individuals. These feed into education, practice and future research. Carrying out research may be comparatively easy, but ensuring it is accessed, appraised and applied by others is much more of a challenge (Ilott 1999).

Developing and testing assessment instruments

Assessment is the starting point for most interventions and there are many different tools around, some of which are shared by different health care disciplines. Patients can often be subjected to unnecessary repetition of assessment and duplicate results are kept. Interdisciplinary communication and rationalisation of procedures may lead to more effective use of time and less intrusion for patients. Therapists

who are tempted to devise their own instruments or amend existing ones might find time could be more profitably spent by building on knowledge of those procedures already well established. One example of meeting this aim of better information, which would be in patients' interests, is the interrater reliability study carried out by Drever & Nicol (1994) into the Revised Elderly Person's Disability Scale, for the Scottish Office Home and Health Department. This study, using a correlational design, suggested that qualified members of staff achieved slightly higher levels of interrater reliability compared with unqualified staff members. While the results must be treated with caution, in view of the small number of subjects, the conclusion remains that no instrument gives results so valid and comprehensive that treatment decisions can be based solely on that information. 'The best practice in assessing elderly populations is the integration of standardised assessments and clinical judgement' (Bond 1985 as cited in Drever & Nicol 1994).

Another recent study relating to assessment instruments established normative data for the Chessington Occupational Therapy Neurological Assessment Battery (COTNAB) by Laver & Huchison (1994). The COTNAB was originally developed for people between 16 and 65 years of age who had suffered head injuries or strokes. Its application to those over 65 years has been limited, in that raw data alone provide little information about the individual's performance in relation to what might be expected for people of similar age. Laver & Huchison's research not only accumulated performance data from a group of normal, healthy elderly people, but also sought comments on their experiences and perceptions of the tasks, with the result that a less physically demanding task has been incorporated for the written instructions subset. This research is a good example of how a gap in knowledge is tackled. Where reliability and validity have been found wanting, modifications have been recommended by the researchers and taken on board by the manufacturer of the battery of tests, to the benefit of the service.

Consumer perceptions and effectiveness of the service

Surveys of patients' satisfaction with the service are increasingly common as part of quality audits and are dealt with elsewhere (see Ch. 9).

Aspects of management: who does what?

With regard to the effectiveness of treatment and who is the best trained person, or which discipline is most appropriate, for carrying out a particular intervention, there are many studies which have examined overlapping roles and their effectiveness. These are considered within the relevant chapter (see Ch. 10).

Community care and empowerment

These are two very topical issues at the beginning of the new millennium. The questions of social inclusion and of patients taking more control are closely related to what different groups of people understand by independence. The independent living movement views independence as a state of mind rather than a physical ability (Campbell 1994). It is about having control over involvement, or not, in daily activities, depending on energy levels and aspirations, and about choosing personal lifestyles. Yet is independence the ultimate aim, or is interdependence a more normal state of being? With increasing emphasis on care in the community, there is evidence (Sutherland & Chesson 1994) that people do not want to be passive recipients of care. They are prepared to commit often scarce finances to enhancing the quality of their lives and would like to be able to pursue more recreational activities, given removal of obstacles and/or availability of reliable helpers. The respondents in the above study expressed frustration at the attitudes of able-bodied people. Empowerment issues will require major changes in the way society adapts, and so too must professional staff be prepared for a reversal of power. Roles will be associated more with the giving of advice in order that informed choices can be made, and therefore therapists will be working *with* people rather than for or on their behalf.

These changes will raise many questions worthy of pursuit. Findings may not always reinforce professional beliefs, but the latter must be open to challenge regarding their validity. Beliefs which stem from tradition, prompted by events in history, influenced by contemporary values, widely shared and jealously guarded, have to be subjected to rigorous investigation. This should not be a threat but instead a welcome opportunity to present evidence in order to substantiate those long-held beliefs.

EVIDENCE BASED PRACTICE

A distinction has to be drawn between research and evidence based practice (EBP), in the same way as audit and research differ. Practice has probably always been based on evidence but EBP is a formal approach of assessing that evidence so that clinical decisions are based on the best evidence of effectiveness (DoH 1998). There is a sequence to these three potentially confusing terms, with research preceding EBP, and audit being an evaluation of that practice. Audit is an essential part of monitoring standards (Sealey 1999).

Much has been written on EBP over the past few years. Muir Gray (1997) and Bury & Mead (1998) provide helpful texts that contribute to changing practice, but there are also controversial papers that challenge the appropriateness of EBP to the decision making of therapists (Miles et al 1997, Clemence 1998, Rogers & Perrin 1999). The controversy around automatic acceptance of the EBP approach results from gaps in the evidence and the relevance of that which is available. The fact that a treatment technique has not been researched does not mean that it is ineffective (Bury & Mead 1998).

As mentioned earlier in this chapter, within EBP there is a hierarchy of evidence, from randomised controlled trials at the top down to personal experience. The EBP movement accumulates evidence and carries out comparative analysis of individual research studies. First, the question relating to a patient's problem has to be identified and then a systematic review of the evidence carried out. This requires rigorous procedures to search out all relevant previous studies through the literature, critically appraising that evidence in terms of its reliability, validity of methods, clarity of research questions, appropriateness of the methodology, thoroughness of analysis of the data, and interpretation of results. The identification of weaknesses, and hence inconclusiveness, is critical. Meta-analysis is the summarising and historical listing of data from more than one source. When statistics have been involved and the data are similar, then confidence intervals can be established. Useful findings should then be implemented in practice.

The increasing attention being paid to EBP, or evidence based health care (EBH), helps to develop a culture in which evidence and therapy are interlinked. However, it takes time to access databases and appraise the quality of that evidence, and the volume of information can be unmanageable. Hence the introduction of guidelines such as those from the Scottish Intercollegiate Guidelines Network (SIGN), and the introduction of NHS Research and Development programmes to influence policy through evidence (National Clinical Guideline 1988).

If research and the development of professional effectiveness are to work, individuals need to know what questions to ask about what needs to be done, and who to team up with. There are many individuals and organisations available to help. What will not lead to effectiveness is having a monodisciplinary attitude to research or, worse still, working in complete isolation without discussing your ideas. Therapists must keep up to date and strive for excellence.

RESEARCH IN EDUCATION

Research-mindedness and the excitement that comes with pursuing a question that will lead to improvements for clients must be generated during the would-be therapist's pre-registration education. The focus on research in education is important to the student becoming a consumer of research and being able to handle research methodology. Changes in the delivery of the educational process itself also form the basis for research. The use of narrative and reflection on experience as presented by Molineux and by Fortune (in Ryan & McKay 1999) provide examples of qualitative methodology. Their stories not only inform the reader about the different perspectives of the players but also influence new directions in professional education.

Development of research awareness in students

Within professional syllabi, research methodology tends to be introduced from an early stage in order that students may readily become consumers of research. Indeed, in order to foster research-mindedness as a way of thinking, examples of research or issues surrounding it should be incorporated throughout undergraduate programmes rather than as isolated activities (Timmerman et al 1994). For long-qualified therapists, postgraduate opportunities are offered through professional bodies and local institutions. Some may see these as opportunities for financial advancement, as personal ego trips, as a professional requirement to conform to the current expectations or even to create a false sense of security. Others will see that acquisition of an understanding of the research process is critical to assessing the efficacy of their treatment interventions and their ability critically to evaluate the findings of others' work. Many students become subjects in the research projects of peers and learn through participating before they themselves become the researcher.

Quality assurance, quality assessment and quality audit within education involve students actively from the start in evaluation processes, assessing the effectiveness of learning strategies and use of resources. The methods used draw on the subjective experiences of students, as well as on quantifiable measures of success as reflected through progression or graduation rates, demand from prospective students for places and demand from potential employers for graduates of the institution. At an idealistic level, course planners seek to meet the needs of a wide range of individuals. At a realistic level, the debate about innovation also has to consider political and economic agendas not dissimilar from those taking place in health care.

SUMMARY

There are many questions waiting to be asked, thus giving potential for research projects. This chapter has covered much ground, from research processes to the role of EBP in delivering effective care, and the necessity for rigour in developing and reviewing studies already done. I hope I have stimulated readers into following up their own ideas based on a better understanding of approaches to research.

There is a cautionary note concerning not being pressurised into adopting deductive, scientific methods, which would reduce occupational therapy to controllable specifics at the expense of the art in therapy and the importance of patients' subjective experiences. Nevertheless, the place for integrated research is put forward and the importance of being a sceptical consumer emphasised.

Nullius in verba

REFERENCES

Bailey D M 1997 Research for the health professional: a practical guide, 2nd edn. F A Davis, Philadelphia
Bury T, Mead J 1998 Evidence-based healthcare: a practical guide for therapists. Butterworth Heinemann, Oxford
Campbell J 1994 Independence is a state of mind not a physical activity. British Journal of Occupational Therapy 57(3): 89–90
Christiansen C 1994 Classification and study in occupational therapy. Journal of Occupational Science 1(3): 3–21
Clemence M L 1998 Evidence-based physiotherapy: seeking the unattainable? British Journal of Therapy and Rehabilitation 5(5): 257–260
Compact Oxford English Dictionary, 2nd edn. 1991. Clarendon Press, Oxford
Craik C, Austin C, Chacksfield J D et al 1998 College of Occupational Therapists: position paper on the way ahead for research, education and practice in mental health. British Journal of Occupational Therapy 61(9): 390–392
Crombie I K, Davies H T O 1996 Research in healthcare. Wiley, Chichester
Department of Health 1998 A first class service: quality in the new NHS. Department of Health, London
DePoy E, Gitlin L 1998 Introduction to research: understanding and applying multiple strategies 2nd edn. Mosby, St Louis
Donaldson M 1978 Children's minds. Collins, Glasgow
Drever F, Nicol M 1994 An interrater reliability study of the Revised Elderly Persons' Disability Scale. Occupational Therapy International 1: 233–249
Ernst E 1993 Complementary therapies: scrutinising the alternatives. The Lancet 341: 1626
Finlay L 1998 Reflexivity: an essential component for all research? British Journal of Occupational Therapy 61(10): 453–456
Finlay L 1999 Applying phenomenology in research: problems, principles and practice. British Journal of Occupational Therapy 62(7): 299–306
Frankfort-Nachmias C, Nachmias D 1992 Research methods in the social sciences. Edward Arnold, London
French S 1994 Practical research: a guide for therapists. Butterworth Heinemann, Oxford
Gentry W D, Kobasa S C 1984 Social and psychological resources mediating stress–illness relationships in humans. In: Gentry W D (ed) Handbook of behavioural medicine. Guildford Press, New York
Gliner J A 1994 Reviewing qualitative research: proposed criteria for fairness and rigor. Occupational Therapy Journal of Research 14(2): 78–90
Hagedorn R 1995 Perspectives and processes. Churchill Livingstone, Edinburgh
Hagedorn R 1997 Occupational therapy: foundations for practice 2nd edn. Churchill Livingstone, Edinburgh.
Hart E, Bond M (1995) Action research for health and social care. Open University Press, Buckingham
Ilott I 1999 Back to basics in OT: genericism or specialism. British Journal of Therapy and Rehabilitation 6(7): 320–323
Journal of Occupational Science Australia 1993 Journal of Occupational Science Australia 1(1): 2
Kielhofner G 1981 An ethnographic study of deinstitutionalised adults. Occupational Therapy Journal of Research 1(2): 125–142
Kielhofner G 1992 Conceptual foundations of occupational therapy. F A Davis, Philadelphia
Krefting L 1991 Rigor in qualitative research: the assessment of trustworthiness. American Journal of Occupational Therapy 45(3): 214–222
Laver A, Huchison S 1994 The performance and experience of normal elderly people on the COTNAB. British Journal of Occupational Therapy 57(4): 137–142
Medawar P 1984 The limits of science. Oxford University Press, London
Miles A, Bentley P, Polychronis A, Grey J 1997 (Editorial) Evidence-based medicine: why all the fuss? Journal of Evaluation in Clinical Practice 3(2): 83–86
Mosey A C 1986 Psychosocial components of occupational therapy. Raven Press, New York

Muir Gray J A 1997 Evidence-based healthcare. Churchill Livingstone, Edinburgh

National Clinical Guideline 1998 Management of patients with stroke – pilot edition. Scottish Intercollegiate Guidelines Network, Edinburgh

Popper K R 1972 Objective knowledge: an evolutionary approach. Oxford University Press, London

Reed J, Proctor S 1995 Practitioner research in health care. Chapman and Hall, London

Reed K 1984 Models of practice in occupational therapy. Williams and Wilkins, Baltimore

Reid N 1993 Health care research by degrees. Blackwell Scientific, London

Robertson I H 1994 Editorial: Methodology in neuropsychological rehabilitation research. Neuropsychological Rehabilitation 4(1): 1–6

Rogers P, Perrin P 1999 Truth or illusion: evidence-based practice in the real world. British Journal of Therapy and Rehabilitation 6(6): 275–280

Ryan S E, McKay E A 1999 Thinking and reasoning in therapy: narratives from practice. Stanley Thornes, Cheltenham

Sealey C 1999 Two common pitfalls in clinical audit: failing to complete the audit cycle and confusing audit with research. British Journal of Occupational Therapy 62(6): 238–243

Seedhouse D 1986 Health: the foundations for achievement. John Wiley, Chichester

Short-DeGraff 1994 (Editorial) Critical assessment of qualitative research. Occupational Therapy Journal of Research 14(2): 75–77

Short-DeGraff M A, Fisher A 1993 Nationally speaking: a proposal for diverse research methods and common research language. American Journal of Occupational Therapy 47: 295–297

Silverman D 1997 Qualitative research. Sage, London

Smith M E 1989 Why research? Tales of the unexpected. Australian Occupational Therapy Journal 36(1): 4–13

Stewart A M 1990 Research. In: Creek J (ed) Occupational therapy and mental health. Churchill Livingstone, Edinburgh

Stewart A M 1992 Casson memorial lecture. Always a little further. British Journal of Occupational Therapy 55(8): 296–302

Sutherland A, Chesson R 1994 The needs of physically disabled people aged 16–65 and service usage in Grampian. British Journal of Occupational Therapy 57(5): 171–176

Timmerman L, Schmidt C, Heater L 1994 Increasing occupational therapy research: is it time to try something new? American Journal of Occupational Therapy 48(7): 647–648

Wallace W 1985 An overview of elements in the scientific process. In: Bynner B, Stribley K M (eds) Social research: principles and procedures. Open University/Longman, Harlow

The occupational therapy process

5

Approaches to practice

Jennifer Creek

INTRODUCTION

Chapter 3 described some of the theories that occupational therapists use, and a framework was offered for understanding how theory relates to practice. In this chapter, we will look in more detail at how theory informs practice. The chapter is in four parts: the content of practice; the changing nature of the profession; the process of intervention, and frames of reference used in the field of mental health.

CONTENT OF PRACTICE

A definition of the structure and scope of occupational therapy practice should derive from the philosophy and theoretical base of the profession, not from the constraints and demands of the service setting, although the way the intervention is carried out will be influenced by such external factors. Practice can be defined as the actions taken by the therapist to serve the needs of the client (Agyris & Schon 1974). Only if these actions are based on a coherent philosophical and theoretical framework can the therapist make skilled predictions about outcome.

We will look at the content of practice under four headings:

• professional goals
• the population served
• core skills
• legitimate tools.

Professional goals

A goal is the specific and positive outcome of therapy to be attained by the client as a result of planned therapeutic interventions. The major goal of occupational therapy is to enable the client to achieve life satisfaction, social integration and productivity through the development of skills that will allow him to adapt to changing circumstances and to function at a level satisfactory to himself and to others. The desired outcome of intervention is for the client to be able to meet his own needs, as far as possible, and to have the motivation to continue working towards achieving his full potential. Occupational therapy helps the individual to achieve what is important to him rather than aiming for normality or conformity. This person-centred goal has been called 'enablement' (Stewart 1994).

Sub-goals which lead to the major goal are to:

- assess the client's needs in terms of the occupations which are important to him
- identify the skills needed to support those occupations
- remove or minimise barriers to successful occupational performance
- assist the client to develop, relearn or maintain skills to a level of competence that will allow him to perform occupations to his own satisfaction in a way that is acceptable within his social context
- help the client to achieve a satisfactory balance of activities in his daily life.

The focus of intervention is always the client and his goals, rather than the problem or the method of intervention.

Population served

The premise that people can influence their own health by their actions can be applied to a wide range of problems once the appropriate specialist knowledge and skills to support it have been acquired. Anyone who has problems of doing, whatever the person's age, gender or diagnosis, is a potential client of occupational therapy.

The client traditionally encountered occupational therapy in a medical setting, which predetermined, to some extent, the range of problems seen, the degree of dysfunction the client was experiencing and the amount of time the therapist could spend on treatment. As the profession expands into new areas, clients are also being encountered in other settings, such as social services departments, educational settings, health centres, day centres, prisons, the workplace and people's own homes.

In practice, referrals are often made by a doctor or other professional who makes the initial decision about who needs occupational therapy. The therapist selects clients from these referrals on the basis of information gained in an initial assessment. In some settings, such as long-stay wards, the therapist makes a selection of clients from the entire patient population. In the multidisciplinary team the decision about which professional should work with a particular client is usually made by all the team members. An increasing number of people are referring themselves for occupational therapy, in part due to the increase in private practice.

Core skills

Occupational therapists are characteristically flexible, innovative and responsive to the client with whom they are working and the context within which the intervention is taking place. In order to achieve this flexibility, the occupational therapist requires a wide range of skills. Some of these skills will be common to all therapists, whatever field they are working in, for example analysing and adapting activities. Other skills will be developed for a specific field of practice. An example of a specific skill is stress management, which is mainly used in the field of acute adult mental health.

Skills which are common to all occupational therapists are called 'core skills'. The College of Occupational Therapists in the UK (COT 1994) defined core skills as 'the expert knowledge at the heart of the profession'. These core skills were identified as:

- the use of purposeful activity and meaningful occupation as therapeutic tools
- ability to enable people to explore, achieve and maintain balance in daily living tasks and roles
- ability to assess the effects of, and then to manipulate, physical and psychosocial environments to maximise function and social integration
- ability to analyse, select and apply occupations as specific therapeutic media.

Hagedorn (1997) suggested that core skills can more usefully be described as core processes, which are complex, integrated forms of skill. The seven core processes in occupational therapy are:

- case management
- assessment and evaluation
- therapeutic use of self
- activity analysis and adaptation
- environmental analysis and adaptation
- intervention
- resource management.

Legitimate tools

The occupational therapist uses various techniques and media during the treatment process. Mosey (1986) described the permissible means of carrying out occupational therapy as the profession's 'legitimate tools'. These tools are: purposeful activities, the environment and the self.

Purposeful activities

Purposeful activities are actions that are directed towards a goal or end result, therefore, purpose organises behaviour towards a particular goal (Creek 1998). The purpose or goal is a part of the activity (for example the main goals of walking to the supermarket are to keep fit and to do the shopping). However, the meaning that a person attaches to an activity is individual (a young housewife with small children may see supermarket shopping as a chore that has to be endured, while an elderly person who lives alone may see it as an opportunity to meet people and have a chat).

The occupational therapist uses skills in analysis and reflection to select or synthesise activities which will both meet therapeutic goals and have purpose and meaning for the client.

Analysis is an objective, systematic review of the mechanics of activity: the skills required for its performance, the sequence of steps that make up the activity and the demands that the activity makes on the person carrying it out. Occupational therapists analyse skills, tasks and activities.

Reflection is a subjective awareness and appreciation of the meaning of activity for the individual and the impact that action has on the self and on the environment. It is a process of self-monitoring and self-regulation leading to an ability to understand what has happened, is happening and might happen to the client through the performance of activity.

Environment

People function within a human and non-human environment which Jenkins (1998, p. 29) called the 'lifeworld context'. Aspects of the client's normal environment must be taken into account when planning treatment. The goal of intervention may be to help the client to adapt to his environment, or to adapt the environment to suit the client's needs and abilities. The occupational therapist analyses the environment in terms of:

- content – the physical and human elements in the environment
- demands the effect the environment has on behaviour
- potential for adaptation (Hagedorn 1995a).

The therapeutic encounter also takes place within an environment which can be manipulated to achieve the desired result, whether it is a specialised treatment setting or the client's own home or workplace.

Therapeutic use of self

The relationship between the therapist and client is an important part of the therapeutic process, from first meeting a newly referred client, through coping together with the successes and setbacks of the intervention process, to ending the programme on a positive note. Ideally, the relationship is a partnership or collaboration between therapist and client in which the goals and methods of intervention are negotiated throughout the therapeutic process. If a client is unable to take a full part in the process because of illness or disability, the therapist has a responsibility to facilitate that client's involvement as far as possible and to protect his interests to the best of her ability.

Mosey (1986) identified 11 elements which contribute to the therapist's ability to relate effectively to clients, as follows:

- a perception of individuality – recognition of each person as a unique whole
- respect for the dignity and rights of each individual
- empathy – ability to enter into the experience of another person without losing objectivity
- compassion or sympathy
- humility – recognition of the limits of one's own knowledge and skill
- unconditional positive regard – concern for the client without moral judgements on his thoughts and actions
- honesty – telling the truth to clients is an aspect of respect for persons
- a relaxed manner
- flexibility – ability to modify behaviour to meet the demands of a situation
- self-awareness – ability to reflect on one's own reactions to the world and on the effect one is having on the world in any given situation
- humour – a lightness of approach, used appropriately, can facilitate the therapeutic process.

Peloquin (1998) described the occupational therapist as *being with* the client by *doing with* the client, and identified empathy as the most important element of the therapeutic relationship. Empathy involves turning to the client in a genuine attempt to make a positive relationship, recognising what the therapist and client have in common, recognising the client's uniqueness, entering into the experience of the client, connecting with the client's feelings and being able

to recover from that connection so that the therapist is not damaged by the therapeutic encounter.

The therapist can use interpersonal skills to deal with a whole range of needs, such as engaging the initial interest of someone with a volitional disorder, supporting a bereaved client through the grieving process, helping someone to express difficult feelings appropriately, valuing a client with chronic low self-esteem and helping carers to work out how best to balance their own and the client's needs. The therapist herself can be the most valuable resource in an intervention.

THE CHANGING NATURE OF THE PROFESSION

The profession of occupational therapy is not static but changes gradually over time. Theories are continually being added or discarded as new knowledge becomes available. Philosophies also change, though more slowly, under the influence of what is happening in the wider society.

In a constantly changing profession, what remains constant? Several occupational therapists have written about a 'hard core' which consists of the consistently present, though slowly changing, elements of the profession. These are:

- the values, beliefs and principles that occupational therapists hold about their practice, the common world view shared by members of the profession known as the philosophy of occupational therapy (Baum & Christiansen 1997)
- an understanding of the relationship between occupation and health (Wilcock 1998)
- the process of practice (Hagedorn 1995a)
- the skills of the therapist.

Hagedorn (1995b) suggested that the core of occupational therapy is like a genetic template that gives rise to new individuals in each generation who are different from the therapists who came before but who remain true to the original type. Each generation of therapists will be influenced by changes in the outside world and will help to influence the way in which the profession changes.

External influences on the profession

There are few internally defined limits on the growth of occupational therapy as a profession, but external factors influencing growth include:

- new knowledge emerging from different disciplines
- the changing roles of other professions
- changing social values
- the national and international political climate
- economic pressures.

The great expansion of knowledge in the 20th century changed how we see the world and how we conceptualise health and disease. For example, the theories of Freud, whether or not we agree with them, have been incorporated into Western thinking so thoroughly that they have shaped, and continue to shape, in a very fundamental way, the way we see ourselves (Spinelli 1994). Vast areas of new knowledge have been incorporated into the theoretical base of the profession and will continue to be absorbed. Technological advances too inevitably influence the ways in which we deliver our services.

Occupational therapy has not established clear boundaries to its field of practice. To some extent, the role of the profession is defined by the other professions operating within the same areas. Some of the traditional roles of occupational therapists have been taken over by other professions, such as clinical psychology and physiotherapy, while our domain of concern has expanded into new fields, such as legal work.

Social values have also changed since the beginning of the 20th century, when occupational therapy took on a distinct identity, partly due to the experience of two world wars, partly to the technological revolution and partly to demographic and economic changes. Modern health care and modern medicine have conquered many life-threatening diseases so that more and more people are living with impairments that would have killed them in an earlier age. For the first time in history, in some countries, old people outnumber children, posing new economic and moral dilemmas. New diseases are occurring, such as auto-immune deficiency syndrome (AIDS), or old ones spreading in new patterns, such as Creutzfeldt-Jakob disease (CJD). More people are developing cancer and circulatory disease due to environmental factors and the fact that we are living longer. Occupational therapy, with its commitment to achieving quality of life, has a major role to play in caring for the chronic sick in society, in carrying out social policies for elderly or disabled people and in influencing those policies.

Social values are reflected in the political climate of a country, and health care policies are defined by politicians. At both the level of national government and at the level of service provision the degree of power and autonomy allowed the different professions is a political decision. National service frameworks are an example of a recent policy development in the UK. The national service framework for mental health (DoH 1999) sets national standards for promoting mental health and treating mental illness, puts in place programmes to support local delivery of services and establishes performance indicators. The aim is to improve the quality of service provision and remove local variations in quality.

Economic pressures also have an effect on the quality of health care in any country. When money is freely available there is an expansion of training and posts, but when times are harder it is necessary to justify the existence of a profession and the employment of therapists in economic terms as well as social or humanitarian ones. In times of economic recession occupational therapists may find themselves employed to meet the need of hospital managers for a quick turnover of patients rather than to meet the needs of their clients.

All these external pressures are experienced by the profession and help to influence the way it develops. Other influences arise directly from our professional practice and the way we perceive its effectiveness.

Internal influences on change

Professional activity is in three main areas: clinical, educational and professional. Feedback from these three areas directs change within the profession.

Clinical

The type of feedback an occupational therapist receives in the clinical setting includes:

- the results of intervention with individual clients
- the effectiveness and efficiency of the service as a whole
- the role and status accorded to the therapist by colleagues
- the number and grade of occupational staff employed.

This feedback comes from evaluation of interventions, outcome measurement, clinical audit and research. There is an expectation that clinical interventions should be based on evidence of what has been shown to be effective, therefore occupational therapists should be able to read about, and assess critically, the different types of evidence available.

Consideration of evidence can bring about changes in:

- the goals of intervention
- the theories, approaches and techniques used
- the way the service is organised
- the location of the service, for example moving from a hospital to a community base
- the areas in which occupational therapists choose to work and, therefore, their range of clinical roles.

Educational

The quality and style of education of occupational therapy students has an influence on:

- the way that practitioners view their role and function as professionals
- the extent to which occupational therapists are prepared to be autonomous, proactive practitioners

- standards of professional practice
- the quality of the theoretical base of the profession and the consistency with which it is used
- the direction and amount of research carried out into professional practice
- recruitment of students
- retention of staff
- the status of the profession, nationally and worldwide.

Professional education is being continually upgraded, from diploma to degree status and now towards postgraduate qualifications. Occupational therapists are expected to engage in continuing professional development throughout their careers, building up a portfolio of experience and skills that will ensure they are able to respond flexibly to changing demands. The *Code of Ethics and Professional Conduct for Occupational Therapists* (COT 2000, p. 13) states that 'Occupational therapists shall be personally responsible for actively maintaining and developing their personal professional competence, and shall base service delivery on accurate and current information in the interests of high quality care.'

Professional

Professional activity takes place at local, national and international levels through professional associations. The function of these associations is to:

- give the profession its public image and market its services
- act as the voice of the profession in negotiating professional issues
- negotiate professional boundaries and protect professional interests
- provide a forum for discussing matters of professional importance
- collect and disseminate information within the profession
- facilitate interdisciplinary communication
- set standards for and regulate education and professional practice
- interface with other bodies concerned with the education and registration of occupational therapists
- protect the interests of members.

A strong professional association can act as an agent of change, controlling and directing the way in which the profession prepares itself for the future.

THE OCCUPATIONAL THERAPY PROCESS

Occupational therapy is a process, in the sense that intervention and change take place over time. In many cases, the process of carrying out a programme of purposeful activity is more important than the goal of the programme. Life itself is more usually experienced as a process rather than as a series of steps or goals to be achieved.

Occupational therapy is also a process in the sense that the therapist's actions follow a recognisable sequence. Mosey (1986) said that 'Principles for sequencing various aspects of practice refer to the way in which a profession goes about the process of problem identification and proceeds through to problem solution relative to assisting the client.' There is an accepted first step to occupational therapy intervention, followed by a logical second step, and so on. There is general agreement on the steps that make up the occupational therapy process, although not all the steps are carried out in every case. In some settings the occupational therapist does not go through the whole process but merely assesses the client and passes the results to others to carry out the intervention.

Clinical reasoning

The process of intervention includes the way occupational therapists make decisions about what to do at each stage. This thinking process is called 'clinical reasoning'. 'Clinical reasoning acts as an internal guide or structure by which the therapist selects from all available information and uses it to understand the patient and make treatment decisions' (Bruce & Borg 1993, p. 33).

Three different types of clinical reasoning can be identified, each used for working through different types of problem. Fleming (1991) described these thinking strategies as:

- **Procedural reasoning**. This is the type of thinking used when considering the patient's disability and how to remediate it. It involves identifying problems, setting goals and planning treatment.
- **Interactive reasoning**. This type of thinking occurs when the therapist is working face-to-face with the client, building a relationship and trying to understand his experience.
- **Conditional reasoning**. This is used when the therapist is thinking broadly about the client in his temporal and lifeworld contexts and about the consequences of possible interventions. The therapist builds an image of the client's past, present and future in order to make predictions about what will work best.

The three main stages of the occupational therapy process are:

- assessment
- treatment/intervention
- evaluation (Fig. 5.1).

Assessment

There are different systems of referral, but an individual who is referred for occupational therapy will first be seen by the therapist and assessed.

Assessment is the basis for all intervention and must be both thorough and valid in order to ensure that treatment is appropriate. Assessment is in two stages:

1. initial assessment
2. detailed assessment.

Assessment begins from the moment a referral is received or, if individual referrals are not made in a particular setting, from the moment the therapist starts to identify those clients who could benefit from occupational therapy.

The initial assessment is a screening process to determine the main areas of need of the client and whether or not occupational therapy can be of any value in this case. Factors influencing whether or not a referral is accepted include:

- the needs of the client
- the client's goals and expectations

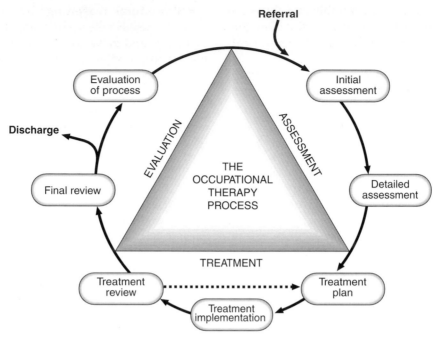

Figure 5.1 The stages of the occupational therapy process.

- the resources available, including manpower and expertise
- the client's personal support systems and social network
- the reason for referral
- the treatment contract.

Once accepted for treatment, a detailed assessment is carried out to determine the client's needs, strengths, interests and goals. Effective assessment will lead directly to setting measurable goals or defining expected outcomes of intervention, and to choice of appropriate treatment methods.

Methods of screening, assessment and goal-setting are discussed in Chapter 6.

Treatment

There may be no clear division between assessment and treatment in occupational therapy, where clients are often assessed by being observed participating in activities which also have therapeutic value. However, at some stage the therapist and client will establish goals and agree

on a treatment plan. Treatment is in three stages which may be repeated as necessary, depending on the client's progress:

1. formulation of treatment plan
2. treatment implementation
3. treatment review.

The preliminary treatment plan should be formulated by the therapist and client together, if the client is capable of making a contribution to the process at this stage. Other significant people, such as carers, may also be involved. The plan will include goals of treatment or desired outcomes, methods to be used, an individual programme and a list of the people who need to be informed about the programme.

The process of occupational therapy has a purpose, which is to achieve a satisfactory outcome. An outcome has been defined as 'the result of the objective of therapeutic intervention or treatment following the activities or treatment processes' (Booth 1995). In other words, the outcome of intervention is the extent to which the goals of the intervention have been met.

Outcomes should be measurable and the easiest way to achieve this is to link them to the objectives of treatment. An objective is a precise statement of the desired change in terms of measurable behaviour. It should include the conditions under which the behaviour will occur and the level of performance expected. For example, an objective for a woman referred for agoraphobia might be: at the end of treatment the client will be able to complete her weekly supermarket shopping within an hour, by herself, without having a panic attack.

A review date should be set at the time when the expected outcomes of treatment are defined. This is the date when measurement occurs. For example, linked with the objective given above, the expected outcome of intervention can be stated as: ability to shop independently at the supermarket. The decision is taken to review the client's progress in one month and a review date is set.

Treatment implementation involves putting the plan into action and continually monitoring the client's process, both during treatment sessions and over time. Minor changes can be made without having to organise a full review or alter the plan. A close liaison is maintained with other disciplines involved so that any changes or problems can be shared. If the treatment setting allows for a long period of intervention, regular reviews are held to evaluate the need for more radical programme changes. Clear and regular records of treatment sessions are kept to assist in the review process (see Ch. 8).

The treatment review serves several purposes:

- It gives the therapist, the client and the team an opportunity to review what progress has been made and to judge the success or otherwise of the programme.
- It gives everyone involved in treatment an update on the client's progress. Review meetings may be multidisciplinary, in which case everyone has a chance to discuss the client's progress, they may be within the occupational therapy team, or they may be between a single therapist and client.

- It is an opportunity to set new short-term goals or objectives and to adjust intermediate and long-term goals in the light of new information or changes in the client's circumstances.

There are three possible results of intervention:

- the expected outcome is achieved
- the outcome falls short of what was expected
- the outcome is better than expected.

After the review the treatment plan is updated and other team members are informed of the new plan. If it is discovered that the goals of intervention have been met, then the discharge procedure may be started. If goals have been partially met, then the treatment programme may be upgraded. If goals have not been met, then the goal setting and treatment planning stages may have to be repeated.

Treatment planning and implementation are discussed in more detail in Chapter 7.

Evaluation

The circular process of occupational therapy is completed by the two stages of evaluation:

1. final treatment review
2. evaluation of the process.

The final review of the client's progress is used to evaluate the success of the intervention and to reach decisions about discharge or referral to other agencies. Major decisions are not usually made during one meeting but it can be useful to meet to formalise decisions. The client and therapist can compare the present state of affairs with the position before intervention so that progress is obvious and termination of treatment is seen as a positive step.

Evaluation is essential to demonstrate the effectiveness of intervention for the client, the therapist, the referring agent and other interested parties. Evaluation should be a part of the whole occupational therapy process, but formal evaluations of particular aspects of the service, such as groups, or of the service as a whole may be carried out at intervals in the form of an audit.

Clinical audit is discussed in more detail in Chapter 9.

Evaluation of the service should be carried out by occupational therapists themselves against their own criteria of performance. Such evaluation may lead to changes in skill mix in a department, to a request for improved resources, to a restructuring of the way the service is delivered, or to a complete change of focus, such as relocating staff away from a hospital base to community settings.

FRAMES OF REFERENCE

In Chapter 3, a frame of reference was defined as selected theories that are compatible with each other and that can be applied within a particular field of practice. As the knowledge base of occupational therapy has expanded, theories have been organised into an increasing number of frames of reference, approaches and models. In 1946, a textbook on the theory of occupational therapy (Haworth & MacDonald 1946) described one approach to therapy (rehabilitation) and offered one chapter on occupational therapy in the treatment of mental disorders which focused on engaging patients in activities to improve or maintain health. In 1997, a textbook on the theory of occupational therapy (Hagedorn 1997) described five frames of reference used by occupational therapists in the field of psychosocial dysfunction: behavioural, cognitive-behavioural, analytical, group work and humanist. Different textbooks suggest different ways of classifying frames of reference, although most of them include the same selection of theories. For example, Finlay (1997) described four psychological approaches: psychodynamic, cognitive-behavioural, humanistic and social.

There is little consensus about how to describe and classify the frames of reference or approaches in general use. Practising clinicians may not be able to say what theories they are using or what their approach is called. Different writers use various terms to describe occupational therapy frames of reference and classify them in different ways. The classification offered in Table 5.1 is not intended to be definitive. It is simply one way of describing how theories are organised for use in practice.

Table 5.1 Occupational therapy frames of reference for mental health

Frame of reference	Main focus
Rehabilitative	Improving function in the activities of everyday life
Psychodynamic	Resolving unconscious conflicts and strengthening ego defence mechanisms
Behavioural	Learning skills to support appropriate behaviour
Occupational behaviour	Learning skills to support a balanced range of activities and occupations
Human developmental	Facilitating normal development to an age-appropriate level
Cognitive-behavioural	Identifying and modifying negative cognitions affecting mood and behaviour
Cognitive disability	Assessing level of cognitive function and providing tasks appropriate to that level

The name of each frame of reference is a general heading that refers to the major theories and goals used in that approach. Each one incorporates a number of models, developed by different occupational therapy theorists, which share most of the theories and goals that make up the frame of reference. For example, occupational behaviour encompasses the occupational performance model (Law et al 1990), the model of human occupation (Kielhofner & Burke 1980) and adaptation through occupation (Reed & Sanderson 1992). All these models share basic assumptions about the occupational nature of people, they all draw on theories of occupation and role theory, and they all have the goal of improving occupational performance. The frame of reference delineates the field and the theoretical base for practice. Models give more precise directions for putting theory into practice.

Seven frames of reference are listed in Table 5.1. The theories, models and approaches associated with each frame of reference are described in different chapters of this book. The rehabilitative approach is described in Chapter 20; cognitive-behavioural and cognitive disability models are described in Chapter 13; some behavioural theories and techniques are outlined briefly in

Chapter 16; this frame of reference is not covered in depth because many of the assumptions about people and motivation which underpin it do not sit comfortably with the person-centred philosophy of occupational therapy. The model of human occupation (Kielhofner & Burke 1980), Mosey's adaptive skills approach (1986) and adaptation through occupation (Reed & Sanderson 1992) are also outlined in Chapter 16 and the model of creative ability is described in Chapter 15.

Three frames of reference are described below: psychodynamic, occupational behaviour and human developmental. Each one is described in terms of: the basic assumptions about the nature of people that underpin the approach, the knowledge base, how function and dysfunction are conceptualised, how change occurs, the client group, the goals of intervention, and techniques for assessment and intervention.

PSYCHODYNAMIC FRAME OF REFERENCE

In the 1950s, Azima & Wittkower (1957), two psychiatrists at McGill University in Canada, carried out a survey of psychiatric occupational therapy in 15 departments in Canada and the USA. They concluded that 'too much emphasis has been put upon the diversional and occupational aspects of activities to the neglect of psychodynamic problems of the individual receiving occupational therapy.' Two years later, Azima & Azima (1959) published their outline of a dynamic theory of occupational therapy. This paper suggested a theoretical base for occupational therapy, drawing on psychodynamic theory and, in particular, the concept of object relations. This theory was taken up and expanded by Fidler & Fidler (1963) in their book *Occupational Therapy: A Communication Process in Psychiatry*. This was the first systematic attempt by occupational therapists to develop their own knowledge base.

Basic assumptions about people

Psychodynamic theory and the psychodynamic approach developed from the work of Sigmund Freud and his followers. Freudian thinking views people as having both a conscious and an unconscious mind. Behaviour is largely influenced by material in the unconscious mind, therefore people are usually not aware of why they act in particular ways and their actions are not under conscious control. Actions are taken to gratify needs, but not necessarily the needs of which the individual is consciously aware.

Fidler & Fidler (1963) described basic assumptions about the relationship of people with activity. People are seen as having an innate drive to be active that is directed towards achieving gratification of basic needs and towards making satisfactory relationships. Action is used to express and communicate feelings and thoughts. It arises from mental images and feedback about the results of action allows these images to be modified to match external reality.

The infant strives for competence in actions that will both meet his needs and increase his sense of personal identity and integrity. A sense of self-worth comes from the intrinsic satisfaction in doing well in the particular areas of life that he values. The more situations and actions the child is able to experience, the greater will be his knowledge of his own potential and limitations, leading to greater adaptability. A knowledge of what patterns of action are most useful and acceptable in the individual's culture are learned through interaction with the social environment.

Knowledge base

A vast number of different psychodynamic theories evolved, as many of Freud's followers developed their own approaches to psychotherapy. The occupational therapist working within a psychodynamic frame of reference will have a knowledge and understanding of:

- psychiatry
- psychoanalytic theory
- psychopathology
- group dynamics
- the symbolic potential of activities and materials
- object relations theory.

One of the most important psychodynamic theories for occupational therapists, and one that was taken up by Fidler & Fidler (1963), is object relations theory: 'The term "object relations" refers to the investment of emotions and psychic energy in objects for the purpose of satisfying needs ... Objects are any human being (including the self), abstract concept, or non-human thing which has the potential for satisfying needs or interfering with need satisfaction' (Mosey 1986).

Object relations theory describes the relationship between the self and other human and non-human objects. The new-born child cannot differentiate between himself and his environment, therefore he cannot have any conscious relationship. As he grows he becomes aware of the mother or mother figure as a separate but vitally important person who is the source of satisfaction of his needs. The relationship is one of total dependence and the baby is 'in love' with the mother to the exclusion of everyone else. This type of dependency is called an anaclitic relationship. Gradually the child realises that he can gratify some of his own needs and this leads to a narcissistic relationship with his own body. More mature object relationships are formed as the child grows and develops a stronger sense of identity that allows him to relate to people and things in a variety of ways other than using them for immediate gratification.

Function and dysfunction

There are several ways of conceptualising dysfunction, depending on which psychodynamic theory is being used. For example, in Freudian theory, the ego has to balance the conflicting demands of reality, the id and the superego. Conflicts that are not dealt with as the individual grows and develops may be retained in the unconscious mind and surface as anxiety. The ego defends against anxiety by using ego defence mechanisms. This takes up psychic energy so that it is no longer available for other uses. Dysfunction occurs when the individual is unable to contain the anxiety because the conflicts are too great, or ego defence mechanisms

are not working effectively, and material from the unconscious interferes with function.

In object relations theory, as applied to occupational therapy by the Fidlers (1963), dysfunction is characterised by immature object relationships which may be the result of a failure to develop healthy object-concepts or may be due to psychopathology and regression. For example, a person experiencing psychological disorganisation in severe psychosis may have difficulty recognising himself as separate from others or may have anaclitic object relationships. A functioning individual is one who has an integrated self-identity and a realistic concept of others, who continues to grow and develop throughout his life, who is able to satisfy his basic needs and who contributes to the welfare of others. A well-organised personality has a positive and realistic sense of self and good object concepts.

How change occurs

Since dysfunction is believed to arise from unresolved conflicts located in the unconscious mind, change can be initiated by bringing these conflicts into the conscious mind so that they can be verbalised and shared. Once the difficult or painful material has been accessed, the therapist can help the client to find alternative ways of coming to terms with the feelings it arouses or dealing with it in a more adaptive way. Alternatively, the therapist may decide not to engage in exploration of the unconscious mind but deal with anxiety by supporting the client's existing coping mechanisms and finding new ways of gratifying needs.

Mosey (1986) pointed out that resolution of conflicts does not necessarily lead to the client spontaneously learning the skills needed for successful functioning. The psychoanalytic frame of reference may have to be used in conjunction with, or followed by, a more pragmatic approach to facilitate the acquisition of these skills.

Client group

The psychodynamic approach is appropriate for use with people of all ages and for treating a wide range of psychosocial disorders. It has been most widely used with adults and adolescents with acute disorders but is also appropriate for children and people with chronic illness. It requires that the client participate actively in the intervention process, therefore it is less suitable for severely handicapped clients. Traditional forms of psychotherapy require good verbal skills but occupational therapists can use non-verbal media, such as paint, to facilitate expression and communication.

Goals

There are two main approaches associated with this frame of reference. An explorative approach assumes that the content of the unconscious mind can best be dealt with by bringing it into the conscious so that it can be shared and examined. The individual can then find ways of resolving conflicts and accepting difficult or painful feelings so that more adaptive ways of meeting needs can be achieved. A supportive approach aims to keep unresolved conflicts and painful feelings hidden in the unconscious mind and to strengthen the client's ego defence mechanisms so that material does not 'leak' into the conscious mind and cause problems.

Whichever approach is used, the goals of intervention may be to:

- assist in finding ways to gratify frustrated basic needs
- reverse psychopathology
- provide conditions for normal psychosexual and psychosocial development
- facilitate the development of a more realistic view of the self in relation to action and to others
- help to build a more healthy and integrated ego.

Assessment and intervention

Activity analysis is in terms of the psychodynamics of activity, the symbolic potential of materials and actions, interpersonal aspects and sociocultural significance.

The two main approaches to psychotherapy are supportive and explorative. In either approach, the therapeutic elements of occupational therapy are:

- actions of the client
- objects used in, or resulting from, the action
- human and non-human objects in the environment
- interpersonal relationships.

The process of intervention begins with the collection of relevant data about the client, including the general goals of the multidisciplinary team. Data analysis allows a tentative treatment plan to be drawn up or a preliminary programme devised for the further collection of data. Close liaison with other team members is essential, especially if an explorative approach is being used. Treatment planning takes account of the amount of support and structure available to the client outside treatment sessions. Activities are selected for their symbolic potential as well as the potential to provide an appropriate level and type of social interaction and to match the client's needs. The choice of activities may be made by the therapist or by the client, depending upon the client's needs. However, the client must be an active participant in the therapeutic process if it is to be of value to him.

Treatment may be individual or in groups but the group should always be small enough to allow the individual to relate closely to everyone in it (8–10 members is usually considered to be the optimum size).

A supportive psychotherapy group would aim to:

- offer encouragement
- provide opportunities for mutual support
- provide a forum for exchanging information about resources
- provide a place to air problems
- help to relieve anxiety
- give opportunities to consider new ways of dealing with problems.

Explorative psychotherapy was traditionally a talking therapy, either one-to-one or in small groups. Occupational therapy has contributed activity to the process, with the development of projective techniques. These can be used for assessment and treatment.

The ego defence mechanism of projection allows unacceptable feelings to be put outside the individual, onto another person or object. For example, instead of admitting that there is a problem in my relationship with you because I don't like you, I think that we are having difficulties because you don't like me. Projective techniques refer to:

- the presentation of stimuli to which the client can respond with feelings or thoughts (e.g. a piece of music or a poem), or to
- the creation of a piece of work through which the client can express feelings or thoughts (e.g. a painting or a piece of free clay modelling).

Within a psychodynamic frame of reference there may be no clear distinction between assessment and treatment. The activities that help to bring unconscious material into the conscious mind allow for a clearer understanding of underlying conflicts while at the same time beginning the process of resolving those conflicts. The client's progress is apparent in the way he responds to the activities provided as treatment.

Some occupational therapists working within a psychodynamic frame of reference have moved away from the use of activities towards talking therapies. Since activity is the goal of occupational therapy intervention, it might be argued that talking is a valid tool for occupational therapists to use in pursuit of that goal. However, talking is only a legitimate tool for occupational therapists if it is used to support activity.

HUMAN DEVELOPMENTAL FRAME OF REFERENCE

A developmental approach to human function and dysfunction fits well with the temporal perspective taken by occupational therapists. The two names most closely associated with the human developmental frame of reference in occupational therapy are Anne Cronin Mosey and Lela A. Llorens. Mosey's 1968 paper

'Recapitulation of ontogenesis: a theory for the practice of occupational therapy' outlined a developmental model which can be used in the field of mental health. She subsequently expanded and developed the model, drawing out general principles of a human developmental frame of reference. Llorens (1970) wrote a paper entitled 'Facilitating growth and development: the promise of occupational therapy' for the Eleanor Clarke Slagle lecture in 1969. In it she outlined a framework for intervention, based on developmental theory, that had grown out of her work in the fields of psychiatry, paediatrics and community health. This was followed by a series of publications expanding and clarifying the model and looking at aspects of its application.

This outline of the human developmental frame of reference will draw on the work of both Mosey and Llorens as well as on the work of some other occupational therapy theorists.

Basic assumptions about people

People are seen as dynamic, developing organisms whose life cycles go through predictable stages of growth and decline that necessitate adaptation by the individual. Developmental achievements are not necessarily permanent – regression to an earlier level can occur and maladaptive or incomplete development can be remediated.

Development takes place in a sequence that is common to everyone, although the pace may vary widely. Each stage of development can only proceed normally if the preceding stages have been completed successfully. Incomplete development in one area of skill, or in one life stage, will influence subsequent development. Age ranges can be suggested for particular skills to be mastered but these are not absolute and are mainly useful for checking whether development in all skill areas is proceeding at the same pace. Early patterns of development influence the personality structure of the adult, but growth and development continue into adulthood and middle age, especially in the areas of changing responsibilities and relationships. It may be assumed that some kind of development continues into old age, but not much work has been done in this area.

People's development is influenced by environmental opportunities and barriers and by what they do. Development will not proceed normally if the child is deprived of a normal range of purposeful activities. Fidler & Fidler (1978) proposed that purposeful action 'is viewed as enabling the development and integration of the sensory, motor, cognitive, and psychological systems'.

Llorens (1970) based her model of human growth and development on ten premises, as follows:

1. A person develops in parallel the areas of neurophysiological, physical, psychosocial and psychodynamic growth, social language, daily living and sociocultural skills.
2. All these areas continue to develop throughout the person's life.
3. Mastery of skills to an age-appropriate level in all areas of development is necessary to the achievement of satisfactory coping behaviour and adaptive relationships.
4. Such mastery is usually achieved naturally in the course of development.
5. Intrinsic factors and external stimulation received within the family environment interact to promote early growth and development.
6. The later influences of the extended family, community and social groups assist in the growth process.
7. Physical or psychological trauma can interrupt the growth and development process.
8. Such interruption will cause a gap in the developmental cycle resulting in a disparity between expected coping behaviour and the skills necessary to achieve it.
9. Occupational therapy can provide growth and developmental links to assist in closing the gap between expectation and ability through the skilled application of activities and relationships.
10. Occupational therapy can provide growth experiences to prevent the development of maladaptive behaviour and skills related to insufficient nurturance.

Knowledge base

This frame of reference is based on theories of human development in the areas of physical, cognitive, psychological, emotional and social growth. Developmental theories are outlined in Chapter 3 but readers are recommended to read the original sources for details.

The developmental frame of reference is flexible enough to work compatibly with other theories, such as learning theory.

Function and dysfunction

Function and dysfunction are a continuum. Growth and development can be disrupted or delayed by congenital or acquired disease or injury, or by absence of the conditions for normal growth and development. A functioning individual is one who achieves satisfactory coping behaviour and adaptive relationships by developing appropriate skills, abilities and relationships at each stage of the lifespan. These adaptive behaviours allow the individual to adjust to both internal needs and external demands.

Dysfunction occurs when the developmental level of the individual, in any area, is unequal to the age-related demands made on him. Some of these expectations will be for skills common to all people, such as walking by a certain age, while others will be culturally determined, such as social skills. Trauma at any age can interrupt the developmental process and inhibit the development of adaptive skills or cause regression to an earlier developmental level. A major disruption in any one area will affect all other areas, and the longer the disruption continues the more gaps there will be in the developmental process. However, Mosey (1986) pointed out that people may complete a delayed developmental stage at a later time, when the conditions are right, or may compensate for developmental delay by learning certain higher level skills without the underpinning of more basic ones.

How change occurs

Skills are learned in the normal developmental sequence so that higher level skills are integrated with lower level skills in the same area and with other skills areas developing in parallel. If higher level skills are not integrated with more basic ones then they may be lost when the individual is under stress, and regression to an earlier level of development may occur.

An individual is able to move from one stage of development to the next when the requirements of the earlier stage have been met and the conditions for further development are in place. As the individual's physical and psychological needs change, and as new environmental demands are made, the person experiences disequilibrium. This motivates him to learn the skills needed to reestablish a state of equilibrium. New skills are acquired through practice of relevant activities in a facilitating environment until mastery is achieved. Once a basic skill has been learned, the individual will refine and elaborate it through use.

Client group

Different aspects of developmental theory will be used with different client groups. For example, the occupational therapist working with children with learning difficulties may draw on knowledge from the areas of language, cognition, emotional, psychosexual, social and sociocultural development. If the child has multiple impairments the therapist may also draw on the areas of physical-motor, sensorimotor and perceptual development. The occupational therapist working with adults in an acute psychiatric setting may use theories of personality, emotional, moral, psychosexual, psychosocial, social and sociocultural development.

Occupational therapists are concerned with promoting development at all ages, therefore this frame of reference is applicable throughout the lifespan. It can be used with people suffering from any kind of chronic or acute mental disorder, as well as those with delay in physical or cognitive development.

Goals

The occupational therapist uses activities and relationships, applied with knowledge and skill, to facilitate growth and development. The overall goal of intervention is to increase skills in all areas, with emphasis being placed on the main area of deficit, so that the gap between expected coping behaviour for the individual's chronological age and actual adaptive ability is closed or narrowed. Short-term goals are to learn the skills needed for the next stage of development.

Occupational therapy is also concerned with maintaining health and preventing maladaptation through early detection of problems and early intervention. This will allow the individual to continue the growth process with a minimum of disruption.

Assessment and intervention

The individual's developmental level in the different skill areas is assessed to find where normal development has been disrupted or has ceased. Appropriate assessment methods include interviews, general observation, observation in tasks designed to elicit specific skills, review of records, projective techniques and testing.

Intervention takes the client's present level of development and ability as the starting point and builds on existing skills. Llorens (1970) stated that it is necessary to meet an individual's needs at his present developmental level if further development is to take place. Bruce & Borg (1993) pointed out that 'confrontation with change creates tension, disequilibrium and stress', but that 'this process is not, of itself, pathological, and in fact is often a necessary part of the change process . . . a history of successful adaptation promotes future success in meeting challenges.'

If development in the different skill areas has proceeded unevenly, so that one or more areas lag behind the others, then intervention is started in the area where development is most delayed. When that area has caught up, attention is transferred to the next most delayed area so that development across the skills areas proceeds relatively evenly. Intervention is continued until the client has attained an age-appropriate level of adaptive skill in all areas, or has attained sufficient skill to be able to function adequately in his expected environment, or has reached what seems to be his highest possible level of achievement.

Treatment techniques include activities and relationships. Activities are analysed and selected for their potential to facilitate the development of particular skills and are combined with a suitable type and level of interpersonal interaction to achieve the maximum benefit.

OCCUPATIONAL BEHAVIOUR FRAME OF REFERENCE

The development of this frame of reference was initiated by Mary Reilly who, from 1959, was chief of the Rehabilitation Department of the Neuropsychiatric Institute at the University of California at Los Angeles (UCLA) (Van Deusen 1988).

Early in her career, Reilly became interested in the relevance of the central nervous system to human performance and, therefore, to the work of the occupational therapist. Through her work on developing patient skills and competence she began to construct a frame of reference that would combine knowledge of the neurosciences with theories of intrinsic motivation and social psychology and with the ideas of Meyer, one of the founders of occupational therapy. As director of occupational therapy studies at UCLA, Reilly was able to influence many generations of occupational therapy students. The occupational behaviour frame of reference has been included in this chapter because it has been researched and amplified by these students and has influenced the development of many new models for practice, such as the model of human occupation and the model of creative ability.

Basic assumptions about people

People are active beings who have an intrinsic need to interact with the environment and achieve mastery through developing competence in skills to support life roles. 'Man has a vital need for occupation and his central nervous system demands the rich and varied stimuli that solving life's problems provides him . . . primary pleasure can be sought through efficient use of the central nervous system for the performance of those ego

integrating tasks which enable man to alter and control his environment' (Reilly 1962).

People function in a variety of occupational roles and their lives are organised as a balance between work, play, rest and sleep.

Reilly (1969) described three aspects of people that are central to the understanding of occupational behaviour:

1. People have an intrinsic drive to achieve.
2. The drive to achieve generates interests, abilities, skills, and habits of competition and cooperation. These are expressed through the developmental continuum of play and work which is called occupational behaviour.
3. People adopt a variety of occupational roles and learn the behaviour appropriate to those roles through the process of socialisation.

Matsutsuyu (1971) described three processes that underpin the development of occupational behaviour:

1. **Occupational choice**. People learn and develop throughout their lives by engaging in occupations. Adult work and social roles evolve from childhood play and work through a process of occupational choice (see Ch. 3). Occupational choice is a developmental process extending over many years.
2. **Occupational role**. Adult roles can be divided into family roles, personal–sexual roles and occupational roles. Occupational roles are identified by the tasks performed and the social position that goes with the role. They include workers, housewives, retirees, students and preschoolers.
3. **Socialisation**. Occupational role behaviours are learned through socialisation. Socialisation enables the maintenance, learning and relearning of roles.

Knowledge base

This frame of reference incorporates knowledge taken from a wide range of disciplines, including medicine, neurophysiology, neuropsychiatry, behavioural sciences, social sciences and social psychology. Reilly (1969) suggested that open systems theory and the concept of hierarchy be used to organise this wide-ranging knowledge.

Specific areas of knowledge required include:

- an understanding of human beings in terms of three systems (biological, personality and social) and three processes (coordination, personality development and socialisation)
- theories of motivation, especially intrinsic motivation and the drives for achievement and competence
- the function of play in human learning and development
- temporal adaptation, balance of occupations, ontogenesis of occupations and the process of change
- general systems theory.

Function and dysfunction

People have the capacity to influence the state of their own health through what they do, and a balance of rest, play and work in daily life is necessary to maintain physical and mental health. People are in a state of function when they have the range of skills and level of competence necessary to support a balanced variety of occupational roles that satisfy their needs and are socially and culturally acceptable.

Dysfunction occurs when people are prevented from being able to act successfully on their environment by disease or injury. Reilly (1969) called this type of dysfunction 'incapacity'.

How change occurs

People can develop the adaptive skills to support occupational roles through playful exploration followed by practice to a level of competence. The task of the occupational therapist is to trigger the individual's intrinsic motivation to act and to create the conditions to support the development of competent performance.

Client group

The occupational behaviour frame of reference was intended to be applicable to the needs of people with chronic disabilities, the population most in need of occupational therapy services. This approach has much to offer this client group because it is concerned with adaptation rather than with freedom from pathology. However, later refinements of the frame of reference have led to it having a very wide applicability.

Goals

Reilly (1969) stated: 'It is the task of medicine to prevent and reduce illness; while the task of occupational therapy is to prevent and reduce the incapacities resulting from illness.' The goal of occupational therapy is to help people to carry out the daily activities required by their social and work roles and to achieve satisfaction from them. This may require habit restructuring and/or making changes to the environment to enable adaptation.

Assessment and intervention

The occupational therapist assesses the client's ability to perform his current life roles and the adaptive skills that support them. Assessment techniques include: structured or semi-structured interviews, occupational role histories, interest checklists, direct observation and skills inventories.

Reilly (1966) stated that a programme of intervention should satisfy the following six criteria:

1. There should be an examination of the client's current life roles and identification of the various skills that support them.

2. The treatment programme should reflect the developmental stages of the acquisition of life skills.

3. Programmes should provide natural and legitimate decision-making opportunities for clients.

4. The treatment milieu must acknowledge competencies, stimulate curiosity, deepen appreciation and require behaviour across the full range of human abilities.

5. The focus of attention should not be on a single activity or on the time spent in treatment, but on the way the client spends his time throughout the week.

6. Programmes must provide opportunities for practising a balanced range of life skills that

match the client's interests, abilities, age, gender and occupational roles.

Smith (1974) proposed four factors in the therapeutic environment that help to activate the client's intrinsic motivation and start the process of learning new skills:

- respectful, close attention to what the client is saying in order to communicate to him that he is being taken seriously
- sustaining faith by the therapist in the client's human potential
- properly paced developmental tasks that pose a challenge for the client and lead to success through his own efforts
- exposure to appropriate role models.

SUMMARY

This chapter looked at the components of occupational therapy practice, other than the knowledge base which was discussed in Chapter 3. It began by outlining the content of practice, including professional goals, the population served by occupational therapy and the core skills and legitimate tools of the profession. Occupations are seen as both the major goal of intervention and the main tool used to bring about change. We then considered what the core of occupational therapy is and what aspects of the profession change in response to internal and external pressures.

The next section of the chapter described briefly the three stages of the occupational therapy process: assessment, treatment and evaluation. (These are discussed in more detail in Chapters 6, 7 and 9.)

The chapter finished by examining the way in which occupational therapy knowledge is organised into frames of reference. Three examples were given: psychodynamic, human developmental and occupational behaviour.

The next chapter looks at aspects of occupational therapy assessment.

REFERENCES

Agyris C, Schon D A 1974 Theory in practice: increasing professional effectiveness. Jossey-Bass, San Francisco

Azima H, Azima F J 1959 Outline of a dynamic theory of occupational therapy. American Journal of Occupational Therapy 13(5): 215–221

Azima H, Wittkower E D 1957 A partial field survey of psychiatric occupational therapy. American Journal of Occupational Therapy 11(1): 1–7

Baum C, Christiansen C 1997 The occupational therapy context: philosophy – principles – practice. In: Christiansen C, Baum C (eds) Occupational therapy: enabling function and well-being, 2nd edn. Slack, New Jersey

Booth M 1995 Practical experiences in measuring occupational therapy outcomes. Unpublished paper presentation, COT Annual Conference

Bruce M A, Borg B 1993 Psychosocial occupational therapy: frames of reference for intervention, 2nd edn. Slack, New Jersey

COT 1994 Core skills and a conceptual framework for practice: a position statement. College of Occupational Therapists, London

COT 2000 Code of ethics and professional conduct for occupational therapists. College of Occupational Therapists, London

Creek J 1998 Purposeful activity. In: Creek J (ed) Occupational therapy: new perspectives. Whurr, London

Department of Health 1999 National service framework for mental health: modern standards and service models. HMSO, London

Fidler G S, Fidler J W 1963 Occupational therapy: a communication process in psychiatry. MacMillan, New York

Fidler G S, Fidler J W 1978 Doing and becoming: purposeful action and self-actualisation. American Journal of Occupational Therapy 32(5): 305–310

Finlay L 1997 The practice of psychosocial occupational therapy, 2nd edn. Stanley Thornes, Cheltenham

Fleming M H 1991 The therapist with the three-track mind. American Journal of Occupational Therapy 45(11): 1007–1014

Hagedorn R 1995a Occupational therapy: perspectives and processes. Churchill Livingstone, Edinburgh

Hagedorn R 1995b Casson Memorial Lecture 1995. An emergent profession – a personal perspective. British Journal of Occupational Therapy 58(8): 324–331

Hagedorn R 1997 Foundations for practice in occupational therapy, 2nd edn. Churchill Livingstone, Edinburgh

Haworth N A, MacDonald E M 1946 Theory of occupational therapy, 3rd edn. Ballière Tindall and Cox, London

Jenkins M 1998 Shifting ground or sifting sand? In: Creek J (ed) Occupational therapy: new perspectives. Whurr, London

Kielhofner G, Burke J P 1980 A model of human occupation, part 1. Conceptual framework and content. American Journal of Occupational Therapy 34(9): 572–581

Law M, Baptiste S, McColl M, Opzoomer A, Polatajko H, Pollock N 1990 The Canadian Occupational Performance Measure: an outcome measure for occupational therapy. Canadian Journal of Occupational Therapy 57(2): 82–87

Llorens L A 1970 Facilitating growth and development: the promise of occupational therapy. American Journal of Occupational Therapy 24(2): 93–101

Matsutsuyu J 1971 Occupational behaviour – a perspective on work and play. American Journal of Occupational Therapy 25(6): 291–294

Mosey A C 1968 Recapitulation of ontogenesis: a theory for the practice of occupational therapy. American Journal of Occupational Therapy 22(5): 426–438

Mosey A C 1986 Psychosocial components of occupational therapy. Raven, New York

Peloquin S M 1998 The therapeutic relationship. In: Neistadt M E, Crepeau E B (eds) Willard and Spackman's Occupational therapy, 9th edn. Lippincott, Philadelphia

Reed K L, Sanderson S N 1992 Concepts of occupational therapy 3rd edn. Williams and Wilkins, Baltimore

Reilly M 1962 Occupational therapy can be one of the great ideas of 20th century medicine. American Journal of Occupational Therapy 16(1): 1–9

Reilly M 1966 A psychiatric occupational therapy program as a teaching model. American Journal of Occupational Therapy 20(2):61–67

Reilly M 1969 The educational process. American Journal of Occupational Therapy 23(4): 299–307

Reilly M 1971 The modernisation of occupational therapy. American Journal of Occupational Therapy 25(5): 243–246

Smith M B 1974 Competence and adaptation. American Journal of Occupational Therapy 28(1): 11–15

Spinelli E 1994 Demystifying therapy. Constable, London

Stewart A 1994 Empowerment and enablement: occupational therapy 2001. British Journal of Occupational Therapy 57(7): 248–254

Van Deusen J 1988 Mary Reilly. In: Miller B R J, Sieg K W, Ludwig F M, Shortridge S D, Van Deusen J Six perspectives on theory for the practice of occupational therapy. Rockville, Aspen

Wilcock A A 1998 A theory of occupation and health. In: Creek J (ed) Occupational therapy: new perspectives. Whurr, London

6

Assessment

Jennifer Creek

INTRODUCTION

Assessment is an integral part of the occupational therapy process. An initial assessment is used to evaluate the client's strengths, identify problem areas, determine whether or not occupational therapy intervention is appropriate and establish a database prior to beginning programme planning. Ongoing assessments show any changes that have taken place during treatment and demonstrate when goals have been reached. Later assessments provide a picture of residual problems, which can be measured against the client's life demands in order to make recommendations about discharge and to plan follow-up.

Assessment is measurement of the quality or degree of the various factors in a situation or condition. In clinical practice it is used to measure the assets and deficits of the client that relate to his referral for therapy. The process of assessment is invoked when a client is referred to the occupational therapist because some change is judged to be necessary in the person's situation.

Assessment is not something that is done to the client. It involves the client's active cooperation, both in providing information and in helping to interpret it.

This chapter will discuss the part that assessment plays in the occupational therapy process, what is assessed, methods of assessment and how to determine the validity of results.

THE ASSESSMENT PROCESS

The process of assessment, as shown in Figure 6.1, relates to the occupational therapy process as a whole.

Assessment techniques are designed to work within particular theoretical perspectives or frames of reference. When assessing clients we do not take account of every factor in their situation, rather, we select certain factors as being important, depending on our philosophical and theoretical bias.

INITIAL ASSESSMENT

Initial assessment can be described as the art of defining the problem to be tackled or identifying the goal to be achieved. When a referral is received, the first step in the occupational therapy process is to collect and organise information about the client from a variety of sources in order to plan treatment effectively.

The initial assessment has four main functions:

1. It gives the therapist an opportunity to judge whether or not the client will benefit from

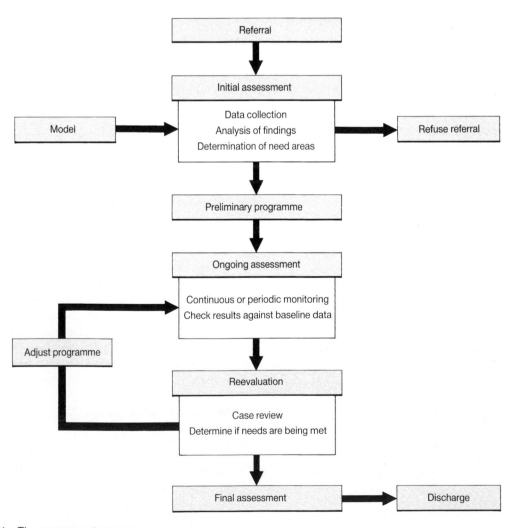

Figure 6.1 The assessment process.

occupational therapy intervention (screening).

2. It provides an opportunity to begin to establish rapport and elicit the client's interest and cooperation.
3. It gives a picture of the client's overall functional ability.
4. It produces a database.

Methods of data collection will be discussed in more detail in the section on methods of assessment.

Recording the results of investigations not only provides a baseline from which to measure change, but is also the starting point for interpretation. Methods of recording data are discussed in Chapter 8. The process of organising information, which should be carried out as far as possible with the active cooperation of the client, is used to:

- produce a list of problems and strengths
- identify goals of treatment
- suggest strategies and methods of intervention.

This process is part of treatment planning and is described in more detail in Chapter 7.

Screening referrals

The outcome of an initial assessment may be a decision *not* to provide an occupational therapy programme. The main reasons why this decision might be taken are as follows:

- The client's problem does not come within the domain of concern of the occupational therapist.
- The client could not benefit from occupational therapy intervention at this particular time (for example, a person with alcoholism needs to acknowledge that he has a drink problem before he can benefit from intervention).
- The resources of the department cannot meet the client's needs at this particular time.

Occupational therapy intervention only contributes directly to the treatment process when the programme is based on an assessment procedure that clearly indicates the need for such intervention (Gillette 1968).

Establishing rapport

Establishing a rapport with the client in this initial meeting is important to the client–therapist relationship. It can take a great deal of courage for someone to admit he needs help and the experience of attending a hospital or clinic can be very traumatic, particularly if it is a first admission. Older clients may be distressed by having to share their difficulties with a young person and may resent being asked to carry out activities if they cannot see their point. The therapist needs to appreciate these feelings and not feel personally threatened if a client is uncooperative at first.

The essential ingredients in establishing rapport with a client are as follows:

- *Respect* for the person, whatever the problems are. The client is a person first, and a client only temporarily.
- *Empathy*. It is not possible to like everyone we come into contact with, but the therapist should be able to empathise with most of the problems encountered. If there is a real personality clash that cannot be overcome with help from the supervisor, then it may be advisable to pass the client to another therapist.
- *Honesty* on the subject of what occupational therapy is about and what it can offer. It may be tempting to promise great results or to try to sound mysterious and potent, but, in the long run, full cooperation can only be engaged if the client understands the therapeutic process and feels in control.

Analysing function

Function has been defined as 'a person's ability to perform those tasks necessary in their daily life' (Punwar 1994). Occupational therapists consider the activities that the person wants to do, the activities that are necessary and those that are expected of him. The part of the assessment process which looks at how the individual functions in the normal range of daily life activities is called functional assessment or functional analysis.

Functional analysis is a wide-spectrum assessment that allows the therapist to identify the client's strengths, problems, sociocultural environment and personal view of life before beginning more focused assessments of particular aspects of function. Mattingly & Fleming (1994) described functional analysis as an important part of the occupational therapist's whole-person approach:

The functional assessment, which is the occupational therapy equivalent of the doctor's diagnosis, generally requires that the therapist go beyond gathering information and assessing the patient's physiological condition. It requires that the therapist pay some attention to the patient's unique life history and to how the patient sees and understands her or his condition.

Function means different things to different people at different times and must be measured in relation to the client's age, cultural background and expected environment (Mosey 1986).

Functional analysis is a process that takes place in three stages:

1. data collection
2. data analysis
3. identification of areas of dysfunction.

Methods of functional analysis will be described in the next section.

Producing a database

Basic information, such as the client's name, age, sex, marital status, can usually be found in the case notes. Much additional information will emerge during the treatment process, the initial assessment being only a starting point from which the general direction of treatment is determined.

The database is used to:

• determine the need for occupational therapy intervention
• identify the client's needs and assets
• provide a baseline against which to measure the outcome of treatment

• identify which areas need further investigation
• produce a set of treatment objectives
• suggest methods of intervention.

When all the preliminary investigations have been completed, the database can be analysed to produce a list of problems and assets, which is the basis for programme planning.

The therapist and client together produce a set of treatment goals and consider how they may be achieved. A programme is then planned and implemented immediately.

It may be necessary to start with a temporary programme while further data are collected, but this programme should be designed to help elicit the information required (as in the case described in Box 6.1).

ONGOING ASSESSMENT

Ongoing assessment is a part of the treatment process and is used to measure the client's progress, or lack of progress, so that the effectiveness of the treatment programme can be judged. This is sometimes called 'formative assessment' (Opacich 1991). Formative assessment is used to build a dynamic picture of the client's progress and to shape the course of intervention and further assessment in a continuous process.

Assessing and reevaluating progress

During the treatment programme, the therapist has many opportunities to observe the client's level of competence in the skills that the programme is designed to develop. Minor adjustments can be made at any time on the basis of observation and discussion with the client. For example, the therapist observes that a client's concentration span has increased: the client now has no difficulty in staying for a half-hour painting session. The therapist points this out to the client and suggests the length of the session be increased to three-quarters of an hour. The client agrees to try, the relevant people are informed of the change and the new length of session is implemented.

Box 6.1   Case example 1

Jim Manson, a young man with a severe learning disability, was referred for occupational therapy to find out whether any activities that would interest him could be found. The nursing staff felt that he had the potential to do more than wander around the home unit all day, but they did not have time to work with him individually.

It was agreed that for his preliminary programme one therapist would see Jim individually twice a week and try various activities with him, using the therapist's judgement and skill to choose activities and to motivate Jim to stay in the sessions.

After a few weeks, Jim's progress was reviewed. He had spent most of the time in his sessions either walking about, trying to leave or finger-flapping. His therapist noticed two barriers to involvement in activity:

- Jim found it hard to tolerate one-to-one attention.
- He could not concentrate on any one activity for more than a few minutes.

It was felt that Jim would do better in a parallel group where he would not receive the therapist's concentrated attention and where he could take time off from his own task to look at what other people were doing.

Jim continued to see his therapist once a week but they stayed in the occupational therapy workshop where many other people were also working and he was included in a small supportive psychotherapy group for people with severe communication and emotional disorders.

After a few weeks, the staff involved noted that Jim seemed much more relaxed and made no efforts to leave either of these sessions. He was spending almost equal proportions of time involved in the activity, looking at other people and indulging in ritualistic behaviour, a great improvement on his performance in individual sessions.

The new programme was continued with 6-monthly reviews. The preliminary programme, while not successful in involving the client in therapy, gave staff the information they needed to design a more appropriate programme.

More radical programme changes are usually discussed by all the people directly involved in the client's programme, if not by the whole team. A case review may be called by the therapist because she feels the client is ready for it, or the review may be routine. All clients should be reviewed regularly. In an acute setting this may take place weekly but, in a long-stay setting, 6-monthly reviews may be adequate.

The case review

In most departments a regular time each week is set aside for reviews so that all staff can attend, although an emergency review may be called at any time. All staff members are invited to the review. It is important that as many people as possible attend because:

- the observations of everyone who sees the client are important
- a broad discussion may shed new light on the client's needs
- it may be necessary to ask new staff to become involved
- the review can serve as a teaching session.

Invitations may be sent to staff of other disciplines, such as nurses or social workers. The client should also be given the opportunity to attend for at least part of the review in order to give his views in person and to hear what other people think about his progress.

The case review provides an opportunity for 'summative assessment' (Opacich 1991). This is assessment that occurs at predetermined intervals and focuses on the client's progress against treatment goals or expected outcomes. The summative assessment leads to decisions being made about changes in the client's programme.

One person is responsible for preparing and presenting the review, usually the client's key worker. The key worker's task is to collect all relevant information about the client from everyone involved and to organise it into a clear and comprehensible format. It is helpful to have a standard review format so that everyone knows how the material will be presented (Fig. 6.2). This also ensures that no points are missed. The format of the review will be determined by the frame of reference or model that the team uses.

The review will cover the client's: background, reason for referral, occupational therapy programme to date, level of involvement in treatment, progress and current areas of deficit. By analysing this information, the team can

Programme

How often the client attends

What sessions or groups the client attends

Whether or not the client's attendance is regular

Whether or not the client seems satisfied with the programme

Review

Brief recap of original goals and status at last review

Client's level of function in areas that were identified as problematic

Goals reached and progress towards other goals

Any other changes and particular areas of interest, progress or deterioration

Needs

An updated list of needs and goals that the client and therapist have agreed

Priorities for action

Suggested intervention for each goal

Suggestions about who might be involved in helping to meet each goal

Recommendations

A summary of recommendations and who is responsible for ensuring that they are carried out

Figure 6.2   A case review format.

determine what changes, if any, need to be made in the client's programme to meet those needs.

An example of a case review is given in Box 6.2. This example shows how aspects of a programme that are still effective are continued at the same level – for example continuing to attend the women's activity group and relaxation group – while other aspects are upgraded to take account of improvements – for example looking for community-based activities.

TERMINATION OF TREATMENT

The process of treatment, assessment, evaluation and replanning can take place as many times as is necessary for the client to reach his optimum level of functioning. Short-term goals are continually being met and updated and it may be necessary to change long-term goals in the light of new information acquired during therapy or if the client's progress does not match expectations.

At some stage it will become apparent that either the goals have been met, or there are

---

Box 6.2   Case example 2

A 6-monthly review meeting was called to discuss Mrs Joan Wallace, a 46-year-old woman with severe, long-term depression attending a mental health day centre. Joan had been attending the centre on at least two days a week for over 2 years, with short periods of hospitalisation. Some of the other people attending the centre were nervous of her because she made jokes at their expense and some of her remarks were experienced as hurtful. The overall aims of her programme were to improve her mood and ability to cope with depression, to improve her social skills and to encourage her to expand the number and range of activities in her life.

At the previous review, several recommendations had been made:

• Joan should be invited to attend a women's activity group and a relaxation class in addition to the drop-in service and social afternoon she had been using.
• She would continue to see her key worker regularly and be able to contact him when she was feeling upset.
• If Joan's comments had upset other service users, her key worker would talk to her about it and listen to her side of the story.
• She should be encouraged to participate in any outings to use community resources.

The present review showed that Joan's attendance at the centre was more regular on the days when she had a structured or focused activity than on the social days. She had had a short period of hospitalisation but returned to the groups immediately upon discharge. She had been out with the women's group on two occasions out of a possible four, including the Christmas lunch. She had made a close female friend at the centre and was getting on better with other service users in general. She was asking to talk to her key worker less often but used his regular visits to discuss matters of concern and to get feedback on her performance.

New recommendations were made to build on the changes that had occurred:

• Joan should continue to attend the structured groups but reduce her attendance at drop-in and social sessions.
• She should be encouraged to look for activities in the community where she could use some of the skills she was learning in the women's group. Her friend might go with her or a volunteer might be found to support her at first.
• Her key worker would continue to give feedback on how other people responded positively to her more gentle humour.

reasons why no further progress can be made at this time. The decision to terminate treatment is ideally taken by therapist and client together, but it may be a one-sided decision in some cases. For example, the therapist may feel that the client could benefit from further practice in the relatively protected environment of the department, but the client feels ready to take on his social responsibilities again and leaves.

Final assessment and outcome measurement

Planned discharge is the ideal, but many factors may intervene to cause treatment to be terminated before the client has attained maximum benefit. The occupational therapist does not make the final decision on how long a client remains in therapy, whether in the health or social services or in private practice.

If the discharge is planned, there will be time to do a final assessment with the client and write a discharge report. This can serve several purposes:

- It provides an opportunity to measure outcomes against the original goals of the programme. These will have been modified during the intervention, but the final assessment allows both therapist and client to see how much progress has been made overall.
- It allows the client to see what changes he has made so that he can leave feeling positive about himself.
- It gives the occupational therapist an opportunity to evaluate the effectiveness of the treatment programme.
- A record of treatment and outcomes goes into the case notes in the form of the discharge summary.
- Any gap between the client's existing level of skills and the skills he needs to carry out his expected roles and occupations is highlighted so that recommendations can be made for further treatment, or advice given on where to find help.

WHAT IS ASSESSED?

Occupational therapists claim to take a holistic view of people, but this does not mean that we assess every aspect of a person's functioning. The holistic approach allows the occupational therapist to make a general assessment of the client's range of activities and occupations so that areas of need can be identified before a more focused, in-depth assessment is carried out. In some cases, the client will have a clear idea of what kind of help is needed and does not want a broad assessment, indeed, it may be perceived as irrelevant or even intrusive.

It is not possible or necessary to learn everything there is to know about a client, therefore data are collected and organised in the context of the frame of reference being used.

The occupational therapy assessment covers both the client and the client's environment.

THE CLIENT

Aspects of the client which are assessed include:

- abilities, strengths, interests
- areas of dysfunction
- balance of activities in daily life
- roles or occupations and any major changes that have taken place recently
- potential for change
- motivation.

Abilities, strengths and interests

Abilities, strengths and interests influence the range of occupations a person adopts and the way in which these occupations are performed. Ability is the measure of the level of competence with which a skill is performed. Strengths are the skills, personal attributes and support systems that enable the client to function effectively. Interest is the expectation of pleasure in an activity which is aroused by a combination of experience and some degree of novelty – experience tells us that we have enjoyed something similar in the past and novelty arouses in us the urge to try a new experience.

In order to function effectively in a desired range of roles and occupations a person must have a variety of skills and be able to perform them competently.

When assessing clients, it should be taken into account that competence is not an absolute concept; norms for competence vary with age and are to some extent socially defined (Mocellin 1988). Each person develops a repertoire of skills that are refined from the unskilled actions of the baby and young child. New skills are learned throughout the life cycle but they are not selected randomly. Skills are developed specifically to support the life roles that the individual undertakes and to carry out the occupations associated with those roles.

For simplicity, function can be divided into skill areas that are interdependent and interrelated but that can be assessed separately in the early stages of intervention. One example is the three types of skill suggested by Reed & Sanderson (1992), as follows:

- sensorimotor
- cognitive
- psychosocial.

These types of skill can be separated for the purpose of assessment but act together in the performance of activities.

Areas of dysfunction

Function and dysfunction are not opposites but exist on a continuum; there is no clear line with function on one side and dysfunction on the other. Spencer (1988) pointed out that:

Temporary or permanent disability takes on a unique meaning for each individual. Age, developmental stage, previous ability, achievements, life-style, family status, self-concept, interests, and general responsibilities affect attitudes such as understanding, acceptance, motivation and emotional response . . . An accurate analysis of the biopsychosocial context by the therapist is essential to determine the functional implications of the patient's condition.

Satisfaction with function is also very individual, and the therapist may have to accept that a client is happy with his own level of functioning in a particular occupation even though the therapist knows the client has the potential to perform to a higher standard.

During assessment it is important to take a temporal perspective, considering the client's past level of functioning and expected future occupations as well as present capabilities, in order to find out whether he has lost skills or never developed competence in certain areas.

The ways in which function and dysfunction are conceptualised are determined by the frame of reference the occupational therapist is using. For example, using the adaptive skills model mentioned above, dysfunction is seen in terms of lack of mastery of the adaptive skills appropriate to the individual's age and stage of development. Within a behavioural frame of reference, dysfunction is seen in terms of the acquisition of undesirable behaviours and the failure to learn desirable ones. Within a cognitive behavioural frame of reference, dysfunction is seen in terms of faulty information processing, irrational thinking and distorted perceptions.

Balance of activities in daily life

Each individual maintains a changing pattern of self-care, work and leisure activities throughout life. A disruption of that balance can be an indicator of dysfunction, as shown in the example in Box 6.3.

Hagedorn (1995) cautioned against trying to apply rigid criteria of balance to all clients. The most important measure of a successful balance of activities may be the client's own perception, or he may lack insight into what appears to others to be a problem. Functional analysis, as described in the next section, can help to identify the client's level of satisfaction with his daily life activities.

Roles and occupations

Roles are patterns of activity associated with social position. They are defined by society and assigned to individuals on the basis of such attributes as age, sex, relationships, possessions, education, job, income and appearance. Each role

---

Box 6.3 Case example 3

Colin, a man in his late 20s, was referred to the occupational therapist with a diagnosis of depression. He had been unemployed for over 2 years and had a very limited range of activities and interests. Previously he had held down a civil service office job for several years, enjoyed reading and cinema and had relationships with women, none of which had lasted very long.

When the occupational therapist asked Colin about which of the activities previously enjoyed he would like to try again in the future he was unenthusiastic but could not say why he had lost interest. A female patient became interested in him and they went out together a few times. The woman then told the therapist she was anxious about some of the odd things Colin had been saying. Colin became more withdrawn in groups and missed sessions occasionally. The therapist began to suspect that Colin's depression was secondary to a more serious, progressive disorder. She discussed his case with the psychiatrist and he agreed that Colin was probably in the early stages of schizophrenia. Colin's medication was changed and he was not expected to join in any groups which would put emotional pressure on him.

Colin, an intelligent young man, asked the therapist if he had been diagnosed as having schizophrenia. He could see that the difficulties he was having fitted the diagnosis and became very anxious and upset. The therapist was able to offer him emotional support while he came to terms with the implications of his changed diagnosis.

---

carries expectations of performance, which the individual who accepts the role attempts to carry out. A properly integrated role, supported by the skills and habits necessary for its performance, satisfies both society's expectations and the individual's needs. However, when a person is assigned a role that he is unable or unwilling to accept, then dissonance occurs between society's expectations and the person's performance. This can lead to social rejection and stigma.

A role contributes to the individual's sense of social and personal identity and influences the way in which occupations are performed.

In order to support occupations and roles, skills are organised into the routines that are habitually used to carry out the individual's daily tasks – for example brushing one's teeth involves a sequence of actions that becomes habitual so that one does not have to think carefully about every stage of the operation. Habits

mean that the individual can perform everyday tasks without having to remember consciously how to go about them. These routines are developed to suit the individual's needs at any one period of life. New habits are learned and old ones discarded as circumstances change.

The therapist assesses how clients organise their time, that is, whether they have useful habits or have to expend a lot of time and energy in working out ways of performing. Habits may also have become too rigid to allow for necessary changes so that the client's behaviour no longer meets the needs of his situation. It is useful to take an occupational history to assess whether the individual's habits have been disrupted or whether he has never developed good habits. If possible, the therapist will want to identify the point at which habits broke down.

Occupations and roles exist in a balance that normally changes throughout the life cycle. A healthy balance is one that allows most of the individual's needs to be satisfied without causing him to be rejected by society. The balance can be disrupted by illness, disability or bereavement.

The therapist wants to know:

- if the client's needs are being met
- if the client is able to carry out the roles and occupations expected of him, or that he expects of himself
- about any reduction in the expected number of roles and occupations
- about any imbalance between self-care, work and leisure
- the client's occupational role history.

Potential for change

Occupational therapists take an essentially optimistic view of human beings, believing that everyone has the potential to change and to influence the direction of that change by what they do. Seedhouse (1986) argued that health is closely related to human potential:

Except in extreme instances of illness or external control, people possess an indefinite number of potentials depending upon what they do and what happens to them . . . This is true even of terminal patients in hospital, even until the time they finally lapse into unconsciousness . . . people can change themselves and their environments for the better.

The extent of change will be limited by personal factors, such as personal goals, degree of disability and investment in maintaining existing coping methods. For example, Allen & Allen (1987) developed a theory of cognitive disability which describes six levels that relate to the functions the patient is able to perform, the types of assistance required to compensate for dysfunction and the social dysfunction occurring in home and work environments. Change will also be influenced by external factors such as the goals of the family or carers, social support networks and social expectations. All these factors must be taken into account when setting goals.

Motivation and volition

The occupational therapist has traditionally taken an interest in motivation for the purpose of treatment, to assist in engaging clients in therapeutic activity. This aspect of motivation is discussed in more depth in Chapter 7 (p. 129). However, an understanding of the theory of intrinsic motivation can also facilitate assessment of dysfunction.

People have an innate urge to use their capacity to explore and interact successfully with the environment (Reilly 1962). The satisfaction in such action comes from the activity itself, not only from the external rewards that the action may bring. This urge is stimulated by novelty in the environment and is strong enough to sustain action even when the immediate consequences are not pleasant. Intrinsic motivation is discussed in more detail in Chapter 7.

If a client appears not to be motivated to participate in treatment, the therapist will look for factors that may be hindering or blocking the client's intrinsic motivation, such as:

- the level of stimulation and novelty in the environment
- unsatisfied needs that may be distracting the client's attention
- opportunities to act on the environment

- sense of competence or efficacy
- goals the client considers worth working for
- activities the client values
- activities the client finds enjoyable or interesting.

People have a basic urge to act, to test their own potential and to have an impact on their surroundings, but the direction of that action is influenced by life experiences. Volition is the skill which enables a person to choose what activities he does (Creek 1998). It is both the ability to choose and an awareness that the action is voluntary. Various factors determine the extent to which an individual is able to exercise volition.

One important factor in how a person chooses to act is his self-image (Kielhofner & Burke 1980). This is conceptualised in different ways depending on the frame of reference being used, but all theorists agree that this factor influences how the individual performs.

Another factor is the degree of confidence a person has in his own ability. Fidler & Fidler (1978) stated that each person learns his own capacities by 'doing'. Successful doing leads to a sense of satisfaction and a sense of competence. Persistent failure, due to lack of skill or lack of opportunity to do, leads to a sense of incompetence and lack of control.

The model of human occupation (Kielhofner & Burke 1980) also conceptualises self-image as arising from interactions of the human system with the environment during development. The balance of success to failure depends on how much the individual feels that events are within his control and how much they are outside it. This model suggests that three factors determine the actions a person takes:

- values
- goals
- interest.

Values. Values not only influence the actions of the individual, but also influence how an individual interprets and reacts to other people's actions. It may therefore be important for the therapist to understand the values underlying the client's behaviour but this is not easy, particularly if the therapist and client are from different cultural backgrounds.

Goals. Goals are linked to values in that they are based on what the individual thinks is worth doing. In order to elicit the client's full cooperation the therapist must be able to elicit his personal goals through the assessment procedure. The client will not strive to achieve the therapist's goals unless they coincide with his own.

Interest. When we say a client is not interested in an activity we mean:

- the client has tried something similar before and not enjoyed it
- the client has tried something similar before and knows he cannot do it
- the client has tried this activity before and there is no challenge in it
- the client has never tried this type of activity before and has no confidence in his ability to succeed at a new task.

The reason for not being interested has implications for suggesting alternative activities, therefore it is important to assess a client's interests before planning intervention.

THE ENVIRONMENT

People are never independent of their environment but learn how to adapt to it, or adapt it to themselves, to satisfy their needs. Through acting on the environment and receiving feedback about the effect of their actions they learn how best to achieve their own aims. Skilled performance of actions is only developed through exploring the environment and acting on it. Failure to adapt to the environment leads to dysfunction.

Assessing opportunities for exploration and practice

Skills are learned through exploration of the environment and of one's own potential. Competence is developed through practising skills in a variety of situations. Some skills are learned by carrying them out in reality, such as learning to climb trees; competence in this skill can only be acquired by doing it. Other skills are learned by role-playing, for example social roles are rehearsed through childhood play.

Lack of opportunity to practise skills and roles in childhood and adolescence prevents the individual from developing a realistic image of his capacities and from knowing what his interests and values really are.

Reasons for being unable to engage in exploration of the environment and to practise skills for coping with it include:

- physical disability
- impoverished environment
- lack of satisfaction of basic needs, for example emotional insecurity
- overcontrolling or overprotective parental figures
- interruptions to normal development, such as injury or illness.

It should be remembered that the treatment situation itself may block engagement in occupation for several of the above reasons.

Once the problem has been identified, the therapist and client can plan intervention that will include new opportunities for exploration and skill generation with a high chance of success.

Assessing adaptation to the environment

Individuals have the ability to influence their own health through what they do. A healthy environment allows individuals to act in a way that will enable them to meet their needs. Sometimes people find themselves in an environment that they cannot adjust to in a healthy way or that does not give them opportunities to make changes. Various constraints may exist, including:

- social expectations, such as the role expectations for young mothers
- physical factors, such as poor housing
- economic constraints, such as poverty or having to stay in an unsatisfactory job.

A person may become ill because of environmental factors and then discover that the illness allows him to meet his needs, either by removing him from a difficult environment or by changing the attitudes and behaviour of people around him. The costs of being ill are outweighed by the benefits, which then act to maintain the illness behaviour.

METHODS OF ASSESSMENT

Occupational therapists use a wide range of assessment tools, from interviews to assessment batteries. Some depend on the experience and skill of the tester, such as observation of performance in activities, while others are standardised and can, in theory, be applied objectively by anyone who has been trained in their use.

Several factors influence the methods of assessment chosen for a particular client:

- the frame of reference or model being used by the therapist
- the information required
- the client's level of ability
- the nature of the client's difficulties
- the stage of assessment.

The first four assessment techniques described below (review of records, interview, observation and home visits) are used by other professionals as well as by occupational therapists. Techniques more specific to occupational therapy are those that focus on function and involve activity or occupation; functional analysis, checklists, performance scales, questionnaires and projective techniques are also described below.

REVIEW OF RECORDS

The therapist sometimes does not have easy access to case notes and other records, for example if she works in the community. In this case, a well-designed referral form is essential to elicit the desired information before the client is seen.

It is sometimes suggested that therapists should not read clients' records before seeing them as this may influence their perceptions. However, it is very frustrating for clients to have to give the same information to many people – if therapists are aware of the danger of bias, they can consciously try to avoid it.

Looking through medical and nursing records can be time-consuming, especially if the client has a long medical history, but familiarity with the way case notes are organised (and with the handwriting of medical officers!) makes the search easier. Hemphill (1982) suggested that the therapist looks at:

- social history
- admission summary
- nurses' notes
- the psychologist's report
- the physician's reports
- any other pertinent reports.

Hemphill (1982) recommended a checklist to use when reading case notes so that no relevant information is missed.

Information gained from the client's records can be used to plan the initial interview.

THE INTERVIEW

In most treatment settings occupational therapists are in constant, informal communication with their clients. However, a formal interview can often be a useful additional method of communication and assessment.

Interviews can be structured or unstructured. No interview is truly unstructured if it is to be of use but there is a difference between knowing what you want to elicit and having a list of set questions to ask. The structured interview tends to be more popular with less experienced therapists (Kielhofner 1988).

Unstructured interviews

Before the interview, the therapist collects together any information about the client and decides what she wants to find out. Time need not be wasted during an interview in going over what the therapist already knows. The client is informed in advance about the time, place and purpose of the interview. The therapist may expect the client to turn up on time or may collect him, depending on the client's needs.

The interview is carried out in an informal atmosphere without distractions or interruptions.

Attention is paid to details such as height and positioning of chairs, in order to gain maximum rapport. Comfortable but straight-backed chairs, placed at an angle of 90 degrees to each other, are probably ideal since both parties can then see each other without effort. Interruptions can usually be avoided if other staff are informed that the interview is taking place, where it is and how long it will take. It has been known for an entire ward staff to turn out to search for a missing client, only to find him being interviewed by a student who forgot to tell anyone that she was with him.

At the beginning of the interview the therapist calls the client by name and makes sure that the client remembers the therapist's name and the purpose of the interview. The therapist may take a more or less directing role in the interview, depending on the client's mental state and the purpose of the interview, but a warm and accepting manner is usually most successful. The therapist is an active listener, paying respectful attention to what the client says and attempting to reach a good understanding of the client's intended meaning.

The length of the interview may be set in advance, especially if there are many constraints on time, or it may be determined by the course of events. A confused person may not be able to tolerate a long interview whereas a client in acute distress may benefit from the therapist's undivided attention until he feels calmer.

Upon termination of the interview, a brief summary by the therapist of its main points can help the client to continue thinking about it afterwards. The therapist then checks that the client knows where he is going and walks with him if it is appropriate. Notes are usually written up after the interview.

Structured interviews

The structured interview format may be designed for use in a particular treatment setting if the therapist finds it useful to collect the same information about each client. Alternatively, it may be designed as part of a particular model, for example an occupational history is often taken to collect information about a client's performance in past and present occupational roles for use within the model of human occupation.

The structured interview consists of a series of questions designed to elicit the desired information. Such a series of questions could also be administered as a questionnaire if the therapist is confident that the client understands it fully but an interview is more personal and allows rapport to be developed (Florey & Michelman 1982). It is often acceptable to take brief notes during a structured interview.

An interview may also be semi-structured, that is, the therapist has a number of questions to ask but allows for digressions if they seem useful. Florey & Michelman (1982) suggested that, while the questionnaire or structured interview are effective for gathering a history of discrete events such as childhood illnesses, the semi-structured interview is useful for taking a history of more abstract events.

Many of the histories and checklists used by occupational therapists could be administered as interviews, self-assessment instruments or computer programs, depending on the needs and abilities of the client.

Content of the interview

During the interview the therapist can observe the client's:

- verbal and non-verbal communication skills
- sensory deficits (if any)
- quality of self-care
- mannerisms (if any)
- posture
- facial expression.

By asking questions, the therapist can find out the client's:

- level of cognitive functioning
- attitudes to the current situation, in general
- feelings about being involved in therapy
- mood
- expectations from therapy.

Questions can be directed towards exploring a particular aspect of the client (e.g. relationships with other people).

The interview is also an opportunity for giving the client information and feedback. At the initial interview, rules and expectations within the occupational therapy department can be explained, including how violations of the rules are dealt with. A discussion of the general function of the department and its potential value helps the client to make more informed decisions about becoming involved in treatment. Clients frequently complain that they do not see how occupational therapy can help them and a clear explanation can enhance the value of therapy.

During later interviews the client can be given feedback on his performance and on any changes that have been observed. The client may also give feedback on how he feels about the programme. Modifications to the programme are discussed so that the client continues to be actively involved in his own treatment.

OBSERVATION

Observation involves noting and recording the type, frequency and duration of activities by the client and interpreting what is observed according to the model being used.

Mosey (1973) described three steps in using observation as a method of assessment.

1. *Observation.* Noting what the client does without ascribing meaning to it.
2. *Interpretation.* Using observed data to reach conclusions about the reasons for the client's actions.
3. *Validation.* Seeking to confirm the accuracy of interpretations by sharing them with the client or others who know the client well.

There are three main types of observation:

- general observation of the client during activities
- observation of specified performances
- observation of performance of set tasks.

General observation

The range of activities provided by occupational therapy gives opportunities for observing clients under different circumstances so that a picture of their capabilities and deficits can be built up. However, clients' performance in the occupational therapy department is often very different from when they are in the ward, so staff also benefit from spending time out of the department to observe clients. In a small community, where clients are frequently encountered outside the treatment setting, the therapist also has opportunities to observe their social functioning in their normal environment.

Using a checklist to record what is observed can help to ensure accuracy and reduce subjectivity. Checklists make it possible to look at complicated areas of skills without becoming confused, although a description may also be needed to give additional information.

Much can be learned from the physical appearance of the client (physique, posture, facial expression, mannerisms, gait, grooming and dress). Some diseases, such as severe depression, produce a characteristic stooped posture and flat expression. However, the use of certain drugs may mask symptoms of the underlying disorder with an array of side-effects, for example obesity or rigidity may be due to phenothiazine medication.

Form and content of speech provide clues to the client's inner life, including mood, insight, cognitive functioning and thought disorder. A good rapport with the client is helpful in that clients will be more willing to share their thoughts in the context of a warm and trusting relationship.

The client's performance patterns can be observed in different situations to assess energy level, diurnal variations in energy, interaction with others, willingness to cooperate, initiative and skills. The client may respond in totally different ways to peers, junior staff, students and senior staff so that everyone in the treatment setting will have something to contribute to a total assessment.

Observation of specified performances

General observation tends to be descriptive and inevitably misses much of what happens. The occupational therapist is usually a participant observer, making it even more difficult to observe a client's performance. A more precise method of observation is to specify what is to be observed and ignore all other activity. This method is commonly used by psychologists but can be useful for occupational therapists, particularly within a behavioural model. The process consists of:

- deciding what to observe
- selecting an observation technique
- making the observation
- recording the observation
- analysing the recorded performance.

The therapist may wish to observe the number of times a particular activity is carried out (frequency) or the length of time the activity lasts (duration). The observation technique chosen will depend on what is to be observed but the three main methods are (Felce & McBrien 1987, Hogg & Raynes 1987):

- event counting
- time sampling
- duration recording.

Event counting and time sampling are used to count the frequency of activities that are brief, discrete and easily identified, such as head-banging. Duration recording is used for activities that last for longer periods.

Event counting

The therapist specifies the action she wishes to observe, for example the client making eye contact with the therapist. The therapist then counts the total number of times the action occurs either during the whole session or during a specified period of time. If the action occurs infrequently then the whole session may be observed (e.g. the client makes eye contact with the therapist twice during a half-hour session).

Interval recording and time sampling

If the action to be observed occurs frequently it may be more appropriate to take samples than to record it continuously. This can be done by noting the number of times the action occurs during brief, regularly spaced intervals of time, say, for 1 minute in every 10 (interval recording), or by making an observation at fixed intervals and noting if the action is occurring at that moment (time sampling). The results can be noted on a record sheet that specifies the action to be observed and only takes a moment to mark.

Duration recording

This method is used for actions that occur for longer periods or for variable periods of time. The easiest method is to use a cumulative stopwatch to record the total amount of time spent on the action in a given period, for example the amount of time a client concentrates on the task in hand during a 1-hour session.

Set tasks

When further information is required about a particular area of functioning, such as cooking a meal or planning an outing, the client can be asked to participate in a task designed to measure that function. The task may demand practical skills, such as hand–eye coordination, or cognitive skills, such as problem solving. It may be a social task that requires interaction with others or it may be designed to highlight the client's attitudes by making unusual demands.

A careful and detailed analysis of the task ensures that it requires the skills that the therapist hopes to observe. A knowledge of normal performance is also necessary so that the client's performance can be measured against it.

It is rarely possible to reproduce external conditions accurately within the treatment setting and it may be appropriate to visit the client's home or workplace to assess its particular demands or try out skills.

HOME VISITS

Home visits may be made at any stage of treatment for the purpose of assessment or treatment, or both. Within a multidisciplinary team it is necessary to coordinate with other staff to limit the number of people who do home visits and to share information obtained.

Doctors, nurses, social workers and therapists all commonly visit clients' homes but it may not be necessary for all of them to visit the same person.

Purpose

Home visits are an expensive use of staff time so it is important to establish the purpose clearly beforehand. The occupational therapist builds up a picture of the client's assets and needs from an assessment in the treatment setting, which the therapist can use to determine what to assess in the home environment.

The home visit can be used to:

- gain a picture of the client's life demands and role expectations
- observe the client's level of functioning in his normal environment
- carry out specific assessments, such as using the kitchen
- observe the physical environment, including where the house is situated and what type of accommodation it is
- meet the client's family and neighbours on their own territory.

The physical environment includes where the home is situated, whether it is convenient for transport, shops, libraries and open spaces, its distance from the workplace and the character of the neighbourhood. The home itself can be assessed for physical barriers to easy access, amount of space, opportunities for privacy, playing space outside for children, facilities, comfort and noise level.

The emotional environment is more difficult to assess in a single visit since the family dynamics will be changed by the presence of a stranger. However, the therapist may learn something about stresses and supports within the home by observing the number of family members and the amount of personal space each one has. More difficult to assess, but very useful to know, is how emotionally close to each other the family members are, what roles they take within the family, what methods of communication they use and their attitudes to the person who is receiving treatment. Neighbours' attitudes are also relevant, especially if the client lives alone.

Carrying out a home visit

A date and time for the visit are set to suit the therapist, the client and the client's family, taking into account transport. It will be easier to determine the length of the visit if the aims are very clear and specific. Uniform is not normally worn for home visits but the therapist can carry some form of identification for the benefit of the family.

Safety is an important consideration when carrying out home visits to clients and/or their families. It is important to let other staff know where you are going and when you expect to return so that they can check on you if you are late. A mobile phone may be carried so that any change of plan can be reported. If there are any anxieties about safety on a particular home visit, the therapist should take a colleague.

The purpose of the visit is clearly explained to the family, especially if the therapist has not met them before. Many families like to offer a cup of tea to a visitor and this can provide an opportunity for getting to know them in a relaxed way. Further structuring of the visit depends on what the therapist wishes to assess.

After a home visit, the therapist can discuss with the other team members the client's level of functioning against his life demands. They can then help the client to decide if any adjustments can be made to the environment or whether the client needs to make personal changes in order to cope. The visit described in Box 6.4 resulted in Mrs Temple being able to return to her own home with support that would allow her to live independently but safely. It was important that the therapist presented all her observations accurately and objectively to the team so that they could discuss with Mrs Temple the facts of the case, and not the therapist's opinion, in order to reach an acceptable solution.

FUNCTIONAL ANALYSIS

As described in the previous section, functional analysis is the part of the assessment process

Box 6.4 Case example 4

Mrs Temple, an 83-year-old widow, had been admitted to hospital 6 weeks previously in a confused state due to malnutrition. She was expressing paranoid ideas about the neighbours. She made a good recovery and was keen to return home but the team had some doubts about her ability to manage alone. The occupational therapist was asked to do a home visit with her to measure the home environment against her existing skills.

At first, Mrs Temple refused to consider taking the therapist home with her, insisting that she could manage well. She changed her mind when the therapist, knowing that Mrs Temple was a very sociable lady, suggested that they shop on the way home and Mrs Temple could cook lunch for them.

Mrs Temple had some difficulty getting on the bus but managed her shopping without any problems. Her house, which she owned, was a two-up two-down terrace house. It was heated by a gas fire in the living room, which also heated the water, and the old gas cooker had to be lit with matches. Several neighbours dropped in to see Mrs Temple while the therapist was there.

From her observations, the therapist felt that Mrs Temple would be able to continue to manage on her own, with some additional support, but that she needed a new heater and gas cooker. A referral was made to social services with a request for home care and a full occupational therapy assessment. The social worker from the hospital visited Mrs Temple regularly until the new arrangements were in place.

which looks at how people spend their time and at their capabilities and any problem areas. Over 200 different techniques have been devised for collecting data about how an individual functions in daily life (Unsworth 1993), but most of these focus only on activities of daily living (e.g. the Barthel Index and the Rivermead ADL Assessment), and most have been devised for use with elderly people.

The simplest way to collect data about function is probably to ask clients to say what they do in a typical day. The Canadian Occupational Performance Measure (Law et al 1994) recommends the therapist to 'Encourage clients to think about a typical day and describe the occupations they typically do'. A form can be used, dividing the day into half-hour sections (Fig. 6.3), which the client fills in to give a record of a typical day. This can then be analysed in various ways to find out where areas of dysfunction are occurring. The Canadian Occupational Performance Measure

(Law et al 1994) suggests that the client first identifies the activities he needs, wants or is expected to do and then identifies which ones he can do to his own satisfaction. This gives an indication of the performance areas the client is having problems with.

One of the purposes of the analysis is to find what meaning clients place on different aspects of life, what activities are important to them, what purpose they see the different activities serving, what motivates them and what their main goals are for therapy.

Other questions that might be asked about the typical day include:

- Which activities does the client find pleasurable, unpleasant or neutral? This will highlight the balance of pleasurable activities in the individual's life.
- Are there any problems in the overall balance of activities – empty times in the day or times when there is too much to cope with?
- What life roles do the day's activities represent? Is the range of roles appropriate to the client's age/developmental level?

The therapist will also be interested in the social, physical and cultural environment in which the client will be functioning, and whether it will support the client in his chosen roles and occupations.

Functional analysis identifies areas of dysfunction as a starting point for deciding the focus of intervention. The client's own priorities should then be taken as a guide in selecting the area to work on first. Once the functional analysis has been completed, the therapist begins a more detailed assessment.

CHECKLISTS, PERFORMANCE SCALES AND QUESTIONNAIRES

Occupational therapists have always used checklists for assessing skills such as activities of daily living (ADL) and work skills but over the last 20 years there has been an increase in the number of assessment procedures developed for use within particular frames of reference. There has also been more interest in standardising assessments,

NAME :		DATE :	
Night hours			
05.00 am			
05.30 am			
06.00 am			
06.30 am			
07.00 am			
07.30 am			
08.00 am			
08.30 am			
09.00 am			
09.30 am			
10.00 am			
10.30 am			
11.00 am			
11.30 am			
12 noon			
12.30 pm			
01.00 pm			
01.30 pm			
02.00 pm			
02.30 pm			
03.00 pm			
03.30 pm			
04.00 pm			
04.30 pm			
05.00 pm			
05.30 pm			
06.00 pm			
06.30 pm			
07.00 pm			
07.30 pm			
08.00 pm			
08.30 pm			
09.00 pm			
09.30 pm			
10.00 pm			
10.30 pm			
11.00 pm			
11.30 pm			
12 midnight			
00.30 am			

Figure 6.3 Activities in a typical day.

although normative data have still to be collected for many tests that are in regular use.

Some checklists and performance scales measure directly observable performance, for example the ability to dress independently. Others assess functions which are more complex and may be more difficult to observe, for example the ability to participate in a mature group (Mosey 1986). In order to assess these functions they can be tied to behaviours which indicate their presence or to behaviours which indicate their absence. Mosey (1986) suggested that the ability to participate in a mature group is indicated by 'comfort in heterogeneous groups and the ability to take a variety of membership roles'. Lack of the skill is shown by 'preference for same sex or other types of homogeneous groups and excessive preoccupation with task accomplishment or satisfaction of social–emotional need'.

Other skills, such as level of cognitive ability, are not directly observable (Allen & Allen 1987). Again these skills can be assessed by linking them to observable performance. Allen & Allen (1987) suggested that the individual's level of cognitive disability is indicated by the activities he is unable to perform. A battery of craft activities was devised to measure precisely the level of disability.

Checklists can be used to make sure no skill area has been missed. The types of checklist commonly used by occupational therapists include:

- broad assessments, such as the Occupational Therapy Development Analysis, Evaluation and Intervention Schedule (DAEIS)
- assessments of specific skill areas, such as ADL checklists and task inventories
- multidisciplinary assessments, such as the Personal Assessment Chart (PAC).

Performance scales may be norm-referenced or criterion-referenced. Norm-referenced scales are those in which a typical range of performance has been identified by administering the test to a broad sample. The client's performance is compared with this typical, or normative, performance. Criterion-referenced scales are those in which the client's performance is judged against the desired outcome of intervention. A criterion sets the standard of performance which the client hopes to achieve by the end of treatment.

Some of the many areas of performance that can be assessed by the use of checklists or performance scales include adaptive skills, sensory integration, past and present life roles, balance of occupations, motivation, interests, locus of control and time structuring. Three of these will be described here: the Comprehensive Occupational Therapy Evaluation Scale (COTE), the Interest Checklist and the Occupational Questionnaire. Readers are recommended to follow up references at the end of the chapter for details of further methods.

Comprehensive Occupational Therapy Evaluation Scale

This instrument was developed by occupational therapists, working in an acute adult psychiatry unit in the USA, to provide a broad but consistent range of information about clients for the purpose of coordinating occupational therapy programmes with the different approaches of other staff (Brayman & Kirby 1982). The four objectives of developing such an evaluation were specified as being:

Date																
1 GENERAL BEHAVIOUR	1	2	3	4	5	6	7	8	9	10	11	12	13	14	15	16
A Appearance																
B Non-productive behaviour																
C Activity level (a or b)																
D Expression																
E Responsibility																
F Punctuality																
G Reality orientation																

Scale 0 – normal 1 – minimal 2 – mild 3 – moderate 4 – severe

Figure 6.4 A comprehensive occupational therapy evaluation scale. (Taken from Hemphill B J 1982 The Evaluative Process in Psychiatric Occupational Therapy. Slack, New Jersey. Reproduced by kind permission of Slack Inc.)

1. to identify behaviours relevant to the practice of occupational therapy
2. to define the identified behaviours in such a way that they can be reliably observed and rated
3. to record information in a way that can easily be read by the referring agent and that can provide a record of client progress
4. to provide an efficient method for data retrieval to assist in treatment planning and evaluation.

The evaluation scale is divided into three sections, general behaviour, interpersonal behaviour and task behaviour, each of which is subdivided into skills that are given a numerical rating from 0 to 4 (Fig. 6.4). A total of 25 skills has been identified and clear definitions of the behaviour indicative of each skill are given on the back of the rating form. Performance in all the skills can be recorded for 16 days on a grid so that the results can be quickly recorded and compared.

It has been found that the COTE shows up areas of competence and deficiency and is therefore useful for setting priorities in developing a treatment plan. However, some more extreme behaviours or more subtle changes are not reflected on the rating scale and it is recommended that a descriptive note is added in such cases.

The Interest Checklist

The Interest Checklist was developed by Matsutsuyu (1969) to assess clients' interests in order to facilitate the selection of therapeutic activities that would evoke and sustain interest throughout the treatment programme. It includes 80 items that the client can mark under the headings of 'casual interest', 'strong interest' or 'no interest'. These include activities such as cooking, gardening, solitaire, religion and swimming. There is space to add any other interests not included in the list and space for a written report on the client's interests from schooldays to the present.

Matsutsuyu suggested six propositions to describe the properties of the interest phenomenon:

1. Interests are influenced by early experiences in the family.
2. Interests are affective in nature and evoke positive or negative emotional responses.
3. Making choices on the basis of interest leads to commitment to the roles chosen.
4. Interest leads the individual to engage in activities that teach him how to act effectively to achieve his goals.
5. Interest in a task can sustain action after the novelty of the task has worn off.
6. Interests reflect the image a person has of himself.

These six propositions became the theoretical basis for designing an interest checklist.

The data from this checklist can be classified by intensity of interest felt, ability to express personal preference, ability to discriminate type and intensity of interests and categories of interest. All the items on the list can be classified as manual skills, physical sports, social recreation, activities of daily living or cultural/educational.

From this information it should be possible to select activities that will maintain the client's commitment to treatment for the attainment of either short-term or long-term goals.

The Occupational Questionnaire

This questionnaire was developed for use within the model of human occupation (Kielhofner 1988). It consists of a daily timetable in half-hour blocks for the client to fill in to show his typical way of spending time on a working day or a non-working day (Fig. 6.5). Each activity can then be rated by the client as being, in the client's perception:

- work
- a daily living task
- recreation
- rest.

The client is also asked to rate each activity on a five-point scale for:

- how well he thinks he performs it – personal causation
- how important he thinks it is – values

Time	Typical activities	Question 1 I consider this activity to be: Work W Daily living task D Recreation R Rest RT				Question 2 I think that I do this: Very well VW Well W About average AA Poorly P Very poorly VP					Question 3 For me this activity is: Extremely important EI Important I Take it or leave it TL Rather not do it RN Total waste of time TW					Question 4 How much do you enjoy this activity? Like it very much LVM Like it L Neither like NLD nor dislike it Dislike it D Strongly dislike it SD				
5.00 – 5.30 am		W	D	R	RT	VW	W	AA	P	VP	EI	I	TL	RN	TW	LVM	L	NLD	D	SD
5.30 – 6.00 am		W	D	R	RT	VW	W	AA	P	VP	EI	I	TL	RN	TW	LVM	L	NLD	D	SD
6.00 – 6.30 am		W	D	R	RT	VW	W	AA	P	VP	EI	I	TL	RN	TW	LVM	L	NLD	D	SD
6.30 – 7.00 am		W	D	R	RT	VW	W	AA	P	VP	EI	I	TL	RN	TW	LVM	L	NLD	D	SD
7.00 – 7.30 am		W	D	R	RT	VW	W	AA	P	VP	EI	I	TL	RN	TW	LVM	L	NLD	D	SD

Figure 6.5 Sample worksheet from the Occupational Questionnaire. (From Smith N R, Kielhofner G, Watts J H 1986 The relationship between volition, activity pattern and life satisfaction in the elderly (activity analysis, geriatrics, human occupation, personal satisfaction). Copyright 1986 American Occupational Therapy Association Inc. Reprinted with kind permission.)

• how much he likes it – interest.

The questionnaire is designed to provide data about the client's habits, balance of activities, feeling of competence, interests and values and to show up problems in any of these areas. Used in collaboration with the client, it can assist in setting therapeutic goals. The results can be displayed in various ways to give a visual picture that the client will understand, for example a pie chart or a profile, since it is necessary for the client to be involved in interpreting the results.

The questionnaire can also be filled in for a time when the client feels he was functioning effectively, so that a comparison can be made with present functioning.

Other versions of the questionnaire are now being developed to measure different aspects of the client, for example one version highlights the amount of pain and fatigue the client is experiencing.

CLIENT-CENTRED ASSESSMENT TOOLS

Client-centred practice is an approach which has become increasingly popular in recent years and which appears to fit well with occupational ther-

apy's philosophy. Several assessment tools have been designed for use with this approach, most notably the Canadian Occupational Performance Measure (described below).

Client-centred practice has been defined as:

an approach to providing occupational therapy which embraces a philosophy of respect for and partnership with people receiving services. It recognises the autonomy of individuals, the need for client choice in making decisions about occupational needs, the strength clients bring to an occupational therapy encounter and the benefits of client–therapist partnership and the need to ensure that services are accessible and fit the context in which a client lives. (Law et al 1995)

The most important task in client-centred assessment is to ensure that the client understands the key issues of this approach. Understanding allows the client to enter into a partnership with the therapist in which together they discuss and agree the goals of the intervention and methods of assessment (Sumsion 1999).

Client-centred assessment often means using individualised measures of outcome rather than standardised assessment tools. Spreadbury (1998, p 108) wrote that 'individualised outcome measures capture what it is that the client wants out of therapy and what therapists achieve in day-to-day practice'.

Canadian Occupational Performance Measure

The Canadian Occupational Performance Measure (COPM) was designed for use by occupational therapists in a variety of fields of practice. It is an individualised outcome measurement which is appropriate for use within the individual programmes of care provided by occupational therapists (Spreadbury 1998).

The COPM (Law et al 1994) focuses on occupational performance and takes the form of a semi-structured interview. The client is assisted to identify occupational performance problems in the areas of self-care, productivity and leisure. He is then asked to rate each problematic activity for how important it is in his life on a 10-point scale from 1 (not important at all) to 10 (extremely important). The client is then invited to choose up to five activities that seem the most important for intervention. Each of these is rated on two further dimensions: performance and satisfaction. The client is asked to mark on a 10-point scale how well he thinks he performs the activity now, from 1 (not able to do it at all) to 10 (able to do it extremely well). He is also asked to rate how satisfied he is with the way he does the activity now from 1 (not satisfied at all) to 10 (extremely satisfied).

After an appropriate period of intervention, the client is asked to rate the activities again for performance and satisfaction. Changes in the scores demonstrate changes in performance and satisfaction.

The COPM has standardised instructions and methods for administration and scoring but it is not norm-referenced (Pollock et al 1999). It is only intended to measure changes in individual performance and satisfaction.

PROJECTIVE TECHNIQUES

Projective techniques were developed as a method of assessing emotions, motivations and values, none of which could be measured with existing tools. Early techniques included the Rorschach Inkblot Test, Morgan and Murray's Thematic Apperception Test and Cattell's Sentence Completion Test. All these tests present subjects with ambiguous stimuli to which they are asked to give meaning. Projective tests use standard stimuli that allow subjects to make their own interpretations. The theory behind them is that the subject does not know what is expected (i.e. what would constitute a good performance), and therefore performs spontaneously (Cutting 1968).

The material projected by the subject may be one of three types:

1. Projection was described by Freud as an ego-defence mechanism through which painful or unacceptable feelings are ascribed to someone else. This is an unconscious process.

2. Projection can also be a way of giving meaning to situations that are otherwise confusing by seeing them in terms of one's own motives and beliefs.

3. It may also be an unconscious method of wish fulfilment, for example a woman who does not find it easy to attract men may think that all men have designs on her (Munn 1966).

All three aspects of projection are involved in projective techniques.

The use of projective techniques by occupational therapists

Occupational therapists use projective techniques in two ways:

1. Creation of an object by the client, such as a painting, or presentation of a stimulus by the therapist, such as a poem, followed by a period of discussion in which the client is encouraged to express his feelings about the object freely. This is usually done in a group.

2. Presentation of a series of standard activities to the client with an assessment of how he copes with them.

Using projective techniques in groups

The distinguishing feature of occupational therapy as opposed to other therapies is the presence of objects that can be manipulated by the client. These objects may already be available or may be created by the client (Azima & Azima 1959). Thus, projective techniques are an appropriate method of assessment for occupational therapists because they involve doing as well as talking.

Most of the projective techniques used by occupational therapists involve a phase of creating, which can be structured or unstructured, and a phase of talking about the created object or free-associating about it. The technique is used as assessment and as a form of treatment simultaneously, in that therapists help clients to accept projected material as their own and gain insight into how their own perceptions are formed.

The functions that are assessed by the use of projective techniques will vary according to the model being used, but may include:

- motor skills
- cognitive skills
- task skills
- interaction skills
- orientation
- motivation
- ego-organisation and control
- mood
- reality orientation
- level of activity
- self-image
- independence.

Projective tests developed by occupational therapists

Two types of projective tests developed by occupational therapists for individual use are the Azima Battery and the Goodman Battery.

The Azima Battery is a typical projective technique developed by an occupational therapist (Azima 1982). This utilises three tasks: a free pencil drawing, drawings of a person of each sex and a free clay model. These are presented to the client in a standard order and method. The client is given a set period of time to complete each task. During the 'doing' phase of the test the therapist records the time taken, the client's behaviour, any verbalisations and the techniques

used. When the work is finished the client is asked to describe his productions.

An evaluation scale is used to interpret the results of the battery. This includes organisation of mood, organisation of drives and organisation of object relations, all of which are inferred from aspects of the client's observed behaviour and content of speech. Findings are analysed and presented as a summary to be used in differential diagnosis, treatment planning and prognosis (Azima 1982).

The Goodman Battery was developed from the Azima Battery and differs from it in that the tasks given are progressively less structured, thus making it possible to assess cognition and ego functioning under decreasingly structured conditions. It was designed for use with young adults and adults suffering from psychiatric disorders.

The four tasks in the battery are: copying a mosaic tile, spontaneous drawing, figure drawing and free clay modelling. The tester assesses the client's ability to conceptualise, to organise and to plan procedures that will enable him to complete the tasks. The theory underlying this technique is that the individual's ability to carry out practical tasks will be affected by the presence of conflicts and defences that consume energy, and by weak ego boundaries. When ego boundaries are weak, performance may be expected to deteriorate as the external structure becomes looser.

A guide has been developed to help in the recording and interpretation of findings, and rating scales are used for the different aspects of performance. These include ability to organise, independence and self-esteem (Evaskus 1982).

VALIDATING RESULTS

An increasing number of assessment procedures that were originally developed by occupational therapists to meet the needs of their particular setting have now been made widely available. Some have been described in this chapter.

If treatment results in general seem satisfactory, then standardisation may not appear important to the therapist in the field who is working under pressure and simply wants to get through the work as efficiently as possible. However, we cannot justify our assessment results if the test used will not stand up to scrutiny.

In developing new testing procedures, or looking at existing ones, there are seven main points to consider:

1. What aspects of the client does the therapist wish to assess?
2. Have these aspects been identified in such a way that they can be measured accurately? (Reliability.)
3. How can the desired function be elicited for assessment?
4. Does the proposed assessment procedure measure what it is intended to measure? (Validity.)
5. Is there a clearly defined way of administering the assessment? (Standardisation of administration.)
6. How are the results to be recorded and scored?
7. Can the results be compared with the normal results for a comparable population? (Standardisation of results.)

Most of these points have been covered in this chapter. The frame of reference being used determines what is to be assessed, how it is assessed and how the assessment results are interpreted. The method of recording is influenced by who is to read the results and what they will be used for. Reliability, validity and standardisation are discussed below.

Reliability and validity

Vague and inaccurate assessment leads to vague and imprecise treatment. This is unacceptable for both ethical and practical reasons. The occupational therapist has a duty to use treatment that will benefit and not harm the client (see Ch. 11), therefore intervention must be based on accurate knowledge of the client's needs and abilities. The two most important concepts in ensuring accuracy of assessment procedures are reliability and validity.

Reliability

The first concern in legitimising an assessment procedure is whether or not it reliably elicits accurate information. There are two main ways of determining reliability:

1. *Test–retest.* The rater assesses the client and records the results. After a suitable interval to minimise the effect of practice, the test is given again and the results are compared. Obviously, results are more likely to be similar if the aspects being measured have been clearly defined and the testing procedure is standard.
2. *Interrater evaluation.* The assessment procedure is carried out on the same client by two or more raters and their results compared. This method is appropriate for evaluating procedures that involve observation. If possible, the raters observe the client doing the same activity, perhaps by using a videotape. The results are more likely to be similar if the testing procedure is standard and the raters have been trained in its use.

Validity

Establishing the validity of an assessment procedure is more difficult than establishing reliability, so it is only carried out on procedures that are known to be accurate and therefore worth validating.

Validation involves checking that the procedure measures what it is intended to measure – if we want to know whether a client is able to cook a meal on a gas cooker there is no point in assessing the client's performance on the department's electric cooker.

There are three main types of validity:

1. *content or face validity*: analysing the assessment procedure to see if it measures what it purports to measure
2. *criterion-related or concurrent validity*: comparing the assessment results with an external criterion such as data collected from other sources
3. *construct validity*: looking at the accuracy of the assessment procedure in measuring the theories or hypotheses behind the intervention.

Standardisation

If an assessment procedure is found to be both accurate and reliable, then it may be appropriate and useful to standardise it for use in a particular way with the client group it was developed for. Establishing a clear and uniform procedure for applying the test is called standardisation of administration and establishing the performance of a similar group of people for comparison is called standardisation of results, or norming.

Standardisation of administration

This means that the procedure can be repeated in exactly the same way by different people, at different times and on different subjects. This involves defining the functions to be assessed very clearly and giving precise instructions about administering and scoring the test. Objective tests are easier to standardise than tests that require an observer to make a judgement. Observer bias must be minimised by training the rater (Garfield 1982).

Standardisation of results

This is a lengthy procedure and is most likely to be neglected when an assessment procedure is developed. It involves administering a reliable and valid assessment procedure to a large number of people who are matched for such factors as sex, age, cultural background and, possibly, disability. The results can be used to show the normal range of performance for that group, to use as a comparison with the scores of an individual.

SUMMARY

This chapter covered the assessment stages of the occupational therapy process, including initial assessment, ongoing assessment and final assessment. It looked at what is assessed by the occupational therapist; function and dysfunction, motivation, performance, and relationship with the environment. Methods of assessment used by occupational therapists were reviewed, including review of client records, interviewing, observation, home visits, checklists, performance scales, questionnaires and projective techniques. Finally, there was a brief section on validating assessment results.

Chapter 7 covers the treatment planning and implementation stage of the occupational therapy process, which follows assessment.

REFERENCES

Allen C K, Allen R E 1987 Cognitive disabilities: measuring the consequences of mental disorders. Clinical Psychiatry 48(5): 185–190

Azima F J C 1982 The Azima Battery: an overview. In: Hemphill B J (ed) The evaluative process in psychiatric occupational therapy. Slack, New Jersey

Azima H, Azima F 1959 Outline of a dynamic theory of occupational therapy. American Journal of Occupational Therapy 13: 1–7

Brayman S J, Kirby T 1982 The Comprehensive Occupational Therapy Evaluation. In: Hemphill B J (ed) The evaluative process in psychiatric occupational therapy. Slack, New Jersey

Creek J 1998 Purposeful activity. In: Creek J (ed) Occupational therapy: new perspectives. Whurr, London

Cutting D 1968 A review of projective techniques. Unpublished American Occupational Therapy Association Regional Institute report.

Evaskus M G 1982 The Goodman Battery. In: Hemphill B J (ed) The evaluative process in psychiatric occupational therapy. Slack, New Jersey

Felce B, McBrien J 1987 Workshop: challenging behaviour in mental handicap. Stockport

Fidler G S, Fidler J W 1978 Doing and becoming: purposeful action and self-actualization. American Journal of Occupational Therapy 32(5): 305–310

Florey L L, Michelman S M 1982 Occupational role history: a screening tool for psychiatric occupational therapy. American Journal of Occupational Therapy 36(5): 301–308

Garfield M 1982 The principles of developing assessment tools. In: Hemphill B J (ed) The evaluative process in psychiatric occupational therapy. Slack, New Jersey

Gillette N 1968 Principles of evaluation. American Occupational Therapy Association Regional Institute

Hagedorn R 1995 Occupational therapy perspectives and processes. Churchill Livingstone, Edinburgh

Hemphill B J (ed) 1982 The evaluative process in psychiatric occupational therapy. Slack, New Jersey

Hogg J, Raynes N V 1987 Assessment in mental handicap: a guide to assessment, practices, tests and checklists. Croom Helm, London

Kielhofner G 1988 Workshop: the model of human occupation. York

Kielhofner G, Burke J P 1980 A model of human occupation, part 1. Conceptual framework and content. American Journal of Occupational Therapy 34(9): 572–581

Law M, Baptiste S, Carswell A, McColl M A, Polatajko H, Pollock N 1994 Canadian Occupational Performance Measure, 2nd edn. CAOT Publications ACE, Toronto

Law M, Baptiste S, Mills J 1995 Client-centred practice: what does it mean and does it make a difference? Canadian Journal of Occupational Therapy 63(2): 250–257

Matsutsuyu J S 1969 The interest checklist. American Journal of Occupational Therapy 23(4): 323–328

Mattingley C, Fleming M H 1994 Clinical reasoning. Slack, Philadelphia

Mocellin G 1988 A perspective on the principles and practice of occupational therapy. British Journal of Occupational Therapy 51(1): 4–7

Mosey A C 1973 Meeting health needs. American Journal of Occupational Therapy 27(1): 14–17

Mosey A C 1986 Psychosocial components of occupational therapy. Raven Press, New York

Munn N L 1966 Psychology: the fundamentals of human adjustment, 5th edn. Houghton Mifflin, Boston

Opacich K J 1991 Assessment and informed decision-making. In: Christiansen C, Baum C (eds) Occupational therapy: overcoming human performance deficits. Slack, Philadelphia

Pollock N, McColl M A, Carswell A 1999 The Canadian Occupational Performance Measure. In: Sumsion T (ed) Client-centred practice in occupational therapy: a guide to implementation. Churchill Livingstone, Edinburgh

Punwar A J 1994 Occupational therapy: principles and practice, 2nd edn. Williams and Wilkins, Baltimore

Reed K L, Sanderson S N 1992 Concepts of occupational therapy, 3rd edn. Williams and Wilkins, Baltimore

Reilly M 1962 Occupational therapy can be one of the great ideas of 20th century medicine. American Journal of Occupational Therapy 16(1): 1–9

Seedhouse D 1986 Health: the foundations for achievement. Wiley, Chichester

Spencer E A 1988 Functional restoration: preliminary concepts and planning. In: Hopkins H L, Smith H D (eds) Willard and Spackman's Occupational therapy, 7th edn. J B Lippincott, Philadelphia

Spreadbury P 1998 You will measure outcomes. In: Creek J (ed) Occupational therapy: new perspectives. Whurr, London

Sumsion T 1999 The client-centred approach. In: Sumsion T (ed) Client-centred practice in occupational therapy: a guide to implementation. Churchill Livingstone, Edinburgh

Unsworth C A 1993 The concept of function. British Journal of Occupational Therapy 56(8): 287–292

7

Treatment planning and implementation

Jennifer Creek

INTRODUCTION

In Chapter 6 we looked at the assessment stages of the occupational therapy process. This chapter looks in detail at the next stage, treatment planning and implementation, starting from the point where a database has been compiled and the therapist and client are ready to analyse it for the purpose of setting goals for intervention.

The chapter covers the process of analysing assessment data and setting long-term, or overall, goals that can then be broken down into intermediate and short-term goals. This process is illustrated with case examples.

Methods of activity analysis, task analysis and adapting or synthesising activities are described in detail, with an example of a generic activity analysis format and a sample activity analysis.

Theories of motivation are discussed, highlighting their relevance to engaging clients in activity. Three factors determine the selection of activities for treatment: client goals, properties of activities and motivation. These are described, together with a discussion of the four key elements of intervention: the client, the activity, the therapist and the environment. This section gives only an outline of the occupational therapy intervention process; Chapters 12 to 17 describe in detail the therapeutic use of activity.

TREATMENT PLANNING

Treatment planning is a collaboration between therapist and client in which assessment data are analysed and goals are set for intervention. As shown in the previous chapter, data collection is not random. The theory or model being used determines what information is sought and provides an outline for analysing the information collected and for clarifying areas for intervention. The whole process should be made as simple as possible for the client so that he can be genuinely involved. Clients are more likely to become involved in treatment and to make changes if they are involved in setting their own goals and monitoring their own progress (Howell 1986).

Once the long-term goals of treatment have been agreed, they can be broken down into short-term goals that lead, in smaller steps, to the achievement of the major goal. Long-term hospitalised clients may have difficulty accepting the overall goal of the treatment team, which usually involves major changes in their way of life, but they can move towards it in stages that they can accept (Drouet 1986).

Therapists use their expertise in activity analysis, task analysis and adaptation of activities to identify appropriate activities for attaining goals, but clients must find meaning and value in the activities chosen. The final decision as to whether to become involved in the activity rests with the client.

The treatment planning process is shown in Figure 7.1. The treatment plan should be put in writing and copies given to the appropriate people, for example the client and the client's key worker.

DATA ANALYSIS

Analysis of data obtained from the initial assessment produces three key areas of information:

1. the client's expected environment and occupations
2. areas of dysfunction that might interfere with the fulfillment of these occupations

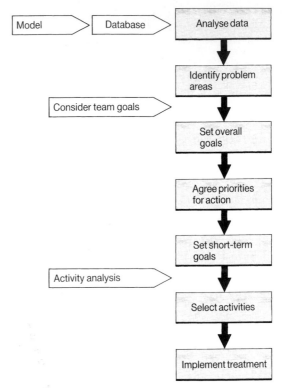

Figure 7.1   The treatment planning process.

3. skills already available in the client's repertoire.

Environment and occupations

The client cannot be considered in isolation from the expected physical and social environment, since the skills required are determined by the demands of that environment, the roles the client adopts within it and the support available. The client may expect to return to his previous environment and previous level of functioning if the problem requiring intervention is an acute one. He may have recently been diagnosed with a serious illness, in which case there will be a lot of unknowns in his future. He may have a chronic disability that necessitates making changes in the occupations that make up his life.

The therapist needs to be clear about what the client expects to do in the future and what skills he will need to cope.

Areas of dysfunction

Clients usually require intervention because they are unable to meet the demands of their physical or social environment, either because the demands have changed, the client has changed, or he has never been able to cope adequately.

The therapist's task is to identify areas of dysfunction where there is a gap between the skills the client needs and the skills the client has. It may be a general deficit across several skill areas, as often occurs in learning disabilities, for example, or it may be a specific deficit, such as inadequate social skills. Dysfunction can only be defined relative to the client's expected environment; there is no universal standard of achievement for all clients.

Skills in the client's repertoire

Skills must be learned in the developmental sequence so that higher level skills are founded on lower level skills, otherwise stress will cause regression to earlier modes of performance. The therapist tries to assess what level of skills the client has reached developmentally and starts intervention from that point. Isolated skills will easily be lost.

As well as looking at the range of skills the client has, the therapist assesses whether or not he has achieved a sufficient level of competence to carry out his expected occupations and whether skills have been organised into habits that allow for efficient use of time and energy. This analysis highlights the skill areas that must be developed if the client is to fulfil his expected occupations, and leads on to setting goals for achieving those skills.

SETTING GOALS

Goals are the targets that the client hopes to reach through involvement in occupational therapy. They define both the skills to be learned and the level of performance that is acceptable. Goals must be within the client's capabilities and he must adopt them as his own. The involvement of clients is crucial in setting occupational therapy goals because they are the experts in their own lives and know both what they want to achieve and what they need to achieve in order to live those lives.

When goals have been set, the client should be absolutely clear about what is expected of him and how he is to reach them. The client and the therapist can easily see what progress has been made by measuring the outcomes of therapy against the goals that were set. Goals must be couched in clear and specific terms so that the therapist, the client and any other interested parties understand the purpose of the intervention and know when it should be terminated. For example, 'getting fit' is too vague to be a goal, but 'walking the dog for at least 2 miles twice a day' is specific and measurable.

Attaching a performance marker to the goal allows both the client and the therapist to see when it has been reached. For example, a woman with severe anxiety and social phobia has the overall aim of feeling less anxious in company. Her immediate goal is to be able to walk into a room with people in it and not feel anxious. The performance marker she identifies, that will enable her to tell when the goal has been attained to a standard that is satisfactory for her, is to be able to walk into the group room and talk to someone within the first 15 minutes.

Levels of goals

Client goals are usually set on two or three levels (see also Fig. 7.2):

1. long-term goals
2. intermediate goals (these will not be necessary in all cases)
3. short-term goals.

Long-term goals

These are the overall goals of the intervention process, the reasons why the client is being offered help and the expected outcome of intervention. They usually take account of:

- where the client might live after discharge
- the level of independence the client might be expected to achieve
- the degree of support that is likely to be needed

Short-term goals	Intermediate goals	Long-term goals
Identify skills to be developed	Practise new skills to a level of competence	Use skills for performance of chosen occupations
Review existing experience, knowledge and skills	Move on to next skills in hierarchy	
Be aware of the consequences of learning new skills	Practise using skills in a variety of situations until they become habitual	
Engage in playful or explorative activities as the first stage of learning new skills		
Practise new skills		

Figure 7.2   The goals of intervention.

- any necessary changes in occupations and the skills required to support them.

Long-term goals can be described as occupational performance goals (Mosey 1986).

Intermediate goals

These may be clusters of skills to be developed or barriers to be overcome on the way to achieving the main goals of therapy. In a crisis intervention or other acute treatment it may not be necessary to use intermediate goals; the fluid nature of the problem and the short intervention time allow problems to be tackled rapidly.

Short-term goals

These are the small steps on the way to achieving major goals. The short-term goal is usually to learn a sub-skill or skill component of the adaptive skill that is needed for successful occupational performance (Mosey 1986). Short-term goals are organised into a hierarchy, with the most basic goal to be tackled first; they can be expressed in performance terms or subjective terms; and they are measurable. Some therapists find it useful to identify performance markers for achieving the goal, making some progress but falling short of full achievement and doing better than expected (Ottenbacher & Cusick 1988).

Setting long-term goals

As discussed in the previous chapter, the occupational therapist and client will produce from the initial assessment a general picture of the client's life roles, balance of occupations, areas of skills deficit and future needs. These data, together with information from other team members, should suggest overall aims of intervention.

Whenever possible, the client's own perception of his needs is the guiding principle in setting aims, since he is the person who must achieve them. However, certain problems impair the ability to make rational decisions about the future. These may be temporary, as in severe depression, or permanent, as in dementia. In such cases the therapist may take a stronger lead in establishing goals, while recognising that these are subject to review as the client changes during treatment and becomes able to express his opinions. If the therapist takes a strongly supportive role in the early stages of treatment it may be difficult to pass personal responsibility back to the client at a later stage, so one of the stated goals of intervention should be for the client to take responsibility for his own progress.

In many cases the client will be expecting to return to his previous occupations, so treatment is designed to restore lost skills, teach additional skills or improve performance of existing skills in order to prevent recurrence of problems. In other cases the problem that caused the client to seek treatment is unlikely to be completely overcome, so that a change in occupations and the skills needed to support them can be anticipated.

The overall goals of the treatment team will also influence the occupational therapist's goals. The therapist's programme is a part of the wider treatment programme and will play a greater or lesser part in achieving its aims.

The setting of long-term goals is illustrated in Box 7.1.

Setting intermediate goals

Long-term goals may not take a long time to reach, particularly in an acute treatment setting. However, in some cases they can take months or years to attain and may be modified to a greater or lesser extent during the treatment process. In the latter case, it may be difficult for the client to see himself ever attaining his ultimate goals and it can be useful to set intermediate goals, which can be seen as easier to reach. These are smaller goals that lead towards attainment of the long-term goals.

Certain disorders, such as dementia, interfere with the ability of clients to take a temporal perspective and therefore with their ability to plan for the long-term future. These clients will have difficulty in setting realistic long-term goals but may become involved in treatment planning by setting smaller goals. The acute phase of illness may also interfere with a person's perception of his own potential and make his involvement in long-term goal setting impossible, although intermediate goals can still be discussed. For example, the therapist might feel that it is appropriate for a severely depressed client to aim to return home once the acute phase of the illness is over. During the acute phase, the client feels utterly hopeless about the possibility of ever leaving hospital, but is able to accept intermediate goals of attending a supportive psychotherapy group twice a week and a creative activities group once a week.

Box 7.1 Case example 1

Lynn suffers from chronic anxiety of such severity that her performance of even simple tasks is seriously impaired. Most of her fear is focused on magic and hypnotism; she is terrified of people being able to make her do things against her will. She also fears change, meeting new people, going out and failing in anything she attempts. These fears cause her to limit her sphere of activity to a few comforting rituals, such as overeating and bouncing a ball.

Lynn first received treatment for hyperactivity at the age of 18 months. Now, at the age of 32, she has experienced several admissions to hospital, various diagnoses and many different treatments. She lives at home and attends a day hospital 5 days a week, with occasional short admissions to give her parents a break. This situation is expected to continue for as long as her parents can keep her at home.

The team hopes to introduce Lynn gradually to a broader range of daytime activities without provoking further anxiety. She is expected to need long-term care eventually, preferably in a community setting such as a group home.

Lynn has insight into her present problems but is unrealistic about the future. She would like to marry, eventually, and to have children, or to look after her parents in their old age. She is able to give much more practical goals that she can start working towards now, which suggests that she recognises her long-term plans to be over-optimistic. She would like to start going out and meeting people, and doing the things other young adults do; to be helped to do more for herself so that she is less of a burden on her parents; to be able to visit the local shops, in company; and to have an interesting hobby such as cooking or sewing.

Taking all these factors into account, the long-term goals set by the occupational therapist in consultation with Lynn are:

- to become independent in self-care
- to perform simple household tasks, such as making coffee, washing up, making beds
- to walk regularly to the local shops with a companion
- to learn simple embroidery.

Achievement of these aims would satisfy Lynn, enable her to live at home longer, and help her to cope with life in a group home.

Three main factors determine what the intermediate goals should be:

1. any barriers to performance that need to be overcome, for example, fear of going out (agoraphobia)
2. the need to learn skills in a developmental sequence
3. the client's wishes.

An example of setting intermediate goals is shown in Box 7.2.

Setting short-term goals

When long-term and/or intermediate treatment goals have been agreed they can be broken down into a hierarchy of smaller steps. Each short-term goal needs to be realistically within the client's reach and a decision must be made about where to start. Each goal should also be measurable, so that client and therapist know when it has been reached (Box 7.3).

Once short-term goals have been agreed, a programme of activities that will lead to their achievement is planned. Knowledge of activity analysis and synthesis enables the therapist to identify or modify activities to incorporate all the skills, personal factors and environmental factors that will best bring about change.

ACTIVITY ANALYSIS, TASK ANALYSIS AND ACTIVITY ADAPTATION

Activity is the tool that occupational therapists use to bring about changes in function. In order

---

Box 7.2   Case example 2

Lynn and the therapist spent some time discussing what skills would be needed to obtain the long-term goals already agreed. They then decided which skills to tackle first. The factors taken into account in this process were:

- Lynn's fear of going out, which had to be overcome before going out to the local shops
- the need to build up Lynn's confidence by starting with goals that could be attained easily
- Lynn's strong interest in food and drink, which helped her to tolerate a certain amount of anxiety
- Lynn's request to be allowed to progress at her own pace in treatment.

It was decided to work towards all the long-term goals simultaneously, using small intermediate goals so that Lynn would develop a sense of achievement. These would be reviewed regularly but no pressure would be put on Lynn to perform any particular tasks in a set period of time. The first set of intermediate goals was:

- to learn to tolerate a certain amount of anxiety while performing tasks
- to learn to comb her own hair
- to learn to make a cup of instant coffee independently
- to learn to wash up crockery independently
- to go to the local cafe with the therapist without being overwhelmed by anxiety
- to learn some simple embroidery stitches.

Box 7.3   Case example 3

Lynn's first aim, to learn to tolerate a certain amount of anxiety while performing tasks, is broken down into steps that are given in the order in which they will be tackled. It is felt that Lynn would quickly learn to perform even the most complex task if not immobilised by anxiety. The aim is to enable her to perform despite her fears. The steps are:

1. to feel at ease with the therapist
2. to identify occupations that she enjoys
3. to give each task its due importance and not take it too seriously
4. to remember to think through each task before beginning
5. to attempt simple tasks, such as combing her hair, with supervision
6. to stop and think about the task in hand if she starts to become anxious.

Some of the above stages are more easily measurable than others. Therapists may prefer to put all their goals into the form of measurable behavioural objectives to make evaluation of results easier. These six goals can be rewritten in objective format as follows:
At the end of treatment, Lynn will be able to:

1. remain in the company of the therapist for the duration of a treatment session without asking to leave
2. state three activities that she has enjoyed in the past and would like to do again
3. state why she is carrying out each task
4. outline the stages involved in each task before beginning it
5. comb her hair, with verbal prompting
6. respond to anxiety by stopping what she is doing and reviewing the stages of the task in hand.

to select the most suitable activity to bring about the desired change, we need to know exactly what demands an activity will make on the client, what skills are required for the performance of the activity and how activities can be adapted to change those demands and skills.

'Activity analysis' is the process of identifying the various components of an activity and the demands that it makes upon the performer.

A task can be defined as a constituent part of an activity. Identifying the tasks that make up an activity is known as 'task analysis'.

'Activity adaptation' is the process of designing an appropriate activity or altering an existing activity by bringing together the desired components.

'Grading activities' is a form of adaptation. The activity is adapted progressively in order to increase or decrease the demands that it makes on the individual.

Activity analysis

An activity can be analysed for all its component parts that come within the domain of the occupational therapist. Mosey (1986) called this the generic approach and pointed out that there is no universally accepted framework for doing this.

An alternative approach is to study only components that are relevant to the model or frame of reference being used, for example a psychodynamic model focuses on the psychological functions and psychosocial interactions involved in performing an activity (Katz 1985).

The format presented here is a generic one that was developed from several different frameworks (Fidler & Fidler 1963, Llorens 1976, Mosey 1986, Hopkins & Tiffany 1988).

Activities are composed of many skills that can be divided for the purpose of analysis into:

- physical
- cognitive
- psychological
- interpersonal.

In order to understand the effect an activity will have on the client, the therapist needs to break it down into these skill areas and look at each one in detail.

Activity analysis also includes any potential for adapting the activity in order to allow for change in the client. This is called 'grading'. Grading allows the client to progress from exploration, through acquisition of skills, to attainment of goals. It also allows the client to move on to the next stage once a skill has been learned. Grading may involve a gradual change in the nature of the activity by changing one or two components, or a complete change of activity.

Analysing an activity enables the therapist to:

- understand the demands the activity will make on the client, that is, the range of skills required for its performance
- assess what needs the activity might satisfy
- determine the extent to which it might inhibit undesirable behaviour
- determine whether or not the activity is within the client's capacity
- discover the skills the activity will develop in the client; these may be specific skills, such as threading a needle, or more general, transferable skills, such as balancing on one leg
- provide a basis for adapting and grading activities to meet particular ends.

Figure 7.3 shows a generic activity analysis format, and Figure 7.4 shows how it was used to analyse a particular activity, ice-skating.

Task analysis

Any activity is made up of steps or tasks that are performed in sequence. For example, in making a clay pinch pot the tasks are:

- cut an appropriately sized piece of clay
- wedge the clay
- shape clay into a ball
- push thumb into clay
- pinch the clay to the required thickness all over
- smooth the inner and outer surfaces
- add any embellishments or decoration
- leave to dry out.

Name of activity
Timing/length of time/number of sessions
Environment
Brief description

Appropriateness for different ages and sexes
Social and cultural value
Preparation
Precautions

Requirements of activity

Physical

sensation
sensory integration
perception
spatial awareness
motor planning
gross motor
mobility
balance
fine motor
repetition
rhythm
coordination
strength
endurance
range of movement
posture
types of movement

Cognitive

attention
concentration
discrimination
generalisation
use of symbols
perceiving cause and effect
abstract thinking
reality testing
choice
language
following demonstration/directions
reading
writing
numbers
orientation
awareness of time
memory
range of knowledge
goal setting
planning
organisation
number of processes
speed
imagination
creativity
logic
problem solving

Psychological

expression of feelings
control of feelings
frustration tolerence
coping with pressure
sublimation
playing/exploring
tolerating risk
trust
independence
passive or active
creativity
reality testing
exploration of feelings and motives
responsibility
involvement
sharing
self-image
body image
identification
sexual identity
end product
contrived or real experience

Interpersonal

individual or group/size of group
mixed or segregated sexes
communication
cooperation
competition
negotiation
compromise
leadership
structure
rules
interaction
isolation
variety of relationships
involvement
role opportunities

Potential for grading

Materials and equipment
Environment — human and non-human
Method
Related activities

Figure 7.3 Activity analysis guidelines.

Name: Ice-skating
Duration: 1 to 3 hours
Timing: An energatic activity so not after a meal
No of sessions: Can be done once or on a regular basis
Environment: Requires a special ice rink or very cold weather and a saftey frozen stretch of water

Brief description:

Ice-skating involves wearing a pair of boots with blades on and attempting to glide around on a flat ice surface. Skilled skaters can perform a variety of moves, some very energetic

Appropriateness:

This activity is appropriate for any age above about 3, because good balance and walking skills are a prerequisite. Reasonable physical fitness is required and an older person may be more at risk of breaking a limb if he or she falls. It is equally suitable for men and women.

Social and cultural value:

Ice-skating is a popular spectator activity and a popular sport with young people because it develops physical fitness and is sociable. The ice rink is a good meeting place for friends

Preparation:

If a large group is to go skating, it may be advisable to book in advance. Ensure that everyone is dressed suitably and knows how to get to the ice rink

Precautions:

Enough staff should be taken to ensure that the group will be safe. If anyone has unpredictable or violent behaviour they may need a one-to-one escort. This sport is not suitable for people who are very unfit or frail

Requirements of Activity

Physical:

Fine motor skills needed for fastening boots
Good standing and walking balance for standing on blades and moving on the ice
Motor planning, sensory integration and good general coordination for mastering the art of moving on skates
Visual–spatial perception to avoid bumping into other skaters or barriers
Good muscle strength required in back, neck, abdomen, legs and arms for maintaining an upright posture, walking, balancing and holding on
Rhythmic and repetitive activity
Range of movement may be limited to mid-range of walking movement in back, hips, knees, shoulders and arms in a skilled skater. Movement of ankles is limited by boots.
Mainly upright or forwards leaning posture except when dancing or performing acrobatics.
Endurance required for a long skating session. Some people find the stiff boots painful at first.

Cognitive:

Need to pay attention to surroundings to avoid bumping into another skater or the barrier
Concentration required for a beginner to master the art of skating
Ability to perceive what effect certain movements have on style of skating.
Ability to work out how to skate from watching others
Spatial orientation for moving round the rink without bumping into anyone
Long-term memory to learn and remember how to skate
Ability to set a series of goals towards achieving the full skill of skating
Ability to react quickly to avert accidents
Ability to visualise oneself skating

Psychological:

Tolerance of the pain of stiff boots
Tolerance of the frustration of not being able to skate at first
Courage to venture onto the ice, then to let go of the barrier and skate freely
Tolerance of risk of falling and injury
Control of anger and frustration when other skaters get in the way
Active involvement
May require trust in others if skating in a chain

Allows for playful exploration of own physical capacities and ability to take risks
Independent movement can be achieved gradually or sought quickly
Responsibility to skate in an orderly manner and not put self or others at risk
Requires image of the self as a skater
Real experience
No concrete end product

Interpersonal:

May be an individual or group activity
Necessity to share space with others and interact physically in order to do so. Risk of physical contact
Usually mixed sexes
Cooperation required in sharing the space equitably, especially when people of mixed ability are on ice together. May require compromise
Obey rules of skating in one direction only and not skating in long chains
May be competitive or cooperative
Physical interaction, which may or may not involve contact, in sharing the ice with others. No requirement for close involvement with others
Opportunity for more experienced skaters to help beginners

Potential for grading

Materials or equipment:

Music could be played

Environment:

Number of people on the ice at any one time
Group or individual skating
Indoor or outdoor

Method:

Formal teaching of how to skate or allow people to try for themselves
Simple skating or more advanced techniques such as speed skating or ice dancing

Related activities:

Roller-blading
Skate-boarding
Snow-boarding

Figure 7.4 A sample activity analysis.

Any one of these steps could be analysed into a further series of tasks. For example, there is a sequence of steps involved in wedging a ball of clay. Task analysis is carried out for a purpose, and the extent to which an activity is analysed into smaller and smaller tasks will depend on the purpose of the analysis. If a person has very specific difficulties it may be necessary to carry out a detailed task analysis to isolate the precise problem. On the other hand, if the therapist is analysing a fairly simple activity in order to teach it to a client it may only be necessary to identify the main steps of the activity.

Task analysis may be carried out in order to:

1. select an appropriate teaching method for an activity, for example, forward or backward chaining
2. select an appropriate activity to meet a therapeutic aim
3. adapt an activity to meet client needs by changing or eliminating a step
4. identify the precise part of an activity a client is having difficulty performing.

The therapist should be cautious about concentrating on a single step in the sequence of actions that make up an activity. Clients should be given opportunities to practise whole activities rather than single tasks because 'performance does not occur normally in a step by step approach but rather as an integrated continuous flow of behavioural performance. Failure to provide practice in the whole sequence may result in halting, awkward performance' (Reed & Sanderson 1992).

Activity adaptation

Activities can be adapted to match the needs, abilities and interests of clients. The two tools the therapist may use to adapt an activity are 'grading' and 'sequencing'.

Grading an activity means gradually increasing or decreasing the demands made on the client by changing elements of the activity in small increments.

Sequencing activities means finding or designing a sequence of different but related activities that will increase the demands on the client as his performance improves or decrease them as his performance deteriorates. For example, there are many different methods of printing on paper that can be organised into a sequence of increasing or decreasing complexity or difficulty, including: sponge printing, leaf printing, stencilling, potato printing, lino cutting and screen printing.

The different elements in an activity that have potential for change are:

- the materials and equipment used (media)
- the environment, including other people involved
- the method of carrying out the activity.

These three dimensions can be manipulated to achieve the desired therapeutic result.

Therapeutic media

Some activities, such as woodwork, centre on the materials and equipment used while in others, such as drama, these are of secondary importance. Certain skills can be more easily assessed and developed using activities that are materials/tools orientated; for example, to develop hand–eye coordination it would be more appropriate to use woodwork than drama. A variety of tools can be used to develop both physical and cognitive skills.

Materials can be selected for their power to evoke feelings (e.g. wet clay may evoke the feelings of lack of control associated with the anal stage of development, as described by Freud). Materials can also influence the outcome of the activity (e.g., good quality paints and paper will make it easier for a client to achieve a satisfactory painting than would poor quality materials).

Within a single activity, a whole range of skills can be upgraded by changing the materials or equipment used. For example, if the chosen activity for developing cognitive skill (Mosey 1986) is pottery, the client may start by exploring the medium of clay by using the hands only, progress to simple hand tools and eventually work on a wheel.

Therapeutic media are discussed in more detail in Chapters 12 to 17.

Therapeutic environment

The environment includes both human and non-human elements. The physical environment in which therapy is carried out is often the aspect of treatment least amenable to manipulation because of external constraints; the therapist works in the space she is able to negotiate, rather than selecting an ideal environment for each activity. However, some environmental factors may be used to change the activity, such as being indoors or outdoors, working with groups or individuals, staying in the treatment setting or going out into the community, using public transport, a car or taxi. Smaller changes within the work setting can be brought about by using background music, altering the level of lighting, adjusting temperature or ventilation. Large or small alterations in the environment influence sensory stimulation, perception, concentration, work tolerance, enjoyment of the activity and social contact.

We could change the environment in which the client is doing pottery by introducing more stimulation or distraction. The client could start by working one-to-one with the therapist, then another person might do pottery in the same room and eventually the client might work in a group.

Other environmental factors are discussed in more detail under treatment implementation (p. 136).

Therapeutic method

The method the therapist uses to direct an activity is usually the simplest element to manipulate. She can be directive or *laissez-faire*, supportive or demanding, involved or an onlooker. As a general rule, when starting a new activity the therapist will be more active herself, gradually taking less part as the group or individual develops and matures. Sensitivity and experience allow the therapist to make subtle adjustments to her approach as the need arises, without delay or preparation. The process of making these decisions during the therapeutic process is called 'clinical reasoning'.

Many adjustments could be made to the method of teaching pottery to the client as his cognitive skills develop. For example, the sessions could become longer as the client's concentration improves, the therapist could start by giving a lot of support and instruction then gradually withdraw, or more choices could be introduced.

TREATMENT IMPLEMENTATION

Throughout the occupational therapy process described in Chapter 5 and earlier in this chapter, the therapist attempts to involve the client fully, to engage his interest, elicit his cooperation and earn his trust. If she succeeds, she will avoid problems in the implementation of treatment. However, some clients will come this far through the process and still not feel able to participate actively in treatment. It is therefore necessary to have an understanding of motivation in order to be able to select appropriate activities that will engage the client.

In this section we look at two theories of motivation:

1. intrinsic motivation
2. Maslow's hierarchy of needs,

and how they can be applied in therapy. We then look at the four key elements of occupational therapy intervention:

- the client
- the therapist
- the activity
- the environment,

highlighting the relationships between them.

MOTIVATION

An understanding of the theory of motivation is necessary to successful treatment implementation because the success of occupational therapy intervention is dependent on the client being actively engaged in treatment, not passively receiving it from the therapist. There are many different theories of motivation but the most important one for occupational therapists is the theory of intrinsic motivation.

Intrinsic motivation

Intrinsic motivation is the urge to use one's capacity to have an effect on the environment, independent of any external reward. Every child is born with this urge but life experiences influence how it is used and developed.

What is intrinsic motivation?

Human beings have an inherent urge to be active and to explore the environment. In doing so they find out that they can have an effect on it and this, in turn, leads to an urge to influence the environment in a controlled way, to act competently to bring about desired changes. There is an inherent satisfaction in being able to act competently, independent of any extrinsic rewards action may bring. This satisfaction can be strong enough to sustain action even when the activity itself causes pain, for example the marathon runner keeps going despite physical exhaustion.

Exploration is prompted by something in the environment that is novel, different from usual in some aspect, puzzling or not understood for whatever reason; this arouses curiosity. The urge to try out one's capacities in new ways on the environment is so strong that people will seek or create puzzles to solve if there are none readily available. Intrinsic motivation prompts the individual to seek and master new skills throughout the life cycle.

Pawns and origins

When a child acts on the environment he receives feedback about the effect his action has had. If the result is satisfactory his self-respect is enhanced and he begins to build an image of himself as a competent performer. This increases the likelihood of him acting again to seek further satisfaction and proof of competence. A high proportion of satisfactory to unsatisfactory outcomes leads to the development of a positive image of the self as a 'doer'. Such a person's sense of competence is enhanced by his successes but he has the confidence to learn from his failures. The result is a benign spiral of action, feedback and satisfaction leading to more action (Fig. 7.5).

If the child frequently experiences unsatisfactory outcomes when he acts, or fails to have any impact at all in the environment, his self-image will develop as an incompetent performer or passive observer of external events. Failure in action leads to a reduction of the urge to act, therefore the child receives less feedback and has reduced opportunities to build up a positive self-image. The process is a vicious spiral, as shown in Figure 7.6.

People with a positive image of themselves as competent actors who can influence events in their environment are known as 'origins'. They have an internal locus of control, or belief that power to make changes lies with them.

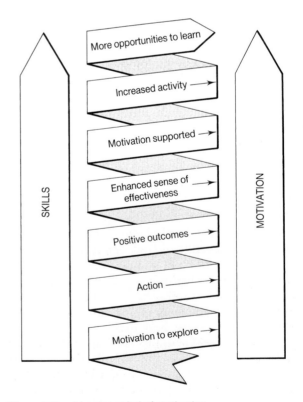

Figure 7.5 A benign spiral of motivation.

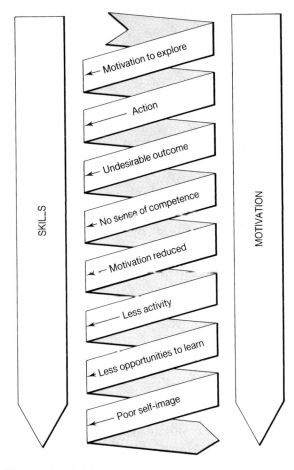

Figure 7.6   A vicious spiral of reduced motivation.

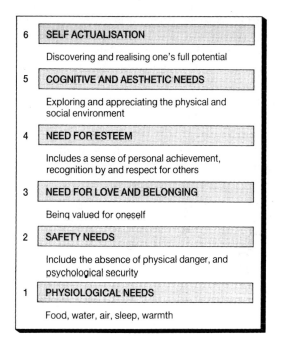

Figure 7.7   Maslow's hierarchy of needs.

People who have no sense of being able to control events are called 'pawns'; they have an external locus of control (DeCharms 1968, Florey 1969, White 1971, Smith 1974, Burke 1977, Robinson 1977).

Maslow's hierarchy of needs

This is an example of a theory of external motivation, that is, it views people as acting to attain ends rather than gaining intrinsic satisfaction from action.

Maslow (1968) suggested that people are motivated by the drive to satisfy physical and psychological needs. Needs exist in a hierarchy, with physiological needs at the bottom and the drive to self-actualise at the top (Fig. 7.7).

The lower needs, including physiological needs and safety needs, provide deficiency motives, that is, the individual acts to remove discomfort. For example, someone who is hungry will take action to procure food. Only when the lower needs are largely satisfied will the person become concerned about satisfying higher needs.

Higher needs do not help the individual to survive; they are concerned with developing each person to his highest potential and are called growth motives. Each of these growth motives leads towards the ultimate goal of self-actualisation, which is the need to use one's capabilities and achieve one's unique potential. Maslow suggested that very few people become self-actualised but that life satisfaction depends on striving towards that goal.

Motivation in therapy

Intervention necessitates motivating the client to voluntary action. Lack of motivation to act is rarely due to lack of interest in attaining valued personal or social goals; it is more likely to be a sense of hopelessness about the possibility of influencing whether or not they are attained. Every therapist has encountered clients who put their faith in drugs or electroconvulsive therapy (ECT) and see occupational therapy as a way of filling in time between treatment sessions.

There are various ways in which the therapist can increase the likelihood of a client being motivated to participate, for example by:

- involving the client fully in all stages of the treatment process, from assessment, through goal setting and treatment planning to implementation
- providing a stimulating environment with objects for the individual to act on and people to interact with
- maintaining enough novelty in the environment to arouse curiosity without causing fear
- providing opportunities for the environment to be explored and actions to be repeated
- ensuring that competent role models are available, either peers or therapists
- helping the client to build up a feeling of efficacy by starting with playful exploration, allowing time for skills to be learned thoroughly, and providing opportunities for skills to be used realistically
- selecting tasks that are appropriate to the individual's age, sex, cultural background, educational level, etc.
- ensuring that lower level needs are met before moving onto higher level needs
- using activities the client sees as being personally and socially valuable
- allowing people to use their particular talents
- ensuring that there is a high probability of success in the activity by using activities that the individual is capable of completing and by providing the correct materials, equipment and instructions
- setting tasks that offer some challenge but are not so difficult that they frustrate
- maintaining motivation by grading activities as the client progresses
- considering the individual's interests when setting a task

- allowing the individual to be responsible for the outcome of his actions
- ensuring that feedback is available so that the individual knows when he has succeeded
- treating each person as someone who can attain valued goals
- showing respect for the client as a person, believing in his potential for change, and listening to what he says.

In order to motivate a client successfully, the therapist must try to eliminate inhibiting factors as well as incorporating positive factors into the programme. Curiosity can be inhibited by:

- physical deprivation or stress, such as hunger, thirst, cold
- too much novelty or too many changes in the environment, which evoke fear rather than curiosity
- lack of stimulation or challenge in the environment.

By following these guidelines it should be possible to engage any client in therapy and to help him to develop a more positive self-image as an active and influential person (Florey 1969, White 1971, Smith 1974, Stewart 1975, Burke 1977, Robinson 1977, Mocellin 1988).

KEY ELEMENTS OF INTERVENTION

The client, the therapist, the activity and the environment are the four elements available to the occupational therapist for assessing and motivating the client and for carrying out treatment programmes. Mosey (1986) called these the 'legitimate tools' of occupational therapy.

Each of these elements is in a dynamic relationship with the others:

- The client's active participation in treatment rather than passive reception of it is the factor that brings about change.
- The quality of the relationship between the client and therapist is a crucial factor in motivating and engaging the active cooperation of the client, thus determining the outcome of intervention.

- The ability to analyse and understand activity allows the therapist to select appropriately for individual clients' needs.
- The context of treatment has a major influence on both process and outcome.

The client

Clients who receive occupational therapy for mental health problems can be of any age. They live in a variety of places and are seen in different settings. Each person has a unique problem or set of problems and each individual brings his own personality, life experience and abilities to the therapeutic encounter.

When a client sees an occupational therapist for the first time, he may already have received psychiatric treatment, perhaps for many months or years. His expectations of the type of help he will receive and of the behaviour expected of him will be coloured by that experience. It may take clients a while to adjust to the different approach that occupational therapists use, with its emphasis on active involvement and on giving responsibility for health to the individual. Some people are unable to accept this type of treatment and prefer a more passive role while others are relieved to be allowed to take control of their own lives again.

Client-centred practice is an approach to intervention which 'recognises the autonomy of individuals, the need for client choice in making decisions about occupational needs, the strength clients bring to an occupational therapy encounter and the benefits of client–therapist partnership' (Law et al 1995). When a client-centred approach is used, the client and therapist 'work together to achieve the agreed goals' (Sumsion 1999) rather than the therapist taking a lead.

Engaging the client in activity

If an activity is to have meaning for the client it must engage his resources and fit in with his value system, therefore an understanding of the client's existing skills and beliefs is essential to treatment planning. The client will not become engaged by an activity that does not match his needs, interests, values and abilities.

The initial assessment of the client includes those factors that influence the choice of therapeutic activity. These are:

- sex and sense of sexual identity
- chronological age
- any sensory deficits, perceptual problems or physical disability
- special aptitudes, such as musical talent
- stage of cognitive development
- any specific cognitive problems, such as short attention span
- educational level
- emotional needs
- stage of psychosocial development
- sense of personal and social identity
- personal values
- social skills and social preferences
- cultural and subcultural background
- communication and language skills
- any contraindications arising from specific problems or other treatment in progress.

In matching activity to client, the therapist needs to be aware of the relative importance of all these factors to the individual and of the personal meaning that engagement in the activity has for the client. This meaning will be different for different people, and for the same person at different times, so the therapist must listen carefully to what the client says about the activity.

The therapist

The occupational therapist can be her own most powerful therapeutic tool. Two important skills which allow the therapist to work effectively are 'clinical reasoning' and 'reflection'.

Clinical reasoning

Clinical reasoning is what therapists think about in the clinical situation, how they perceive their clients, what they focus on as the central problem, what they ignore, how they describe the client's problem and how they see the client as a person. An American occupational therapist, Fleming (1991), described three types of clinical reasoning: procedural, interactive and conditional.

Procedural reasoning is used when the therapist is thinking about the client's disease or disability and deciding what media and methods to use. This equates to thinking about body functions and structures in the international classification of functioning, disability and health (ICIDH-2, WHO 2000; see Fig. 3.1, p. 33).

Interactive reasoning takes place during encounters between the therapist and client when the therapist is trying to understand the experience of the individual. This equates to thinking about activity in the ICIDH-2 (see Fig. 3.1, p. 33).

Conditional reasoning is used when the therapist is thinking about the client within his broader social and temporal context. This equates to thinking about participation in the ICIDH-2 (see Fig. 3.1, p. 33).

Reflective practice

An important tool in the therapist's understanding of her own practice is reflection. Reflection is subjective awareness and appreciation of action and its impact on the environment. It is a process of self-awareness and self-regulation alongside a perception of what is happening or might happen to the client. Reflection is about interpreting experience rather than analysing it. A knowledge of one's own qualities, strengths and weaknesses, gained through reflection, allows us to respond effectively to clients.

The therapist is constantly making interpretations of the client's performance and responses to activity. These interpretations influence how a therapist works with a client and any decisions made on the spot about what to do next. This process of observation, interpretation and decision making during intervention is called 'reflective practice'.

The skilled therapist is able to respond immediately and appropriately to what is happening during a treatment session because of her awareness of her own motivations and the client's likely motivations that underpin the way he responds to the activity. This contextuality and flexibility in carrying out a programme of intervention is characteristic of good occupational therapy.

The effective therapist also helps the client to reflect on the meaning that activity has for him and on how the activities he does and the skills he develops during therapy can be put into practice to improve his everyday life.

Personality

Personality is important. The therapist who chooses to specialise in psychotherapy is likely to be a very different person from the one who works contentedly in the long-term rehabilitation of institutionalised psychiatric patients, and they would not happily exchange positions. Personality also plays a part in determining the therapist's style of therapeutic interaction and the treatment techniques chosen.

An understanding of her own needs, foibles and ways of relating to others will allow for more appropriate selection of roles in the therapist's relationship with the client.

Experience and skill

The experience and skill of the therapist also determine which treatment techniques are used. Some techniques, such as psychodrama, require specialist postgraduate training. Basic occupational therapy training can only teach a limited number of activities, so the qualified therapist will add on new techniques to suit her interest and field of practice. Using a computer to encourage a child with learning disabilities to communicate, or helping a group of adults to explore causes of anxiety with projective art, is a long way from teaching basket weaving, although the same principles are used in selecting the treatment media.

The more skills the occupational therapist has in her repertoire, and the more theories she is able to draw on, the better able she will be to work in a person centred way and respond to individual needs and environmental demands.

Therapeutic relationship

There are many different kinds of therapeutic relationship, from a warm, mutual sharing of experience to a less personal relationship that allows the client to project feelings onto the therapist without fear of retaliation or rejection. The type of relationship developed will depend on:

- *The therapeutic setting*. For example, it is usually considered inappropriate for staff to share personal information with clients in an analytical psychotherapy unit.
- *The needs of the client*. These needs change as treatment progresses, so the therapist may start by being supportive and readily available but withdraw as the client becomes more independent.
- *The age and experience of the therapist*. Newly qualified staff may feel more comfortable with a sharing relationship. It takes experience and confidence to allow clients to project feelings, particularly negative feelings, without taking them personally.

The therapeutic relationship is a dynamic one, affecting the therapist as well as the client. In order to maintain objectivity and to avoid feeling threatened it is useful to have supervision from another occupational therapist. Even an experienced therapist can benefit from being able to discuss feelings and problems as they arise.

Staff availability

When planning treatment programmes to achieve both quantity and quality of treatment, the therapist takes account of several factors, including the number of staff available and their experience. Some activities cannot be used by a therapist working single-handed, either because of the nature of the activity, for example psychodrama, or because of the degree of disability or disturbance of the client. When working alone it may be necessary to reduce either the intensity of treatment or the number of clients in order to ensure safety.

The activity

Activity is at the core of occupational therapy practice. If the therapist cannot engage the client in activity that has meaning and value for him, then there is no assessment and no treatment implementation. Engagement is achieved by involving the client at all stages of the treatment process, by understanding the factors that will motivate the individual, as described on page 132, and by establishing an expectation that clients attending the occupational therapy department will be active in their own treatment processes.

The functions of activity for the individual have been described in this chapter and elsewhere in the book, and will only be summarised here.

Summary of activity functions

- Activity is essential for the normal development of the individual. Without activity no personal development can take place, and inability to perform activities competently leads to maladaptive development.
- People use activity to explore the environment and to test their own position in it.
- We become embedded in our social and cultural context through activity.
- Activity helps to build a healthy personal and social identity.
- Activity is intrinsically satisfying.
- Activity is used to learn and practise skills that can be used for occupational performance.
- People are able to adapt to changing circumstances through activity.
- The individual can construct purpose and meaning in his life and gratify his needs through activity.
- Relationships with others can be made through shared activity.

The process of analysing activities into their component parts and synthesising therapeutic activities was described in the previous section. Details of how various activities are used can be found in Chapters 12 to 17.

The environment

People cannot be considered in isolation from their environment, and treatment cannot be considered separately from the environment in which it takes place. In this section we will look at the elements that make up the therapeutic environment, and at how they can be manipulated to achieve therapeutic goals.

What is the therapeutic environment?

The therapeutic environment consists of human and non-human elements that can, to a greater or lesser extent, be manipulated by the therapist to facilitate engagement in tasks and the achievement of goals. Some elements in the environment are physically or emotionally closer to the individual and some are further away.

The human environment consists of:

- the therapist
- other clients
- other staff
- relatives and friends
- neighbours
- peers.

The non-human environment consists of:

- the treatment setting (for example hospital, community centre, clinic)
- the occupational therapy setting (for example department, client's own home)
- the physical space where treatment occurs
- the home
- the workplace
- the neighbourhood
- the resources and facilities within the environment
- non-human objects within the environment, including aids to independent performance.

There are various ways of looking at both the human and non-human environment to assess the effect it might have on clients. One such system is PASS 3 (Program Analysis of Service Systems), devised by Wolfensberger & Glenn (1975) to examine and rate 50 variables in the therapeutic environment. It was designed for use on services for people with learning disability but the authors claim it can be applied to other settings without adaptation. Examples of some of the factors evaluated by this system are:

- physical resources
- age-appropriate facilities, environmental design and appointments
- staff development
- model coherency
- culture-appropriate labels and forms of address.

Many of these items are outside the control of the occupational therapist, such as location of the treatment centre, but other items are relevant, such as forms of address used with clients. The quality of the therapeutic environment gives the client a powerful message about how much he is valued as a person.

Manipulating the environment

The first task of the therapist is to ensure that the therapeutic environment is so designed that it meets the needs of the client. As far as possible, the client is involved in this process. Dunning (1972) suggested that there are three environmental variables to be considered by the occupational therapist:

1. space
2. people
3. the task,

and that the therapist should not neglect any one of them:

- space can be arranged to promote stimulation
- people can be organised to encourage social interaction
- tasks can be designed to develop skills.

It may be appropriate to teach people how to manipulate their own environments by:

- physically moving objects (e.g. moving the furniture around at home to give more privacy)
- changing the function of rooms (e.g. turning the spare bedroom into a study)

- changing the way the house or workplace looks (e.g. by decorating or buying house plants)
- using space differently (e.g. by going out more)
- learning methods of communication and assertiveness
- learning new social skills
- going out to practise new skills in new social settings
- attending evening classes or community college to learn new skills.

SUMMARY

This chapter looked at the treatment planning stage of the occupational therapy process. This includes data analysis, goal setting, activity analysis and activity synthesis.

Data analysis includes looking at the client's environment and occupational roles, areas of dysfunction and available skills. Goal setting is in three stages, short-term, intermediate and long-term goals, which were illustrated by a case example.

Activity analysis can be generic, taking into account as many factors as possible, or specific to a particular model for practice. The format given here is for a generic activity analysis, and was illustrated by a sample activity, ice-skating.

Activity adaptation involves manipulating the three elements of activity – media, environment and method – in order to achieve the desired therapeutic result.

The chapter also considered the ways in which therapists can engage clients in treatment by evoking the intrinsic drive to be active and by ensuring that basic needs are met.

The four elements of intervention – client, therapist, activity and environment – were discussed. The contribution that each element makes to the therapeutic process and the relationships between them were highlighted.

Therapeutic techniques used by occupational therapists are discussed in Chapters 12 to 17, and treatment implementation with specific client groups is covered in Chapters 18 to 29.

REFERENCES

Burke J P 1977 A clinical perspective on motivation: pawn versus origin. American Journal of Occupational Therapy 31(4): 254–258

DeCharms R 1968 Personal causation. Academic Press, New York

Drouet V M 1986 Individual behavioural programme planning with long-stay schizophrenic patients, part 1. British Journal of Occupational Therapy 49: 7

Dunning H 1972 Environmental occupational therapy. American Journal of Occupational Therapy 26(2): 292–298

Fidler G S, Fidler J W 1963 Occupational therapy: a communication process in psychiatry. Macmillan, New York

Florey L L 1969 Intrinsic motivation: the dynamics of occupational therapy theory. Papers: Research and development in occupational therapy, Southern California

Hopkins H L, Tiffany E G 1988 Assessment and evaluation: an overview. In: Hopkins H L, Smith H D (eds) Willard and Spackman's Occupational therapy, 7th edn. J B Lippincott, Philadelphia

Howell C 1986 A controlled trial of goal setting for long-term community psychiatric patients. British Journal of Occupational Therapy 49(8)

Katz N 1985 Occupational therapy's domain of concern: reconsidered. American Journal of Occupational Therapy 39(8)

Law M, Baptiste S, Mills J 1995 Client centred practice: what does it mean and does it make a difference? Canadian Journal of Occupational Therapy 62(5): 250–257

Llorens L A 1976 Application of a development theory for health and rehabilitation. American Occupational Therapy Association, Maryland

Maslow A H 1968 Towards a psychology of being. Van Nostrand, New York

Mocellin G 1988 A perspective on the principles and practice of occupational therapy. British Journal of Occupational Therapy 51(1): 4–7

Mosey A C 1986 Psychosocial components of occupational therapy. Raven Press, New York

Ottenbacher K, Cusick A 1988 The significance of clinical change and clinical change of significance: issues and methods. American Journal of Occupational Therapy 44(6): 519–525

Reed K L, Sanderson S N 1992 Concepts of occupational therapy, 3rd edn. Williams and Wilkins, Baltimore

Robinson A L 1977 Play: the arena for acquisition of rules for competent behaviour. American Journal of Occupational Therapy 31(4): 248–253

Smith M B 1974 Competence and adaptation. American Journal of Occupational Therapy 28(1): 11–15

Stewart M C 1975 Motivation in old age. Physiotherapy 61(6): 180–182

Sumsion T 1999 The client-centred approach. In: Sumsion T (ed) Client-centred practice in occupational therapy: a guide to implementation. Churchill Livingstone, Edinburgh

White R W 1971 The urge towards competence. American Journal of Occupational Therapy 25(6): 271–274

Wolfensberger W, Glenn L 1975 PASS 3 Program Analysis of Service Systems. National Institute on Mental Retardation, sponsored by the Canadian Association for the Mentally Retarded, Toronto

World Health Organization 1997 International classification of functioning, disability and health. WHO, Geneva

8

Record keeping

Mary Booth

INTRODUCTION

Good record keeping can be considered an essential foundation which underpins excellence in health care planning and delivery. Accurately and adequately recording patient information, assessments, interventions, treatments and outcomes is time consuming. In all areas of health and social care, but particularly in the mental health field, recording an activity can take as long as performing it. However, it is vital to the provision of good quality care that this time is both available and effectively used. Occupational therapists, like other health and social care professionals, are required to keep a range of records relating to patient activity. These can generally be considered to fall into two main categories:

1. statistical information
2. patient records.

Why records are important

Keeping records is important because:

• Patient records provide a detailed account of patients from the time they enter the care of a health facility until they are discharged. They can show whether the care has been appropriate, timely and effective.

• This type of recording is essential to individual health care workers, who should rely on the record, rather than their own memories, with regard to the planning and progress of interventions with the patient.

• The existence of records means that all team members involved with the patient's care can, subject to confidentiality, immediately have an overview of the patient's and other care providers' aims, goals, progress and outcomes.

• Occupational therapists have a statutory duty to maintain records which is placed on their employing organisations. Records should be kept for a minimum of 7 years for adults and 25 years for children.

• As occupational therapists, our *Code of Ethics and Professional Conduct* states that 'Accurate, legible, factual, contemporaneous and attributed records and reports of occupational therapy intervention must be kept in order to provide information for professional colleagues and for legal purposes, such as client access and court reports.' It also makes reference to the purpose of records and secure and confidential storage and disposal of records (College of Occupational Therapists 2000, p. 6).

• Records can be useful tools in audit and research which lead to effective practice based on evidence.

• Good record keeping safeguards the patient as it gives a visual record of the quality of care provided. It also safeguards the occupational therapist, and the employing organisation, in situations where complaints are made or litigation becomes an issue.

This chapter examines the different types of records and recording used, the professional and legal implications of poor record keeping and the essential components for occupational therapy case notes.

STATISTICAL RECORDS

Occupational therapists working in the health service will be required by their employing organisations to keep statistical records. These records will be demanded of the organisation for government information and by the health authority for commissioning and purchasing purposes. From 1 April 1999, information is increasingly required by primary care groups as they take on commissioning of services under recent legislation (DoH 1997).

National Health Service (NHS) Trusts will have differing methods of recording the necessary information but all are increasingly likely to be linked to an organisation-wide information system. Some occupational therapists will be required to use a paper based system which is then input into the information system by data clerks, others will directly input into the system themselves from a networked personal computer, and some may record information on small, hand held computers which they then download to the main computer on a regular basis.

A major aspect of the strategy for information for the NHS in England is the development of a common information infrastructure including a thesaurus of agreed clinical terms known as Read codes. There is now a national set of agreed clinical terms expressed in the language of health, including those relevant to occupational therapy, which can be computer coded. While occupational therapists do not need to know the detail, they should be aware of the code's existence to help them understand and to cooperate when they are asked to code in a certain way (DoH 1986).

The information collected in this way will include the following patient details:

• Patient identification number
• Patient's name, address, date of birth
• Diagnosis codes
• Consultant and general practitioner
• Service and contract identification codes
• Codes relating to clinical activity and contacts.

In some organisations one system will collect all data relevant to the occupational therapist's daily work, and the patient data collection sheet will also act as a time and attendance sheet and record travel claims. In other organisations these types of records are collected separately.

From these records the organisation can provide the statutory information demanded by the government, such as Körner reports which, for the allied health professions, are compiled of a minimum data set and other information relating to the professional group or geographical area. For England these are collected on the Department of Health annual return KT26 and published annually.

Information will also be collated to show the amount and type of patient activity required by commissioners of services and, increasingly, the funding and monitoring of occupational therapy services will be based on this information. If the occupational therapist does not accurately record this information on the IT system it could result in penalties for the organisation and eventual loss of services to patients. In addition, if the government and commissioners cannot obtain statistical reports which include occupational therapy, they will not see the need to fund future occupational therapy services. It is important that occupational therapists understand the need to record accurately this information even though it often seems distant and not relevant to busy daily clinical practice.

Most information systems are also capable of recording and later providing analysis of other information which is helpful to both clinicians and managers. Individual occupational therapists and the service can obtain useful information from such records, which will help them to plan and organise their work. This can include case lists, frequency and type of contact with patients, waiting list times, average contacts per case, length of time of intervention and a range of other information, depending on the records collected.

PATIENT RECORDS

Patient records are kept by all professionals who are working with the patient. It is still normal practice for any one patient to have several sets of notes, and all relevant sets should receive information about the patient's occupational therapy intervention. The main sets of notes will include:

- *Case notes*. These are generally the psychiatrist's notes which relate to both in-patient and out-patient episodes of care. Occupational therapy assessments and reports should be copied to these.

- *General practitioner notes*. These are retained in the patient's general practitioner's office. Depending on local policy and procedure, occupational therapy reports and assessments may be sent directly to the general practitioner or may be included in team reports.

- *Nursing notes*. These may be in-patient nursing notes or community psychiatric nurse notes. Again, it is essential that occupational therapy reports are copied to nursing colleagues.

In addition, the mental health patient may have psychology notes, occupational therapy notes, notes from the other allied health professionals and may also have separate sets of notes relating to physical ailments.

There is a move towards having a single set of case records for each patient and it is clearly sensible, within mental health settings, for this to occur where practical. In time, single electronic records are likely to come into use, but the confidentiality aspects of electronic records have not yet been fully addressed. Electronic records will overcome the practical problem of several people, often in different locations, wanting to access the same notes. Meanwhile, occupational therapists should be aware of the policy towards single case notes in their working area and follow this.

Paper based records

Most patient records are still based on paper and, as mentioned above, one patient is likely to have several records kept by different professionals. The main set of case notes will probably be called the medical notes and will contain the doctor's day-to-day notes, tests and test results, assessments, care plans, letters, reports, prescriptions and discharge summaries. Occupational therapy notes are also likely to be paper based. Paper based notes contain a variety of typed and handwritten entries.

Storage of paper based records

Records, while current, will be stored in a secure place, usually within the working area of the health care worker. This might be a ward, a department or an office and can be in a hospital or community based setting. Once the record is no longer active, the hospital case notes and medical notes will generally be sent to the medical records department for storage. However, in a community setting such as a community mental health team, and in departments such as occupational therapy, the records not actively in use may be stored at the base.

Health organisations have different practices and policies relating to the storage of records. Some will convert the paper file to microfiche which lasts longer and takes up less storage space. However, the process of recording and retrieving such records can be time consuming. Many organisations today use outside companies which offer secure, safe storage with a rapid retrieval time of the original paper record. In this case the record will be stored in a sealed, numbered box and it is the box which will be recalled, for reasons of confidentiality.

Computer records and the Data Protection Act 1984

The Data Protection Act of 1984 addresses the use of information kept on computer. It aims to protect information about individuals and enforce standards on the processing of information kept on computer. Health care workers should be aware that:

• Organisations must register computers holding personal information about an individual. This means patient based information, such as letters and reports, must not be stored on the hard disk of the occupational therapy department computer unless it is appropriately registered. Most organisations will have policies on this.

• Data must be relevant, accurate and up to date, and the person concerned has a right to be told that the information is held and the right of access to it.

• Security measures to ensure confidentiality – such as personal passwords for occupational therapists who input and access data – must be in place.

The main current use of computers in record keeping has been discussed above, under statistical records. There is, however, a move towards the introduction of a single electronic patient record, accessible on a need-to-know basis. It is important to remember that an occupational therapy department should not keep *any* information about patients on the hard disk of a personal computer unless it is registered with their employer's data protection officer (College of Occupational Therapists 1990a). Organisations employing occupational therapists in the mental health field will have policies on the use of computer data and the individual occupational therapist should be familiar with these policies.

In today's health care environment, the needs and care of clients are inextricably linked to the need to collect and utilise information from the client record. With the advances in computers it becomes more feasible to capture and use client information through electronic means. There is still much work to be done by systems designers and clinicians before integrated clinical workstations are a part of everyday recording practice. The Integrated Clinical Workstation (ICWS) project is a vehicle to make terms collected under the work of the Clinical Terms (Read Codes) project available to clinicians at the point of care (College of Occupational Therapists 1996). An integrated clinical workstation will offer access to shared computer terminology in everyday clinical language, with software to support professional practice, and will be capable of both linking to a single patient electronic record and gathering necessary statistical information.

The Care Programme Approach and Supervision Register discussed below are likely to be maintained by the employing organisation on a computer.

Photographs and videotapes

Occupational therapists may wish to take photographs or videotapes to record patient changes and, while this is more usual in the physical setting, it is sometimes used in mental health, for example to record body posture, eye contact or other social interaction. The occupational therapist must ensure that the patient gives consent both to the photograph and to the uses to which it will or may be put. When a record is made in this way, a written note should be entered into the patient's written record. Permission should always be gained before using photographs or videotapes of clients for staff training or reproduction in a textbook to show treatment methods.

Confidentiality of records

The importance given to confidentiality of computer based records was discussed above. The confidentiality of records stored on other media such as paper, videotapes and photographs is equally important. The College of Occupational Therapists' *Code of Ethics and Professional Conduct* (1995) states that 'Occupational therapists are ethically and legally obliged to safeguard confidential information relating to clients' and that disclosure of confidential information is normally only permissible where:

- 'The client gives consent (expressed or implied)
- There is legal compulsion (by statute or Court order)
- It is considered to be in the public interest in order to prevent serious harm, injury or damage to the client, carer or to any other person.'
- The code also states: 'Disclosure to third parties (which may include the relatives, police, lawyers and the media) regarding the client's diagnosis, treatment, prognosis or future requirements should only be made where there is valid consent or legal justification to do so (College of Occupational Therapists 2000, p. 3). In addition it directs 'All shall be kept securely and made available only to those who have a legitimate right/need to see them' (College of Occupational Therapists 2000, p. 3).

Employing organisations will also have policies and procedures relating to confidentiality of records. In practical terms, confidentiality of records means:

- Records must be kept secure, for example in a locked filing cabinet, and not left unattended when in use.
- Discussions relating to patients should be confined to those colleagues involved in their care.

OCCUPATIONAL THERAPY PATIENT RECORDS

Occupational therapists must make themselves familiar with the College of Occupational Therapists' guidelines for documentation (College of Occupational Therapists 1990b) and with the operational policies and guidelines on documentation and record keeping of their own service and employing body.

It is good practice for an agreed set of notes to be used throughout an occupational therapy service. The patient record should be well thought out and designed to keep general information, history, assessments, treatment plans, progress notes and evaluations in a logical and easy to follow order:

1. *Information sheet.* Details about the patient such as name, address and next of kin, legal and care programme status, other professionals involved and an outline of any precautions to be taken.

2. *Details of referral to and registration with the service.*

3. *History sheet.* This will include a diagnosis or diagnostic label. The history sheet can be designed to give prompts or reminders of what to include.

4. *Occupational therapy assessment.* All formal assessments, both standardised and observational, are recorded.

Assessments recorded will vary depending on the model of occupational therapy used but are likely to include some of the following:

- Self-maintenance
  — personal activities of daily living
  — sleep
  — neglect/self-harm
  — rest

— finance
— accommodation
— coping strategies (e.g. alcohol, drugs)

- Productivity
  — domestic activities of daily living
  — education/schooling
  — work/employment
  — budgeting
  — insight/future aspirations

- Leisure
  — hobbies/pastimes
  — social resources
  — satisfaction

- Motor sensory skills

- Cognitive skills
  — concentration
  — motivation
  — orientation
  — insight
  — problem solving/decision making

- Psychosocial skills
  — intrapersonal
  — interpersonal relationships
  — religion/spiritual
  — social support.

5. *Treatment plans*. The way in which a treatment plan is structured will depend to some extent on the model of occupational therapy followed. It should include a reference to the model being used and the problems identified for occupational therapy intervention. The aims of the patient, and/or carer, if appropriate, should be recorded, together with the therapist's aims, objectives and actions. A review date should be included. The treatment plan should be discussed and agreed with the patient.

6. *Evaluation of treatment plan*. A section which allows for evaluation of the treatment plan and may include a record of outcome and further action required should be included.

7. *Progress notes*. Sections within the notes should be organised for correspondence and reports. A well designed set of patient records that includes prompts (eg. 'Date and sign all entries') will help to ensure that the record meets

quality requirements. See Boxes 8.1–8.8 for examples of occupational therapy records used in one NHS Trust for community mental health, acute adult mental health, learning disabilities, forensic services, psychiatry of old age and child and family mental health services.

The sample notes for occupational therapy have been designed to use either as a set of stand alone occupational therapy notes or within a set of multidisciplinary or single case notes. When used in multidisciplinary or single case notes, the parts used are the occupational therapy assessment sheets, the occupational therapy treatment plan and the occupational therapy evaluation sheets. The patient information and history sheets are the general sheets shared by the team. Progress notes are chronological, either as an overall progress record or as progress sections for each professional group involved with the patient's care, such as doctors' progress notes and nursing progress notes.

Access to health records

Since November 1991, in response to the Access to Health Records Act 1990, patients have had the right to see their records. They may request access formally in writing or may ask the occupational therapist to go through the notes with them. Subject to the occupational therapist's employing organisation's policy, it is good practice to respond to a request to show the patient the occupational therapy records. However, the occupational therapist is only at liberty to show the patient the occupational therapy records. Other requests must be passed on to the professional concerned. All organisations will have forms for the formal request to view notes and can charge a set fee.

RECORDING OF CARE PROGRAMME APPROACH, SUPERVISION REGISTER AND SECTION 117 AFTERCARE

The Care Programme Approach, Supervision Registers and Section 117 of the Mental Health

Box 8.1   Example of a patient information sheet (reproduced with kind permission from Tees and North East Yorkshire NHS Trust (South Locality))

OCCUPATIONAL THERAPY PATIENT RECORD
Location...

Part 1: Patient Information Sheet

Completed by..   Signature...

Designation..   Date................./...................../......................

NHS Number (if known):	Marital Status: married/single/divorced/widowed
Name:	Male/Female
Prefers to be known as:	DOB:
Address:	Occupation:
Cultural/Religion:	
Postcode	Legal Status:
Tel. No:	CPA Status: Full/Minimal/N/A
Carer Name:	CPA Coordinator:
Relationship:	Next of kin name:
Address:	Address:
Tel. No:	Emergency contact number and name:
GP:	Consultant:
Address and Tel. No:	Address and Tel. No:

Details of other professionals involved:

Precautions – history of aggression, medical conditions, family members with physical/mental health problems, risk of self-harm

Act 1983 are strategies to ensure communication between agencies and services involved in the care and management of people with mental health needs.

Care Programme Approach

The Care Programme Approach (CPA) was introduced in the UK on 1 April 1991. It was described as the new cornerstone of the government's mental health policy and it remains a critical tool in the care of people receiving mental health services. CPA is intended to ensure a systemic approach to, and coordination of, assessment, care and review of all persons over the age of 16 years who are receiving any care/treatment in the community from specialist mental health services (South Tees Community and Mental Health NHS Trust 1999).

While this chapter does not concentrate on this approach in detail, the recording of the CPA underpins the process.

Box 8.2 Example of referral and registration details (reproduced with kind permission from Tees and North East Yorkshire NHS Trust (South Locality))

Referrer	Date of admission	Date of referral	Date first seen
....	....	....	....
....	....	....	....
....	....	....	....
....	....	....	....
....	....	....	....
....	....	....	....

Comwise Date

Registration	........./........./.........	........./........./.........	........./........./.........	........./........./.........
Discharge	........./........./.........	........./........./.........	........./........./.........	........./........./.........
Registration	........./........./.........	........./........./.........	........./........./.........	........./........./.........
Discharge	........./........./.........	........./........./.........	........./........./.........	........./........./.........

O.T. Service Information Leaflet Given/Sent

Dates: ..../........./.........   ..../........./.........   ..../........./.........   ..../........./.........

Named O.T...

Keyworker/Named Nurse...

Box 8.3 Example of history sheet (reproduced with kind permission from Tees and North East Yorkshire NHS Trust (South Locality))

OCCUPATIONAL THERAPY PATIENT RECORD

HISTORY SHEET

Part 2

Patient Name.. Date of Birth..

Date, Time and Sign all entries

Diagnosis/Diagnostic label

History:
(e.g. history of current admission/referral, psychiatric history, forensic history, medical history, birth, development, education, family structure, social, work, previous OT involvement, where information obtained from, medication)

Box 8.4 Example of assessment sheet (reproduced with kind permission from Tees and North East Yorkshire NHS Trust (South Locality))

OCCUPATIONAL THERAPY PATIENT RECORD

ASSESSMENT

Part 3

Patient Name.. Date of Birth...

Date, Time and Sign all entries

Patient/Carer's understanding of problems/condition

Occupational Therapy Assessment
(e.g. reason for referral to OT, patient's account of difficulties, physical problems, psychological assessment, ADL, financial, social, occupational, insight, outcome of assessment)

Box 8.5 Example of treatment plan sheet side 1 (reproduced with kind permission from Tees and North East Yorkshire NHS Trust (South Locality))

OCCUPATIONAL THERAPY PATIENT RECORD

TREATMENT PLAN

Part 4

Treatment Plan Number...   Date............/........../.........

Patient Name...   Date of Birth..

OCCUPATIONAL THERAPY MODEL – Tick Selected Process Driven Problem Based Models of Occupational Therapy and associated approaches to be used. Approaches appear under models.

DEVELOPMENTAL	REHABILITATION	EDUCATION	ADAPTATION
Sensory Integration	Biomechanical	Developmental	Biomechanical
Neuro-developmental	Neuro-developmental	Student Centred	Organisational (e.g. time)
Interactive	Interactive	Interactive	Activity Analysis
Behavioural	Behavioural	Behavioural	Cognitive Behavioural
Cognitive	Client Centred	Client Centred	Client Centred
	Cognitive	Cognitive	Sensory Stimulation
			Ergonomic
			Analytical
			Architectural

(Hagedorn 1995)

Date, Time and Sign each Section

Problems Identified for O.T. Treatment:

Box 8.6 Example of treatment plan sheet side 2 (reproduced with kind permission from Tees and North East Yorkshire NHS Trust (South Locality))

Patient/Carer Aims (if appropriate)

Therapist Aims

Objectives/Actions

Review Date

"The Occupational Therapist has discussed this treatment plan with me":

Signed ....(patient/carer)   Date.............................

Box 8.7   Example of evaluation of treatment plan (reproduced with kind permission from Tees and North East Yorkshire NHS Trust (South Locality))

Part 5

Treatment Plan Number..   Date............/........../.........

Patient Name...   Date of Birth..

Date, Time and Sign each entry

Outcomes:

Further Action:

Box 8.8 Example of Progress Note Sheet (reproduced with kind permission from Tees and North East Yorkshire NHS Trust (South Locality))

OCCUPATIONAL THERAPY PATIENT RECORD

PROGRESS NOTES

Part 6

Relating to treatment plan number... Date........./........./........ Page No...............

Patient Name.. Date of Birth..

Date, Time and Sign each entry

The essential elements of CPA are:

- systemic assessment of health and social care needs, including an assessment of risk
- an agreed care plan
- allocation of a Care Programme Coordinator (CPC)
- regular review – monitoring of needs and progress and of the delivery of the care programme.

Mental health services are the joint responsibility of both health and social services and it is important that CPA, for which health authorities are responsible, and Care Management (CM), for which Social Services are responsible, work in harmony. To achieve this, organisations within health and social care will have locally agreed Care Programme Approach policies and procedures with which the occupational therapist must be familiar and should implement or participate in where appropriate. For patients who are receiving both the Care Programme Approach and Care Management, local agreements are likely to provide a single shared care plan, a single care programme coordinator and a single shared review process.

Health authorities have minor differences of implementation allowed within the original guidance (HC(90)23/LASSL(90)11). Some areas will have two levels of CPA, minimal and full, and others will have three levels. Locally designed documentation for recording the CPA process will be in use and it is this the occupational therapist must use. Care Programme Approach documentation currently tends to be additional documentation which appears within records and, where appropriate in accordance with local policy, should be copied to the occupational therapy notes.

The CPA will apply to all occupational therapists working for a health organisation within the mental health setting. It is vital that occupational therapists know the CPA status of patients they are working with and occupational therapy records should record both the Care Programme Coordinator and the patient's Care Programme Approach status. Occupational therapy intervention should form an integrated part of the care plan and be recorded in this as well as in the occupational therapy records.

An occupational therapist may be the care programme coordinator, a role which holds specific responsibilities over and above the provision of occupational therapy intervention. The extent to which occupational therapists act as Care Programme Coordinators varies with the teams they work within. Occupational therapists acting as Care Programme Coordinators will find the College of Occupational Therapists' (1997) guidance on occupational therapists undertaking a key worker role helpful. This guidance confirms that occupational therapists have the skills to be Care Programme Coordinators and recommends this is most appropriate when occupational therapy forms the major part of the care plan (College of Occupational Therapists 1997).

Supervision Register

Supervision Registers were introduced by the Department of Health on 1 April 1995 (HSG (94)5). These are local registers which are intended to identify people with a severe mental illness who may be at significant risk to themselves or others. The purpose is to ensure that services focus effectively on people who have the greatest need for care and follow-up. The decision to place a patient on the register must be based on a thorough and careful multidisciplinary risk assessment and the outcome of that risk assessment should be recorded within the Care Programme Approach. It is the responsibility of the consultant psychiatrist to place the patient on the Supervision Register within the Care Programme Approach process. Similar procedures are required for removal from the register.

Section 117 Aftercare

Section 117 of the Mental Health Act 1983 requires health and social services to provide aftercare for certain categories of detained patients. Patients subject to Section 117 Aftercare will meet the Care Programme Approach indicators and the implementation of the full Care Programme Approach will ensure these statutory obligations are met.

GOOD RECORD KEEPING

Over a number of years the Audit Commission (1995) invited a varied group of health care professionals to distil a set of good practice principles from a number of organisations which have issued guidance on standards for record keeping. These should be incorporated into the design of any occupational therapy format for record keeping, as they have within the sample set of notes. The guidance is shown in Box 8.9.

It is important that occupational therapists are proactive in maintaining an up-to-date knowledge of any changes in legislation that may impact on record keeping. For example, at the time of writing, draft outline proposals are being consulted on a review of the Mental Health Act 1983 which may have implications for recording (Scoping Committee 1999).

While documentation can be well planned to aid the clinician, since the introduction of the Access to Health Records Act 1990 there is an increased emphasis on the responsibility of health care professionals to record in a clear, concise and professional manner. Organisations will usually have their own record keeping guidelines and the occupational therapist should ensure that these, together with the professional body's guidelines, are followed. Should the employing organisation not have an official policy, the guidelines shown in Box 8.10 will help occupational therapists to ensure that their record keeping fulfils all legal requirements, protects both patients and staff and minimises the risk of litigation.

It is important that occupational therapists, like other health care workers, write all patient records in the knowledge and understanding that a treatment record is a crucial piece of evidence around which legal action can turn (Schulmeister 1987, cited by Bradshaw 1999). Health care records should be completed as if every note will be examined in a court of law. If this seems unrealistic, it is important to understand that some claims are successful not because sub-standard care was proved but because there was no evidence in the record that any care

---

Box 8.9 Audit Commission: principles of good practice for case notes (Audit Commission 1995)

- The patient should be clearly identified and the case notes should set out diagnosis, history, treatment, results and care plans.
- Case notes should be kept neat and tidy with legible entries signed and dated, preferably in black ink.
- They should be kept up to date and filed in chronological order with the most recent on top.
- Case notes should have a clear structure which is agreed with users and should be organised into sections.
- There should be a policy determining which documents should remain in the case notes after discharge (culling).
- There should be one set of notes for each patient.

Box 8.10 Record keeping guidelines (adapted with kind permission from Tees and North East Yorkshire NHS Trust)

All entries must be legible
All entries must be written in black ink
All entries must be signed when written
All entries must be timed when written
All entries must be dated when written
Alterations to entries must be scored out with a single line followed by initials, date and time
Additions to existing entries must be individually dated, timed and signed
Organisation policy on the use of abbreviations must be known and followed
All statements must be free from ambiguity
All statements must be factual and objective
All records must be in chronological order
The patient's/client's name and hospital number, where applicable, must be written on each sheet of their records
Written sheets must not be erased
Correction fluid must not be used
If there are lines between entries or entry and signature, this space must be scored with a straight line
Ditto lines must not be used
The professional prescribing the plan/care must print their name, sign and state their professional qualification on the record, and it is good practice for all names to be printed followed by a signature after each new entry
All records must be kept in a secure place to exclude unauthorised access and breach of confidentiality
All records in regard to medication must be completed according to the Trust/organisation's drug policy
Individual records must not be tagged/coded for recognition purposes
Highlighter pens can only be used if the highlighter does not erase or partially erase records when they are photocopied
Auxiliary staff and students' signatures after entries in records must be countersigned by qualified staff

had been given (Schulmeister 1987, cited by Bradshaw 1999).

Audit of record keeping

It is good practice to audit records regularly to maintain quality and to provide a continued emphasis on the importance of good record keeping. Organisations will have formal audit procedures which will include the audit of records, however, occupational therapists are recommended also to adopt a regular peer review of records. One example would be, on a monthly basis, for a colleague to select randomly five records which could then be audited against a record keeping audit tool. Box 8.11 shows the tool used for auditing the record keeping guidelines given in Box 8.10.

SUMMARY

This chapter has addressed the importance attached to record keeping in the modern health service. Throughout, the emphasis has been on occupational therapists working in the field of mental health being conversant with, and implementing, the record-keeping policies and procedures of the professional bodies and of their employing organisation. Accurate, defensible record keeping protects the patient from poor care and the occupational therapist from complaints and litigation.

Box 8.11 Audit tool for measuring record keeping criteria (adapted with kind permission from Tees and North East Yorkshire NHS Trust)

Is the record legible throughout?
Are all entries written in black ink?
Are all entries signed?
Does each entry include a time?
Is each entry dated?
Are alterations scored out by a single line followed by initials?
Date and time corrected?
Are additions to existing entries individually dated, timed and signed?
Are all abbreviations explained?
Is the record free of ambiguity?
Is the document free of subjective statement?
Does the record read in chronological order?
Is the patient's name and ID number, where appropriate, identified on each sheet?
Is there evidence of erasure?
Is there evidence of the use of correction fluid?
Are there lines left between entries and/or between entry and signature?
Are ditto marks used?
Are all records kept in a secure place to exclude unauthorised access and breach of confidentiality?
Is the Trust's drugs policy followed?
Are records tagged/coded?
Are highlighter pens used correctly?
Are unqualified/student's signatures countersigned by qualified staff?

REFERENCES

Audit Commission (1995) Setting the records straight: a study of hospital medical records. Department of Health, London
Bradshaw T 1999 Clinical treatment recording practice: still a cause for concern. British Journal of Therapy and Rehabilitation 6(1): 627
College of Occupational Therapists 1990a Guide to the Data Protection Act 1984. College of Occupational Therapists, London
College of Occupational Therapists 1990b Standards policies and procedures 145 statement on guidelines for documentation. College of Occupational Therapists, London
College of Occupational Therapists 2000 Code of ethics and professional conduct for Occupational Therpists. College of Occupational Therapists, London
College of Occupational Therapists 1996 The integrated clinical workstation (ICWS): user requirements of

occupational therapists. College of Occupational Therapists, London
College of Occupational Therapists 1997 Guidelines for occupational therapists working in mental health who are key workers. College of Occupational Therapists, London
Department of Health 1986 An introduction to the NHS centre for coding and classification. NHS Executive, Department of Health, HMSO London
Department of Health 1997 The new NHS – modern – dependable. Department of Health, HMSO, London
Department of Health (issued annually) Occupational therapy services: summary information for (year) England. Government Statistical Department, Department of Health Statistics Department 2B. HMSO, London

Hagedorn R 1995 Occupational therapy perspectives and processes. Churchill Livingstone, Edinburgh

South Tees Community and Mental Health NHS Trust (now part of Tees and North East Yorkshire NHS Trust) 1999 c/o St. Luke's Hospital, Marton Road, Middlesbrough

Care Programme Approach policy and procedures. Sections 2, 19, 20

Scoping Committee 1999 Review of the Mental Health Act 1983. Department of Health, London

ACKNOWLEDGEMENT

I would like to thank occupational therapy staff working in Tees and North East Yorkshire NHS Trust (South Locality) for sample Occupational Therapy Record Sheets and Assessment protocol.

9

Clinical governance and clinical audit

Sarah Cook   Penny Spreadbury

INTRODUCTION

In the document *The New National Health Service* (DoH 1997), what was formerly called quality assurance was replaced by the umbrella title 'Clinical governance', which has an emphasis on:

- quality
- financial responsibility
- building on good practice
- professional self-regulation
- assessing and minimising risks.

In the White Paper *A First Class Service* (DoH 1999), clinical governance is described as 'a framework through which National Health Service organisations are accountable for continuously improving the quality of their services and safeguarding high standards of care by creating an environment in which excellence in clinical care will flourish'.

This chapter will look at quality through clinical governance, with particular reference to clinical audit and outcomes of the occupational therapy process. The audit process is described, ways of measuring the outcomes of therapy are outlined, and an example of clinical audit is given.

Clinical audit in health focuses on the standards that are set within an organisation which concern the delivery of care. Information about what is actually happening is collected and compared with standards in order to check that those standards are being met (this is sometimes called auditing). Clinical audit involves collecting information about the local clinical service in order to identify gaps, failings and strengths. This information is then used to generate practical ways forward which will improve the service for clients. When changes have been implemented the service is reevaluated to see if it has improved as planned.

Clinical audit and other quality initiatives should not be confused with research, although they may share some methods. The purpose of research is to try and discover truths that can be generalised to a large population of people. For example, treatments are tested to prove or disprove their effectiveness. There is also more exploratory research which helps gain a deep understanding about a specific situation. Clinical audit has altogether a different purpose. A local service is investigated, not to test new innovations but to check that the service reaches required standards (Firth-Cozens 1993). There is also a commitment from the start that the clinical team will identify gaps and deficits and act on what they find. Research is different because the results may not necessarily be acted on, only published with recommendations.

Clinical audit has progressed since it was formally introduced in the UK in the late 1980s. Before then all manner of activity was being carried out by occupational therapists and other health professionals which is now formally recognised as audit, for example peer review and case load management. These are now widely practised, with differing levels of support and enthusiasm. The drive from the centre of the National Health Service is to spread audit into all areas of the service under the umbrella of clinical governance (Fig. 9.1).

It is important that senior managers and clinical staff see audit and clinical governance as part of their remit. This responsibility is clearly specified in section 3 of the government White Paper *A First Class Service* (DoH 1999). Managers, in conjunction with their professional colleagues, are expected to reexamine all areas of work to identify the most cost-effective use of profession-

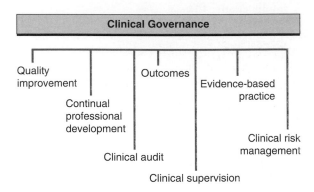

Figure 9.1 Clinical governance.

al skills. This may involve a reappraisal of traditional patterns and practices.

Outcome measurement

Donabedian (1980) proposed a threefold approach to measuring the quality of care, involving structure, process and outcome. This approach still applies today, but the emphasis must now be on the measurement of outcome rather than the measurement of process, if we are to understand the effects our service has on its users.

Florence Nightingale, in the 19th century, was one of the first to attempt to measure health outcomes. She devised a simple classification of patient outcome following a period of hospitalisation. On discharge from hospital patients were classified as being:

- relieved,
- not relieved, or
- dead.

This classification was still being used in some teaching hospitals until the late 1960s.

Now that clinical governance is high on the agenda for all health workers and managers, more useful measures of quality should be available to all. Learning about outcomes, and providing proof of that learning process, will be a component of continuing professional development, that is, lifelong learning. Monitoring will be via clinical supervision, peer review and annual performance reviews. All interventions with patients and users of the service should be based on evidence of effectiveness, and clinical risk management should be part of all aspects of clinical work. All of these will be useful when judging the quality of clinical care. Information on outcomes is also needed to supplement information concerning process.

CLINICAL AUDIT AND QUALITY

Quality assessment and quality assurance have been topics of concern to occupational therapists for many years. Interest in the quality of occupational therapy practice has come from a drive from within the profession to provide quality care, from external pressures such as the *Patient's Charter* (DoH 1991) and from the demands of purchasers such as primary care groups to evaluate and demonstrate the quality of care provided. Quality assurance initiatives in the past tended to focus on the delivery of health care (structure and process) and often produced long lists of quality standards that were set at the minimum level that was acceptable. For instance, quality standards for an outpatient department might concern the décor of the waiting room, signposts in the hospital, behaviour of reception staff and the length of time patients waited to see their therapist. Now the emphasis is on 'Continuous Quality Improvement' and clinical audit cycles can be seen to reflect this more dynamic focus. It is an activity that continually seeks improvement and is committed to the implementation of changes in practice and patient outcomes (Morrell & Harvey 1999).

As part of the government's drive to improve the National Health Service and put quality back at the top of the political agenda, in 1999 it funded the National Institute for Clinical Excellence (NICE). The role of NICE is to produce information on clinical good practice and cost-effectiveness. NICE will gather information on new interventions and products at the earliest possible stage and research their impact on health services. NICE has encompassed the National Centre for Clinical Audit (NCCA).

ASPECTS OF QUALITY

The following discussion concerning the components of a quality service has been adapted from Firth-Cozens (1993), Strong & Robinson (1988) and *A First Class Service* (DoH 1999).

Effectiveness

Effectiveness concerns the service as a whole, as well as an individual's treatment, and should result in a beneficial outcome. The outcome should meet standards of effectiveness that have been suggested, where possible, by research. Where evidence of effectiveness has not been produced by research the local service can still set standards. For example, the expected levels of independence to be reached by a group of clients in a community rehabilitation programme of therapy can be specified. Questions that need to be asked concerning effectiveness include the following:

- Does the intervention meet the set objectives?
- Who is defining the objectives? (Client, carer or therapist?)
- Is the intervention justified, or is it better not to intervene at all?
- Is the outcome a result of the intervention? (Or of other factors?)

Efficiency

Efficiency is where the intervention and outcome are achieved with the optimal use of all resources available. Resources should be used to achieve a high quality service for as many people as possible. Factors to be considered include: an efficient choice of skill mix (expertise and grade of health worker); the cost of travelling to clients; the length and frequency of therapy needed for a desired outcome, and the choice or combination of group and individual therapy.

Fair access

This is the access to and delivery of health care across geographical locations, age, gender, social and cultural background. Everyone should have equal quality of service, including referral and choice of treatment.

Access

Everyone should have sufficiently prompt access to an appropriate level of service. Access includes: physical access to buildings; transport to get to services; languages and methods available to enable communication; referral to, and treatment from, the appropriate grade and profession of health worker, and realistic waiting times for referral and treatment.

Appropriateness

The service must meet an individual's needs and preferences. This includes provision and delivery of health care which is sensitive to the complexity of an individual's needs, including their dignity. Treatment should be carried out using appropriate therapy (for example, creative therapy, counselling, skills training), in the appropriate setting (such as home, community centre or hospital), either with the individual or as part of a group.

CLINICAL AUDIT

Clinical audit is used to ensure that the above aspects of quality are being adequately delivered by local services. Clinical audit is an opportunity to do something about an aspect of practice, or the quality of a service, that needs improving.

Clinicians, through their daily experience, often suspect that something is not working as well as it should but feel powerless to change it. By getting together as an audit group staff can unite in leading and owning a process of positive change and take pride in their own professional development.

The audit can be carried out by one professional group, such as occupational therapists, and is then called a uniprofessional audit. When audit is carried out by people from more than one profession it is referred to as a multiprofessional audit (Fig. 9.2).

This is very much a team exercise, carried out by the staff involved in providing the service. Teams often wish to involve their service users to help them identify problems and improve their service. They may wish to bring in people with expertise from other areas. Most organisations have audit staff who can help with the audit design and the collection and analysis of information.

The audit process is cyclical, as shown in Figure 9.3, using stages adapted from the recommendations of the NCCA (1997). The process involves getting all the people on board who influence the day-to-day delivery of services. These stakeholders meet to select a suitable topic and plan the audit (design). Once the necessary data have been collected and analysed (measure), the results are compared with good practice or agreed standards (present and analyse). If standards are met, this is fed back to stakeholders and the service continued. If the standards are not met changes are made to improve clinical services (act to improve). These changes must be re-audited to check that good practice has been achieved (repeat audit).

Design

Stakeholders

It is important that everyone in the team is committed to using the information collected in an audit to develop improvements that are actually carried out. This is helped by:

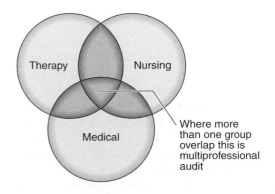

Figure 9.2 Uniprofessional and multiprofessional audits.

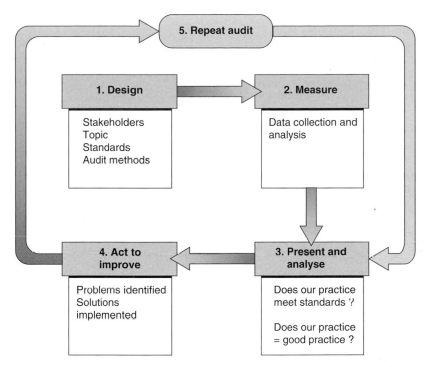

Figure 9.3 The clinical audit process: repeated cycles.

- including all the people who have the power to change practice
- a team that is committed to examining its own practice and making improvements for the benefit of its clients
- a team that is able to make decisions and carry out agreed changes in policy and practice
- an audit coordinator who will keep the audit process on track towards fulfilling the agreed purpose
- a management structure that supports the audit process and the recommendations that may arise from individual audits.

Topic

If staff are going to spend time and effort collecting information and attending audit meetings, it is imperative that they select a topic that is relevant to local needs and has a clearly defined purpose.

The audit team can brainstorm issues to generate a list of topics that they are keen to audit in order to improve the service. Having generated a list of areas that are of local concern, the next step is to select one topic to audit. The following suggestions for selecting a suitable topic have been adapted from the criteria proposed by Walshe (1994):

1. *Start small.* If inexperienced, or intimidated by the audit process, start small. Focus on a small area of work that requires minimal data collection over a short period of time. The audit group will then be able to analyse the data quickly, suggest a way forward and implement their solutions to see prompt results.

2. *Get advice.* The local clinical audit or quality department will advise on the feasibility of favoured topics. They will help with the selection and planning of each audit and the resources needed to investigate different topics (staff time, effort, administration and computer software).

3. *Focus on an important area of practice.* This may be something that concerns many clients, or is very costly, or involves a high risk to clients.

4. *Check that improvements are possible.* Ensure that practical solutions can be found that will not be dependent on factors outside the control of the audit group.

5. *Check that colleagues agree.* The standards that are required for a quality service in this area of practice need to be agreed. If not, there may be a need for research, rather than audit, to be carried out to ascertain what is considered to be good practice.

6. *Reflect current concerns.* Choose a topic that reflects the current concerns of user groups, commissioners and providers. These concerns may include, for example, whether a particular group in the local community has equitable access to the service, whether an expensive service is worth continuing, or whether a recent innovation is providing an acceptable and effective service and should therefore be expanded.

The purpose of the audit should be defined in writing. At the end of the audit process it will then be possible to evaluate whether or not the purpose was fulfilled. The defined purpose needs to specify:

- the quality area
- the client group
- the service.

In a mental health service, the purposes of audit may be, for example:

- to increase the effectiveness of occupational therapy in improving the daily living skills of people attending a rehabilitation programme in a day service
- to ensure that people with enduring mental health problems who are homeless, or in temporary accommodation, have fair access to community services
- to ensure that activity based groups in the community are acceptable to, and meeting the needs of, elderly service users.

Once the purpose has been defined and a suitable topic chosen, the next stage is to set the standards and plan the audit.

Standards

Explicit standards are agreed formally by the audit group, after they have studied recommendations from research, clinical guidelines, user views and professional experts. For the level of the standards a choice is made between:

- *minimum*: lowest acceptable standard of performance
- *ideal*: attainable under ideal conditions with no local constraints, and
- *optimum*: the performance most likely to be achieved under normal conditions of practice (Irvine & Irvine 1997).

When an audit relies on implicit standards that are not stated in advance but exist in the minds of clinicians (for instance in a peer review of case notes), the danger is that practice will be viewed more favourably than it merits (NCCA 1997).

Audit methods

There are three aspects to selecting the audit methods: formulating an audit question, choosing an audit method and deciding what measures to use.

Formulating an audit question involves specifying exactly what information is needed so that staff do not waste their time. Any question concerning audit investigates one or more of the following aspects of the service (Donabedian 1980):

- *structure*: organisation, resources, communications, staff training
- *process*: referral system, assessment procedures, therapeutic techniques and relationships
- *outcomes*: the benefits of therapy experienced by the client.

Sometimes it will be most useful to collect information about the past (*retrospective* data collection), or information is needed about present clinical work (*concurrent* data collection), or future practice may be audited (*prospective* data collection).

The method selected for collecting and analysing data should be the most suitable and practical. This will depend on:

- who will be investigated: the sample of clients or staff (for example a random sample of 50 out of all the 200 people treated last year, or a convenient sample of the last 50 cases to be referred to the service, or a total sample of all the occupational therapy staff currently employed)
- how the data will be collected (for example by studying existing referrals or client records, or by using an instrument, such as questionnaire, interview guide or standardised test).
- how the data will be analysed (quantitatively, for example, using averages and percentages displayed in tables, graphs or charts, or qualitatively, seeking emerging themes, patterns and ranges of opinion)
- who will do it
- what the time frame will be.

A common audit method is the Criterion Based Audit in which performance is compared to standards. Other methods include Retrospective Case Load Analysis, Adverse Occurrences (used to audit and improve undesirable practice), and Patient Surveys of satisfaction, needs, quality of life and usefulness of communications (Sealey 1998). Further methods of audit are: Peer Review or review of clients' cases by colleagues; Critical Path Analysis of care pathways; Activity Analysis, quantifying all the major service processes, and Confidential Enquiries, investigating significant events such as suicides (Irvine & Irvine 1997). All methods are strengthened by the inclusion of standard setting. Some examples of appropriate methods of data collection and analysis to suit different purposes are shown in Table 9.1.

Outcome measures have been developed to assist in the process of evaluating interventions. These can be classified into standardised and individualised measures (Cook 1995).

Standardised outcome measures

Measures used in research can be used for the purposes of clinical audit. These tools have been developed to measure the same aspect of illness or

Table 9.1   Methods of collecting and analysing data in clinical audit

Purpose	Data collection	Data analysis
To check that documentation meets required standards (process)	Review case notes (retrospective)	Use a checklist and score each set of notes against a list of criteria that meet the standards. Identify which criteria are not being met
To check standards of care meet the minimum standards required in clinical guidelines (process)	Review case notes in peer review meetings (concurrent)	Identify deficits and the causes of these
To prevent suicide attempts during admission (structure, process and outcomes)	Adverse event screening. Investigate past suicide events and collect data from staff, clients and carers on why they happened (retrospective)	Identify causal factors and items of service delivery and communication that need changing
To ensure effectiveness of group therapy. Standards set in accordance with evidence based practice: using published outcomes for the same population of clients experiencing the same therapy (outcomes)	Criterion audit. Measure clients' outcomes with a standardised test administered before and after the course of therapy (prospective)	Test for statistical and clinical significance, compare with standards
To increase clients' satisfaction with the service (outcomes)	Patient satisfaction questionnaire, group interviews with clients, or in-depth interviews with a purposeful sample of clients	Quantitative and qualitative analysis to identify current levels of satisfaction and to suggest improvements to aspects of the service

well-being across a large population of people. Standardised measures can be concerned with very generalised aspects of health, such as the SF 36 Health Status Questionnaire (Ware 1993) or the Quality of Life Scale (Malm et al 1981, Fabian 1990). The Health of the Nation Outcome Scale (HoNOS) is a popular tool for auditing within mental health services (Royal College of Psychiatrists 1994). Standardised measures are also available to measure more specific aspects of health, such as: symptomatology, for example, the Brief Psychiatric Rating Scale (BPRS) (Overall & Gorham 1962) and the SCL-90 R measure (Derogotis et al 1973); changes in specific emotional states, such as the Hospital Anxiety and Depression (HAD) Scale (Zigmond & Snaith 1983) and changes in social function (Birchwood et al 1990). The effects of specific therapies or rehabilitation are measured with scales such as the Therapy Outcome Measure (TOM) (Enderby 1997) which includes scales for people with anxiety, cognitive difficulties or a diagnosis of schizophrenia.

If standardised outcome measures are used, the results of previous research will be available to show the scores that suggest a level of success for a particular therapy or service to be judged as effective. These results can be used to set standards for a local clinical audit. It is then possible to use a standardised measure to audit whether clients have achieved clinically significant outcomes according to evidence based practice. An example is given in Box 9.1.

Individualised outcome measures

Individualised measures have the advantage of defining each outcome according to what is pertinent to the individual client. The desired outcome is either the solving of particular problems or the attainment of specific goals. Having defined the starting point and the content and level of the desired outcomes, progress can be measured either by auditing whether the outcomes have been achieved, 'yes' or 'no' (Spreadbury & Cook 1995), or by assessing progress on a scale (Milne & Learmonth 1991). This may be a scale of indicators (Le Roux 1993) or a scale of performance and satisfaction, such

---

Box 9.1   Use of a standardised measure

A community mental health team used the SCL-90-R to audit the following:

- The number of users of anxiety management groups whose scores changed from above the normal level of symptomatology before therapy, to within the normal range of symptomatology after therapy. This showed that the proportion of clients with this successful outcome was comparable with the proportion in published research.

- Whether the scores of people presenting with anxiety, who attended a set number of group sessions, were comparable to the scores reported in research for similar clients who had attended the same number of individual therapy sessions. The scores were very similar and it was concluded that group sessions were more efficient in terms of cost.

---

as the Canadian Occupational Performance Measure (COPM; Law et al 1991).

Individual problems or goals are specified by, or at least negotiated with, the client. If this is not possible then a carer may be consulted. Problems or goals need to be carefully defined so that they are measurable by the client's self-reporting (COPM) or by observation. In order for an outcome to be observed, some individualised measures require each outcome to be operationalised into an item of behaviour (Ottenbacher & Cusick 1990). For example, the goal 'to feel more confident in meeting new people' may be operationalised by a client into 'join the darts team at the local pub'. These measures can be integrated with clinical records so that no extra data collection is required.

Measure

Having involved the stakeholders in the audit team and designed the audit, the next task is to collect and analyse the measurement data. It is important that this stage is done reasonably quickly, otherwise the audit team will lose interest and lose motivation to use the audit to improve services. It may be necessary to pilot the audit methods, measures and data collection forms and to check that reliable and accurate data are generated. When a measurement involves judgement of what is done or achieved it is important to check that those doing the assessment agree with each other. Ethics and confidentiality must be respected as rigorously as in a research project. This may require advice from the local ethical committee prior to carrying out the audit.

Analysis of data may require the use of a handwritten spreadsheet or computer software programmes such as Microsoft Excel or the Statistical Package for Social Sciences (SPSS). Often, the amount of data collected falls short of the desired size of the sample. This needs analysing so that it is clear how representative the results are, for instance, a 35% response rate to a patient satisfaction survey does not give an adequate picture of clients' views. Descriptive statistics, such as counts, mean averages and percentages, are often sufficient for an audit, and easily understood by all staff, managers and clients.

Present and analyse

The audit team now meets and collaborates in a systematic problem solving process in order to utilise the data that have been collected. The steps are as follows:

1. Present the audit results in clear, accessible formats using charts and diagrams and summary reports. Remember, busy staff do not have time to read a long document.
2. Compare the results with the pre-set standards, reveal failings and gaps, and then identify the causes of these deficits. Results can also reveal successes which identify good practice and the need to resource the continuation of the service.
3. Generate creative solutions to the identified problems and ways of building on good practice.
4. Decide which solutions are practicable and most likely to fulfil the purpose of the audit. These may require changes to practice or to a service, staff training and professional development, different skill mix and staff roles or staffing levels, changes in resources and commissioning of services or the development of policy.

Act to improve

The next stage is to change day-to-day practice in the local service. This is a challenging process for everyone but, if those who have to make the changes are the people who have been involved in the audit from the beginning, there will be enthusiasm rather than resistance. The steps to implement improvements include:

1. Decide on who is responsible for carrying out the improvements and set a time frame for implementation.
2. Ensure the necessary resources are available.
3. Inform and consult with all staff and clients on why and how things are going to improve.
4. Make the changes and improvements.
5. Plan the repeat audit.
6. Confirm or re-set a standard to be met concerning the required improvement.

Repeat audit

A repeat audit is essential to check that changes have been implemented, that the new standards have been reached and that there is a genuine improvement in the clinical service. If standards are still not being met, the audit cycle needs to be repeated until the clinical practice and service are satisfactory. It is important that those involved are kept on board during these repeated cycles and have clear, frequent communication about audit results and the achievements of staff and the service. Positive feedback is vital to maintain staff morale. Even if a desired standard is not yet met, the efforts of staff and moves towards improvement can be praised.

EXAMPLE OF CLINICAL AUDIT

The following study is an example of clinical audit being used for a clearly defined purpose which concerns the quality of care. Aspects of this example have been taken from actual clinical audits, but the example in its entirety is fictitious in order to preserve anonymity.

EXAMPLE: A MULTIDISCIPLINARY AUDIT OF CARE PROGRAMMES FOR PEOPLE WITH SEVERE AND ENDURING MENTAL HEALTH PROBLEMS

Design

Representatives of the different professions in a community mental health team met with clerical staff and user representatives to design a clinical audit (Phillips 1996, Sainsbury Centre 1996). They realised that care programming and the delivery of care is complex and multifaceted (DoH 1995), and that several aspects could be audited (NHS Executive 1996). They decided to prioritise a few aspects that urgently needed improving so that staff would stay motivated. These concerned clients' satisfaction, documentation and outcomes of care. The chosen audit method was a criterion audit. Optimum standards were set with reference to external sources such as research evidence (Irvine & Irvine 1997). For example, the outcome standard was set with reference to similar investigations in which 68% and 85% of treatment goals were fully achieved (Macpherson et al 1999). Criteria and standards were set as in Box 9.2.

Measure

All care programme meetings within a 3-month period were audited. After each care programme meeting, the care programme coordinator dis-cussed the meeting with the client and asked for feedback using a brief, client satisfaction questionnaire.

Goals were defined and measured using the Binary Individualised Outcome Measure (Spreadbury & Cook 1995) and a scale developed by Eames and colleagues (1999):

0. Goal not fully achieved
   0.1 information/education given to patient/carer for action
   0.2 awaiting service from another agency
   0.3 plan/treatment discontinued
1. Goal fully achieved

One of the clerical staff examined the care programme documentation which included a goal achievement section. She created data checking sheets that listed the audit criteria. Data were entered onto a spreadsheet using Microsoft Word Excel computer software. The data were analysed quantitatively with descriptive statistics, and displayed in charts. The results of the first audit were presented to a meeting of the audit group.

Present and analyse

The audit group was presented with the results of the first audit (Table 9.2). During the 3-month period, 115 care programme meetings were held. Satisfaction data were gathered after 82 (71%) meetings and only 95 (56%) of the surveyed clients were satisfied on all three criteria. From

---

Box 9.2 Criteria and standards for care programming

Structure:
Criterion: The client is satisfied with the care programming meeting. **Standard = 80%**
Satisfaction with: 1. Place of meeting; 2. Who attended the meeting; 3. Whether his or her views were listened to.

Process:
Criterion: Care programme documentation is fully completed. **Standard = 75%**
Components: 1. Client, key worker, main carer, and those attending meeting named;
2. Previous period and the goals achieved reported; 3. Goals defined, action planned
and those responsible for achieving them; and 4. Time frame and next meeting planned.

Outcome:
Criterion: Goals fully achieved within planned time frame. **Standard = 70%**

Table 9.2 Current practice compared with standards (first audit)

	Percentages		
	Client satisfaction	Documentation	Goal achievement
Standard	80	75	70
First audit results	56	50	57
Shortfall	*24*	*25*	*13*

112 (97%) sets of care programme documents, all five criteria were met in only 56 (50%) documents. Goal achievement was reported in only 62 (55%) documents, with an average of 3.8 goals having previously been set per client (236 goals in total). Within this incomplete sample, 135 (57%) goals were fully achieved. When compared with the standards, major shortfalls were identified.

Act to improve

The audit group learned from the satisfaction survey that clients did not like coming to the community mental health team building for their care programme meetings. They wanted somewhere more local and familiar, such as their GP surgery or the new healthy living centre where some of the therapeutic groups met. Although less convenient for staff, it was decided to try and vary the venues for meetings. The occupational therapist agreed to approach the healthy living centre, and the community mental health nurse reported that two GP surgeries (frequented by many of the clients) were keen to host care programme meetings. A few clients requested meetings in their own homes. It was decided to add 'place of next meeting' to the documentation.

The standard of documentation was good for names and arrangements, which was pleasing as this had previously been a problem. The group were also pleased that goal setting was being recorded fairly well, following recent training of all staff. The problem was that staff were not recording adequately the recent experiences and achievements of clients. Everyone agreed that

these were being discussed in the meetings but often the discussion went off on a tangent. It was decided to:

1. have a designated chair of each meeting whose job it was to make sure goal achievement was reported
2. provide a half-day training for staff to improve their recording skills
3. circulate an example of how the documentation should be completed.

This was the first period when the community mental health team had tried to record outcomes of care in a systematic way, so they were very interested in the results. The goal achievement results suggested that outcomes were particularly poor when clients and carers were expected to act on information and education that they had been given by staff. Failed outcomes included: clients rejecting medication changes, family tensions not being resolved, and clients not pursuing opportunities in the community for leisure, social contact and work. A meeting was held with the whole community mental health team at which research evidence and local practice were discussed.

The consensus from this meeting was that, although the team had access to a great deal of information, they were not spending enough time sharing it in accessible ways with clients. Action that was agreed was:

1. Three staff (two nurses and one social worker) who had additional training in psychosocial interventions for people with psychosis to have their case loads trimmed so they could spend more time offering psycho-educational approaches with clients and their families (Fadden 1998, Pharoah et al 1999).
2. The senior 2 occupational therapist together with one of the patient representatives to set up a sharing information group for people with psychotic experiences (Buccheri et al 1996).
3. The employment of two part-time support workers to spend time helping clients to make use of information and opportunities in the community (Sainsbury Centre 1999). The support

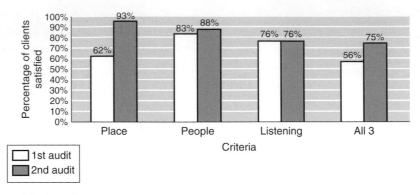

Figure 9.4 Clients' satisfaction with care programme meetings.

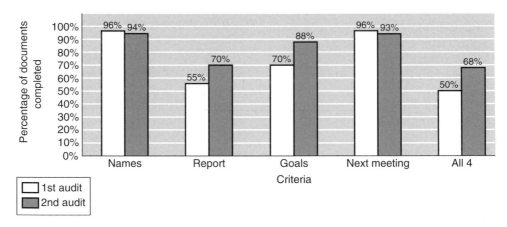

Figure 9.5 Documentation of care programme meetings.

workers would be supervised by the senior occupational therapist.

It was decided to implement these changes over the next 3 months and then re-audit over the following 3 months.

Repeat audit

The audit team and the community mental health team were presented with charts that clearly showed changes between the first and second audits (Figs 9.4, 9.5 and 9.6). The second audit showed that improvements had been made but further developments were still needed, as shown in Table 9.3.

Clients were happier coming to care programme meetings in places of their choice. There was no improvement, however, with how clients felt they were listened to (Fig. 9.4).

Table 9.3 Current practice compared with standards (second audit)

	Percentages		
	Client satisfaction	Documentation	Goal achievement
Standard	80	75	70
Second audit results	75	68	72
Shortfall	*5*	*7*	*+2*

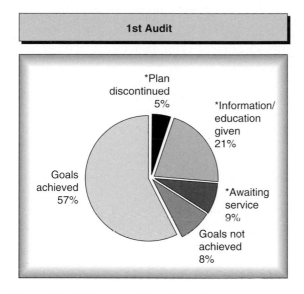

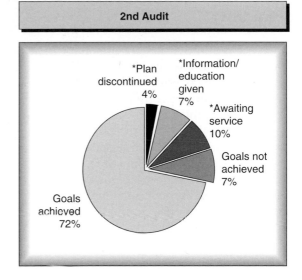

Figure 9.6   Achievement of goals set in care programme meetings.

It was decided to set up training of staff by mental health service user/trainers (NHS Executive Mental Health Task Force User Group 1994). It was agreed that the new user involvement development worker would be asked to help organise this.

Documentation had mostly improved. There were a few problems with recording the place of the next meeting, and reporting on progress and goal achievement still needed to improve (Fig. 9.5). Not all staff had attended a half-day training on recording goals, so it was decided to include it in the formal induction of new staff, and instigate regular small group peer review meetings to discuss individual cases and goal setting and evaluation.

Outcomes in terms of overall goal achievement had improved from 57% to 72%, which was just above the standard of 70%. Goals *not* fully achieved had decreased, including when information/education had been given to patients or carers for action (Fig. 9.6).

The audit group evaluated the audit process (Walshe & Coles 1993) and commented that the process itself was educational and motivated staff to focus on areas of their daily work that needed improvement. Staff enjoyed the positive feedback on their achievements as they often felt under-appreciated. Someone said it was the first time that they had ever been told the results of an audit. Previously, they had collected data for managers and never had any feedback. The clerical worker was thanked for all her data gathering. Limitations of the audit methods were noted, including:

- the reliability and validity of the data were compromised
- clients may have felt they had to please staff when asked to complete the satisfaction questionnaire
- the sample for the first and second audits did not contain exactly the same clients
- outcome data relied on the goal achievement that was recorded and may not have accurately reflected what was actually achieved
- although the expectation was that goals would be achieved through a programme of therapeutic interventions, the attainment or lack of achievement may have been due to external factors experienced by people in their daily lives.

Despite these drawbacks, the audit group felt that their clinical audit had reflected staff's clinical practice and clients' experiences and, most importantly, had led to real improvements in practice.

SUMMARY

Quality and effectiveness are important issues in health care, and are here to stay under the umbrella of clinical governance. The drive to re-assess clinical interventions constantly and to improve service delivery must become an important part of the occupational therapy process. It is imperative that clinical audit cycles are repeated until necessary improvements are achieved, rather than the audit carried out just once and then forgotten.

Issues of quality concern the service as a whole, as well as the individual's treatment.

Quality assurance and clinical audit can be combined to practise continuous quality improvements in clinical care, as well as making real changes to the service.

Outcomes of intervention should meet the standards of effectiveness that have been suggested by research or through local consultation with staff and users. Methods of recording and measuring the effectiveness of interventions are becoming more sophisticated and more user-friendly, both to therapist and client. Outcome measurement (using standardised and individualised tools) should be part of routine clinical practice as well as being useful for clinical audit.

REFERENCES

Birchwood M, Smith J et al 1990 The Social Functioning Scale: the development and validation of a new scale of social adjustment for use in family intervention programmes with schizophrenic patients. British Journal of Psychiatry 157: 853–859

Buccheri R, Trygstad L, Kanas N, Waldron B, Dowling G 1996 Auditory hallucinations in schizophrenia: group experience in examining symptom management and behavioural strategies. Journal of Psychosocial Nursing 34(2): 12–26

Cook 1995 The merits of individualised outcome measures within routine clinical practice. Outcomes Briefing 6: 15–18. UK Clearing House on Health Outcomes, Leeds

Department of Health 1991 The patient's charter: raising the standard. HMSO, London

Department of Health 1995 Building bridges. Department of Health, London

Department of Health 1997 The new NHS. Modern. Dependable. Department of Health, London

Department of Health 1999 A first class service: quality in the new NHS. Department of Health, London

Derogotis L R, Lipman R S, Covi 1973 SCL-90: an outpatient rating scale: preliminary report. Psychopharmacology Bulletin 9: 13–23. The SCL-90-R is available from NCS Assessments, 27 Church Road, Hove, East Sussex BN3 2FA

Donabedian A 1980 The definition of quality and approaches to its assessment. Health Administration Press, Michigan

Eames J, Ward G, Siddons L 1999 Clinical audit of the outcome of individualised occupational therapy goals. British Journal of Occupational Therapy 62(6): 257–260

Enderby P 1998 Therapy outcome measures, physiotherapy, occupational therapy, rehabilitation nursing. Singular, London

Fabian E 1990 Quality of life: a review of theory and practice implications for individuals with long-term mental illness. Rehabilitation Psychology 35(3): 161–169

Fadden G 1998 Family intervention in psychosis. Journal of Mental Health 7(2): 115–122

Firth-Cozens J 1993 Audit in mental health services. Lawrence Erlbaum, Hove

Irvine D, Irvine S 1997 Making sense of audit, 2nd edn. Radcliffe, New York

Law M, Baptiste S, Carswell-Opzoomer A, McCall M, Polatajko H, Pollock N 1991 Canadian Occupational Performance Measure. Canadian Association of Occupational Therapists, Toronto

Le Roux A A 1993 TELER: the concept. Physiotherapy 79(11): 755–758

Macpherson R, Jerrom B, Lott G, Ryce M 1999 The outcome of clinical goal setting in a mental health rehabilitation service: a model evaluating clinical effectiveness. Journal of Mental Health 8(1): 95–102

Malm U, May P R A, Deneker S J 1981 Evaluation of the quality of life of the schizophrenic outpatient: a checklist. Schizophrenia Bulletin 7(3): 476–485

Milne D, Learmonth M 1991 How to evaluate an occupational therapy service: a case study. British Journal of Occupational Therapy 54(2): 42–44

Morrell C, Harvey G 1999 The clinical audit handbook: improving the quality of health care. Baillière Tindall, London

National Centre for Clinical Audit 1997 Key points in the audit literature related to criteria for clinical audit. National Centre for Clinical Audit/NICE

NHS Executive Mental Health Task Force User Group 1994 Building on experience: a training pack for mental health service users working as trainers, speakers and workshop facilitators. Department of Health, London

NHS Executive 1996 An audit pack for monitoring the Care Programme Approach. Department of Health, London

Ottenbacher H, Cusick A 1990 Goal attainment scaling as a method of clinical evaluation. American Journal of Occupational Therapy 44(6): 519–525

Overall J E, Gorham D R 1962 The brief psychiatric rating scale. Psychological Reports 10: 799–812

Pharoah F M, Mari J J, Streiner D 1999 Family intervention for schizophrenia. Cochrane Database of Systematic Reviews (2)

Phillips P 1996 How to plan your own care review meeting. The Advocate: Journal of the United Kingdom Advocacy Network late summer (1): 13

Royal College of Psychiatrists 1994 Health of the nation outcome scales: 4th draft. Royal College of Psychiatrists, London

Sainsbury Centre 1996 Mental Health Quality Assurance Network. Special issue: User involvement in quality improvements. Q-Net 3. Sainsbury Centre for Mental Health, London

Sainsbury Centre 1999 More than a friend: role of support workers in community mental health services. Sainsbury Centre for Mental Health, London

Sealey C 1998 Clinical audit information pack: a resource pack to assist occupational therapists with clinical audit and clinical effectiveness. College of Occupational Therapists, London

Spreadbury P, Cook S 1995 Measuring the outcomes of individualised care: the binary individualised outcome measure. Occupational Therapy Department, Nottingham City Hospital NHS Trust, Nottingham

Strong P, Robinson J 1988 New model management: Griffiths and the NHS. Nursing Policy Studies Centre, University of Warwick, Warwick

Walshe K 1994 Making audit work: guidelines on selecting, planning, implementing and evaluating audit projects. CASPE Research and Brighton Health Care Department of Research and Clinical Audit, Brighton

Walshe K, Coles J 1993 Evaluating audit: developing a framework. CASPE Research. 22 Palace Court, Bayswater, London W2 4HU

Ware J 1993 Measuring patients' views: the optimum outcome measure. SF 36: a valid, reliable assessment of health from the patient's point of view. British Medical Journal 306: 1429–1430

Zigmond A S, Snaith R P 1983 The Hospital Anxiety and Depression scale. Acta Psychiatrica Scandinavica 67: 361–370

The context of occupational therapy

10

Roles and settings

Cathy Ormston

INTRODUCTION

Mental health care has undergone immense changes over the past decade, with its shift in focus from hospital based services to care in the community following the National Health Service and Community Care Act 1991 (DoH 1990). Further radical reforms for mental health services were outlined by central government in *Modernising Mental Health Services* (DoH 1998). This sought to address some of the problems of inequity of service provision across the country, the lack of investment in appropriate in-patient care, and the failure of community care to deliver consistently high standards. A keystone to implementing the reforms was the development of the National Service Framework (NSF) for mental health (DoH 1999). The NSF determines service models and standards for future mental health care, and provides a united vision for all key members of the multidisciplinary team. With its emphasis on multiprofessional and multiagency partnership, and in engaging service users through respectful collaboration, it impacts on the roles of all mental health service providers.

Modern mental health services provide a comprehensive range of services in the community and focus on the individual's needs specific to their own home context. NSF standards demand local, timely and consistent provision that is based on the best available evidence. Intervention goals are as much about helping people achieve optimal function within their community setting, and providing practical support, as it is about treatment of symptoms. With the increased priority given to user involvement, outreach, day care, and home based support, and the elevation of quality of life and functional ability as priorities for care, the role of the occupational therapist has never been so germane.

The decade of development of a community focus to health has, in turn, impacted on the roles and functions of hospital based care. People for whom even the extended range of home treatments, long-term supports, crisis intervention and outreach still cannot prevent relapse severe enough to warrant hospital admission are, by default, likely to be a more disturbed, distressed and vulnerable population than previously. Acute admission stays are shortening, and the proportion of people who are compulsorily detained is rising (Sainsbury Centre, 1999). Similarly, longer-term in-patient services have to address the needs of a much more disabled and challenging group than before – not because mental illnesses have become worse, but because many of those who previously faced years of hospitalisation can now sustain community living; people with needs that make community living unrealistic and who still require hospital care are concentrated in the much reduced hospital wards. Occupational therapists based in in-patient settings will need to adapt to the changing needs of this new hospital population.

Now there is a wider acceptance of the need to address people's ability to function in their home environment, other professionals are embracing roles traditionally seen as particular to the occupational therapist. If the occupational therapist's role and identity is defined by goals and purpose, then it should be acknowledged that this is shared with a wide number of professionals who all aim to enhance independence and function, assist meaningful engagement in community settings, and improve quality of life, as well as decrease people's distress and vulnerability to symptoms. Defined this way, the occupational therapist adopts a number of roles generic to any mental health worker in a contemporary service context. However, if occupational therapists' roles are defined by the specific part they play,

that is, what they do to contribute to the team as a whole, then it is easier to distinguish their profession-specific roles.

Occupational therapists working in multidisciplinary teams, in widely dispersed settings, have to respond flexibly to a client-centred approach in which a number of generic skills are needed. This chapter therefore aims to explore the balance of generic and specialist, core, acquired and required roles of occupational therapists, in various mental health settings. It focuses on the occupational therapist as an individual professional, and on the interface with other team members.

INFLUENCES ON THE OCCUPATIONAL THERAPIST'S ROLE

As we view each service user as a unique individual with a wide repertoire of roles, so every occupational therapist has a unique part to play in their distinct setting with a similar diversity of roles and functions, influenced by a complex interplay of intrinsic and extrinsic factors. Some roles are inherently accepted as core to occupational therapy, others are aspired to and achieved through growing competence and credibility, and some are thrust upon the therapist by colleagues, employers and service users.

EXTRINSIC FACTORS

National policy and local implementation

The contexts in which occupational therapists operate influence both the roles available to them and those demanded of them. The priorities of each service are determined by both national and local health and social strategies. For example, national mental health policy has focused on improving community responses to people with severe, long-term mental health problems who do not traditionally engage with services. The Sainsbury Centre for Mental Health's influential report *Keys to Engagement* (Sainsbury Centre 1998) reviewed care for this client group, and made recommendations targeted at central and local government, and the NHS, regarding the developments needed to achieve the right mix of day-to-day engagement and active health care and rehabilitation. The *National Service Framework for Mental Health* (DoH 1999) supported the recommendations, and included the availability, in all localities, of services based on an assertive outreach model, as a milestone in monitoring progress towards delivering elements of standards 4 and 5 of the framework (the standards relating to developing effective services for people with severe mental illness). These teams have a definitive model of operation (Stein & Test 1980, Sainsbury Centre 1998) based on growing evidence of effective practice for work with people with psychoses (Lehman et al 1997, Marshall & Lockwood 1998). The model includes the use of bio-psycho-social interventions, cognitive therapy, family psychoeducational interventions, team responsibility rather than key-worker relationships, extended hours of availability, intensive contact over months or years, and rights for direct hospital admission. Thus the shaping of the role of an occupational therapist employed in such an environment can be demonstrably linked to central government policy, local priorities and strategic planning within health and/or social services, research evidence, as well as the strategic planning of the employing NHS Trust.

Roles and work setting

There is an ever growing range of settings where occupational therapists may work, all of which are subject to the same complex array of defining influences as that cited above. Though service patterns and configurations vary regionally, the following are some common examples:

- *In-patient services*
    acute admission wards
    rehabilitation units
    services for people with 'challenging behaviour'
    long-term and continuing/intensive care wards
    specialist services, e.g. forensic/medium secure; drug and alcohol; mother and baby; eating disorder
    elderly services – short-term assessment/continuing care
    child and adolescent units

- *Day services*
    day hospitals/partial hospitalisation programmes (NHS)
    day centres (Social Services)
    combined day services (NHS/Social Services/non-statutory)
    employment and training projects
    mobile day hospitals/services

- *Community services*
    community mental health centres/teams
    assertive outreach services
    home treatment teams
    specialist services, e.g. drug and alcohol; homeless; dual diagnosis; child and adolescent mental health services
    primary care services
    hostels and group homes
    residential care homes (social services).

The particular constellation of roles the occupational therapist will fulfil in each of these will be influenced by a wide range of factors that may include:

- the client group at whom the service is targeted and the purpose for which the team exists
- the skill mix of the particular team – the personal qualities and skills of the particular team member, and the mix of professionals
- team resources – roles may need to be more flexible in a team with few resources
- the clarity (or otherwise) of the team's individual job descriptions and the effective use of performance management to craft the team roles to meet shared service objectives
- particular service philosophies, operational models and the dominance of a specific treatment or intervention framework
- the management style and background of the team leader
- the existence of the post as a single-handed occupational therapy practitioner or as part of an occupational therapy team

- the status afforded to the occupational therapist and degree of resultant autonomy
- cultural norms and historical expectations that predetermine accepted roles within a pre-existing team.

INTRINSIC FACTORS

Though the tangible roles and functions of an occupational therapist will be outlined in a job description, a whole number of issues individual to each therapist will influence role performance. This includes essential personality traits, professional philosophy and internal schema regarding her role as an occupational therapist working in mental health as well as individual interest.

Experience

The scope and depth of therapist's previous experience will have a direct bearing on the roles they comfortably undertake. Clearly, an occupational therapist with several years' experience is more likely to seek out – or be offered – opportunities to act as project leader, supervisor, or chair of a management group than someone new to a field or recently qualified.

As individuals amass a greater body of knowledge, based on a widening body of experience, the complexity of their clinical reasoning develops and will have consequent impact on their occupational therapy role. As Schon (1991) puts it: 'as a practitioner experiences many variations of a small number of types of case, he is able to "practice" his practice. He develops a repertoire of expectations, images and techniques. He learns what to look for and how to respond to what he finds.' Hagedorn (1995) refers to the 'value of experience in building the therapist's mental "database" ', leading to the development of a sound cognitive construct of occupational therapy, and an ability to visualise a possible sequence of events leading to actions based on multiple hypotheses. Proficient practitioners with this advanced repertoire of expectation demonstrate greater flexibility, creativity and an increased ability to consider wider issues when finding solutions than their less experienced

colleagues, whether other occupational therapists or members of the multidisciplinary team. These personal characteristics of therapists will affect the roles and status afforded them.

Personal traits

In addition to the roles described within the occupational therapist's job description, the therapist's personality and preferred working roles will influence the contributions she makes within a team. An example is Belbin's (1981) work on teams which characterises members' preferred behaviours and roles demonstrating the very different strengths people bring to the overall functioning of the team. He postulates that effective teams need a wide range of personality types, and advocates the use of team role analysis in recruitment, selection and development. A team needs innovators, lateral thinkers and people to generate enthusiasm and creativity, but must also have a body of people able to focus on a task, seek out resources, and complete projects. The individual occupational therapist's own preferred work style will undoubtedly affect the role she undertakes within her team.

Another example of actively recruiting particular people with particular attitudes and personal attributes for the role they may then contribute is in selecting staff who can sustain low levels of 'expressed emotion' (EE) in their relationships with service users into teams working with people with severe mental illness. Work by Kuipers (Kuiper & Moore 1995) suggests that relapse rates in people with psychosis are positively influenced by family or care groups who demonstrate low EE; it is suggested that this knowledge be utilised when recruiting and training staff for this client group so as to maximise the likelihood that staff will not become frustrated in the face of repeated failure, and will not generally blame service users for their difficulties (Ball et al 1992, Shepherd 1998).

The person's level of professional autonomy will also be a key factor influencing the occupational therapist's role. Many occupational therapists work single-handedly in a multidisciplinary team. The expectations of their colleagues, and demands from managers of different professional backgrounds, can lead to the therapist's role moving away from their core competencies and priorities as an occupational therapist (Peck & Norman 1999). Therapists may embrace generic roles that are seen as valuable to the team as a means of gaining acceptance within the group, providing the same interventions as their colleagues regardless of whether this makes best use of their occupational therapy skills.

Sometimes occupational therapists take on roles because the other team members are reluctant to take them on, without analysis of whether this is appropriate. Individuals need sufficient professional autonomy with the scope to define their occupational therapy priorities, and a robust internal schema of their occupational therapy role.

Individual values and interests

Therapists' personal and professional interests will contribute to their assumed role. For example, one occupational therapist may believe strongly in preventive work and the contributions occupational therapy can make in promoting healthy lifestyles with a broad range of clients, offering an 'open door' policy for referrals; another believes it important to target services for people whose illness has a severe impact on function. Meeson's (1998) study of the factors influencing the practice of a group of community occupational therapists demonstrated that the therapist's personal interest in a specific area (for example anxiety management, creative therapies, supportive counselling and problem solving) was a key factor influencing her choice of intervention with an individual, and hence the team role she assumed. Meeson noted that personal preferences seemed to be linked also with familiarity, knowledge and previous experience rather than with a particular theoretical perspective.

Occupational therapists who have undertaken postgraduate training in a specialist area are likely to use it to develop the role they play within a team, perhaps acting as researcher, family worker, or advisor/supervisor for a specific approach, for example cognitive therapy.

INTRINSIC AND EXTERNAL INFLUENCES ON ROLE – IN PRACTICE

Other chapters describe the contribution occupational therapy makes in many of the work settings in detail, but it is interesting to take an overview of the similarities and differences in the potential roles of occupational therapists doing very different jobs. The influences discussed above interact to shape the roles of four individual therapists presented here. A summary of their work is followed by an examination of some of the contextual influences on the therapist's role.

Case studies

Anna: working as part of an urban community mental health team...

Anna is a Senior I occupational therapist working from an office base in a busy urban centre. Having been part of the team since its formation 4 years ago, she is perceived by her colleagues as highly skilled, and her advice is often sought by those working with clients with complex needs.

Her mixed caseload reflects clients with a range of problems, but more than half have a long-standing diagnosis of psychosis. Much of her work is with individuals, and their families, in their homes. Her work often involves problem-solving issues concerned with people's day-to-day activities, reflecting on achievements, and talking through plans for the days ahead. She may visit people several times a week if it is felt they are at risk of relapse, and uses part of her visit to help an individual construct coping strategies to deal with triggers that seem to increase their symptoms. Most clients are seen on a weekly basis, or as part of a group.

Anna makes use of local shops and cafes, the market, pub and YMCA with individuals and groups of clients, who are socially isolated, anxious about public spaces, or who are wanting to develop new interests and skills, or for whom simply getting the rent paid and the shopping done is an ordeal. Anna works as a single-handed occupational therapist, but regularly takes students for fieldwork placements. She meets with the head occupational therapist, who manages a number of dispersed community based staff, on a monthly basis, and is currently working with her on a proposal for an additional therapist to relieve the strain of increasing referrals.

Discussion

Without the facilities available in a day centre or occupational therapy department, Anna's work relies less heavily on creative and expressive activities than hospital based colleagues, and more on the productive, leisure or self-care activities connected with people's everyday life. The urban community setting gives Anna opportunities for activities to occur in ordinary, valued settings, and the chance for her clients to feel included in community life as an ordinary citizen. Anna's work as enabler and facilitator is a shared role – other multidisciplinary colleagues also assist people to participate as full citizens as this is a key objective within the team's operational philosophy. Her role in using psychosocial interventions and relapse prevention strategies is also generic to the team, who all operate within a similar theoretical framework.

Her specialist occupational therapy role is more evident in her attention to her clients' needs for meaningful daily occupations: her concern in developing people's life skills, the manner in which she assesses and explores people's occupational goals, and the graded application of activities that are relevant to each person's lifestyle.

Anna's focus on working with people with psychosis can be directly connected to her role as an occupational therapist – the head occupational therapist believes that people with the most severe mental health problems experience the greatest interruption in their role performance and a significant deterioration in their quality of life. As these are key concerns for occupational therapy, Anna's work, like that of the other community occupational therapists under the head occupational therapist's supervision, is directed towards this priority group.

As an established team of 4 years, members are comfortable with role overlap and respect individual skills and experience, thus Anna's role is autonomous, accepted, and advisory to colleagues working with challenging clients.

Additional important roles include supervisor, fieldwork educator, counsellor and family supporter, researcher (preparing information supporting the need for additional resources and gaining information on effective practice), manager (of her own time workload) and administrator.

Tony: working in a rural community mental health centre...

Tony is a senior therapist working in a community mental health team (CMHT) in a rural market town. Tony sees a number of people in small groups, particularly those with depression and anxiety problems. He supervises a support worker, who works with people in their home facilitating self-care activities and providing social activities in church and community halls in the local towns and villages.

Tony has a particular interest in cognitive therapy and is currently undertaking specialist training in this area. He regularly leads anxiety management and relaxation courses in response to the large numbers of referrals he receives from colleagues and believes that this is seen as a highly valuable skill he can contribute to the work of the team.

Once every fortnight, Tony acts as a duty worker for the team, responding to requests for emergency assessments and queries from GPs and other referrers. He holds care coordinator responsibilities within the Care Programme Approach (CPA) for the small number of clients he sees who have more severe and long-term needs, coordinating input from other workers and services, and convening case reviews. Tony works with a community psychiatric nurse (CPN) colleague on a weekly basis at a local GP practice providing a stress clinic and liaising with the primary health care team over a number of clients whose care they share.

Tony is managed by the CMHT manager, with access to the head occupational therapist for advice. He meets with other community occupational therapists throughout his area and receives specialist supervision from a psychologist for his cognitive therapy work.

Discussion

Tony's caseload mix is very typical of many occupational therapists working in community mental health teams. The high demand for work addressing problems connected with anxiety and/or depression is reflective of its high incidence within the spectrum of mental health problems, and echoes the experiences of many community based occupational therapists reported by Meeson (1998) and Harries (1998).

People in rural communities are statistically less likely to suffer from severe mental illness (DoH 1995) and Tony's close contact with primary care has also been significant in shaping his role. General practitioners are pressured by the high number of consultations by people with depression and anxiety-related problems, and hence demand that mental health services provide for this group.

Many of Tony's roles are generic to his community team, for example care manager, group leader, crisis worker, assessor. The duty worker role arose from a team decision that all senior staff would provide duty cover as all were perceived to have the core skills, and sufficient experience, to respond to crises, provide an initial assessment, and coordinate an appropriate first-line response.

Tony is valued for his specialist knowledge within cognitive therapy, and his work is noted for being evidence based (Roth & Fonagy 1996). The team have a pragmatic approach to client allocation: staff take on new referrals according to space within their caseload and to match client need with specific skills (for example expertise in family work, eating disorders, cognitive behavioural therapy), rather than directing clients towards a particular professional. Tony's role as an occupational therapist is made particular use of when he acts as co-worker with a colleague, sharing the care of someone with complex needs who, in addition to CPN support, can particular-

ly benefit from an exploration of their occupational performance and needs, and provision of activity based interventions. As supervisor for the support worker, he can delegate some of this work, extending the number of people he can work with, and enabling him to develop his other roles.

The Care Programme Approach (CPA) ensures that people with severe or enduring problems receive a high quality care plan and a coordinated service, organised by an identified professional with an ongoing responsibility to assess and review ongoing needs and broker a range of services on the client's behalf (DoH 2000). While acting as care coordinator is a role undertaken by all the professionally qualified team members, Tony most often undertakes this function for people who have clear problems in daily living skills, or who want to develop their work skills, two areas which remain identified with occupational therapy (Peck & Norman 1999). Thus he combines a generic role (coordinating care, linking with families and carers, initiating the review process, monitoring progress over an extended period) with that of a specialist assessor and provider of occupational therapy.

CMHTs are typically managed by one person to whom all staff, regardless of profession, are accountable (Ovtrevit 1993) Their effectiveness as a multidisciplinary resource has been the focus of much debate (Onyett & Ford 1996, Shepherd 1998, Norman & Peck 1999). There is clearly a balance to be struck: on the one hand ensuring the sensible cooperation of a group of professionals towards common priorities and ensuring appropriate core generic skills are available in the team as a whole, while on the other hand maintaining a healthy tension between the differing approaches and varied theoretical frameworks contributed by the professions, enabling the distinct professional skills to remain available to clients who really need them (Sainsbury Centre 1997).

As Peck surmised: 'The relative professional isolation of OTs within CMHTs makes them vulnerable to group pressure, and pressure from CMHT managers towards generic working' (Peck & Norman 1999). The need to be accepted by the team, and a readiness to undertake those tasks seen as valued rather than retaining professional distinctness can result in roles becoming so merged as to be indistinguishable. This may not be in the interests of clients who, consequently, have access to a reduced range of potential responses to a given problem. In this instance, Tony clearly identifies with the benefits of being fully integrated within the team, though he often debates with his colleagues the relative merits of specialist versus generic worker. The head occupational therapist contributes to this debate, and gives guidance to his developing role, but ultimately has to defer to the CMHT manager who has the final say on Tony's work priorities and team function.

Sally: working in an acute in-patient setting...

Sally is a basic grade occupational therapist working in an acute admission unit of a psychiatric hospital with a countywide catchment area. Often the clients she sees are in hospital only for a week or two, though some stay for longer, especially those who have been formally detained.

With access to a wide range of facilities within the occupational therapy department, Sally's work may include creative, expressive or domestic activities. There are clients whose distress is such that Sally needs to see them for very short periods, two or three times throughout the day. They work on small, achievable tasks that help rebuild a sense of competence during this very confusing and disempowering period. Others take part in groups targeted at shared problems and issues, or work steadily on plans connected to their goals following discharge. Sally uses the Canadian Occupational Performance Measure (Law et al 1994) to identify priorities for intervention, and to monitor progress towards the goals clients set. Sometimes the goals her clients see as the most important do not coincide with what the multidisciplinary team views as priority. Sally sometimes faces pressure from her colleagues who want her to work to change a person's daily routines.

Team members recognise that, seeing clients in a different context, Sally witnesses different behaviours, emotional responses, strengths and emerging vulnerabilities. She reports how symptoms affect an individual's roles, volition, routines and skills, and describes the progress she sees as people become less symptomatic, or develop ways of coping with residual illness or problems.

Sally shares an office with the team of three occupational therapists and receives fortnightly formal supervision from the senior therapist, who guides her work and provides support, development and training. She supervises the work of an occupational therapy support worker.

Discussion

Sally's role is most influenced by the speed at which people move through the acute admission unit, and by the degree of distress and disturbance people face during this period. She has to focus on short-term goals, yet needs to keep a view to the person's home context, and the longer-term goals as prioritised by the client and identified by the wider team. Sally's role may be catalytic in that she may provoke the beginning of a change in the person's coping strategies and self-esteem and the development of more successful and satisfying roles that she herself never sees to completion but hands over as an ongoing package of care on discharge.

Sally's role is clearly differentiated as an occupational therapist, providing a range of graded, personally tailored activities, and using group processes to achieve occupational goals. The environment in which she works can offer access to many different types of creative, domestic, expressive and work based activities. She often acts as a motivator when acute illness or distress has directly affected people's volition, habits and routines and skills. Sally believes the distinct contribution occupational therapy provides within an acute admission setting is offering an environment in which people can achieve or retain a sense of mastery (for example over materials, media, the purpose and scope of their occupational therapy sessions) when so much else seems out of their personal control.

Sally is perceived as having an important contribution to assessments of strengths and interests and her approach can be more oriented towards solutions than problems (de Shazer 1991, Cade & O'Hanlon 1993). The team are particularly interested to hear feedback on changes in levels of performance in the various activities and interactive settings which may be a significant indicator of the person's overall response to interventions and treatments, or, alternatively, represent relapse indicators (Birchwood et al 1998). Sally similarly needs to glean as much information as possible from her nurse colleagues, who spend a much more intense period of time with the clients, to keep abreast of significant changes, responses to treatment and safety issues.

Sally's nursing colleagues have to exercise differing roles with in-patients, particularly those who are formally detained. Sally has, like any other member of the team, to work towards agreed team objectives expressed in each individual's care plan, and work with close attention to safety and risk, but does not have to cope with the complexities that nursing, medical and social work staff face when they have been directly involved in detaining someone without their consent or giving treatment that is not wanted by the client. This facilitates her role as a collaborator in working with the client, and supports her preference for client centred practice.

Having an insight into what are the primary motivations for individual clients, and exploring their preferred roles, personal performance goals and typical daily routines, Sally sometimes acts as an advocate for clients if the team sets priorities that do not reflect the client's personal drives. This is a difficult role and she has to be ready to recognise the difference between those times when the team can and should be urged to review their plans, and when issues of safety, or a client's unrealistic expectations, require her own view to be revised. As Sally does not have a long history with the team, or extensive personal experience, she has to work carefully to sustain and develop their confidence in her while not unduly compromising her position or her professional viewpoint.

As Sally's clients often experience distressing symptoms (e.g. hallucinatory voices or destructive and compulsive thoughts) which can be alleviated by becoming absorbed in an activity, she often finds herself being asked to 'occupy the clients with something'. At first she worried that her role could be seen as diversional and was reluctant to fulfil this element of the team's expectations of her. Over time, however, she has begun to identify those occasions when specific activities can be graded and applied as a powerful coping mechanism, with the potential for it to become integrated into the person's repertoire of skills for managing residual problems.

Her position as a junior member of a broader occupational therapy team helps Sally consolidate her skills and build on her knowledge. Work requiring greater expertise and development work can be taken on by the senior therapist, or she works alongside her supervisor as a co-therapist. Regular supervision, and the identification of an appropriate role model or mentor is key to sustaining the morale and confidence of staff at all grades (Allan & Ledwith 1998, Blair 1999), but has particular pertinence for Sally as a newly qualified occupational therapist (Rugg 1996).

Karen: working in sectorised elderly services ...

Karen is a head occupational therapist in a sectorised service for older people in an inner city. She has a small caseload of people with functional illnesses, but specialises in working with people with dementia, particularly in its early stages. Some of her time is within an assessment ward in the local hospital; her base is a shared office with her nursing and social work colleagues.

Much of her clinical work is around supporting people during the difficult time when they first are diagnosed as having dementia. Karen plans with individuals how they can maintain as much independence as possible, especially in the areas they place as highest priority, and teaches memory retraining techniques. A lot of time is spent supporting carers and providing them with information to aid their understanding of dementia, as well as working together with families and carers building up portfolios of photographs, personal stories and memories, and information connected to the person's past and current interests and important life events. Karen sometimes assesses for simple adaptive equipment and advises on physical problems that are impeding the person's independence in daily living skills.

Karen leads a team of four occupational therapists and a support worker and regularly takes students for clinical placements. She is a visiting lecturer for the local occupational therapy course. She feels passionate about the value of working with older people and wants to influence new graduates' attitudes to this area of work.

Karen is recognised as having considerable experience in her field and is a member of the Trust's elderly services' strategy team. She is working on a current research project with the consultant psychogeriatrician and nurse specialist looking at practice within the in-patient assessment ward.

Discussion

Karen's complex range of roles stems from her position of seniority, and the combination of managerial responsibilities with those of an expert clinician. Karen's leadership role requires her to plan, support or review the work of others, develop their skills and potential, ensure the quality of the occupational therapy she and her staff provide, lead the development of occupational therapy within elderly mental health services, and champion occupational therapy's contribution within this field among her multidisciplinary colleagues.

Karen's colleagues' expectations of the broad contributions she can offer are based on their respect for the level of experience she has gathered. As a clinician, she has reached the degree of mastery where she can tackle complex and challenging work with a minimum of support and with insightful awareness and autonomy (Stoltenberg & Delworth 1987). Her practice has matured to the level where she can focus on specialist issues for occupational therapy and is shaped by theory, for example early interven-

tions in dementia, based on theories of well-being and the maintenance of personhood (Kitwood & Bredin 1992).

Karen's work context also permits her to develop her role as a teacher and mentor – both in the workplace, and, specifically, within the local university. This satisfies her own interest in passing on knowledge, and is supported as a role seen to provide a useful academic link and promote the organisation's credibility as a centre of excellence.

Karen's organisational position, her research interests, and the opportunities for multiprofessional initiatives, lead to her inclusion within strategic planning groups and into roles that extend beyond her core team, into the organisation as a whole. Her role as an agent of change within the elderly services is heavily relied on.

COMPLEMENTARY TEAM ROLES

Having looked at the ways in which the roles of *individual* occupational therapists may develop, the following case vignette demonstrates the effective use of the *complementary* roles and skills of a multidisciplinary team:

Case study

Stewart's story

Stewart's first psychotic episode occurred in his late teens. Now aged 38, he is preparing to leave the hospital in which he has been resident for the past 19 years. Many of the people he had shared a ward with left the hospital several years ago as the Health Trust developed new community services.

Despite years of in-patient treatment, Stewart had, until about 2 years ago, continued to experience disturbing hallucinations. Delusional ideas made him unpredictable, paranoid and occasionally in danger of harming his closest family members. He showed many of the negative symptoms of schizophrenia (American Psychiatric Association 1997) and was isolated, had very poor self-esteem and impoverished social and daily living skills. His behaviour and presentation were often bizarre as he responded to the voices that were so often taunting him, further alienating him from others.

Despite Stewart's profound and enduring problems, the team within the rehabilitation service saw it as a collective role to sustain hope that he could make progress – a feature recognised as critical to the success of rehabilitation (Anthony et al 1987, Cnaan et al 1989). When the consultant psychiatrist discussed with the nursing team a new medication regime using clozapine, an atypical antipsychotic drug, great care had to be taken to ensure the dosage did not become toxic and regular blood tests were needed. Stewart discussed the potential benefits and risks with his key-worker nurse and agreed on how his responses to the new drug would be monitored.

The new medication had a remarkable effect on Stewart's symptoms. The hallucinations diminished, and on most days became little more than an irritation. His bizarre responses to his voices disappeared. Stewart began work with a senior nurse with specialist cognitive therapy training. Now that his negative symptoms were a little alleviated he was accessible for work on the positive symptoms – he could be challenged on the strength of his delusional beliefs to the extent that he was less prevented from engaging with activities, his own care, and relationships with others.

Unfortunately, the medication produced some unwanted side-effects. Nursing and medical staff used scaling techniques to monitor the extent to which Stewart was troubled by these and worked to achieve the optimum dose. With help from his key nurse who was trained in motivational interviewing, Stewart looked at the relative advantages and disadvantages of continuing the drug using cost/benefit analysis approach (Rollnick & Miller 1995). He remained willing to tolerate some of the side-effects to retain the relief he was finding from abusive voices and upsetting beliefs about himself.

Though Stewart's psychotic symptoms were becoming less disabling, as his insight grew and his engagement with the people around him

improved, he became quite severely depressed as a reaction to the growing awareness he had about the youth he now felt he'd missed and the paucity of his relationships with his family. He suffered huge guilt as he realised the threat he had posed to his parents, and was anxious during their visits. For a brief time the team were concerned that he might be at risk of suicide. His key nurse played an important role in supporting him through this period, giving him opportunities to express his sadness, confusion and anger and explore his future options. The nurse and a psychologist met over several weeks with Stewart and his family to work through issues arising from his illness, his changing abilities and expectations, and his future relationship with them.

The occupational therapist had worked over several months trying gently to establish a relationship with Stewart. As he became less dominated by hallucinations and distressing beliefs, he became more interested in looking at the skills he needed to develop to move on from the hospital – now becoming a realistic, if long-term, goal. Directed by his main motivating goals ('to feel more like a capable adult and prove I'm not useless'; 'to get out of the hospital'; 'to have a normal life and meet people'), she worked on practical daily living skills as well as exploring his leisure interests and began, gradually, extending his everyday experiences from the confines of the hospital into the local town. During these sessions the demands placed on him inevitably increased Stewart's anxiety. She reinforced some of the cognitive techniques he had learned to cope with stress and with invasive thoughts. She noticed that when participating in activities he enjoyed he did not experience any hallucinations. They worked together on identifying which activities were stress provoking, and which were restorative and absorbing, looking particularly for opportunities to combine those that helped block symptoms with demanding tasks, or to sandwich helpful activities around those he found more anxiety provoking. Stewart created his own menu of effective and discrete additional coping techniques, for example studying favourite magazines, listening to the local pop radio station, cycling, taking digital photographs while out walking and later working on the computer with them. His sense that he was exerting control over the symptoms that had previously dominated him gave him enormous satisfaction and hope.

Forming friendships remained a significant challenge for Stewart, yet his increased insight into the extent of his isolation was a source of distress. The team worked together to identify ways in which Stewart might increase his chances of forming more satisfying relationships with his family, his fellow in-patients and the people he met through his increased use of the town's facilities. He was helped to explore how his social skills, the way he presented himself, and the activities he pursued could be adapted or targeted to help him engage people more successfully.

Stewart has decided that he does not want to live in his parents' home – an option explored during the family sessions – but instead hopes to move to a group home in a nearby area. In preparation for this he was allocated a care manager, a social worker based in a community team. She has begun to discuss with Stewart using a local day service to provide continued therapeutic work and support on his discharge from hospital. The occupational therapist is preparing to hand over her work to the day service occupational therapist and, as Stewart highlights his need for employment, has requested that there is early priority given to assessing and developing his work aspirations and skills.

Discussion

The roles of the different members of the team can be clearly seen to work together to contribute to Stewart's progress. There are *shared* team goals (relief from symptoms, increased level of function and independence, improved quality of life, resolution of family conflicts and development of satisfying relationships within and external to his family) and treatment approaches/models (collaborative rehabilitation models, psychosocial interventions and use of the Stress/Vulnerability model (Birchwood & Tarrier 1992,

Fowler et al 1995). There are also clear areas where *individual* contributions are specifically targeted, sometimes specific to professional role, for example:

- the psychiatrist's review of the appropriateness of continuing with a previous medication regime and prescribing of newer atypical drugs based on a growing evidence base of effectiveness (National Schizophrenia Guideline Group 2000)
- the nurse's collaborative work with Stewart to ensure the unwanted side-effects of his medication were minimised, and that he felt listened to and active in the decision making over continuing with medication using motivational interviewing techniques (Birchwood & Tarrier 1992, Fowler et al 1995)
- the occupational therapist's analysis of activities in terms of their stress/therapeutic effects and development of daily living skills through graded application of domestic and self care activities.

Individual team roles sometimes evolve due to personal interest and development, for example:

- The nurse specialist in cognitive therapy had pursued particular training to be able to offer this approach to people with psychosis.
- The psychologist in this team had particular interest and training in the provision of family based psychosocial interventions and had an accepted role within the team as co-worker and supervisor for this style of work.

In this team, there is also evidence of co-working between the professions to maximise the chances of success, for example the joint family work between the psychologist and nurse, the reinforcement of cognitive strategies taught by the psychologist during occupational therapy sessions, the careful management of the medication's positive and negative effects by the medical and nursing team and the future planning for Stewart's attendance at the day service between the occupational therapist and the social worker. The whole team worked closely together, in collaboration with Stewart, in exploring future options and planning to meet his needs in order that he might be able to move on from the hospital.

The effectiveness of this team required them to have a degree of consensus over what generic roles were required of them, and how to make best use of profession/person-specific roles. Evidence shows that this balance of comfort between generic and specialist function, together with role clarity, is best for service users in terms of effectiveness, and best for staff in relation to morale and maintenance of lower levels of work stress (Onyett et al 1995, 1997).

Stewart's case demonstrates the results of effective team working. It might not always work like that. It is worth thinking about what the result might have been if:

- the occupational therapist did not know what cognitive therapy coping strategies had been found successful with Stewart and believed that cognitive therapy was only appropriate for people with neuroses
- The nurse had used a collaborative approach and taken Stewart's reporting of medication side-effects seriously, but the psychiatrist felt the side-effects were minor and it was not worth the risk of altering medication and ignored the request for review
- There was competition over who should act as Stewart's key worker, and who was best placed to deliver family interventions
- Any part of the bio-psycho-social approach to Stewart's complex needs was neglected.

Role balance and role conflict

Much has been written regarding the balance of necessary roles required from mental health professions, noting both the great value in diversity – the need to match the broad spread of clients' needs with the diversity of professional backgrounds and skills – and the need to develop consistent core competencies and generic abilities and aptitudes. The Sainsbury Centre for Mental Health proposes core competencies for all staff working with people with severe mental illness spanning across the areas of administration, assessment, treatment and care management, and collaborative working, while also describing profession-specific issues connected with the changing roles of mental health staff groups (Sainsbury Centre 1997).

The role balance health professionals are expected to achieve is highly complex. It is possible to see how the network of roles surrounding the individual, described by Merton (1957; cited in Blair et al 1998) as 'role sets', can explode into an elaborate mosaic:

- *Occupational therapist*
  manager – leader, monitor, developer, motivator
  clinician – therapist, researcher, advocate, advisor, administrator
  colleague – supporter, challenger, negotiator
  generic mental health worker – counsellor, care coordinator, carer, supporter/educator

and so on . . .

As modern mental health care becomes increasingly complex, and all the professions across the health and social services are forced to adapt their roles to embrace new structures and practice developments, the opportunities for role rivalries increase. Indeed, the more roles one holds, the greater is the possibility for role conflict, overload or ambiguity. The loss of familiar roles brings its own stresses requiring adaptive responses (Blair 1998) and supportive management.

SUMMARY

Occupational therapists are operating in a complex system of mental health provision that relies on collaboration between service users, health and social care staff and non-statutory agencies and charities. They have to be flexible in their responses to differing client groups, service settings, team skill mixes and management styles and lines of accountability. They must respond to priorities as they emerge from central and local health and social care policy but might celebrate the language of the National Service Framework for mental health: it is liberally peppered with references to meeting service users' occupational, social and leisure needs, and attends to issues of independence in daily living skills.

The actual roles occupational therapists perform depend on the interaction of external demands and intrinsic values, skills, experience, interest and training. Despite potential role strain, ambiguity and competing priorities arising from the wide variety of roles assumed by occupation-al therapists, the place of occupational therapy within the multidisciplinary team is well established. Occupational therapists are well placed to undertake the generic work necessary for a team to be effective, yet must not do so at the cost of their specialist value: using occupation to enhance people's functioning and quality of life, and their development of satisfying relationships and resilience to the effects of mental illness.

REFERENCES

Allan F, Ledwith F 1998 Levels of stress and perceived need for supervision in senior occupational therapy staff. British Journal of Occupational Therapy 61(8): 346–350

American Psychiatric Association 1997 Practice guideline for the treatment of patients with schizophrenia. American Journal of Psychiatry 154(4) (April supplement)

Anthony W A, Farkas, M D, Unger K V 1987 Psychiatric rehabilitation training package: overall rehabilitation goal. Centre for Psychiatric Rehabilitation, Boston University

Ball R, Moore E, and Kuipers E 1992 Expressed emotion in community care staff. Social Psychiatry and Psychiatric Epidemiology 27: 35–39

Belbin R M 1981 Management teams: why they succeed or fail. Butterworth Heineman, Oxford

Birchwood M, Tarrier N (eds) 1992 Innovations in the psychological management of schizophrenia. Wiley, Chichester

Birchwood M, Smith J, Macmillan F, McGovern D 1998 Early intervention in psychotic relapse. In: Brooker C, Repper J (eds) Serious mental health problems in the community: policy, practice and research. Ballière Tindall, London, Ch 10

Blair S 1998 Role. In: Jones D, Blair S, Hartery T, Jones R K (eds) Sociology and occupational therapy: an integrated approach. Churchill Livingstone, Edinburgh, Ch 5

Cade B, O'Hanlon W 1993 A brief guide to brief therapy. Norton, New York

Cnaan R A, Blankertz L, Messinger K, Gardner R 1989 Psychosocial rehabilitation: towards a theoretical base. Psychosocial Rehabilitation Journal 13: 1

Department of Health 1990 National Health Service and Community Care Act 1991

Department of Health 1995 Mental health in England: statistical bulletin. HMSO, London

Department of Health 1998 Modernising mental health services. HMSO, London

Department of Health 1999 National service framework for mental health. HMSO, London

Department of Health 2000 Effective care co-ordination in mental health services: modernising the Care Programme Approach: a policy booklet. HMSO, London

de Shazer 1991 Putting difference to work. Norton, New York

Fowler D, Garety P, Kuipers E 1995 Cognitive behaviour therapy of psychosis: theory and practice. Wiley, London

Hagedorn R 1995 Occupational therapy: perspectives and processes. Churchill Livingstone, Edinburgh, Ch 11, 160–161

Harries P 1998 Community mental health teams: occupational therapists' changing role. British Journal of Occupational Therapy 61(5): 219–220

Kitwood T, Bredin K 1992 Towards a theory of dementia care: personhood and well-being. Ageing and Society 12: 269–287

Kuipers E, Moore E 1995 Expressed emotion and staff–client relationships: implications for community care of the severely mentally ill. International Journal of Mental Health 24(3): 3–26

Law M, Baptiste S, Carswell A et al 1994 Canadian Occupational Performance Measure, 2nd edn. CAOT Publications ACE, Toronto

Lehman A F, Dixon L B, Kernan E, DeForge B R, Pastrado L T 1997 A randomised trial of assertive community treatment for homeless persons with severe mental illness. Archives of General Psychiatry 54: 1038–1043

Marshall M, Lockwood A 1998 Assertive community treatment for people with severe mental disorders. Cochrane Library: Oxford update software, Oxford

Meeson B 1998 Occupational therapy in community mental health, part 2. Factors influencing intervention choice. British Journal of Occupational Therapy 61(2): 57–62

Merton R K 1957 The role set: problems in sociological theory. British Journal of Sociology 8: 106–120

National Schizophrenia Guideline Group 2000 The management of schizophrenia, part 1. Pharmacological treatments. Royal College of Psychiatrists and British Psychological Society, London

Norman I, Peck E 1999 Working together in community mental health services: an inter-professional dialogue. Journal of Mental Health 8(3): 217–230

Onyett S, Ford R 1996 Multidisciplinary community teams: where is the wreckage? Journal of Mental Health 5: 47–55

Onyett S, Pillinger T, Muijen M 1995 Making community mental health teams work: CMHTs and the people who work in them. Sainsbury Centre for Mental Health, London

Onyett S, Pillinger T, Muijen M 1997 Job satisfaction and burnout among members of community mental health teams. Journal of Mental Health 6(1): 55–66

Ovtrevit J 1993 Co-ordinating community care: multi-disciplinary teams and care-management. Open University Press, Buckingham

Peck E, Norman I J 1999 Working together in adult community mental health services: exploring inter-professional role relations. Journal of Mental Health 8(3): 231–242

Rollnick, Miller 1995 What is motivational interviewing? Behavioural and Cognitive Psychotherapy 23: 325–334

Roth A, Fonagy P 1996 What works for whom? Guildford Press, New York

Rugg S 1996 The transition of junior occupational therapists to clinical practice: report of a preliminary study. British Journal of Occupational Therapy 59(4): 165–168

Sainsbury Centre 1997 Pulling together: the future roles and training of mental health staff. Sainsbury Centre for Mental Health, London

Sainsbury Centre 1998 Keys to engagement. Sainsbury Centre For Mental Health, London

Sainsbury Centre 1999 Acute problems: a survey of the quality of care in acute psychiatric wards. Sainsbury Centre For Mental Health, London

Schon D A 1991 The reflective practitioner: how professionals think in action. Arena, England, Ch 2, p. 60

Shepherd G 1998 Models of community care. Journal of Mental Health 7(2): 165–177

Stein L I, Test M A 1980 Alternative to mental hospital treatment: 1. A conceptual model, treatment program and clinical evaluation. Archives of General Psychiatry 37: 392–397

Stoltenberg C D, Delworth U 1987 Supervising counsellors and therapists. Jossey-Bass, San Francisco

11

Ethics

Ian E. Thompson

INTRODUCTION

The current interest in ethics in business, the public services and professional life can be explained in a number of ways. First, it can be related to increasing interest, aroused by the media, in well-publicised cases of corruption or abuse of public resources by public officials (and health care workers all hold public office, with different degrees of responsibility for public resources). Against this background there has been an increase in pressure group activity on behalf of various client interests against the established professions, with growing malpractice litigation and insistent demands for higher standards of probity and accountability in public life (Nolan 1995, 1996, 1997). In this context, there may be some justification for the cynic who sees the rush of those in business and the professions to be ethical as self-interested, and the quest for a code of ethics as a fig-leaf to cover a multitude of sins. Clearly, ethics is on the public agenda, but what is ethics and why is it important?

The purpose of this chapter is to demystify ethics and to remove some of the misconceptions which are around. Having examined what ethics is and is not, it explores the ethical basis of occupational therapy as a profession and the role of ethics in its practice. Thus, the first part of the chapter examines some general questions about moral values and rules, rights and duties, costs and benefits. Next we consider fundamental ethical principles in health care and how we address the questions of interpersonal, cultural and philosophical relativities in practice. We then move from the consideration of these general ethical questions to their application in occupational therapy, and to some specific ethical and moral problems encountered by carers and therapists in day-to-day practice and the management of occupational therapy services. Finally, we raise the question of whether ethical difficulties can be addressed as problems to be solved with appropriate problem-solving methods, rather than mystifying them as dilemmas. There is a glossary of ethical terms at the end of the book (p. 588).

WHAT IS ETHICS?

For many people the term 'ethics' is associated with religion or acceptance of some belief-system and/or a framework of rules of behaviour imposed by authority (see also Box 11.1). It is often associated with negative prohibitions and with disciplinary procedures. Alternatively, ethics may be thought of as something very personal, associated with one's private feelings and attitudes towards other people or one's choice of lifestyle and other personal preferences. Related to these subjective interpretations of ethics is the view that everything in ethics is relative and contestable, that ethical disputes are irresolvable,

or that ethical argument simply amounts to people grandstanding their opinions.

These popularly held views influence the way people think about ethics and judge their own and other people's moral actions, but they can be seriously misleading. In contrast to the above, philosophical ethics has traditionally been concerned with the question of what makes possible the positive health and well-being of people and society. It may be helpful briefly to examine this tradition (MacIntyre 1967).

For the early Greek philosophers, notably Plato and Aristotle, as well as Eastern philosophers Confucius and Buddha, ethics was basically concerned with defining the conditions for human flourishing – with the attempt to clarify what conditions must be created in society if individuals and communities are to flourish (texts by these philosophers are available on the internet – see References). Ethics is also necessarily concerned with identifying what kinds of things or actions can prevent this flourishing or injure or undermine people and communities. The primary ethical question then is: 'What is good for human beings?' or 'What will ensure the happiness and fulfilment of human beings?'

If we interpret ethics in this way, it is profoundly relevant to occupational therapy with its concern to enable people to lead fulfilled and

---

Box 11.1 Defining 'ethics' and 'morals'

In ordinary English usage the terms 'ethics' and 'morals' can be, and often are, used interchangeably. This is not surprising, since their root meanings in Greek (ethos) and Latin (mores) are very similar.

Literally, the word 'morals' derives from the Latin mores, meaning 'established social custom', 'convention' or 'etiquette'. In common usage, it retains the general sense of relating to the personal conduct of individuals or groups of people. When we describe actions as 'moral' or 'immoral', we are usually referring to personal beliefs and actions.

The word 'ethics' derives from the Greek word ethos which, in addition to meaning 'habit', 'custom' or 'usage', also refers to the 'disposition' or 'character' of an individual or to the 'spirit' of a community, or to the customs required for a community to function as a community.

In philosophy the terms tend to have acquired slightly more technical meanings. Ethics is often defined as the

science (or rational study) of the principles of conduct. However, in the formal academic study of ethics we tend to distinguish between the critical study of human conduct at two levels, the applied everyday level, and the theoretical reflective level, namely:

- rational application of moral principles to everyday decision making and action
- rational justification of our general moral beliefs and their coherence as a way of life.

There are various conventions about the use of the terms in philosophy, but in general, philosophers would want to distinguish clearly between the applied and theoretical levels, as follows:

- either using 'ethics' or 'morals' for the former and 'moral philosophy' for the latter
- or, using 'ethics' for the former and 'meta-ethics' for the latter.

Box 11.2 What ethics is and is not (reproduced with kind permission from Thompson & Harries 1997)

What ethics is not	What ethics is
Ethics is not primarily about negative rules and regulations, disciplinary measures or policing misconduct	Ethics is essentially concerned with the conditions for human flourishing, for the health and well-being of individuals and society
Ethics is not simply about matters of a private nature nor mainly about our personal feelings, attitudes and beliefs	Ethics is a community enterprise, based on universal principles and reasoned public debate and negotiation about how they are applied
Ethics is not about mysterious occult processes, feelings in the gut, hearing voices, or privileged access to moral truth	Ethics is about real power relations between people and the responsible sharing of power between them
Ethics is not a business requiring academic study, nor only for experts, for religious authorities, lawyers, philosophers or gurus	Ethics is about participation in a moral community and ownership of the policies it develops (e.g. Code of ethics for OTs)
Ethics is not about endless disputes, disagreements and dilemmas, nor about grandstanding our opinions	Ethics is a problem-solving activity based on knowledge of principles and skills in their application
Ethics is not a matter of innate knowledge, special powers of intuition, nor about supernatural revelation	Ethics is an educational process in which we acquire good habits and discover what it means to be responsible moral agents

---

healthy lives compatible with their abilities. The World Health Organization (WHO) definition of health gives expression to this central ethical concern when it states that: 'Health is complete physical, mental and social well-being and not merely the absence of disease or infirmity' (UNO 1947a).

What ethics is and is not

Let us summarise what ethics is, and what it is not (Box 11.2). Ethics is concerned with what is *good* or *bad* for human beings, that is, with the choice of values and the pursuit of goals that will ensure the flourishing of human societies, and the avoidance of what will cause harm (Ross 1930, Findlay 1970). Ethics is concerned with specifying the conditions for the general well-being, health and happiness of people and determining what standards we should apply in striving to attain our goals.

Ethics is also concerned with defining what is *right* or *wrong*,[1] that is, with such regulation of human society as is necessary to foster a positive environment in which individuals and communities can flourish and with what protective measures or rules are necessary to prevent people from being harmed. Protective rules or regulations defining what is right or wrong, legal or illegal, must be value based and promote personal and social well-being if they are to be fair and ethical.

Thus the study of ethics covers:

1. *Values, goals and standards* – defining what we regard as good and bad for ourselves and others. In life we pursue a wide range of both internal and external, instrumental and intrinsic goods.

2. *Principles and rules* – defining what we regard as right and wrong for ourselves and others. The framework of principles and rules serves to define both our duties or responsibilities, and also our rights and entitlements.

Values are related directly to goals because our choice of values determines both our short-term and long-term life goals. We make our decisions

---

[1] Although the distinction between 'right' and 'wrong' and 'good' and 'bad' has ancient roots in the history of philosophy, the classic work on the distinction between the two is Ross (1930) (compare with the views of Findlay 1970).

'Good' and 'bad' are our terms of widest application to our goals and the things we value. They are called 'teleological' and 'axiological' terms from the Greek words *telos* (end or goal) and *axios* (value).

'Right' and 'wrong' are terms whose scope is defined by principles, rules and duties. They are called 'deontological' terms from the Greek word *deon* (duty).

on how to act by applying our values to the choice of available means to achieve our goals. Values have to be chosen by ourselves. They cannot be imposed on us by others, for we stake our everyday decisions and actions on them and we have to accept responsibility for the outcomes of our actions. We may be called upon to stake our reputations, or even our lives, on our values. People's actions are usually judged to be moral or immoral depending on how their actions square with their own and society's professed values (or those of their profession).

For occupational therapists, as for other people, the values chosen will relate to the pursuit of a wide range of internal and external, instrumental and intrinsic goods that enrich therapists' lives and give satisfaction in their work.

Values related to internal and external, instrumental and intrinsic goods

We are all born into a morally structured world and encounter rules and regulations whichever way we turn. Our parents, the Church, schools, professional groups, and society all lay rules upon us and seek to govern us by regulations of various kinds. Not surprisingly, we may be inclined to say with regard to ethics: 'In the beginning was the Rule.'

However, we may always question whether a rule is a good rule or not. As adolescents, we challenge family rules in this way and will not own a rule unless we feel that it benefits us as well as others. In this sense, judgements of value have to be made about rules, as to whether they are fair, respect the rights of all parties and pro-

tect those who cannot defend their rights. Value judgements are therefore more fundamental than rules. Sound statutory law must be based on, and consistent with, common law and natural justice. Legislation alone does not make a law just or fair, it must serve to promote human well-being.

Being mature and responsible moral agents means that we do not simply do our duty because we are ordered to do so by some authority or because the law says we must. We have to make our own commitment to the law (or conscientiously object to unjust laws) and take full responsibility for our actions. To make conscientious moral choices means that we have internalised the moral law and made it our own. The same applies to the institutions within which we work or to the rules of our profession, the codes of professional conduct. Within the framework of a code of ethics or set of formal rules, actions infringing the rules of a profession are generally described as unethical or illegal.

The 'Russian dolls' model of ethics

Against the prevailing popular tendency to privatise and psychologise ethics, to treat all ethical questions and all ethical discourse as subjective and relative to our personal interests, we wish to emphasise the traditional view, going back to Aristotle (Saunders 1981), that ethics is about power and responsibility, about responsible power sharing and prevention of the abuse of power. This applies to our most intimate relations with our sexual partners, as it does to our relations with our families, parents, siblings and children, and to professional/client relations and employer/employee or manager/staff

Box 11.3	Values related to internal, external, instrumental and intrinsic goods
Internal goods	Pleasure of working with people, respecting, caring for and helping to rehabilitate disabled people, general job satisfaction
External goods	Secure employment, good income, good colleagues and working environment, house and garden, leisure opportunities, transport
Instrumental goods	Knowledge, skills and experience to be able to secure employment and provide competent service to others, power and influence
Intrinsic goods	Happiness, professional competence, personal integrity, good personal and professional reputation, friendship, health

Box 11.4 Ethics at the macro, meso, 'macho' and micro levels (adapted with kind permission from Thompson & Harries 1997)

External stakeholder level – MACRO	Ethics in strategic planning and inter-agency relations
Internal stakeholder level – MESO	Ethics in corporate management of human and financial resources
Team leadership level – 'MACHO'	Ethics in professional life, professional/client relationships, and inter-disciplinary cooperation and teamwork
Individual (clinical) level – MICRO	Ethics in personal decision making, maintaining competence and professional and personal development

relationships. The privatised view of ethics sets up a gulf between the private and public spheres of our lives, between ethics and law or politics, between ethics and business, and between ethics and medical science. If, on the other hand, we recognise that ethics has to do with the checks and balances on power in personal and public relations, then personal ethics and professional ethics, the ethics of caring and the ethics of corporate management, form parts of a continuum governed by the same demands of ethical responsibility and accountability.

The privatisation of ethics has tended to exaggerate the importance of individual ethical decision making and to ignore the many other levels at which ethics enters into our negotiations, planning and action in our professional and institutional life at work. In reality, most of our ethical decisions are not made in isolation: we consult with our partners, family and friends, we discuss options and review the outcomes of our decisions with our colleagues and clients, we work in teams and committees and have to take decisions which hold up ethically. If we are in positions of management, we have to be concerned with the well-being, rights and duties of the hospital or institution, staff and customers, and the wider political ethics of inter-institutional cooperation.

To do justice to this complexity in professional life it is necessary to disaggregate values, ethical decision making and policies applicable at the four levels shown in Box 11.4.

FUNDAMENTAL ETHICAL PRINCIPLES [2]

If ethics is to have any credibility it must be based on principles that are universally acknow-ledged and respected. Here we seem to be up against a real difficulty, for the popular view of ethics is that everyone has different ethical principles and that no agreement is possible. However, is this really true?

In a liberal society, tolerance of religious, moral and cultural diversity is encouraged. We live in a multicultural society and we are taught that:

- everyone is entitled to their own opinions about matters of ethics and politics
- people should not be prevented from expressing these views
- people should not be discriminated against because of the views they hold.

This seems to imply that all points of view have equal validity, or that all moral points of view are relative. If all moral beliefs are just that (points of view) then it would not seem to be possible to talk of moral truth or of universal moral principles. However, arguing that we *ought* to allow everyone the right to express their views on ethical and political matters is based on an unstated ethical principle, namely, that of *respect for persons* and their rights. To argue that we *ought not* to discriminate against people with moral, political or religious views different from our own is based on appeal to the *principle of justice* (Box 11.5).

Linked to these arguments are similar arguments about our duty to defend the rights of those who are too young or weak to defend their own interests, including ethnic and religious

[2] This section and the section which follows it are adapted, with permission, from material copyright to Dr I. E. Thompson's consultancy, Corporate Ethical Services.

Box 11.5 Fundamental ethical principles

Principles	Examples of right derived from principles
Beneficence (protective duty of powerful to weak)	• Duty to do good and avoid doing harm to other people, especially those dependent on you • Duty of care, on the part of the strong, to protect the weak and vulnerable • Duty of advocacy: defending rights of those unable or incompetent to defend their own Like the 'golden rule' (Do to others as you would have them do to you), beneficence or non-maleficence are sometimes referred to as expressing the 'principle of reciprocity')
Justice (Fair and reasonable power sharing)	• Duty of universal fairness: to ensure equality of opportunity for individuals, and fair and equal treatment of people, regardless of race, age, sex, class, gender or religion • Duty of equity: to share power, resources, knowledge and skills in such a way as to ensure equality of outcome for all groups in society • Duty to ensure equality before the law, transparent observance of due process, and to avoid discrimination, abuse or exploitation of people on any grounds (Justice demands that any rule we apply to our own actions, should also be capable of being applied equally to everybody else. Justice is thus based on the 'principle of universalisability')
Respect for persons (duty to empower one another for our mutual benefit)	• Duty to treat people as ends in themselves, never simply instrumentally as means to an end, to respect their individuality, dignity, freedom and rights • Duty to promote the autonomy and general flourishing or well-being of other people, for their benefit, one's own and the common good • Duty to be truthful, honest and sincere with other people (honesty is a demand of respect for persons, for to honour = to respect, and to deceive someone shows contempt for that person) (The concept of 'personhood' is a 'Constitutive Principle of Ethics' (Kant) for in both ethics and law 'a person' is defined as 'an individual who is a bearer of rights and responsibilities (or duties)'

---

minorities. Here appeal is being made to the underlying *principle of beneficence* or protective duty of care the strong owe to the weak. We are all weak and vulnerable at different times in our lives. This means that we must all recognise a reciprocal duty of care to one another, or society could not function at all. It is the basis of the golden rule: 'Do as you would be done by.'

Principles are starting points or beginnings (from the Latin *principium* = beginning). As such, principles simply point a direction. Like navigation instruments, they help us orientate ourselves. They do not provide us with a map nor dictate a course to us. We have to choose our own destinations and routes for getting there. The adoption of our own moral beliefs, values and ethical rules is necessary to enable us to chart a course through life and to achieve our life goals.

The principles of beneficence, justice and respect for persons each deal with different ways that power can be expressed or shared in relations between people. The basis of justice is equitable

power sharing between people. Beneficence has to do with the duty of the powerful to protect those that are weak and vulnerable (e.g. as parents have a duty to care for their children and not to abuse or exploit them). Respect for people's rights has to do with our duty, as members of a moral community, to assist others to achieve their full potential, to empower people to claim and exercise their rights and to express their full potential.

There are many different ways that we can, and do, seek to justify our moral beliefs or commitment to a philosophy of life. It can be argued, however, that different moral theories serve to emphasise different but complementary aspects of human action and different aspects of our moral experience. So, each type of theory has its own validity, thus:

• *Deontological theories* emphasise the importance of principles and rules, rights and duties as necessary to the proper functioning of moral communities.

- *Virtue (or prudential) ethics* emphasises the importance of personal moral integrity and competence in applied ethics in individuals and institutions.
- *Teleological theories* (including Utilitarianism) emphasise the importance of assessment of outcomes and costs and benefits relative to our values and goals.

In justifying specific decisions and actions we generally go no further than to describe the circumstances in which we acted, explaining what principles or rules we applied in reaching our decision, what options and means we considered and what possible outcomes or consequences we anticipated relative to what actually occurred.

ETHICS AND HEALTH

Health is something we value, even if we do not value it properly until we lose it or become ill. Health and disease represent, like good and bad, degrees of perfection and imperfection in a value continuum on which these terms are the polar limits. Because our health is valuable to us, whether we take it for granted simply as enabling us to do other things we value or whether we pursue it as an end in itself, we do make efforts to protect our health, by:

- trying to ensure that we have food, water, shelter and employment
- building relationships of mutual support and cooperation for our common good
- seeking to prevent disease, accidents and mental disorder and avoiding infection
- investing considerable personal and public resources in health care
- engaging in sport and physical development and supporting health promotion.

The United Nations *Universal Declaration of Human Rights* makes the right to health and access to health care a fundamental human right and therefore member states have a responsibility to promote the health of their citizens and to ensure that all citizens have equal access to health care (UNO 1947b):

1. Everyone has the right to a standard of living adequate for the health and well-being of himself and his family, including food, clothing, housing and medical care and necessary social services, and the right to security in the event of unemployment, sickness, disability, widowhood, old age or other lack of livelihood in circumstances beyond his control.

2. Motherhood and childhood are entitled to special care and assistance. All children, whether born in or out of wedlock, shall enjoy the same protection.

(UNO 1947b, Article 25)

(In addition, Article 22 (on Social Security), Article 24 (on work and leisure) and Article 26 (on education) all have a bearing on the wider interpretation of health and well-being.)

To appreciate the ethical principles underlying the World Health Organization definition of health (UNO 1947a), we must first examine the meaning of the words 'health' and 'disease'.

Defining 'health' and 'disease'

Definitions of health and disease have varied over the centuries. Classical medicine saw health as the maintenance of an internal state of homeostasis (or balance) between functioning body systems. Disease was the disturbance or disruption of this balance by trauma, invasion by foreign organisms or mental disorder. No definition can be perfectly free of implied values, however, this classical definition is rather one-dimensional, placing too much emphasis on maintaining the desirable state of homeostasis to the detriment of other aspects of health. Modern attempts to define health in terms of the 'optimum function or dysfunction of an organism' (Oxford Medical Dictionary 1980) are similarly biased towards technical measures of health.

Returning again to the 1947 WHO definition (p. 193), its significance is two-fold: First, it indicates a shift from a predominantly medical model of health, biased towards homeostasis, to one in which behavioural, social and economic factors are more clearly recognised as essential to human well-being. Second, it involves an implicit recognition that questions of meaning and value play an important part in human life and shape our understanding of health.

The ethical basis of occupational therapy

As occupational therapists know only too well from their work in rehabilitative medicine, it is not self-evident to people that they should care for their health or attempt to recover it, especially if they are depressed following injury or serious illness. Motivating people to lead healthy lives, or to cooperate in their rehabilitation, is to assist them to rediscover meaning and value in their lives. The German philosopher Paul Tillich once remarked that 'Man is that being who is essentially concerned with his being and meaning' (Tillich 1957). Our state of physical and mental health is directly related to our ability to make sense of our lives. This quest for meaning and value is something in which occupational therapists attempt to assist people – whether they are healthy or unhealthy, whole or injured, employed or unemployed, institutionalised or living in the community. To empower people to take control of their lives once again, to give meaning to their lives by their decisions, is the fundamental ethical responsibility of the occupational therapist.[3]

The role of occupational therapy, and what is in many ways the justification for its continued existence as a profession, lies in its link with man's basic need for occupation. The value of occupational therapy is, therefore, crucially linked to the role of activity, work and occupation in integrating the physical, psychological and social functions of human beings. Reilly (1962), for example, in a classic paper exploring the justification for the continued existence of occupational therapy, put forward the hypothesis, 'Man through the use of his hands, as they are energised by mind and will, can influence the state of his own health'. She cites the philosopher Fromm (1960), who said that the need to work is an imperative part of man's nature because man has to eat, drink, sleep and protect himself from his enemies and, in order to ensure his self-

preservation, must work and produce. She points to the demoralising effect of unemployment or enforced inactivity in confinement, or the impact of forced retirement on the health and well-being of people, and argues that occupation is a basic human need: 'Man has a vital need for occupation for his central nervous system demands the rich and varied stimuli that solving life problems provides for him. This is the basic need occupational therapy ought to be servicing'.

We can now move on to explain some more direct links between the ethics of health care in general and occupational therapy in particular.

In the ethics of health care, the principles of protective beneficence (or the duty of care), justice (or universal fairness) and respect for persons (or unconditional regard for the dignity and rights of individuals) all have a particular value and importance in practice (Thompson 1987, 1995).

In the literature on bioethics there has been considerable discussion of these principles and it has been argued that other principles such as non-maleficence, truth-telling and autonomy need to be added to the other three. Gillon (1985) described seven principles underpinning medical ethics: respect for autonomy, beneficence (helping others), non-maleficence (not harming others), justice, telling the truth, confidentiality and informed consent. On the other hand it has been counter-argued that non-maleficence is not a separate principle, but is simply the negative form or obverse of the principle of protective beneficence. Further, it has been argued that truth-telling or honesty and respect for the autonomy of patients or clients and informed consent are implied in respect for persons and derivable from this more basic principle. Similarly, the duty of confidentiality can be interpreted as a requirement of the principle of protective beneficence and respect for the vulnerability of the patient or client (Veatch 1981, Beauchamp & Childress 1994).

The value and limitations of codes of ethics

All professions, including occupational therapy, find it useful, indeed essential, to state in writing

---

[3] The French philosopher Merleau-Ponty (1962) observed that 'Man is a meaning-maker'. His contemporary Jean-Paul Sartre makes a similar point in his play *No Exit* (1956), when he says 'Man makes himself by his decisions'.

the general ethical principles that govern practice. These take the form of codes. Codes attempt to:

- state the duties of professionals, and emphasise their role in protecting vulnerable clients
- set limits to professional responsibility, and standards for their public accountability
- protect and maintain standards (for example education and training)
- establish ways of regulating professional conduct (Freidson 1970).

In the positive sense, a code of ethics can also set aspirational standards and can specify rules for the appraisal of professional and unprofessional conduct. Although it can be argued that codes are primarily established to serve the interests of a profession, they do have another purpose, that of informing the public about what standards they can expect of the practitioners whose help they seek. Further, they can become the basis on which clients can seek to hold professionals accountable for their conduct and the standard of their services (Grace & Cohen 1998).

Limitations of codes

Professional codes are undoubtedly useful, but they do have some common failings:

- They have traditionally been developed as a basis for justifying professional intervention in crisis situations. At such times, clients are often in desperate need of help and very dependent. With this crisis or problem focus, codes often ignore the more positive duties of professionals, such as positive health promotion and due regard for patient or client autonomy.
- Codes can perpetuate a patronising attitude towards clients, as recipients of care. Again, this occurs because most codes view the carer as the one in control (in the time of crisis) and the client as dependent. Overprotective care can conflict with the fundamental moral duty underlying rehabilitation, namely promotion of client autonomy (Thompson et al 1994).

In the British *Code of Ethics and Professional Conduct for Occupational Therapists* (COT 2000) there is no clear or explicit statement of the values of the profession; however, these are clearly implied in the specific provisions of the code (Box 11.6).

Thus, occupational therapists seek to apply the following values:

- caring for people in need – recognising and respecting their dignity, autonomy, individual potential and uniqueness as human beings
- sharing with people – using our own power, expertise and authority to transfer knowledge, skills, strength and resources to clients, to enhance their health and well-being as well as our own
- preparing people for a healthy life – whether children or vulnerable adults – and developing people's capacity to help themselves, while protecting, nurturing and developing their potential, thereby empowering them to take greater control of their own lives.

Box 11.6 Values, mentioned and implicit, in the British Code of Ethics and Professional Conduct for Occupational Therapists

Professional values mentioned or implied in the Code:

- To maintain high standards of professional knowledge and expertise
- To provide caring, efficient and effective services and to maintain good records
- To contribute to research and critical appraisal of service delivery to clients
- To exhibit personal moral integrity and legal probity of a high standard
- To model good health behaviour and be agents of positive health promotion

Client-related values of occupational therapists mentioned in the Code:

- To respect and promote the autonomy of their clients and their life choices
- To act as advocates on behalf of their clients, especially those most vulnerable
- To share their skills and knowledge for the empowerment of their clients
- To respect the vulnerability, need for privacy and confidentiality of clients
- To promote the well-being and avoid the exploitation or abuse of clients

CARERS' DUTIES AND CLIENT'S RIGHTS

The caring professions rightly emphasise the duty of professionals to protect clients' interests and ensure that the rights of the latter are not infringed. But what are the principal duties of health care workers and what are the key rights of clients? We should be as specific as possible about this important subject.

CARERS' DUTIES

The principal duties of health care workers include the following:

- They should give people adequate information and resources, enabling them to make responsible choices for themselves and to maintain control over their own lives.
- They should promote people's autonomy, enabling them to develop their full human potential and to enjoy good health (physical, mental and social well-being and not just the absence of disease).
- They should consult people about their needs, sharing power and resources with them to ensure they enjoy equal opportunities and do not suffer discrimination or turn people into dependants.
- They should recognise the need of vulnerable people to have their rights protected.

CLIENTS' RIGHTS

So we return to clients' rights. These include:

- the right to know (i.e. the right to adequate information to make informed choices)
- the right to privacy (i.e. the right to appropriate physical privacy and confidentiality)
- the right to care and treatment (i.e. the right of access to the best available health resources).

Violations of clients' rights

The rights of clients with mental disorder (whether mental illness or learning difficulties) are all too easily compromised. The Mental Health Acts (HMSO 1983, 1984) empower health professionals to detain and treat clients compulsorily, thus abrogating the clients' rights to freedom of movement, to be kept informed and to give voluntary consent (including the otherwise absolute right to refuse treatment). Many other, more subtle rights are also threatened.

Some examples of possible violations of rights are as follows:

- The right to know may be denied to psychiatric clients who have been labelled mentally incompetent merely because they are held under the Act, not because they are actually incapable of understanding.
- Physical privacy may be widely compromised in mixed wards.
- Confidentiality may be violated in team management where extended confidentiality is the order of the day, or by the staff reading correspondence and closely observing visitors and family interactions as part of treatment.
- Consent to treatment, even when given by voluntary or informal clients, can be interpreted so broadly that clients may be constrained to join in group therapy, dance therapy or whatever else is on offer.

Caring staff working in psychiatric settings are very often placed in the difficult position of being required to be at once an advocate of clients' rights and society's agent to control and restrict the client's freedom. They must try to reconcile their commitment to clients' rights with their responsibility to society: a daunting ethical dilemma for occupational therapists.

Each of the fundamental rights of clients mentioned above deserves closer scrutiny, namely, the right to privacy, the right to know, and the right to care and treatment.

The client's right to privacy

Invasion of privacy strikes at the heart of a person's dignity (Box 11.7). The right to privacy has three aspects, which include:

- respect for a person's dignity and physical privacy – his 'body space'

Box 11.7   Issues of privacy of information in a department

The professional staff in the occupational therapy department of a psychiatric day hospital became concerned that a wide range of unqualified staff had access to clients' notes. Because the hospital was situated in a small community, clients and staff often knew each other personally and maintaining confidentiality was a problem.

To help safeguard clients' privacy, some qualified staff refused to write confidential material in the clients' notes, but their managers pointed out that if anything went wrong they could be held legally responsible for withholding information. Staff had to choose between protecting their clients or themselves.

Box 11.8   Does the client have a right to know the diagnosis?

'Brett,' in his early 30s, has three children who are in the custody of his ex-wife. Brett is referred to the occupational therapist for help with anger management. He and his two sisters discovered recently that their father died of Huntington's disease, in a mental hospital, some years after leaving the family. Both sisters have tested positive for the disease. The geneticist refuses to give Brett the test because he thinks he is too emotionally unstable to cope with an adverse result. Brett says he finds the uncertainty of not knowing whether he has the disease unbearable.

- respect for the person's intimate secrets, sexual preferences, psychological experience and social life
- respect for confidential information; professionals should be very cautious about sharing a client's confidences with colleagues, even for the client's own good.

Professionals may demand that these personal areas of privacy be exposed to critical examination as part of the medical, psychiatric and social assessments that precede treatment. They therefore have a particular duty of care to protect the privacy and confidences of vulnerable clients (Sim 1996).

The client's right to know

It is a truism that knowledge is power. However, we often do not recognise that the converse is also true, namely, that to be kept in a state of ignorance is to be kept in a state of impotence and dependency. The ability to control information is a powerful tool. If used responsibly, it can restore dignity and enable clients to share in decision making about their lives and futures.

Sharing of knowledge (skills, expertise) is about sharing power; it empowers others to be more independent. It is not merely about the right to adequate information to make informed choices and to give voluntary consent (to treatment, for example). It includes the rights to be informed of one's diagnosis as a client and the proposed course of treatment – indeed, the right to be informed of one's rights!

Whether clients should always be told everything about their diagnosis is, however, controversial (Box 11.8). Doctors and other carers often feel they have a duty to withhold information for client's own good. Others would argue that the client, having voluntarily sought help, always has the right to be told everything about his condition.

The client's right to care and treatment

In the UK, as in many other countries, we have decided that all citizens have a moral and legal right to free medical care and treatment, but putting this right into practice is not easy. Care and treatment includes everything from highly technical surgery to tender loving care and occupational therapy. Who decides which clients have the right to occupational therapy? On what criteria is it decided how many occupational therapists there should be? Many would argue that society has not satisfactorily resolved the ethical dilemma of how to balance the right of clients to therapy with the responsible use of public resources to employ sufficient occupational therapists (Box 11.9).

Another example shows the difficulties that can be encountered in providing adequate care and treatment. Therapists often make decisions based on their own values. Because they are unaware of this bias in their value judgements they may find it impossible to separate them from their clinical judgements. For instance,

---

Box 11.9 The management of resources and treatment services

An occupational therapy department had a shortage of qualified staff. They faced the choice of insisting on giving effective and specific intervention to a small number of clients or taking the easier path of supplying a diversional service to a larger number.

Pressure was applied from all quarters:

- The managers wanted to keep the numbers up for statistical purposes.
- Nursing staff, also understaffed, demanded that the occupational therapy department accommodate as many people as possible to ease the burden on them.
- Medical staff expected all the people they referred to be offered treatment.
- The clients themselves often complained if they were not included in occupational therapy.
- Occupational therapy helpers complained as well (rather surprisingly) because they felt their role was being undervalued if fewer clients were treated.

In the face of such opposition it was difficult for the small number of therapists to remain convinced of the value of what they were doing and to continue to offer what they saw as effective treatment.

---

what the therapist decides is for the client's own good, regarding the desirable outcome of treatment or the quality of life to be aimed for on the client's behalf, may reflect the values of the therapist more than those of the client.

DEALING WITH ETHICAL PROBLEMS IN OCCUPATIONAL THERAPY

The reader will by now be aware of the difficulties of translating principles into practice. Many of the problems we have mentioned, for example those concerned with client's rights, are shared by all health care workers but working with psychiatric clients places very particular demands on the therapist's ethical and moral code.

The treatment of clients who are mentally disordered may be virtually indistinguishable from that of prisoners, except that their sentences are indeterminate. The deviant behaviour of the mentally ill may result in social sanctions and restrictions on their personal liberty.

The conscientious therapist may feel uneasy when society denies a client his freedom and

may well ask whether society has the right to lock up clients and give them treatment against their will, for their own good, in the belief that it will help restore their autonomy!

The diagnosis of mental disorder as an illness, with labels such as 'schizophrenic', 'psychopathic', 'manic-depressive' or 'neurotic', is both a blessing and curse. It is a blessing because it allows the client access to care and treatment. It is a curse because the client is stigmatised, set apart and regarded as different from other people. Many observers feel it would benefit clients to find ways to take mental illness out of the medical domain, to eliminate medical labels that connote disease. However, such a step could be disastrous if mentally disordered offenders were given penal treatment rather than appropriate medical treatment, nursing care and rehabilitation.

Specific problems and dilemmas

The following problems and dilemmas further illustrate the tensions that can arise between our personal principles, or those of our profession, and the rights of clients:

Discharge of clients from hospital

Here, the conflict is between the duty to protect the client and at the same time respect his rights. The problem is even more acute when the client is a suicide risk or has a history of violent behaviour, or when there is fear that he may be unable to cope with life in the community. Assessments of dangerousness or social competence are notoriously fallible and even arbitrary.

Carers' reluctance to allow clients to take risks or to make mistakes

Overprotectiveness may be rationalised as in the client's interest but may be a form of self-protection for the carer, who does not wish to accept responsibility if things go wrong. People only learn if they are allowed to try and fail and perhaps try again. Clients will never find out whether they can cope outside if they are kept in an artificial, safe environment and never allowed to make mistakes.

Social class attitudes and values in occupational therapy

The therapist's definitions of coping, social skills or self-care may not match the client's social background. There is always a risk that therapists hold up to the client inappropriate social norms, whether in domestic matters, employment or patterns of social and sexual interaction (Freidson 1970).

Methods of sound ethical problem solving

It has become fashionable to refer to every kind of moral difficulty or quandary as a moral dilemma. Strictly speaking, a real moral dilemma involves an irresolvable conflict of duties, so to treat all moral difficulties or problems as irresolvable dilemmas encourages people either to avoid taking responsibility for making difficult decisions or to treat them as simply a matter of personal judgement.

By far the greater proportion of ethical difficulties faced by therapists in everyday practice can be reframed as problems. Because we have methods for dealing with problems, we can generally find solutions to them, provided time is taken to look at them carefully. We can develop competence by learning to apply systematic approaches to dealing with routine ethical problems. However, some difficult dilemmas will remain. Because there can be no general rules for dealing with dilemmas, it requires personal courage to tackle them. We can only attempt to act as wisely as possible in the particular circumstances and be prepared to accept responsibility for the consequences.

In analysing the nature of moral judgements and moral actions, Aristotle suggests that all human acts have the same basic structure:

causes → means → ends

(Aristotle, analysis of Prudence, Book VI). If this is true, it is logical to suggest that in planning a course of action, making a rational decision or acting in a purposeful way we must:

- review the prevailing circumstances and the facts of the specific situation, including what ball-game we are in and what principles and rules apply
- consider what options are available, what expertise, assistance or resources we need and what means or methods we need to solve the presenting problem
- anticipate the likely outcomes of each option, have specific goals and realistic objectives so that we can assess whether or not our actions succeed.

Using the DECIDE model

There are many variants of problem solving that involve reviewing the factors involved in this basic causes → means → ends structure of intentional acts (compare, e.g., Grace & Cohen 1998 and Seedhouse 1988). However, we propose the model shown in Boxes 11.10 and 11.11 because it is not only a tested and tried method of systematic ethical decision making, but it also implicitly

---

Box 11.10   The DECIDE model (adapted from the SPIRAL model in Thompson et al 1994)

Causes (circumstances and rules)		Means (agency and methods)		Ends (goals and outcomes)	
D	E	C	I	D	E
D-etermine the facts	E-stablish the rules	C-onsider the options	I-dentify the outcomes	D-ecide on action plan	E-valuate the results
Deontological ethics (Principles, rights and duties)		Virtue/prudential ethics (competence and integrity)		Teleological ethics (costs and benefits, outcomes)	

Box 11.11 Using the DECIDE model to formulate ethical decisions (reproduced with kind permission from Thompson & Harries 1997)

D = **DEFINE THE PROBLEM/S. What are the key facts of the case and what ethical issue/s demand a decision immediately from you or your team?**

Analysis of a problem situation, using stakeholder analysis, generally reveals that defining the problem [or teasing out entangled problems] is often the most difficult part of the process. However, to define the problem clearly is essential before you can proceed to the next steps.
It is useful to start by identifying all the stakeholders (those people with a direct interest in the outcome of a decision), and then proceed by the following steps:

- Familiarise yourself thoroughly with the key facts of the case
- List the key stakeholders and rank them in order of importance
- Clarify what are the primary rights of the main stakeholders and their contractual duties
- Determine what are your (or your agency's) primary duties in relation to each stakeholder, and what rights you have in the matter.

E = **ESTABLISH THE RULES. Which ethical principles or rules have a special bearing on the decision you have to make, and how do you prioritise these?**

Identify which of the fundamental principles of protective beneficence, justice and respect for people's rights, as well as other requirements of the Code of Ethics and Professional Conduct for Occupational Therapists have a bearing on the case. Then decide which of these principles 'trumps' the others in this situation. (Deciding between the competing demands of different principles is difficult and requires sound value judgement. There is often no obvious 'right' answer, or there would not be a problem in the first place.)

C = **CONSIDER OPTIONS. What are the most reasonable, ethical and practical choices available to you in the specific situation under consideration?**

It is important to brainstorm all the possible things that you could do to deal with the problem, and then to spend some time focusing down on which are the most sensible and practical options. Some options will depend on obtaining further help or resources, or will take longer to achieve a satisfactory result, and some options may be more expensive or risky, etc.

I = **INVESTIGATE OUTCOMES. Given past experience, what are the likely ethical outcomes, costs and benefits, of each choice?**

Having generated a list of options and having ranked these in order of priority from your point of view, it is important to run each option past the three fundamental principles of justice, respect for people's rights and responsible care for others and the public good. If you tabulate the options and score each against the principles it is usually possible to see quite quickly which option is both more practical and ethically acceptable, or, at worst, least harmful.

D = **DECIDE ON ACTION. What is your goal? What are your practical objectives? How do you intend to achieve them effectively?**

Having conducted a careful option appraisal, on both factual and ethical grounds, you should have identified your best option for action. The next step is to develop a specific action plan with clear and achievable objectives, for only if you have clear goals and objectives, can you be said to be acting responsibly, and it is only with reference to your goals and objectives that you can evaluate later whether your action was successful or not. It is then important to commit yourself to resolute action and to execute your plan as efficiently and effectively as possible.

E = **EVALUATE RESULTS. What criteria will you use to judge your success in achieving your goal, practical and ethical objectives?**

No ethical decision can be said to be a fully responsible one if you have not carefully appraised the results of your action and identified what you can learn from your successes or mistakes. Accountability means 'being able to give an account' of what you have done to someone else, e.g.:

- What you perceived the problem to be and what ethical considerations you took into account
- What options you considered and what reasons you had for choosing your course of action
- What your action plan was and what goals and objectives you hoped to achieve
- What the specific outcomes of your action were, and whether these were good or bad.

(To be able to demonstrate what steps you took and to be able to justify them presupposes that you have documented the process and kept records of decisions and outcomes. Only in this way can you compare results on future occasions when you are faced with similar circumstances.)

takes account of the various aspects emphasised by the three broad types of ethical theory discussed.

To develop habits of systematic ethical decision making, individually and in teams, it is useful to practise the use of the DECIDE model (or the others mentioned in this chapter) on the case studies provided in the text. In this way you will develop competence in sound ethical decision making and be able to justify what you do.

SUMMARY

This chapter first set out to demystify ethics and to clarify what it is and is not, then emphasised that ethics is concerned primarily with ensuring the conditions for human flourishing and the responsible exercise of power in human relationships.

The differences between right/wrong discourse about duties and rules and good/bad discourse about values and outcomes, was discussed.

The various aspects of ethics to be considered in health care were distinguished, from the micro to the macro levels. Fundamental ethical principles common to all moral communities were examined.

The meaning of health and disease and the ethics of health care were then investigated, followed by consideration of how ethical principles apply to occupational therapists. The purpose of ethical codes was outlined and their limitations discussed.

The specific duties of the carer and the rights of the client were then considered, with examples of problematic situations.

Finally, specific ethical problems arising in occupational therapy and methods of coping with these dilemmas were looked at, and the DECIDE model for ethical problem solving introduced as a useful tool to aid ethical decision making.

REFERENCES

Aristotle 384–322BC Nicomachean ethics: http://classics.mit.edu/classics/Aristotle/nicomachaen. html

Barnitt R E 1996 Factitious disorders in occupational therapy: sad cases or incorrigible rogues? British Journal of Occupational Therapy 59(2)

Barnitt R, Warbery J, Rawlins S 1998 Two case discussions of ethics: editing the truth and the right to resources. British Journal of Occupational Therapy 61(2)

Beauchamp T L, Childress J F 1994 Principles of bio-medical ethics, 4th edn. Oxford University Press, Oxford

Buddha c 563–480BC Left no written record. See, however: http://www.knight.org/advent/cathen/03028b.htm

Confucius 551–479BC Analects. http://www.human. toyogakuen-u.ac.jp/~acmuller/contao/analects.htm

COT 2000 Code of ethics and professional conduct for occupational therapists. College of Occupational Therapists, London

Findlay J N 1970 Axiological ethics. Macmillan St Martin's Press, London

Freidson E 1970 The profession of medicine. Dodd and Mead, New York

Fromm E 1960 The fear of freedom. Routledge and Kegan Paul, London

Gillon R 1985 Philosophical medical ethics. Wiley, Chichester

Grace D, Cohen S 1998 Business ethics, 2nd edn. Oxford University Press, Oxford

Her Majesty's Stationery Office 1983 Mental Health Act. HMSO, London

Her Majesty's Stationery Office 1984 Mental Health (Scotland) Act. HMSO, London

MacIntyre A 1967 A short history of ethics. Routledge and Kegan Paul, London

Merleau-Ponty M 1962 The phenomenology of perception. Routledge and Kegan Paul, London

Nolan Committee 1995, 1996, 1997 First, second and third reports of the Committee on Standards in Public Life: Cm 2850–1; Cm 3270–1; Cm 3702–1. Stationery Office, London

Oxford Medical Dictionary 1980 Oxford University Press, Oxford

Plato Republic. http://classics.mit.edu/Plato/republic.html

Reilly M 1962 Occupational therapy can be one of the great ideas of twentieth century medicine. American Journal of Occupational Therapy 16(1): 1–9

Ross W D 1930 The right and the good. Oxford University Press, Oxford

Sartre J P 1956 No exit, and three other plays. Vintage Books, London

Saunders T J (ed) 1981 Aristotle, The politics, trans. T A Sinclair. Penguin, Harmondsworth

Seedhouse D 1988 Ethics: the heart of health care. Wiley, London

Sim J 1996 Client confidentiality: ethical issues in occupational therapy. British Journal of Occupational Therapy 59(2)

Thompson I E 1987 Fundamental ethical principles in health care. British Medical Journal, 295 (5 December)

Thompson I E 1995 A corporate approach to ethics in medicine. In: C I Phillips (ed) Logic and medicine, 2nd edn. BMJ Publishing, London

Thompson I E, Harries M 1997 Putting ethics to work. Office of the Public Sector Standards Commissioner, Western Australia

Thompson I E, Melia K M, Boyd K M 2000 Nursing ethics, 3rd edn. Churchill Livingstone, Edinburgh

Tillich P 1957 Systematic theology. Nisbet, London, Vol. 1

UNO 1947a Constitution of the World Health Organization. Chronicle of the WHO 1 (3.1). UN, New York

UNO 1947b Universal declaration of human rights. UN, New York

Veatch R M 1981 A theory of medical ethics. Basic Books, New York, Part 3

WHO 1978 Primary health care. Report. International conference on primary health care, Alma Ata, USSR, 6–12 September 1978. World Health Organization, Geneva

Media and Methods

12

Developing physical fitness to promote mental health

Hazel Bracegirdle

INTRODUCTION

Mens sana in corpore sano

Since ancient times, philosophers have speculated about the relationship between mind and body (Stein & Motta 1992). The idea that the body and mind, or soul, are interdependent but separate is common to many religions (Russell 1945, Ryle 1949, Popkin 1956, James 1960). The debate about whether the mind is an integral function of the body or a discrete entity influences the basic assumptions made by scientists and clinicians. In psychiatry, there is a continuing ideological battle between those who 'insist that all genuine psychiatric disorders rest upon a physical basis' and those who prefer psychosocial, cultural and political explanations of mental illness (Clare 1976). Interestingly, the use of physically demanding occupations, sports and exercise in the treatment of mental illness has a long history (Macdonald 1976). Hippocrates emphasised 'the body–mind link in all treatment' and 'recommended wrestling, riding and labour'. Later, Galen favoured digging, ploughing and building as treatments. During the Renaissance, 'exercises . . . for toughening up and for enjoyment were recommended by physicians and educationalists' alike (Macdonald 1976). In 1705, Francis Fuller wrote a popular treatise on medical gymnastics in *The Cure of*

Several Distempers especially the Hysterick or Hypochondriac Case. His assertion that a sedentary life may result in 'effete and languid . . . nerves' is probably just as relevant today (Hunter & Macalpine 1963). In the 19th century, male inmates were allowed to work in asylum gardens and farms and were taken on regular country walks. Victorian women patients, however, fared less well, being confined to ward-based and sedentary occupations (Bracegirdle 1991).

Thus we see that the benefits of physical exercise in the treatment of bodily illness and disability and the maintenance of health have long been known, but it is only in recent decades that its psychological effects have been studied scientifically (Gleser & Mendelberg 1990). There is a growing literature of 'positive findings for a cause–effect relationship between physical exercise and psychological well-being' (Crocker & Grozelle 1991, Sheridan & Radmacher 1992). Specifically, physical fitness correlates with mental health and well-being and is associated with reductions in anxiety and mild to moderate depression (Morgan & Goldston 1987, Steptoe & Butler 1996). Exercise is associated with a reduction of stress indicators, including heart rate, hormone levels and neuromuscular tension (Morgan & Goldston 1987). Vigorous physical activity is thought to benefit people of both sexes and all ages and is considered a safe addition to other therapies, including psychotropic medicine (Box 12.1; Morgan & Goldston 1987, Ruuskanen & Ruoppila 1995, Steptoe & Butler 1996). Health education campaigns often focus on the health benefits of exercise because about 60% of British and American people engage in little or no exercise (Gloag 1996, Rosellini 1997).

This chapter will present both biomedical and psychological research evidence for the affective benefits of exercise and discuss a number of possible explanations for this. A brief summary of normal motor development will be given, and then the physical difficulties and impairments that can afflict both those suffering from mental illness and those with learning disabilities will be described. Practical guidelines for therapists wishing to use exercise as therapy will be offered, with emphasis on important contraindi-

---

Box 12.1   National Institute of Mental Health workshop

The following consensus statements were issued by the [American] National Institute of Mental Health following a 'state of the art' workshop in 1984 (Morgan & Goldston 1987):

- Physical fitness is positively associated with mental health and well-being.
- Exercise is associated with the reduction of stress emotions, such as state anxiety.
- Anxiety and depression are common symptoms of failure to cope with mental stress, and exercise has been associated with a decreased level of mild to moderate depression and anxiety.
- Long-term exercise is usually associated with reductions in traits such as neuroticism and anxiety.
- Severe depression usually requires professional treatment, which may include medication, electroconvulsive therapy and/or psychotherapy, with exercise as an adjunct.
- Appropriate exercise results in reductions in various stress indices, such as neuromuscular tension, resting heart rate and some stress hormones.
- Current clinical opinion holds that exercise has beneficial emotional effects across all ages and in both sexes.
- Physically healthy people who require psychotropic medication may safely exercise when exercise and medication are titrated under close medical supervision.

---

cations, and a number of activities will be suggested. Finally, the chapter will be illustrated by an account of a gym club for people with learning disabilities, in which the author took part.

THE MENTAL HEALTH BENEFITS OF EXERCISE

BIOMEDICAL EVIDENCE

The endorphin hypothesis

In 1975 Hughes and colleagues isolated the first endogenous opioids (Grossman & Sutton 1985). Endogenous opioids are chemical brain transmitters, comprising a group of opioid peptides including endorphins. Endogenous opioids have a chemical structure similar to that of morphine and its derivatives, which have all been used medicinally – and abused addictively – since ancient times. Endorphins are produced by the brain, pituitary gland and some other cell lines.

Research into endorphin production and function in human beings usually utilises measurements of plasma levels and the demonstration of responses to the opiate antagonist naloxone (Morgan 1985).

The action of endogenous opioids has often been described as 'morphine-like' (Morgan 1985). Although the precise physiological role of the endorphins has yet to be found, and it is likely that endorphins act in conjunction with other transmitters to produce their effects, the following functions of endorphins have been proposed:

- they act as natural analgesics
- they produce a feeling of well-being, sometimes even of euphoria
- they seem to reduce responsiveness to external stimuli
- they reduce levels of tension or anxiety
- they may also be implicated in appetite control, blood pressure control, temperature regulation, pituitary secretions and the control of ventilation.

Because endorphins so closely resemble morphine and its derivatives, that is, drugs which both inhibit pain and produce a sense of well-being, these claims seem plausible. Endorphins may well function to reduce pain during strenuous activity (Phillipson 1987a, Hatfield 1991). Endorphin levels in pregnant women, for example, peak during labour and delivery. There is also much anecdotal evidence of soldiers and athletes being unaware of the pain of injuries sustained during physically strenuous activity, until it has stopped.

The 'runner's high', that is, the achievement of transcendental or 'peak' experiences during exercise, has been described (Houston et al 1989). Mandell described his own altered state of consciousness in this way: 'the running literature says that if you run six miles a day for two months, you are addicted forever. I understand. A cosmic view and peace are located between six and ten miles of running' (quoted by Morgan 1985). However, it must be remembered that a runner's high is distinguishable from that obtained by an injection of heroin, although it may lead to a form of addiction or dependence in

some runners. It may be that people who exercise regularly do develop a positive addiction for their sport, which then enables them to overcome damaging addictions and maintain their well-being (Griffiths 1996).

The common observation that 'improved affective states accompany both acute and chronic physical activity of a vigorous nature' (Morgan 1985) may be explained by the often repeated finding that vigorous physical activity stimulates endogenous opiate production (Wylie 1994). Farrel (1985) reviewed 12 studies, each of which clearly demonstrated a significant increase in β-endorphin levels following running. He concluded that 'exercise activates the endogenous opiate systems'. This effect can be seen both in human subjects and in animal models. Apparently, even laboratory mice can become so 'hooked' on swimming that they develop full blown morphine-like withdrawal symptoms when prevented from exercising (Christie & Chesser, quoted by Morgan 1985).

Other physiological explanations

Hyperthermia

A number of competing, speculative hypotheses have been proposed to explain the somatopsychic effect of exercise. These include the pyrogen hypothesis which suggests that the hyperthermia (overheating) induced by exercise acts through the hypothalamus to modify brain activity and reduce muscle tension, thus reducing arousal in both human and animal subjects (Martinsen 1987a, Gleser & Mendelberg 1990, Hatfield 1991).

Autonomic alterations

Catecholamines are of particular interest in the study of depression, which can be effectively treated by drugs which increase the availability of noradrenaline (Phillipson 1987b). The adrenal medulla releases the hormones noradrenaline and adrenaline in response to stressors including physical exercise (Phillipson 1987b). In the long term, repeated exercise may result in increased adrenal activity, allowing an increased store of corticosteroids which are then available to counter stress (Gleser & Mendelberg 1990, Hatfield 1991).

Neurotransmitter changes

Neurotransmitters, including serotonin (5-HT), noradrenaline and dopamine, mediate communication between adjacent neurons. These neurotransmitters are concentrated within the limbic system and the thalamus, areas of the brain which are implicated in the control of emotion and motivation. In depression, neurotransmitter levels are reduced. Antidepressant drugs raise these levels and can be used to improve mood. A natural increase in dopamine and serotonin has been observed in exercising rats. Mentally ill subjects have been shown to excrete increased levels of transmitter metabolites following a day of increased physical activity. It is likely that the exercise-related 'feel better' phenomenon is, in part, based on complex interactions between changes in these neurotransmitter levels (Hatfield 1991).

Additional hypotheses

It has been suggested that the increased levels of cerebral blood flow and oxygenation associated with exercise may be responsible for improvements in mood (Gleser & Mendelberg 1990). Hatfield (1991) has also described a number of other processes, termed the lateralisation of visceral feedback (the right hemispheric effect), the opponent-process model of affective change and the cardiac influence model (visceral afferent feedback), which appear to be highly speculative and are beyond the scope of this chapter.

It is unlikely that a single physiological change is responsible for the improvements in mood and reduction in anxiety enjoyed by exercisers. A number of processes have been outlined above, and these probably interact in highly complex ways during and after exercise. There is probably also considerable individual variation in physiological response to physical activity and in sensitivity to biochemical change.

PSYCHOLOGICAL EFFECTS OF EXERCISE

Recently, psychological research has demonstrated a significant, positive correlation between vigorous physical activity and improved mood, reduced anxiety and, in some instances, improved behaviour. Although studies have not proved a direct causal relationship between physical exercise and improved mental health, they do suggest that involvement in physically demanding activities is effective therapy. Moreover, improvements resulting from exercise can be shown in a variety of client groups, from behaviourally disordered children to elderly people (Evans 1985, Paillard & Newak 1985, Stacey 1985, Moore & Bracegirdle 1994, Ruuskanen & Ruoppila 1995, Steptoe & Butler 1996).

Exercise and depression

Although the mechanisms of the antidepressant effect of exercise are not clear, numerous studies and review articles have now documented the association between physical activity and improved mood (Simons 1985, Hales & Travis 1987, Martinsen 1987a, 1987b, Raglin 1990, Sheridan & Radmacher 1992). Most studies utilise aerobic exercise which is more effective than placebo and as effective as other treatments, including psychotherapy, but there is also evidence that nonaerobic training can help too (Martinsen 1987a, 1987b, Stein & Motta 1992, Wylie 1994). Some researchers have noted a dose–response effect in that long-term exercisers and those who exercise more vigorously seem to gain most improvement in mood (Dua & Hargreaves 1992). However, in extreme cases, overtraining by athletes, or exercise abuse, can lead to staleness and depression (Raglin 1990). According to Gleser & Mendelberg (1990), the 'antidepressant effect of exercise parallels an increment of fitness'. Exercise sessions should take place at least three times a week if both the physical and mental benefits are to be maintained (Greist 1987). People suffering from mild to moderate unipolar clinical depression are more likely to benefit from exercise than those with melancholia or bipolar disorders (Martinsen 1987b, Wylie 1994).

Anxiety and exercise

There is empirical evidence that vigorous physical exercise can not only lift mood but can also 'alleviate the negative consequences of anxiety and stress' (Simono 1991). Highly anxious people seem to benefit more than others, although there is no evidence that trait anxiety is reduced (Hales & Travis 1987, Gleser & Mendelberg 1990, Simono 1991). Many studies have investigated state anxiety in normal subjects, although the best results were obtained with people whose anxiety resulted from moderate affective disturbance (Morgan 1987, Crocker & Grozelle 1991, Wylie 1994).

There are a number of reports of the successful treatment of phobias through exercise (Hales & Travis 1987, Simono 1991). However, some individuals suffering from panic disorders may find that exercise accentuates physiological symptoms and this may increase anxiety (Wylie 1994).

Exercise seems to affect the physiological manifestations of stress, including heart rate and hormone levels, so that physically fit subjects recover more rapidly from stressful events (Hales & Travis 1987, Sheridan & Radmacher 1992). It has been suggested that exercise 'buffers the effects of stress on illness' and there is evidence that stressful life events are not associated with ill health among those who exercise (Sheridan & Radmacher 1992). The tension reduction associated with exercise usually lasts for up to 4–6 hours (Morgan 1987, Gleser & Mendelberg 1990). Again, exercise must be moderate to provide tension reduction. There is some evidence, for example, that marathon running does not improve stress tolerance (Hales & Travis 1987).

Psychological explanations

Improved self-concept

Exercisers typically report improvements in self-concept and this may reflect their perceptions about their fitter bodies and improved physical appearance (Sheridan & Radmacher 1992, Stein & Motta 1992). People who become stronger, more supple and more attractive as a result of exercise may feel greater self-mastery and control (Connolly & Einzig 1986). Heightened self-esteem and self-knowledge are often associated with this enhancement of self-concept (Gleser & Mendelberg 1990, Wylie 1994). Happiness and increased self-esteem also tend to result from success in reaching exercise goals and realising personal potential (Connolly & Einzig 1986, Reich et al 1997).

Sense of mastery

People have an innate need to overcome obstacles and confront the forces of nature, and doing so gives rise to a feeling of mastery (Connolly & Einzig 1986, Wylie 1994). Attaining mastery on a graded task combats the classic symptoms of helplessness, hopelessness and worthlessness, and probably reduces the self-defeating cognitions of people with depression (Gleser & Mendelberg 1990, Stein & Motta 1992). In this way, physical exercise may easily fit into Bandura's self-efficacy theory (Martinsen 1987b, Griffiths 1996).

Group participation

'When exercise takes place in a group setting, the effects of the therapist, the group, mutual support and encouragement' contribute to its beneficial effect (Wylie 1994). An important confounding variable in one study was that subjects made friends with one another and exercised together informally (Moore & Bracegirdle 1994). Participation in sport gives many opportunities for the development of team spirit, group participation and cooperation (Connolly & Einzig 1986, Gleser & Mendelberg 1990).

Diversion

The exercise session offers 'simple distraction or a cognitive time out' from day-to-day stressors, and some researchers suggest that this in itself reduces anxiety (Gleser & Mendelberg 1990, Hatfield 1991). An example of this form of diversion can be seen in the treatment of phobias through exercise (Wylie 1994).

Creativity and self-expression

People can express their feelings by moving and dancing and can communicate effectively through body language. Physical activities may meet a basic human need for aesthetic and creative endeavour (Connolly & Einzig 1986). Certainly, sport is widely believed to provide an outlet for both aggressive and affiliative impulses.

PHYSICAL DIFFICULTIES AND MENTAL HEALTH

NORMAL MOTOR DEVELOPMENT

Neurodevelopmental approaches to the treatment of motor control problems are based on the principle that motor development occurs sequentially. Some theorists claim that motor ontogeny recapitulates phylogeny, that is, an individual's development follows the evolution of the whole species. Generally, voluntary control of gross, mass or total movements is achieved before that of fine and discrete movements. Voluntary control of the body and limbs proceeds cephalocaudally, proximally to distally, and, in the hand, ulnarly to radially (Trombly & Scott 1977).

Although the sequence of normal motor development is roughly similar from individual to individual, there are normal exceptions. Some children, for example, never crawl but proceed from sitting through to 'bottom shuffling' to walking. All the developmental milestones described below may occur at any time within a broad range, so only the average age of each accomplishment is given (Sheridan 1973).

The movement and posture of newborn babies are dominated by primary reflexes. Head control is poor so there is marked head lag when the baby is pulled into a sitting position. Gradually, the strength of the primary reflexes diminishes as the baby gains increasing control of neck and shoulder muscles by the age of 3 months. By 5 or 6 months most babies can lift head and chest when prone, supporting their weight through extended arms. They will also grasp their toes when supine and sit with support. By 9 months babies can roll over, pull themselves up to sit and sit without support. Some may have started to pull themselves up to stand (supported) and many will begin to crawl.

Babies become increasingly active and mobile as they approach their first birthday. Most by then are fast crawlers, some have even tried the stairs and most will have taken their first few steps unaided. By 18 months many toddlers can walk well independently and run safely. They will be tumbling less frequently and can usually crawl upstairs and down again, backwards, without mishap. These toddlers can elegantly pick up objects from the floor without toppling over and can sit down upon small chairs.

Two-year-olds have become graceful and competent movers. They can run well, stopping and starting safely, and some will walk upstairs unaided. By the age of 3 most children can walk downstairs (two feet onto each step) and will clamber about happily on nursery climbing apparatus and manage toy cycles. Some 3-year-olds can walk on tiptoe and jump with two feet together. The average 5-year-old appears to be far more graceful, athletic and coordinated than his parents! Five-year-olds can run up and down stairs, demonstrate various party tricks (such as handstands and forward rolls) and can hop and skip beautifully.

We need to know about normal motor development so that we can tailor exercise programmes to suit individual developmental needs.

PHYSICAL PROBLEMS ASSOCIATED WITH MENTAL DISORDERS

Psychiatry is a relatively young branch of medicine and so there is still much disagreement among practitioners about the underlying causes of mental illness. Biological, psychological and social explanations have all been given for the abnormal behaviour. Richard Hunter, a neuropsychiatrist, carefully researched the history of psychiatry. He found that abnormal posture and movements among the mentally ill occurred before the introduction of neuroleptic medication (Hunter & Macalpine 1974). His observation that 'the high incidence of dystonic and dyskinetic syndromes explains why mental hospital patients the world over look and move alike, and appear to have done so since pictorial records began' tends to support his contention that all mental illness has an organic basis, though this is yet to be established.

Institutional neurosis

However, Barton (1976) claimed that many motor and postural abnormalities were the direct result of a syndrome he named 'institutional neurosis'. This comprises passivity, submissiveness, apathy and inactivity, together with deterioration of posture, gait and physical condition. People may be mute, losing motivation and interest in the outside world and ceasing to care for their appearance. They may lose all sense of individuality as a result of living in overcrowded 'total institutions' where browbeating, petty restrictions and enforced idleness are the norm (Goffman 1961).

Whatever the cause, it is well known that psychiatric in-patients and, in particular, those with a diagnosis of schizophrenia, score well below normal on measures related to physical activity and physical fitness (Chamove 1985).

Effects of drugs

Movements may also be affected by the side-effects of commonly prescribed medicines. The fatigue and drowsiness associated with the use of antidepressants and tranquillisers may reduce some people's drive to exercise (Eriksson et al 1990). According to Martinsen (1987a, 1987b), the neuroleptics have a wide range of effects on the body and some of these, including weight gain, interfere with the capacity and motivation to exercise. The most recently developed antipsy-

chotic drugs do not have the same range of side-effects, but they are not always prescribed because of the cost.

The drug-induced dyskinesias

Dopamine is a chemical messenger implicated in the integration of motor function and dopamine levels can be affected by various drugs (Lees 1985). Amphetamine addicts develop abnormal movements, as do Parkinsonian clients who are treated with L-dopa, but it is the effect of neuroleptics that concerns us here. These drugs are widely used in psychiatric practice, often in heavy doses, for controlling psychotic symptoms.

In 1949, Charpentier first synthesised chlorpromazine, a neuroleptic in the phenothiazine family, which was found to induce a state of affective indifference and to reduce drive and aggressiveness without impairing memory or cognition. In 1952, Val de Grace et al concluded that chlorpromazine possessed antipsychotic properties. Since then it has been partly responsible for reducing the numbers of long-stay clients in institutions and has enabled general practitioners to manage acute psychotic relapses in the community.

Unfortunately, a range of distressing extrapyramidal side-effects frequently occurs, sometimes persisting long after drug withdrawal. These include the following, commonly observed disorders:

Acute movement disorders. These start within the first few days or weeks of treatment, or after an increase in dosage, and are usually reversible. They include:

- *Acute dyskinesias*. These typically affect children and young adults and have an incidence of 3–10% in routine practice. Symptoms include painful dystonia, choreoathetosis and Pisa syndrome (a postural disturbance).
- *Akathisia*. This affects 10–20% of people of all ages. It consists of dysphoria and distressing motor restlessness, often seen as shuffling or foot tapping while the person is sitting down.
- *Parkinson's syndrome*. Again, 10–20% of people will be affected, particularly those who are

middle-aged or elderly. They show rigidity, bradykinesia and rest tremor.

- *Rabbit syndrome*. Middle-aged and elderly people may be afflicted more rarely by these perioral 'nibbling' movements (Lees 1985).

Late-onset movement disorder. Finally, a late-onset and potentially irreversible disorder may occur up to 5 years after medication is started:

- *Tardive dyskinesia*. This afflicts 10–20% of elderly people. Symptoms include buccolingo masticatory dyskinesia, limb choreoathetosis and dystonia (Lees 1985).

The occupational therapist's responsibilities

The occupational therapist is likely to have very much more face-to-face contact with the psychotic client than the psychiatrist who prescribes for him. The responsible therapist remains alert to the possibility of these disabling side-effects and is quick to report their occurrence so that drug dosages may be modified or anticholinergic medication given.

Lees (1985) reported that the cosmetic impact of orofacial dyskinesias can be modified by chewing gum or sucking sweets. He also stated that, because the abnormal movements are often at their worst during inactivity and stress, 'physical activity and relaxation techniques should also be encouraged'.

PHYSICAL IMPAIRMENTS ASSOCIATED WITH LEARNING DISABILITY IN ADULTHOOD

Answar (1986) stated that 'mentally handicapped people have consistently been found to be inferior to non-handicapped subjects on measures of physical development, gross motor and fine motor abilities'. More severe learning disabilities are often associated with more severe physical disabilities, while moderately and mildly learning disabled people still have more physical difficulties to contend with than the average person.

Psychological research has established that there is a strong relationship between cognitive development and motor performance. Even simple actions have to be planned in advance, the individual making predictions and inferences, based on specific cues and past experience, to coordinate motor behaviour.

Motor planning seems to be an intellectual function. A person uses information received from a variety of sensory receptors in order to learn new motor skills. This sensory input must be encoded and stored in a format that allows movement planning, execution and evaluation to occur. Kinaesthetic and other sensory cues are compared to inner mental representations or body schemata. These representations become increasingly differentiated as the child develops and gains mastery of his bodily movements.

The complexity of this mental process perhaps explains the common observation that even people with moderate learning disability who have no obvious organic damage are often slow and clumsy in their movements. Furthermore, simple automatic movements such as walking and running, which are thought to present little challenge to motor planning, are well executed by this group but complex or intellectually challenging tasks cause them to become increasingly awkward and clumsy. Sporting activities can be used to engage these people's competence in gross motor performance, thus proving more successful and pleasurable than activities that demand fine motor coordination. For this group, it is important to break down directions into simple steps that can be learned sequentially. Repetition, demonstration and a 'hands-on' teaching approach are also useful (Maisto & Stephens 1991).

Many people with severe learning disabilities are limited physically, not only by their cognitive deficits but also by specific areas of brain impairment. For example, the physical handicaps associated with cerebral palsy in the adult ambulant population include deformities that result from the interplay of gravity, abnormal movements and lack of muscle usage over years. Mild or moderate spasticity may make one or more limbs stiff and difficult to move, with a marked springiness at the extremes of joint movement. This leads to characteristic abnormal postures and gait. Individuals suffering from spasticity may have sudden, unpleasant spasms if roughly handled or exposed to unexpected noises. Pathological tonic reflexes may also persist into adulthood and can seriously impede voluntary movement (Golding & Goldsmith 1986).

THERAPEUTIC EXERCISE

How can we help clients to benefit from vigorous physical exercise? How do we get them up out of their chairs? Each therapist needs to develop her own dynamic, individual approach, and the following guidelines may help.

Setting up therapeutic exercise and sports programmes

In an ideal world, the physical activities chosen for an individual would be geared precisely to his needs and capabilities and would meet the aims and objectives of his treatment. Unfortunately, financial, organisational and social factors also affect the selection of activities. A compromise is usually made between the individual's requirements, the demands of the group, the therapist's talents and, of course, the facilities, equipment and money available.

The astute therapist gains access to all the space and equipment that is available in her department, clinic or hospital. She also establishes links with local community sports and swimming facilities and liaises with appropriate charitable organisations (see Useful addresses, p. 225). The therapist must also keep an up-to-date file of local resources so that she can advise discharged clients about local clubs and facilities.

Contraindications to vigorous exercise

A study of anatomy, physiology and kinesiology equips the occupational therapist with an understanding of the body in action. However, it is also necessary to be aware of the many contraindica-

tions to physical exercise and to be ready to consult medical colleagues if a client's capacity to participate is in doubt. Such contraindications include the following:

- Vigorous physical exercise is contraindicated in heart disease, hypertension, musculoskeletal conditions and, more rarely, bone cancers.
- Poorly controlled epilepsy may make the use of sports equipment especially dangerous.
- Some people with Down's syndrome have atlantoaxial instability and may risk neurological damage through subluxation (Collacott 1987).
- Young women suffering from anorexia nervosa a refusal to eat combined with distorted body image – tend to abuse exercise in order to lose weight and should be excluded from sports programmes. Recent research suggests that bulimia sufferers also exercise to control weight and to counteract the effects of binge eating (Pruitt & Kappius 1991).
- People on phenothiazine medication are likely to have highly photosensitive skin and need to be protected from exposure to sunshine. Protective clothing and sunscreen lotions should be used (Eriksson et al 1990).

ELEMENTS OF THERAPEUTIC EXERCISE

The therapist's role

The therapist must, of course, be physically fit to lead exercise and sports groups. These activities are physically demanding and the therapist needs considerable strength and stamina.

Simple activities such as folk dancing, soft play, keep fit or running will be well within the capabilities of most occupational therapists. However, ideally, the therapist will have additional experience or training in chosen activities. For example, it may be necessary to rescue a floundering swimmer or to instil the discipline needed for safety on a trampoline.

The therapist should be aware of health and safety requirements and be a competent first-aider. She should be a good model, therefore her style of leadership should allow for her own participation in the activity. The effective occupational therapist is suitably dressed for action and ready to communicate her own enthusiasm for, and enjoyment of, the activity. The skilled therapist will also recruit other expert or talented staff, such as nurses and physiotherapists, to help her.

The location

Ideally, clients should carry out sports and exercise programmes in purpose-built buildings or on special playing fields, tracks or pitches. This usually involves having to leave the clinical setting and seek out appropriate community facilities (Fig. 12.1) with all the benefits of improved social integration and reduced dependence on the health care setting that this brings. However, playing fields, large halls and hydrotherapy pools are sometimes available within hospitals and are invaluable for those who are too fragile or ill to venture far.

Health and safety criteria must be met, whether the location is inside or outside the health care setting, and the environment should be well ventilated, warm and clean. The condi-

tion of the floor is particularly important; a clean, non-slip surface is imperative and special care should be taken to avoid slipping at the swimming baths.

Equipment

Many activities do not require special equipment but most sports do. Cheap and simple items such as mats, skittles, bean bags, skipping ropes and balls should be available in every department, although the therapist may need to argue her case before larger and more expensive items such as punch bags and table-tennis tables are obtained. Highly specialised equipment is also highly expensive, so if people want to use trampolines and ski slopes they will almost certainly have to seek them outside the hospital or day centre!

All equipment should be well maintained, kept clean and stored safely. Broken, shoddy equipment is uninspiring and unattractive. A technical instructor is usually recruited to help maintain and repair such things as bicycles, and may even make simple equipment.

Kit

Everybody should be appropriately dressed for sports and exercise. Clothes should be loose-fitting, warm but absorbent and easily washed. Track suits, shorts and T-shirts are relatively inexpensive to buy and hardwearing. Most are easy to put on and take off and will fit people who are not standard shapes and sizes. People who are resident in hospitals and other institutions may need to go on a special shopping trip to obtain kit. Care should then be taken that it does not disappear in the laundry.

Adequate footwear is extremely important. Advice may be obtained from the chiropodist or physiotherapist if a client has fitting problems. No one should go running without wearing proper running shoes, and pumps or lightweight sports shoes will help prevent slipping and tripping in the gym. In some activities, notably dance and yoga, the best footwear is no footwear. Finally, the client's kitbag should also contain

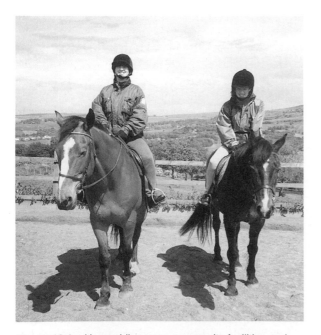

Figure 12.1 Horse-riding uses community facilities and can boost social skills and client morale.

soap, shampoo, towel and a comb or brush, so that he may take a shower after exercise.

Interpersonal processes

The competent therapist organises activities to give opportunities for satisfactory social interaction and to promote social skilfulness. Social aspects of exercise groups include the following:

- The therapist manages the social factors involved in sports and exercise sessions to promote social integration and thereby enhance the individual's self-esteem.
- There is social psychological evidence to suggest that being part of a team gives rise to intra-group cooperation and identification, which produces a sense of belonging.
- Creative movement and dance groups, in particular, encourage contact and help to develop nonverbal communication skills.
- Competitive activities channel aggressive feelings productively and improve motivation to achieve and to participate.

Almost all clients who suffer from mental illness or learning disability have some degree of impairment of social function and most have little social confidence. By focusing on the team effort and on the physical activity itself, rather than upon specific communication skills, the client's social competence is developed relatively painlessly. In the course of the sports activity he simply becomes a little closer to his team-mates and is more able to express himself and to be playful with them.

RECOMMENDED ACTIVITIES

The activities described below have all been successfully incorporated into occupational therapy programmes for people with mental illness or those with learning disabilities. Each requires a minimum of specialised equipment and little expenditure, although most demand that the occupational therapist has a little extra training and experience. All can be adapted to meet the needs of individuals with a range of abilities and nobody needs to be particularly fit before attempting any of them. None of the activities needs to stress competitiveness and all are suitable for groups.

Relaxation training is a valuable addition to physical exercise, therefore this is included.

Relaxation training

Vigorous physical activity undoubtedly prepares the mind and body for relaxation. While reminding us that relaxation still appears to defy definition, Keable (1985a) states that it is usually considered to be a mixture of reduced awareness of the environment and feelings of drowsiness and well-being. These responses are accompanied by decreases in breathing rate, skeletal blood flow, sweat output and blood pressure, and are thought to be the result of parasympathetic autonomic activity.

A variety of relaxation training methods is successfully used by both therapists and clinical psychologists:

- The physiological techniques, pioneered by Jacobson, emphasise learning to 'turn off' tensions as a muscular skill. This is achieved by, first, recognising the presence of minute amounts of tension, then releasing it, proceeding muscle group by muscle group.
- Meditative techniques require a peaceful environment, the cultivation of a passive attitude and, usually, some form of mantra (repetitive subvocalisation). Benson's method, for example, resulted from his observation that ancient teachings or prayer and meditation had common features (Keable 1985a). His subjects were asked to subvocalise the word 'one' with every exhalation.
- Hypnotic techniques rely on the therapist's suggestion that the subject should concentrate on peaceful thoughts, experience warmth and heaviness in the muscles and witness his own thoughts in a detached way. The actual mechanism of suggestion is unknown but many techniques include hypnotic elements, such as repetitive phrases and visualisation exercises.

Dance

Minas (1978) claimed that dance has considerable therapeutic value, whether or not it is used in conjunction with traditional talk therapies, for the following reasons:

- Dancing enables the individual to become efficient and well coordinated and to function better in his environment.
- Most dance-and-movement therapy is based on the belief that free movement is a powerful medium for the expression of emotion. The body and its movements become the instrument of expression, thus allowing the release of feeling.
- Dance therapy fosters spontaneity and gives opportunities for self-exploration through creativity.
- It teaches the art of differential relaxation, enabling the client to master anxiety and tension in everyday life.
- Dance is a social activity that involves developing the ability to communicate nonverbally and through touch.
- It encourages participants to be aware of their use of space, including the socially important personal space.
- It gives people an opportunity to have fun together without demanding skilful verbal communication of them.

Swimming

The value of hydrotherapy in the treatment of people with physical disability has long been recognised. Less formally, swimming sessions at the local baths have much to offer people with learning disability or mental illness (Fig. 12.2).

Swimming is a great leveller. Once in the water, people with moderate physical handicaps can participate as freely as the able-bodied. Everybody can enjoy the vigorous physical pre-swimming exercises, even if they cannot yet swim. Swimming is especially suitable for those who have arthritis, back pain or are overweight.

Most local authorities provide modern swimming pools, complete with changing rooms and snack bars. Swimming should be inexpensive; special rates may be available and swimming

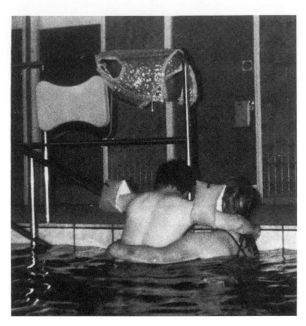

Figure 12.2 Using local community swimming facilities. (Source: Offerton House, Stockport.)

instruction may be available from trained attendants. The occupational therapist in charge must, however, be a good swimmer and have passed her life-saver test. Trips to the swimming baths also encourage institutionalised people to use public transport and give the opportunity to practise self-care skills such as dressing.

Research has shown that, in the short term, both men and women 'swimmers are less anxious, depressed, angry, and more clear minded and vigorous after swimming than before', with both beginning and intermediate swimmers reporting benefits (Berger 1987, Wylie 1994).

Yoga

Gellharn reported that electroencephalogram changes accompany yoga trance states where 'unusual degrees of mental concentration and corresponding levels of cortical excitation may be attained during complete muscular relaxation' (quoted by Keable 1985a). Anderton & Winterbane (1979) stressed that yoga does not require special philosophical or religious belief and, when practised, increases the individual's ability for mental and physical relaxation. Mastery of the yoga asanas (postures) and breathing techniques is said to increase concentration, stimulate interest and improve body awareness.

Occupational therapists giving instruction in yoga should be adequately trained themselves but there is no shortage of yoga teachers and clients who develop an interest in the occupational therapy department can usually be directed to local classes.

Yoga is non-competitive, requires a peaceful atmosphere and emphasises relaxation, therefore it is of great value to the frightened and fragile mentally ill person who cannot face more boisterous activity.

Keep fit

Keep fit has been, for more than half a century, the most popular and accessible form of exercise for many people. Most clients will recognise the term, and both men and women of all ages can easily be persuaded to participate. Basic occupational therapy training equips the therapist with sufficient knowledge to run classes safely.

The keep-fit session should be well organised and disciplined but geared to the individual's needs and abilities. Recently, keep-fit teachers have introduced simple props such as balls, hoops and ribbons, and it may be appropriate to use lively music.

Again, having gained a reasonable degree of fitness and confidence in the occupational therapy department, clients can be directed to locally available classes including 'Look after yourself' courses and over 60s groups.

Walking, jogging and running

Walking is the simplest and most natural form of exercise, even for those who are very unfit. Walking trips encourage people to explore their neighbourhoods and a bus ride to the countryside offers an opportunity to enjoy nature. No special equipment is needed (except for hill walking) other than a pair of stout shoes and warm socks. Ramblers' Associations may meet locally and offer undemanding social contact, especially for older people.

As fitness increases, walking and jogging may be alternated, provided that proper running shoes are worn and care is taken to prevent overuse injuries. Jogging and running are extremely popular, cheap and fun, and need not be solitary activities. Athletic clubs welcome runners and joggers and may organise competitive events and 'fun runs' locally for the keen runner.

A GYM CLUB FOR PEOPLE WITH LEARNING DISABILITIES

Finally, there follows an account of a gym club for people with learning disabilities that the author helped to run for $1\frac{1}{2}$ years. The club catered for 12 clients and enjoyed a high staff: client ratio (about 1:2.5). Apart from the trained staff (one charge nurse and one senior occupational therapist), there were up to three auxiliary nurses, additional help from students (nurses and occupational therapists) and occasional help from basic grade physiotherapists on short placements.

The club met each Friday afternoon for sessions lasting about $2\frac{1}{2}$ hours, which included walking to and from the gymnasium which was about half a mile from the hospital. The gym was well equipped with mats, wall bars and apparatus. Changing rooms, showers, toilets and a drinks machine were made available to club members.

The clients

A group of 13 people, 10 residents and three day clients, was selected initially. Nine were men, and four women; five people had moderate learning disabilities and the rest were diagnosed as 'severely subnormal'. The latter group included two people who had mild spasticity and associated deformities but all were ambulant. At least four participants suffered from mood disturbance and one woman had severe anxiety. Another woman had arthritis and one man suffered from frequent episodes of occulogyric crisis. Everybody else was in reasonably good health and most of the club members were in their thirties. Two men had Down syndrome. Only one participant had to be dropped from the programme because of incontinence, which was difficult to manage in a public place.

Of the 12 remaining club members, not every person could attend every week (because of home visits, staff shortages or other treatments) but most had about three sessions each month. Just over half of the group received at least one occupational therapy session per week and most of the others were engaged in activities run by nursing staff. Three clients were involved in no other activities at all during the week.

Aims and objectives

Individual clients could be given their own, short-term objectives which could be met in the gym club context; for example, 'Bill will tolerate being with the group for the duration of the activity and will not leave the gym during the session' or 'John will put on his own trainers, independently, in response to verbal prompts'. Most people in the group also liked to have their own exercise targets and personal-best records and were applauded for their efforts to do 'just one more' sit up or, perhaps, their first proper seat drop on the trampoline.

In addition to these goals, staff formulated the following broad aims of treatment:

Social aims

These were:

- to give residents a break from institutional life
- to teach clients how to find their way around the locality and use a community facility
- to promote communication (including the use of sign language)
- to develop a sense of belonging by increasing group cohesion.

Physical aims

These were:

- to improve coordination and spatial awareness

- to improve general physical condition and increase cardiovascular fitness
- to develop strength and suppleness and to improve posture and gait.

Personal aims

These included:

- to improve mood and reduce anxiety
- to provide an outlet for aggressive impulses
- to improve confidence and enhance self-image
- to encourage independent personal care (especially dressing and grooming)
- to provide opportunities for clients to face challenges and achieve success.

The procedure

Clients were asked if they wished to attend and arrangements were made for their kit to be provided. It was determined from the beginning that only those who could be appropriately clad in the gym might attend. The party assembled at the same time and place each week and walked to the gym, following precisely the same route each time so that no one got lost. One qualified member of staff assumed responsibility each week for the safety and well-being of club members. Once at the gym, clients and staff changed in the changing rooms, with only minimal help given.

The session began with keep-fit exercises. With everybody seated on gym mats, all joints were put through a full range of movement and muscles were warmed up and stretched. This was followed by a brief jog of five laps around the gym, then more strenuous exercises were done in a standing position. Individuals were encouraged to demonstrate or choose favourite exercises and people were asked to pair off to help each other, for example, to do sit ups. This was followed by a faster jog around the gym and, sometimes, a brisk game of tag. If there were sufficient staff to provide safe supervision, clients could then clamber up wall bars or balance on bars. The gym club members then took turns on the trampoline. Care was taken that there were enough people to 'spot' and nobody got on to the trampoline alone until he had demonstrated adequate caution when partnered by a staff member. Finally, the participants relaxed on the gym mats.

Afterwards, everybody showered, dressed and had a hot drink before heading home.

Leadership

Staff used a democratic leadership style because institutionalised people are, unfortunately, often subjected to authoritarian approaches. Qualified staff took turns to explain and to demonstrate exercises and all staff joined in throughout. A playful and accepting group atmosphere was thus created and clients were encouraged to tease and cajole staff who failed to meet their own targets.

Results

Eighteen months is a relatively short period for a project involving people with severe learning disabilities, and yet some improvements were noted. Among the severely handicapped group, the following changes were observed:

- Two men showed a decrease in unacceptable behaviours (spitting and yelling), even outside the gym.
- Everybody in the group turned up on time each week and each exhibited a readiness to set out for the gym.
- Most people were mute and socially withdrawn but during the course of the workout they smiled and made eye contact more often, and also made more frequent verbal utterances than usual.
- One man only began to join in consistently each week after attending for 11 months. Results were slow in coming but very worthwhile.

Most impressive were the responses of three men who were usually to be found rocking or exhibiting other stereotypic behaviour on their own during the week, but who came alive in the gym. They frequently demonstrated greater comprehension of the spoken word and a greater willingness to interact with others during the session than at home.

Of the less handicapped group, most of whom could, and would, express themselves verbally, nearly every person took a great deal of pride in his accomplishments. It was particularly delightful to see people who were once afraid of, for example, the trampoline, developing confidence and surprising themselves by overcoming their fears. These people all said they enjoyed coming to the gym and clearly looked forward to the sessions. One woman reported feeling less anxious as a result of doing her weekly workout, and all learned to relax more. Our results were similar to those reported by Schurrer (1985).

SUMMARY

Historically, there have been many attempts to understand the mind–body relationship and from ancient times the notion that bodily and mental fitness are interdependent has prevailed. This chapter reviewed recent literature on the scientific study of exercise, anxiety and depression. Both physiological and psychological explanations for the well established association between physical fitness and mental health were outlined.

Normal motor development was briefly described. The chapter described the motor impairments which are often associated with mental illness, with drug treatments and with learning disability. Simple guidelines were given for running safe and effective sports and exercise programmes and contraindications to treatment were listed.

The chapter was illustrated by an account of the author's work with a group of institutionalised people with learning disabilities.

REFERENCES

Anderton F, Winterbane A 1979 Yoga in a short stay psychiatric unit. British Journal of Occupational Therapy 42(8): 191–193

Answar F 1986 Cognitive deficit and motor skill. In: Ellis D (ed) Sensory impairments in mentally handicapped people. Croom Helm, Kent

Barton R 1976 Institutional neurosis, 3rd edn. Wright, Bristol

Berger B G 1987 Stress levels in swimmers. In: Morgan W P, Goldston S E (eds) Exercise and mental health. Hemisphere, Washington

Bracegirdle H 1991 Two hundred years of therapeutic occupations for women hospital patients. British Journal of Occupational Therapy 54(6): 231–232

Chamove A S 1985 Exercise improves behaviour: a rationale for occupational therapy. British Journal of Occupational Therapy 49(3): 83–86

Clare A 1976 Psychiatry in dissent. Tavistock, London

Collacott R A 1987 Atlantoaxial instability in Down's syndrome. British Medical Journal 294(6578): 988–989

Connolly C, Einzig H 1986 The fitness jungle. Century Hutchinson, London

Crocker P R E, Grozelle C 1991 Reducing induced state anxiety: effects of acute aerobic exercise and autogenic relaxation. Journal of Sports Medicine and Physical Fitness 32(2)

Dua J, Hargreaves L 1992 Effect of aerobic exercise on negative affect, positive affect, stress and depression. Perceptual and Motor Skills 75: 355–361

Eriksson B O, Mellstrand T, Peterson L, Renstršm P, Svedmyr N 1990 Sports medicine, health and medication. Guinness Publishing, London

Evans W H 1985 The effects of exercise on selected classroom behaviours of behaviourally disordered adolescents. Behavioural Disorders 11(1)

Farrel P A 1985 Exercise and endorphins: male responses. Medicine and Science in Sport and Exercise 17(1)

Gleser J, Mendelberg H 1990 Exercise and sport in mental health: a review of the literature. Israel Journal of Psychiatry and Related Sciences 2: 99–112

Gloag D 1996 Campaign aims to make the British more active. British Medical Journal 7034(312): 799

Goffman E 1961 Asylums. Penguin, Harmondsworth

Golding R, Goldsmith L 1986 The caring persons guide to handling the severely multiply handicapped. Macmillan, London

Greist J H 1987 Exercise intervention with depressed outpatients. In: Morgan W P, Goldston S E (eds) 1987 Exercise and mental health. Hemisphere, Washington

Griffiths M 1996 Behavioural addictions. Psychology Review pp 9–12

Grossman A, Sutton J R 1985 Endorphins: what are they? How are they measured? What is their role in exercise? Medicine and Science in Sport and Exercise 17(1)

Hales R E, Travis T W 1987 Exercise as a treatment option for anxiety and depressive disorder. Military Medicine 152(6): 299–302

Hatfield B D 1991 Exercise and mental health: the mechanisms of exercise-induced psychological states. In: Diamant L (ed) Psychology of sports, exercise and fitness: social and personal issues. Hemisphere, New York

Houston J P, Hammen C, Padilla A et al 1989 Invitation to psychology, 3rd edn. Harcourt Brace Jovanovich, Orlando, Florida

Hunter R, Macalpine I 1963 Three hundred years of psychiatry, 1535–1860. Oxford University Press, Oxford

Hunter R, Macalpine I 1974 Psychiatry for the poor. Dawsons, Kent

James W 1960 The varieties of religious experience. Collins, London

Keable D 1985a Relaxation training techniques: a review. Part 1. British Journal of Occupational Therapy 48(4): 99–102

Keable D 1985b Relaxation training techniques: a review. Part 2. British Journal of Occupational Therapy 48(7): 201–204

Lees A J 1985 Tics and related disorders. Churchill Livingstone, Edinburgh

Macdonald 1976 Occupational therapy in rehabilitation, 4th edn. Ballière Tindall, London

Maisto A A, Stephens J R 1991 Mental retardation and recreational fitness programs. In: Diamant L (ed) Psychology of sports, exercise and fitness: social and personal issues. Hemisphere, New York

Martinsen E W 1987a Exercise and medication in the psychiatric patient. In: Morgan W P, Goldston S E (eds) Exercise and mental health. Hemisphere, Washington

Martinsen E W 1987b The role of aerobic exercise in the treatment of depression. Stress Medicine 3: 93–100

Minas S C 1978 Dance as a therapy. British Journal of Occupational Therapy 41(3): 101–103

Morgan W P 1985 Affective benefience of vigorous physical activity. Medicine and Science in Sports and Exercise 17(1): 94–100

Morgan W P 1987 State anxiety following acute physical activity. In: Morgan W P, Goldston S E (eds) Exercise and mental health. Hemisphere, Washington

Morgan W P, Goldston S E (eds) 1987 Exercise and mental health. Hemisphere, Washington

Moore C, Bracegirdle H 1994 The effects of a short term low intensity exercise programme on the psychological well being of community dwelling elderly women. British Journal of Occupational Therapy 57(6): 213–216

Paillard M, Newak K 1985 Use exercise to help older adults: clients in acute care benefit from exercise/relaxation plan. Journal of Gerontogical Nursing 11(7)

Phillipson O T 1987a Endorphins. In: Gregory R L (ed) The Oxford companion to the mind. Oxford University Press, Oxford

Phillipson O T 1987b Catecholamines. In: Gregory R L (ed) The Oxford companion to the mind. Oxford University Press, Oxford

Popkin R 1956 Philosophy made simple. W H Allen, London

Pruitt U A, Kappius R V 1991 Sports, exercise and eating disorders. In: Diamant L (ed) Psychology of sports, exercise and fitness: social and personal issues. Hemisphere, New York

Raglin J S 1990 Exercise and mental health: beneficial and detrimental effects. Sports Medicine 9(6): 323–329

Reich J, Diener E, Meyers D G, Michalos A C 1994 The road to happiness. Psychology Today 27(4): 32

Roselli L 1997 How far should you go to stay fit? US News and World Report 123(18): 95

Russell B 1945 A history of western philosophy. Simon and Schuster, New York

Ruuskanen J M, Ruoppila I 1995 Physical activity and psychological well-being among people aged 65 to 84 years. Age and Ageing 24: 292

Ryle G 1949 The concept of mind. Hazell, Watson and Viney, Aylesbury

Schurrer R 1985 Effects of physical training on cardiovascular fitness and behaviour patterns of mentally retarded adults. American Journal of Mental Deficiency 90(2)

Schutz W C 1967 Joy. Grove Press, Houston

Sheridan C L, Radmacher S A 1992 Health psychology: challenging the biomedical model. Wiley, New York

Sheridan M D 1973 From birth to five years: children's developmental progress. Nelson, London

Simono R B 1991 Anxiety reduction and stress management through physical fitness. In: Diamant L (ed) Psychology of sports, exercise and fitness: social and personal issues. Hemisphere, New York

Simons A 1985 Exercise as a treatment for depression: an update. Clinical Psychology Review 5(6): 553–568

Stacey C 1985 Simple cognitive and behavioural changes resulting in improved physical fitness in persons over 50 years of age. Canadian Journal on Aging 4(2)

Stein P N, Motta R W 1992 Effects of aerobic and nonaerobic exercise on depression and self-concept. Perceptual and Motor Skills 74: 79–89

Steptoe A, Butler N 1996, Sports participation and emotional well being in adolescents. The Lancet 347: 1789

Takagi H, Simon E J 1981 Advances in endogenous and exogenous opioids. Elsevier, Amsterdam

Trombly C A, Scott A D 1977 Occupational therapy for physical dysfunction. Williams and Wilkins, Baltimore

Wylie K 1994 Benefits of exercise in affective illness. Psychiatry in Practice 13(1): 18–20

FURTHER READING

Cotton M 1981 Out of doors with handicapped people. Souvenir Press, London

Health Education Council and Sports Council. Exercise: why bother? Health Education Council, London (suitable for clients)

Iyengar B K J 1976 Light on yoga. Allen and Unwin, London

Levette G 1982 No handicap to dance. Souvenir Press, London

Thompson N 1984 Sport and recreation provision for disabled people. The Disabled Living Foundation and the Sports Council, Architectural Press, London

USEFUL ADDRESSES

Association of Swimming Therapy, Treetops, Swan Hill, Ellesmere, Shropshire SY12 0LZ

Central Council for Physical Recreation, Francis House, Francis Street, London SW1P 1PQ

Cerebral Palsy International Sports and Recreation Association, c/o Capability Scotland, 22 Corstorphine Road, Edinburgh EH12 6HP

British Sports Association for the Disabled, Hayward House, Harvey Road, Aylesbury, Buckinghamshire HP21 8PP

Duke of Edinburgh's Award Scheme, 5 Prince of Wales Terrace, London W8

Handicapped Adventure Playground Association, Fulham Palace, Bishop's Avenue, London SW6

National Association of Swimming Clubs for the Handicapped, 219 Preston Drove, Brighton, East Sussex BN1 6FL

Scottish Sports Council, 1 St Colme Street, Edinburgh EH3 6AA

SHAPE, 9 Fitzroy Square, London W1P 6AE

Society for Horticultural Therapy and Rural Training Ltd, Goulds Ground, Vallis Way, Frome, Somerset, BA11 1DA

Sports Council, 16 Upper Woburn Place, London WC1 0QP

United Kingdom Sports Association for People with Mental Handicap, c/o the Sports Council, 16 Upper Woburn Place, London WC1 0QP

13

Cognitive approaches

Marjorie Gardner

INTRODUCTION

Cognition is a global term used to describe the mental processes by which we acquire, transform, organise, store and retrieve information. Cognition is the ability to bring past experience to bear on current situations, to reason, to plan and to solve problems; or 'knowledge, apprehension, knowing in the widest sense, including sensation, perception' (Schwarz 1992).

Cognition has a major influence on human functional performance. This can be clearly seen in injuries and disorders which primarily impair cognitive functioning, such as brain injury or dementia. Cognitive skills form part of the network of component skills which underpin effective occupational performance, therefore they have always been a focus for assessment and treatment in occupational therapy, to a greater or lesser extent.

Over the last 20 years there has been a 'cognitive revolution' in experimental psychology and this has had an impact on mental health practice, just as experimental behavioural psychology did in the 1950s and 1960s. Increasingly, cognitive explanations are used to understand psychopathology and cognitive methods of intervention have been developed for many psychiatric disorders (Hawton et al 1989). Cognitive approaches focus on how an individual structures and makes sense of his world and how that in turn affects his mood, behaviour and functional abilities.

The causes, effects and assessment of cognitive dysfunction are looked at in this chapter. Occupational therapy for cognitive dysfunction is then examined in the context of three models of practice:

1. occupational performance
2. cognitive disability theory
3. cognitive therapy and cognitive behaviour therapy.

COGNITIVE DYSFUNCTION

Cognitive dysfunction is a temporary or permanent failure to process, store and retrieve the information necessary to perform ordinary activities safely or at a level commensurate with a person's age, educational background and culture. Everyone is likely to experience temporary cognitive dysfunction sometime during their lifetime, due, for example, to the effects of extreme fatigue, influenza, fever, or drugs and alcohol. Overall functioning is affected for a period of time but, providing the cause of the dysfunction is attended to, there are no long-term consequences.

Causes of cognitive dysfunction

The causes of cognitive dysfunction seen in mental health practice can be divided into three categories:

1. organic syndromes
2. affective disorders and neuroses
3. major psychoses.

Organic syndromes

Organic syndromes are a group of disorders characterised by anatomical or physiological disturbances to the brain which disrupt brain function. They are caused by trauma, tumours, genetic factors, degeneration (as in senile dementia), infection, metabolic disturbances and toxins (such as alcohol and heavy metal poisoning).

A variety of physical and mental effects may occur, depending on the nature and extent of the damage. Damage to the brain before, during or soon after birth leads to many of the conditions known as learning difficulties. The causes, effects and treatment of learning difficulties are covered in Chapter 23. In adults whose brains have developed normally, organic syndromes can be either acute or chronic.

Acute organic syndromes are temporary disorganisations of brain function resulting in a state of delirium. They are often the result of infection, physical trauma or intoxication, for example delirium tremens. The main clinical feature of mild delirium is clouding of consciousness; this is a global impairment of cognitive function such that the patient cannot maintain effective communication between himself and his environment. Acute organic syndromes are usually reversible with treatment but can lead to chronic focal organic syndromes such as Korsakoff's syndrome (profound short-term memory loss and confabulation) which is associated with past episodes of delirium tremens.

Chronic organic syndromes are either generalised (affecting the whole brain) or focal (affecting part of the brain, as in Korsakoff's syndrome, above). Generalised degeneration of the brain results in the chronic organic syndrome known as dementia. This is an irreversible, insidious and continual loss of mental faculties (Ch. 21). Chronic focal organic impairment is also seen in people with head injuries and tumours. For example, a temporal lobe tumour in the dominant hemisphere typically impairs learning and the ability to retain verbal material, as well as being associated with a high risk of affective disorder.

Affective disorders and neuroses

The affective disorders are primary disorders of mood such as depression and mania. They can range from mild states to life-threatening conditions. The neuroses are a varied range of disorders characterised by the presence of anxiety.

Cognitive function can be affected during an acute or severe episode of depression, mania or anxiety. The effect on functioning is usually temporary, and normal functioning resumes once the period of severe emotional turmoil subsides. For example: during an acute anxiety attack an individual's ability to attend to events in the environment may be limited; this will affect their information processing, and subsequently their memory of the event may be impaired.

People suffering from anxiety and depression frequently complain about impaired attention and concentration and difficulty with decision making. Thought content is also affected by mood. Depressive thought content is pessimistic and negative; suicidal ideas are common. Manic thought content is expansive and positive.

In severe mania and depression, mood-congruent delusional beliefs can occur, for example a severely depressed widower believing he is responsible for the death of his wife (delusional guilt).

The presence of delusions in depression or mania results in the condition being classified as 'psychotic', that is, out of touch with shared reality.

Major psychoses

This term usually refers to the conditions of manic-depressive psychosis and schizophrenia. The effects of mania and depression on cognitive functions are described above.

Schizophrenia is a complex and varied syndrome. Acute schizophrenia is associated with a variety of cognitive symptoms as well as many other phenomena (Rose 1988). Characteristic disorders of thought content and thought processing are diagnostic of schizophrenia. In chronic schizophrenia the more florid symptoms of the syndrome may have subsided leaving enduring social and cognitive disability. Attentional deficit and associated poor concentration is recognised as a 'core cognitive deficit of schizophrenia' (Tryssenaar & Goldberg 1994, p. 199).

Assessment of cognitive dysfunction

Assessment of cognitive dysfunction forms an important part of the mental state examination used by psychiatrists to gather information to aid diagnosis.

While the psychiatrist primarily uses questions and verbal tasks to determine cognitive functioning, the occupational therapist observes an individual's task performance during individual and group activities. It is important, therefore, for therapists to be aware of the cognitive requirements of the activities they are using, particularly in terms of attention, concentration, information processing and problem solving. The assessment of cognitive function forms an important part of the occupational therapist's overall assessment of occupational performance. Standardised psychometric tests are available to measure aspects of cognitive function, for example the Clifton Assessment Procedures for the Elderly (CAPE) and the Wechsler Adult Intelligence Scale-Revised (WAIS-R).

Therapists working with particular client groups need to develop expertise with standardised assessments relevant to their client group needs.

OCCUPATIONAL THERAPY FOR COGNITIVE DYSFUNCTION

Cognitive skills are fundamental to our functioning as human beings. The range and complexity of our cognitive processes set us apart from other animals. They are necessary for effective occupational performance and as such are the target of interventions across all areas of occupational therapy practice. In the field of mental health, cognitive skills are assessed in order to understand fully the causes of functional deficits. They are the subject of direct intervention (retraining, practice, compensation) in order to improve functioning and, particularly in the practice of cognitive therapy, cognitive processes themselves are used as the means to effect change.

The role of cognition is explored in the following three different approaches:

1. occupational performance
2. cognitive disability
3. cognitive therapy.

OCCUPATIONAL PERFORMANCE

Occupational therapists believe that what people do affects their physical and mental well-being. A focus on occupation and the balance of the activities of life – that is, self-care, work, play and sleep – is central to the philosophy of occupational therapy. Man's occupational nature was recognised during the early years of occupational therapy, but this view was submerged during the 1950s, 60s and 70s as interventions became more focused on symptomatology within the medical model of care. In recent years the focus on occupational behaviour has returned, and recent models of occupational therapy reflect this (Reed & Sanderson 1980, Kielhofner 1985, Canadian Association of Occupational Therapists 1991).

Within these models cognition is seen as a performance component or skill which contributes, along with many other performance components, to a person's ability to function competently, and to their own satisfaction, in a given occupational area. For example, Reed & Sanderson's (1980) human occupation model includes cognitive skills which, together with sensory, motor, interpersonal and intrapersonal skills, interact to underpin effective functioning in the occupational areas of self-maintenance, productivity, leisure and relationships. The therapist first assesses the individual's overall functioning and adaptation to his environment and lifestyle, and then looks more closely at functioning in the four occupational areas (Box 13.1).

Problems with functioning in the occupational areas may be due to impairments at the level of performance components. Reed & Sanderson (1980) identified five types of skill as performance components:

1. motor
2. sensory
3. interpersonal
4. intrapersonal
5. cognitive.

The last two of these performance components can be considered under the broad category of 'cognition'.

The cognitive requirements for effective occupational performance include the following:

• Intrapersonal skills include: the ability to identify one's own needs and goals; accurate perception of self and others; insight into areas of difficulty; a set of beliefs which are congruent with an image of oneself as a competent performer, and values which motivate learning.

• Cognitive skills include: ability to attend to, select, store and retrieve relevant information from the environment; ability to reason, plan and solve problems; numeracy and literacy skills.

Individuals may show similar problems in occupational performance which are caused by different impairments at the performance component level, or they may be due to environmental constraints. Information must be gathered from a number of sources before the causes of occupational dysfunction can be identified. These sources will include:

• the psychiatrist's initial assessment and interview results (which include non-standardised verbal tests of cognitive function)

Box 13.1 The four occupational areas	
Self-maintenance	Includes personal care, mobility, independence and community skills
Productivity	Includes tasks such as home management, work (paid or voluntary) and education
Leisure	Includes self-directed activities for pleasure, personal growth or socialisation, and quiet and active recreation
Relationships	Includes social relationships, such as at work, and close relationships with family and friends

- the client's own report
- significant others' reports
- standardised assessments, for example psychometric testing of cognitive function by a psychologist
- observation of task performance in occupational therapy
- functional assessments
- formalised self-report, for example the Beck Depression Inventory
- social reports
- nursing reports.

The Reed & Sanderson model emphasises the importance, to the individual involved, of functional independence. It also takes into account two other broad influences on occupational performance.

- *Values and beliefs*. Developed through our culture, family and individual experience, these influence which skills are learned and maintained, which occupational behaviours are valued, and what level of functioning is acceptable to each individual.
- *Environment*. This is considered to be the physical and social context in which we operate, our roles and the expectations of others.

The model has been further developed by Reed (1984) as the 'adaptation through occupation' model, and by the Canadian Association of Occupational Therapists (1991) as the 'model of occupational performance'. In each model, cognition is identified as a performance component.

Interventions to improve cognitive functioning take three different forms:

1. treatment of cognitive impairment
2. adaptation of environment and task requirements
3. treatment of occupational dysfunction.

Treatment of cognitive impairment

This involves creating opportunities through carefully graded activities for an individual to develop or maintain his cognitive skills, in particular the skills of attention, concentration, memory, language, planning and problem solving.

Brown and colleagues (1993) compared the effectiveness of two different therapeutic programmes in improving attention in people with schizophrenia. These were a cognitive rehabilitation programme of the type developed for people with acquired brain injury, which contained five levels of tasks specifically targeting different levels of attention, and a programme of task orientated activities of the type traditionally found in occupational therapy departments. They found that both groups improved on simple cognitive tasks, with specific gains in attention and memory. Both groups also showed improvement in efficiency, motivation and self-confidence. The authors identified the common therapeutic elements shared by both treatment programmes as:

- graded activities with a gradual increase in complexity
- one to one working with therapist
- an environment that minimises excess sensory stimulation not related to the task
- frequent feedback, including concrete feedback on performance (e.g. time taken on tasks)
- activities that are structured, concrete, easily learned and visual
- active teaching by therapists of information processing techniques (e.g. how to organise task, use of cues).

Group activities can give opportunity for less specific work on cognitive deficits. They are most useful for maintaining skills, developing an individual's confidence in their skills and for the less severe cognitive impairments seen in people suffering from anxiety and depression. For example:

- *Play reading* requires attention to the text at any given moment, and sustained concentration in order to follow the theme of the play. Subsequent discussion can prompt recall of the plot/key events. The process of reading aloud can develop verbal fluency and language skills.
- *Quizzes, table games and computer games* can be used to develop concentration, recall from short- and long-term memory and problem-solving skills.
- *Problem-solving or goal-planning groups* provide a structure to help the development of

problem-solving skills, and practice and support in their application.

• *Creative activities* can free individuals from their normal modes of problem solving in order to develop a new appraisal of a situation (see also the section on the use of imagery in cognitive therapy, p.242).

For many patients suffering from anxiety or depression, cognitive skills will improve as the acute phase of their condition resolves. However, a continued lack of confidence in their skills is common. Opportunity to practise and have some objective assessment of, for example, concentration and memory is an important aspect of treatment for these patients.

Adaptation of environment and tasks

If a particular cognitive skill, such as memory, is assessed as being severely impaired and unlikely to improve, adaptation of work tasks and environments may compensate. For example, with memory impairment, visual cues in the environment may be useful. These can either label parts of the environment (e.g. 'Toilet') for those who are severely disorientated, or give cues/instructions for action; for example, a label 'Switch off all electrical appliances' may be placed on the front door, to be seen on leaving the house. The use of lists and diaries can also help those with mild memory loss.

The environment in which we operate also includes friends, spouse, carers, and so on. They may be involved in helping compensate for cognitive impairment by taking over some tasks and by helping to cue and simplify others.

Treatment of occupational dysfunction

If opportunities are given to practise the occupational tasks that an individual needs to be competent in, then all the necessary performance components (skills) required to complete that task will also be practised. Many occupational therapists (Allen 1985, Canadian Association of Occupational Therapists 1991) believe that engaging in occupational tasks in the normal environment is the most effective way to learn new skills, maintain old skills and achieve occupational competence. Certainly this approach needs to be used in conjunction with any work on specific cognitive deficits in order that any improvements can generalise to a person's real life environment.

COGNITIVE DISABILITY THEORY

There has been a growth in interest and research into cognitive models in occupational therapy over the last 5 years. Increasingly, the role of cognition is seen as central to the occupational therapy process rather than as a component skill. Allen's cognitive disability theory (Allen 1985) is so far the most established in occupational therapy. It was originally developed in relation to psychiatric patients and has been applied to patients suffering from brain injuries, learning difficulties, cardiovascular accidents and dementia; that is, to all patients who may have difficulty in acquiring new information and adapting to change.

Central to the theory is the importance of assessing learning ability.

To the extent that a therapist's services depend on the therapist's ability to teach a person how to do something, the therapist should evaluate that person's ability to learn. Therapists have a tendency to assume that learning ability is within normal limits, and that assumption is often wrong. (Allen 1992a)

Cognitive levels

Allen's hypothesis is that cognitive disability can be assessed by observing task performance, that is, the ability to function in specific tasks reflects information-processing capabilities.

After observing the patient carrying out functional activities (such as activities of daily living or crafts), or by using a standardised evaluation tool, such as the Allen Cognitive Level (ACL) test, the patient is classified as being on one of six cognitive levels. These range from level 1, which represents profound cognitive disability, to level 6 which represents normal functioning.

Allen emphasised the importance of the patient's being willing to do the task, in order to rule out motivational variables. Therapists use the descriptions of the cognitive levels to classify observed task performance for patients unwilling or unable to complete the ACL test.

Box 13.2 gives a descriptive profile of the cognitive levels.

Allen suggested diagnoses which are likely to lead to functioning at each cognitive level. However, the main emphasis of Allen's theory is on how cognitive disability cuts across

---

Box 13.2   Allen's six cognitive levels (adapted from Allen & Allen 1987, Allen 1988, Allen 1992b)

Level 1 Automatic actions
- Conscious but unable to attend to stimuli for more than a few seconds.
- May be able to eat and drink but fluid and food intake needs monitoring.
- Requires 24-hour nursing care.
- Appears unaware of people, objects and the passing of time.
- May be able to communicate fear or pain by sound, expression or gesture.

Level 2 Postural actions
- Can adjust posture in response to discomfort.
- May attempt to repeat or imitate gross body movements.
- Aimless pacing or wandering may occur.
- Transient awareness of the environment.
- Can focus attention for brief periods, requires continuous prompting or direction, e.g. when walking, going to the bathroom, eating.
- Can follow simple spoken directions (1–4 words) if spoken slowly and repeated.

Level 3 Manual actions
- Spontaneous manual actions occur, e.g. picking up and examining objects. May demonstrate normal use of object (writing with pencil, drinking from cup) many times. Responds to tactile cues.
- Can carry out daily grooming tasks such as dressing, washing hands and face, brushing hair, brushing teeth, and simple household tasks such as dusting, but may require prompting and supervision in order to perform tasks at correct time and to the required quality.
- Listens to short phrases or sentences relating to immediate needs or environment.
- Communicates in short sentences but may stray from topic.
- May get lost in unfamiliar or large areas.
- Requires supervision with medication, money management and household management. Some people on this level will require 24-hour supervision.

Level 4 Goal-directed actions
- Purposeful action occurs; the individual can follow steps to achieve a goal. Concrete, visible aspects of the environment are attended to successfully while less obvious features are not.
- Can listen to and communicate information relating to very familiar topics or past experience.

New information may be ignored or misinterpreted.
- May be able to work on simple, repetitive procedures with a standard procedure and demonstrated steps. May not be able to follow written or verbal instructions.
- May not be able to generalise from one situation to another or use own judgement to deal with unpredictable events.
- May not be aware of own disabilities, and requires social support on a daily basis.

Level 5 Exploratory actions
Level 5 may be the usual level of functioning for about 20% of the population.

- Exploratory actions are performed spontaneously. The individual can use trial-and-error learning and inductive reasoning to understand cause and effect. New learning can occur and be generalised.
- No evidence of difficulty with personal care.
- Listens to and communicates information related to present and past experiences.
- Problems may arise at home, within relationships and at work because of difficulties with:
  — anticipating events
  — planning and prioritising
  — understanding consequences of own behaviour
  — using abstract concepts and deductive reasoning.
- Although many people maintain jobs and relationships at level 5, considerable distress can result from continued level 6 demands. This is particularly relevant to individuals who have previously functioned at level 6 and whose lifestyle reflects this. Job loss, divorce and separations may occur.

Level 6 Planned actions
Level 6 represents, theoretically, absence of cognitive dysfunction and is the level at which the majority of the population normally functions.

- Uses symbolic cues to formulate plans that guide actions.
- Can consider hypothetical possibilities. Can use deductive reasoning.
- Verbal and written directions can be followed, demonstration of tasks no longer necessary.
- Future events are anticipated. Behaviour is planned and organised.

diagnostic categories; it is relatively independent of the severity of traditionally assessed psychiatric symptomatology, which relies heavily on verbal interviews and observation of gross behaviour changes. The cognitive levels are assessed by detailed attention to what patients do rather than what they say. This is especially important for patients with good educational background and verbal fluency which can disguise problems with day-to-day functioning.

Allen's approach is supported by researchers in other areas. Townes et al (1983) found that the level of impairment as measured by a variety of cognitive tests was independent of the severity of psychiatric disorder. They suggested, as did Allen, that looking at patients' competencies is a better guide, when planning discharge and treatment, than psychiatric diagnosis.

Allen (1982) conducted research with the ACL on samples of normal, depressed and schizophrenic people. 20% of the normal group showed some cognitive disability (18% at level 5 and 2% at level 4) and 72% of the depressed group showed some cognitive disability (25% at level 5 and 47% at level 4). However, people suffering from schizophrenia showed the greatest level of cognitive disability, with 83% scoring at level 4 or below.

In terms of learning ability, Allen believes that if a person is functioning at level 4 or below, they will not be able to generalise learning from one situation to another. Some generalisation occurs at level 5 but only at level 6 does it occur reliably.

Implications for treatment

Assessment and monitoring

Assessment of cognitive levels can be used during the acute phases of a disorder to monitor progress and response to treatment. Allen noted that changes in cognitive level are often related to effectiveness of medication. They can be used to identify when a stable state has been reached and when a patient is ready for discharge, in which case they can help to predict the level of support required.

Planning activities and optimising functioning

For each cognitive level, a corresponding task analysis details the complexity of activity the patient is able to perform. This gives the therapist guidance on how to design and structure an activity so that it is within a patient's ability range. Activities which are challenging and enjoyable, but within an individual's capabilities, allow for the experience of interacting successfully with the environment. These experiences provide feedback, build confidence and maintain skills.

Allen believes that cognitive disability, as measured by the ACL, is a result of brain pathology, and therefore interventions do not change a person's cognitive level once a stable state has been achieved. The aim of intervention is to identify accurately an individual's stable level of cognitive disability and optimise his functioning within those constraints. This will include:

- identifying activities the patient is able to perform
- identifying ways in which the patient can be helped to compensate for disabilities, for example
  — visual and verbal prompts
  — adapted work tasks
  — adapted environment
  — support from carers/community staff
- avoiding undue stress by placing too few or too great demands on the patient
- identifying whether new learning is possible (usually level 4 and above) and creating optimum conditions for it to occur.

The process of intervention involves the occupational therapist in the support and education of relatives and carers so that realistic expectations are fulfilled.

Allen's theory suggests that when new tasks are to be learned, training will be more effective on the job or at home, that is, the specific activity needs to be taught in the situation in which it is required, as it may not be generalised effectively from a treatment setting. Similarly, Allen doubted the effectiveness of teaching component cognitive skills, such as memory and concentration, for patients functioning below level 5 as these may not be generalised to real activities.

Rehabilitation and community support

Given that 83% of Allen's (1982) sample of people suffering from schizophrenia scored at cognitive levels 4 and below, there are clear implications for how rehabilitation and community support programmes are designed.

Many people who are supported by community mental health workers have long histories of mental health problems, most commonly schizophrenia and chronic affective disorders.

Allen's theory would suggest that community support for people functioning at levels 4 and 5 should involve practical help, demonstration of tasks, use of role play to learn new behaviours and clear written information to follow any verbal advice.

Raweh & Katz (1999) conducted a pilot study into the effectiveness of a treatment programme for people in the post-acute stage of schizophrenia based on Allen's cognitive disability model. They found evidence of increased performance of routine tasks and improved cognitive functioning within the study group.

COGNITIVE THERAPY

Cognitive therapy is a form of psychological treatment based on the premise that the ways in which an individual structures his experiences will affect his mood, behaviour and attitude towards the world.

Like behaviour therapy, cognitive therapy is based on an experimental or scientific attitude to treatment and shares much in common with behaviour therapy in the ways in which therapy is structured. Some practitioners prefer the term 'cognitive behavioural therapy' which emphasises the use of both behavioural and cognitive techniques.

All psychological treatments share the assumption that psychological factors have contributed to the causation, maintenance or exacerbation of an individual's presenting problems. Specific psychological treatments are developed from an underlying explanatory model of psychological functioning.

Cognitive therapy is based on a cognitive model of the emotional disorders which provides a consistent rationale for treatment.

Rationale of cognitive therapy

The cognitive model of emotional and behavioural disorders has been most refined and researched in relation to depression and anxiety, although more recent work has explored the usefulness of this approach with people suffering from schizophrenia (Drury et al 1996, Tarrier et al 1998).

Within the cognitive model, cognitions or thoughts are seen as the mediators of behaviour and mood; the way we think about an event affects the way we feel about it, which in turn modifies the way we behave in response to that event.

Beck (1976) has researched and identified the typical distorted and negative evaluations of events found in people suffering from depression. This cognitive triad consists of:

- a negative view of the world
- a negative concept of self
- a negative appraisal of the future.

These negative evaluations occur because of dysfunctions in cognitive mediation which contribute to the development and maintenance of depression and anxiety. Cognitive mediation operates on three levels: schemata, cognitive processes and content of thoughts.

Schemata

These stable knowledge structures represent our beliefs, theories and assumptions about people, ourselves and the world. They affect what aspects of a situation we attend to and what we remember, they influence our cognitive processes and subsequently our thoughts.

The schemata of depressed and anxious people tend to be rigid and undifferentiated. They are often personal and associated with powerful emotions. They are normally not immediately available in consciousness.

Cognitive theory proposes that such schemata are acquired during childhood or adolescence (or later during particularly traumatic or emotional episodes) via the experience of events such as the loss of a parent, a succession of traumas or rejection by significant others. They remain immature and are not moderated by subsequent experiences. They become activated when a situation similar to the one in which they were learned occurs. They then have an effect on information processing, behaviour and emotions.

There are parallels between the cognitive model of depression and social theories of depression which also identify the importance of early loss as a vulnerability factor and subsequent perceived loss or stress as a precipitating factor in depression.

Cognitive processes

There is a tendency for all of us to process information to fit into a readily available schema, especially when under stress or in familiar circumstances. This occurs to a much greater extent in the emotional disorders, so that information is continually distorted to fit into rigid, dysfunctional schemata. Therefore, depressed people process information so as to confirm negative schemata and anxious people process information so as to confirm anxiogenic schemata. In terms of Piaget's concepts of accommodation and assimilation, people suffering from emotional disorders tend to overassimilate into preexisting schemata and resist accommodation to new information. Typical information-processing errors are outlined in Box 13.3.

These information-processing errors produce the profoundly negative thoughts found in depression. For example, a man buying a house finds he has been gazumped. A person who is not depressed may feel angry, frustrated or disappointed at first, but will eventually come to terms with the experience by considering all aspects of the situation. For example, he might think: 'It is typical of the state of the housing market at the time', 'There were inefficiencies in the manner in which the sale was conducted', 'The house was very desirable'. However, a

---

Box 13.3 Typical information-processing errors in depression and anxiety

Selective abstraction
A conclusion drawn on the basis of one aspect of a situation ignoring other relevant elements, e.g. 'I made a complete mess of that presentation'.

Overgeneralisation
A general conclusion is drawn on the basis of one experience and applied across the board, e.g. 'I always fail'.

Catastrophising
Magnifying of negative aspects of a situation and minimising positive aspects. Error in evaluating the significance of an event, e.g. 'If I mess up this presentation, I'll be fired'.

All-or-nothing thinking
Tendency to place all experiences in one of two opposite categories, e.g. flawless or defective, calm or out of control. Patient places himself in the extreme negative category, e.g. 'If I don't stay completely calm during this presentation I'll go out of control'.

Personalisation
Relating to external events to self without justification, e.g. 'It's my fault','I can tell they are looking at me', 'They think I'm a fool'.

---

depressed person might conclude that the deal fell through because the sellers had taken a dislike to him (personalisation), he may feel as a result that he is an absolute failure at everything (overgeneralisation) and he might conclude that he will never be able to move house (catastrophising).

Content of thoughts

'Content of thoughts' is what is going on during thinking. It refers to the thoughts and images in consciousness which are readily accessible. It reveals the patient's assessments of his problems.

The negative cognitive triad of depression is readily seen in a patient's content of thoughts. Automatic thoughts or self-talk (often referred to as negative automatic thoughts) are habitual involuntary thoughts which can be difficult to pin down and identify. They occur most readily at times of increased emotion or crisis. They often reflect the information-processing errors that are occurring at the time and the underlying assumptions. Identifying negative automatic thoughts is an important element of cognitive therapy.

Treatment at the three levels of cognitive mediation

The cognitive model of emotional disorders attributes the observed disturbances in thoughts, mood and behaviour in conditions such as depression and anxiety to dysfunctions in the three levels of cognitive mediation. Treatment is therefore directed at remedying these dysfunctions by:

- identifying thoughts and testing them against reality
- identifying and changing information-processing errors
- identifying dysfunctional assumptions and beliefs which increase vulnerability to emotional disorder, and reconstructing more adaptive schemata.

Characteristics of cognitive therapy

Cognitive therapy is a directive, structured and time-limited approach to the treatment of psychiatric disorders such as depression, anxiety and phobias. It uses a variety of cognitive and behavioural techniques to help the patient, which include (Beck et al 1979):

- monitoring negative automatic thoughts (cognitions)
- recognising the relationship between thoughts, feelings and behaviour
- examining the evidence for and against the patient's cognitions
- substituting more reality-orientated interpretations for biased cognitions
- identifying and altering the dysfunctional beliefs that predispose patients to distort their experiences.

The rationale for cognitive therapy, together with an explanation of the treatment process, is discussed with the patient at the start of therapy. The whole process of therapy is conducted in this educative and collaborative manner.

The treatment techniques of cognitive therapy fall into two broad categories: cognitive and behavioural.

Cognitive techniques

These are primarily verbal techniques used by the therapist and taught to the patient during one-to-one treatment sessions.

Initially the task is to help the patient identify negative thoughts, which will give opportunities to examine the faulty information processing and help pinpoint underlying beliefs and assumptions.

Negative automatic thoughts can often be accessed by using moments of strong emotion. If the therapist detects a change in mood, for example the patient suddenly becomes tearful, the therapist will ask a question such as 'What is going through your mind right now?' and encourage the patient to identify the thought or image which has produced the emotional reaction. Thoughts accessed in this way are sometimes referred to as 'hot cognitions'.

However, perhaps the central technique of cognitive therapy is the use of inductive questioning or guided discovery to identify key cognitions and their meaning:

the therapist uses inductive questioning, sometimes called 'guided discovery', to help the patient trace the thoughts which maintain his dysphoric mood. This technique is probably the key technique of cognitive therapy and requires a great deal of skill. The therapist needs to be very attentive, so as to be able to ask a series of appropriate questions without actually putting words in the patient's mouth. The questions will lead the patient to recreate a situation in his mind and to gain an understanding of what was really going on. Moreover, this style of questioning constitutes a model for the patient which helps him to acquire the skills of monitoring his thoughts. (Blackburn & Davidson 1990)

The therapist uses open questions such as:
'What do you mean by . . . ?'
'What happened next?'
'Was anything else going on at the same time?'
'Did you have any thoughts or images in your mind at the time?'

The use of behavioural tasks in homework is used to create situations which can subsequently be examined in this way. Patients are often asked to keep diaries of their activities, moods and accompanying thoughts to be examined in the treatment session. Once negative automatic thoughts are identified, the patient is helped to understand the relationship between his thoughts, mood and behaviour. Further questioning explores the information-processing errors which produce negative thoughts.

Patients are encouraged to take an objective, scientific view of their thoughts and, once distanced, to assess how plausible they are. Questions guide them to examine evidence for and against their thoughts, consider alternative interpretations, determine how probable each interpretation is and consider specific information-processing errors, such as those described in Box 13.3.

Underlying beliefs and assumptions are identified through recurring themes in therapy, and also by using the 'downward arrow' technique, asking the questions:

'What if that were true?'
'What if that did happen?'

until the underlying belief system is reached. Once identified, treatment can be targeted to restructuring dysfunctional belief systems.

This questioning technique accepts the thoughts that the patient presents as true and examines the consequences for the patient.

Behavioural techniques

Cognitive therapy utilises many behavioural techniques similar to those used in behavioural therapy. However, as Beck et al (1979) stressed, they are used within a cognitive model:

Many of the techniques...are also part of the repertoire of the behaviour therapist. The impact of the therapeutic techniques derived from a strictly behavioural or conditioning model is limited because of the restriction to observable behaviour and selective exclusion of information regarding the patient's attitudes, beliefs and thoughts – his cognitions. Hence, even though the behaviour therapist induces the patient to become more active, his pessimism, self-disparagement, and suicidal impulses may remain unchanged. For the behavioural therapist, the modification of behaviour is an end in itself; for the cognitive therapist it is a means to an end – namely, cognitive change. (Beck et al 1979)

Behavioural techniques are used most commonly at the beginning of treatment. The severely depressed or anxious patient may be more easily engaged with active techniques while he is still learning about the cognitive techniques. In addition, the reduction in normal daily activities often seen in these patients causes problems with day-to-day functioning which need to be addressed early in treatment.

Typical behavioural strategies include a weekly activity schedule in which the patient logs hour by hour everything he does. Filling in the schedule focuses the patient on a purposeful activity and gives accurate feedback on what he does. Using this as a baseline, the therapist can encourage the patient to schedule activities in advance. This type of planning can help with problems of motivation, disorganisation and indecisiveness, and demonstrates to the patient that he can take some control over his time and his life.

The activity schedule can be adapted to include graded task assignments. These, as the name suggests, involve grading tasks so that the patient will not experience failure and setbacks. Activities are rated on a 0–5 scale for mastery and pleasure. Mastery refers to the sense of accomplishment associated with an activity and pleasure to the feelings of enjoyment associated with it. Patients are encouraged to recognise small degrees of success or enjoyment as opposed to all or nothing grading.

Behavioural techniques are used to tackle specific behavioural problems associated with anxiety and depression (Table 13.1). They are presented as behavioural experiments in which the patient can find out for himself whether his assumptions about his functioning are accurate or not. Actual skill deficits may still need to be addressed, for example training in relaxation techniques, stress management, assertiveness training and problem-solving skills.

Table 13.1 Behavioural techniques in depression and anxiety (adapted from Blackburn & Davidson 1990)

Behavioural target	Techniques
Inactivity Indecisiveness and/or procrastination	Scheduling activities in advance Keeping weekly activity log Grading introduction of activities especially in terms of time and effort
Low mood	Distraction Identification of previously pleasurable activities Grading activities for mastery (M) and pleasure (P)
Anxious mood Physical tension	Distraction Relaxation Exercise scheduling
Loss of interest Loss of pleasure in life	Scheduling pleasurable activities Grade for mastery and pleasure
Poor concentration	Graded activities
Poor motivation	Graded activities
Panic attacks	Respiratory control Distraction
Avoidance	Graded exposure Respiratory control
Specific problem situation	Practice in relevant coping strategies, e.g. assertiveness training

A COGNITIVE THERAPY APPROACH TO OCCUPATIONAL THERAPY

A number of prerequisites have been identified for competent practice as a cognitive therapist (Beck et al 1979, Blackburn & Davidson 1990):

- A good understanding of the clinical syndromes treated, in particular skill in assessing suicide risk, is needed.
- An aspiring cognitive therapist must first be a good psychotherapist.
- The therapist must have an understanding of the cognitive model of the emotional disorders.
- The therapist must have an understanding of the framework of cognitive therapy.
- Formal training at a centre of cognitive therapy, with continual supervision or training from a trained cognitive therapist, is necessary.

Training is necessary in order both to understand the application of the cognitive model and to develop skill in the specific treatment techniques. The verbal questioning technique in particular needs to be developed under supervision

in order to become an effective treatment tool. Research into the effectiveness of psychological treatments suggests that the professional group to which a therapist belongs is less important than that she has received training in the intervention she is offering (NHSE 1996).

Cognitive behavioural techniques are being found to be effective with a range of client groups and, as a consequence, there are now increasing opportunities for health and social care professionals to access postgraduate training.

Some aspects of the treatment repertoire of cognitive therapy are very familiar to occupational therapists and are consistent with the practice of occupational therapy. They include:

- educator/facilitator role
- use of activities to facilitate change
- use of images in therapy.

The educator/facilitator role

The role of the therapist as an educator, and as a collaborator with the patient to achieve agreed goals, is common to both occupational therapy and cognitive therapy. The client centred approach within occupational therapy is best developed in the Canadian Occupational Performance Model (Canadian Association of Occupational Therapists 1991).

Much of occupational therapy is directed to enabling patients to learn new skills, new ways of interacting with others and new ways of viewing the world. Our role as facilitator is one of improving access to appropriate environments in which learning can occur.

The use of activities to facilitate change

It is in this area that there is most overlap between the techniques used by cognitive therapists and those used by occupational therapists. The interventions in Table 13.1 are used by many occupational therapists in mental health practice, though not always within a cognitive model. There is also a difference in emphasis: in cognitive therapy, activities are often used as homework assignments which are then discussed in the next therapy session. In occupational therapy, activities are the 'real' work, the focus of therapeutic effort.

Beck et al (1979) reflected that it is impossible to talk a severely depressed person out of his beliefs of worthlessness and inadequacy without some evidence to work on, hence the need for behavioural experiments. Occupational therapists working within a cognitive model place these behavioural experiments at the centre of their work and use activities as the experimental melting pot in which individuals can experience success, pleasure, learning and a sense of competence. Activities provide opportunities for 'hot cognitions' to be caught and challenged. Group activities can be particularly useful in that the individual client's perception of his performance can be measured against that of other group members as well as that of the therapist.

Activity scheduling

This involves finding out an individual's baseline activity schedule by keeping a weekly log and then building on it by incorporating an increasing range of activities. This can be very useful for any patient suffering from inactivity, poor motivation or difficulty in initiating activity.

It is useful to start by finding out about past and current interests so that suggested activities are meaningful. This can be done by structured interviews in which patients are asked about what they are doing now which interests them or gives them pleasure, or about activities enjoyed in the past. Alternatively, a checklist such as the Interest Check List (Matsutsuyu 1969) or the Pleasant Events Schedule (Lewinsohn et al 1978) can be used.

Occupational therapists are familiar with the concept that an activity must have meaning for, and be interesting to, the patient in order to be of value. Similarly, the patient must be involved in the activity under his own volition, otherwise he will not credit himself with any achievements made.

Activity scheduling involves building on the activities a patient can do and enjoys doing, however small, and gradually extending the repertoire. Grading activities for mastery and pleasure enables the patient to reflect with the therapist on their involvement in the activity and achieve a realistic appraisal.

Activity grading

Activity grading is related to activity scheduling and involves ensuring that the demands of an activity at a given time are within a patient's capabilities. Occupational therapists have always been involved in prescribing, designing, monitoring and evaluating activity interventions. Core skills of occupational therapy, such as activity analysis and assessment of task performance, are central to the process of grading activities from simple to more complex tasks.

Occupational therapy and activity within a cognitive model

As occupational therapists we have an advantage in that we are often with patients while they are engaged in activity, be it in in-patient, day patient or community settings. We are therefore well placed to assess functional ability and match activities accordingly. We can ensure that vulnerable individuals do not have damaging experiences of failure. Similarly, we can design activities in which anxious and depressed patients can experience success and competence.

Beck (1976) cited an earlier experiment by Loeb et al (1971) on the effects on mood of a simple activity. Given a simple card-sorting task, depressed patients in a psychiatric clinic were significantly more pessimistic about their chances of success than a matched control group of nondepressed patients. During the task both groups performed equally well. The depressed patients who succeeded in reaching their stated goals were much more optimistic on a second task and they subsequently outperformed the nondepressed patients. This and similar studies have been repeated, and a consistent finding is that a successful experience in depressed patients leads to an increase in self-esteem and optimism which spreads to other areas of the patient's life.

How can occupational therapists extract added therapeutic value from their use of activities within a cognitive model?

* They can monitor for automatic thoughts and 'hot cognitions' during the activity.
* They can turn disadvantages to advantages (a core concept in the practice of cognitive therapy), using situations such as poor motivation or non-attendance to explore issues with the client in an information-gathering, objective manner (see the advantages–disadvantages analysis, in Figure 13.1).
* They can set specific, achievable goals with patients before activity begins.
* They can use activities as behavioural experiments in which patients can find out whether or not their assumptions are accurate.
* They can give feedback and encourage accurate perception of performance.
* They can use activities to the full by exploring the experience fully afterwards; they can encourage grading for mastery and pleasure, and reframe dysfunctional and inaccurate

	Advantages	Disadvantages
Joining the group	Might enjoy it. Might succeed at something. Might meet others in similar situations	Might fail. Might be criticised. Might not enjoy it
Not joining the group	Can stay at home/on ward. Don't have to make the effort	Bored at home/on ward. Nothing changes

Figure 13.1 Advantages–disadvantages analysis, using the example of attending a cookery group in the occupational therapy department.

perceptions, then and there, to avoid the experience subsequently being distorted to confirm negative beliefs.

* They can encourage patients to see that achievements during activities are due to their own efforts.

Diversion

Diverting patients from their anxious, depressive or obsessional thoughts and directing their attention towards more enjoyable activities was one of the original aims of occupational therapy. In recent years this has been rejected as too trivial an enterprise for trained occupational therapists. Perhaps because, too often, patients have been bombarded with meaningless stimuli or grouped together for activities with no regard to individual abilities, diversion has been given a bad name. In fact, if a patient is truly diverted, he is actively engaged. Being asked to 'keep people occupied' is another horror of occupational therapists, but distraction, diversion and occupation are valuable treatment techniques which have been rediscovered in the practice of cognitive therapy and stress management. Friedland (1988) argued that diversion has a small but important place in occupational therapy and that a reconsideration of diversional activity is in keeping with the current philosophy of occupation being necessary to health.

Relaxation and distraction are important in helping to control anxiety. Anxious patients often need to learn a quick distraction technique to use in any situation, for example focusing on a particular object, doing mental arithmetic, using a positive thought. Upsetting thoughts can be controlled by keeping fully occupied in activities one enjoys such as physical activity, crossword puzzles or listening to music. The use of distraction and diversional activities offers ways in which a patient can gain some control over his symptoms. They serve as valuable coping strategies, allowing more in-depth work to be started.

Role play

Role play is used in specific skill training such as assertiveness training and anxiety management. In cognitive therapy it is used in a more impromptu manner in order to play out and gain understanding of particular problem situations. This is usually done in a purely verbal mode, although occupational therapists used to more active techniques could employ them in the same way.

Role playing is used to shed light on faulty information processing going on within the problem situation and the beliefs and assumptions which underpin it. When patients take on the role of other significant people in the situation they are able to distance themselves and consider their interpretations more objectively.

The use of images in therapy

Since the earliest days of cognitive therapy, imagery has been used as a potent way to access beliefs and assumptions. Negative automatic thoughts are not always verbal; they may occur as brief images in the mind. Images can encapsulate a whole network of beliefs and are often emotionally laden, making them particularly useful to the cognitive therapist. Working with images can be useful with patients who do not readily verbalise but are natural visualisers. At the other extreme, imagery is a useful technique with the patient who is too good with words,

who intellectualises and avoids identifying key cognitions.

Guided imagery

Edwards (1989) provided a useful review of guided imagery techniques. Patients are asked to provide as much detail as possible (prompted description) and to consider what happens before and after the particular moment that the image has frozen. The patient can be guided to take different perspectives within the image, for example as himself, as another person or object within the image or as an observer, in order to challenge beliefs and assumptions within the image. The therapist may prompt dialogue between the figures in the image and ask the patient to speak for himself or another, in much the same way as role play techniques are used. The aim is to understand the idiosyncratic meaning the image has for the patient and how it encapsulates his beliefs and assumptions about the world. Cognitive restructuring can then be facilitated by image restructuring.

Use of creative media

Therapists who use creative media, such as art, clay or drama, will be familiar with the power of imagery, the creation of an image which can then be worked with. In the creative therapies, the image is visible and often permanent as opposed to being within the patient's head. Restructuring can be seen as the patient develops a theme over time, for example in a series of paintings. To be creative means to make a new appraisal, to have a new look at a situation.

Creative media are so called because they can provide new ways of looking at a problem. These media are not creative per se; they work creatively because they free individuals from more ordinary ways of thinking, and hence an artist may not find art a therapeutic medium because it is too familiar.

Creative media are used by occupational, art and drama therapists for the same reasons that cognitive therapists use imagery: they provide an effective alternative to verbal techniques and allow dysfunctional beliefs and assumptions to surface. Many therapists who use art, both individually and in groups, will have experienced this happening. An image can combine current preoccupations, future hopes and fears and underlying beliefs.

Once an image has been created it is accessible to reality testing, perspective taking, restructuring, 'what if . . . ' questioning and detailed analysis, and not only by the therapist. In art groups, patients are often very skilled at examining the detail of each other's paintings and challenging faulty interpretations. These can be extremely useful interventions, as fellow patients are not seen as having the same vested interest in recovery as the therapist.

The cognitive model offers a valuable framework for the creative therapist. Many therapists who work with image-making materials, while they may not ostensibly use a cognitive approach, will recognise in it some aspects of the way in which they work.

DISCUSSION

In the literature on cognitive dysfunction in mental health, and its treatment, two themes emerge. First, to what extent is cognitive dysfunction the result of neuroanatomical or neurochemical changes in the brain? Second, to what extent can cognitive dysfunction be treated?

Certain signs, such as confusion, disorientation, visual hallucinations and memory impairment, are accepted in psychiatry as indicating possible organic causes. These may be neuroanatomical, as in dementia, or due to a change in the neurochemistry of the brain, as in a toxic confusional state. Broadly speaking, neuroanatomical changes to the brain are thought to give rise to permanent deficits, while neurochemical changes are potentially reversible. However, for much of the cognitive dysfunction seen in mental health practice, little is known about what is going on within the brain. The two themes identified earlier are interrelated, in that if there is an assumption of damage to the neuroanatomy there is a corresponding assumption that there is

little potential for improvement. These assumptions underpin Allen's cognitive disability theory.

Beck's cognitive model operates at the level of cognitions and information processing. There is a strong assumption within the model that dysfunctional information processing can be changed by cognitive therapy and there is now a large body of research to support that assumption. However, Beck did not see the neurochemical approach to the study of depression as being in conflict with the cognitive model, rather that they represent different levels of analysis:

the biological changes and the cognitive changes do not represent different 'systems', rather they represent different levels of analysis of the *same* system. . . . the results of a successful cognitive intervention will be reflected in a change in the neurochemistry of the brain, *or* in the cognitive structures, depending on whether one is sampling blood levels or reports of introspectual experiences. (Beck 1984) [emphasis as in the original text]

Beck's work supports the view that non-physical therapy can affect brain functioning, as does the work of Katz & Ziv (1992), on occupational therapy within a Piagetian framework, and the work of Raweh & Katz (1999) using Allen's cognitive disability model.

The combination of cognitive approaches with activity interventions offers a strong theoretical framework for treatment entirely in keeping with the core skills of occupational therapy:

Through experience with materials and objects, the patient will acquire logical, objective and deductive operations. Concrete experience is essential to the logical organisation of an adult's performance. *This is occupational therapy's unique and special contribution to mental health.* (Katz & Ziv 1992) [emphasis as in the original text]

SUMMARY

This chapter has taken a broad look at the range of cognitive dysfunction seen in mental health practice. Three approaches to treatment have been covered. The first looks at cognitive skills and deficits in much the same way as motor or sensory skills and deficits, and at their impact on occupational performance. The next two approaches place cognition at centre stage, with considerable emphasis on the quality of an individual's information processing. They differ in the extent to which they believe that information processing skills can be modified or improved.

New approaches to the study of cognition and its central role in mental health practice are being developed rapidly. An individual's learning capability is central to the practice of occupational therapy; this practice is enhanced by a fuller understanding of cognition.

REFERENCES

Allen C K 1982 Independence through activity: the practice of occupational therapy (psychiatry). American Journal of Occupational Therapy 36(11): 731–739

Allen C K 1985 Occupational therapy for psychiatric diseases: measurement and management of cognitive disabilities. Little, Brown, Boston

Allen C K 1988 Occupational therapy: functional assessment of the severity of mental disorders. Hospital and Community Psychiatry 39(?): 140–142

Allen C K 1992a Cognitive disabilities theory. In: Katz N (ed) Cognitive rehabilitation: models for intervention in occupational therapy. Andover Medical, Boston

Allen C K 1992b Workshop material

Allen C K, Allen R E 1987 Cognitive disabilities: measuring the social consequences of mental disorders. Journal of Clinical Psychiatry 48(5): 181–191

Beck A T 1976 Cognitive therapy and emotional disorders. International Universities Press, New York

Beck A T 1984 Cognition and therapy. Archives of General Psychiatry 41: 1112–1114

Beck A T, Rush J A, Shaw B F, Emery G 1979 Cognitive therapy of depression. Guilford Press, New York

Blackburn I, Davidson K 1990 Cognitive therapy for depression and anxiety. Blackwell Scientific, Oxford

Brown C, Harwood K, Hays C, Heckman J, Short J E 1993 Effectiveness of cognitive rehabilitation for improving attention in patients with schizophrenia. Occupational Therapy Journal of Research 13(2): 71–86

Canadian Association of Occupational Therapists 1991 Occupational therapy guidelines for client-centred practice. CAOT, Toronto

Drury V, Birchwood M, Cochrane R, Macmillan F 1996 Cognitive therapy and recovery from acute psychosis: a controlled trial 1. Impact on psychotic symptoms. 2. Impact on recovery time. British Journal of Psychiatry 169: 593–607

Edwards D J A 1989 Cognitive restructuring through guided imagery: lessons from gestalt therapy. In: Freeman A, Simon K, Arkowitz H, Beutler L (eds) Comprehensive handbook of cognitive therapy. Plenum, New York

Friedland J 1988 Diversional activity: does it deserve its bad name? American Journal of Occupational Therapy 42(9): 603–611

Hawton K, Kirk J, Clark D, Salkovskis P 1989 Cognitive behavioural therapy for psychiatric problems: a practical guide. Oxford University Press, Oxford

Katz N, Ziv N 1992 A Piagetian framework for occupational therapy in mental health. In: Katz N (ed) Cognitive rehabilitation: models for intervention in occupational therapy. Andover Medical, Boston

Kielhofner G (ed) 1985 A model of human occupation: theory and application. Williams and Wilkins, Baltimore

Lewinsohn P M, Munoz R F, Youngress M A, Zeiss A 1978 Control your depression. Prentice Hall, New Jersey

Loeb A, Beck A T, Diggory J 1971 Differential effects of success and failure on depressed and non-depressed patients. Journal of Nervous and Mental Disease 152: 106–114

Matsutsuyu J S 1969 The interest checklist. American Journal of Occupational Therapy 23(4): 323–328

Raweh D, Katz N 1999 Treatment effectiveness of Allen's cognitive disabilities model with adult schizophrenic outpatients: a pilot study.

Reed K L 1984 Models of practice in occupational therapy. Williams and Wilkins, Baltimore

Reed K L, Sanderson S 1980 Concepts of occupational therapy. Williams and Wilkins, Baltimore

Rose N (ed) 1988 Essential psychiatry. Blackwell Scientific, Oxford

Schwarz C (ed) 1992 Chambers maxi paperback dictionary. Chambers, Edinburgh

Tarrier N, Yusupoff L, Kinney C, McCarthy E, Gledhill A, Haddock G, Morris J 1998 Randomised controlled trial of intensive cognitive behaviour therapy for patients with chronic schizophrenia. British Medical Journal 317: 303–307

Townes B D, Martin D C, Nelson D, Prosser R, Pepping M, Maxwell J 1983 Neurobehavioural approach to classification of psychiatric patients using a competency model. Journal of Consulting and Clinical Psychology 53(1): 33–42

Tryssenaar J, Goldberg J 1994 Improving attention in a person with schizophrenia. Canadian Journal of Occupational Therapy 61(4): 198–204

ACKNOWLEDGEMENT

I would like to acknowledge the help and support of Netta Jennison, occupational therapist and cognitive therapist, Oxford Brookes University, for sharing her clinical expertise.

14

Groupwork

Linda Finlay

INTRODUCTION

Human development is powerfully shaped by our experiences in groups. Therefore, groups can be seen as the foundation of society. Groups help us develop our sense of personal and social identity. Through interaction with others we acquire skills, attitudes and ways of behaving. When we are in a group we respond to the expectations of others and adopt different roles. We gain strength as we share with others, both giving and receiving support. In a real sense, as Leary puts it, 'In groups people experience life' (Leary 1994, p. 203).

In group therapy we harness these special characteristics of a group and aim to select the learning and supportive experiences which will benefit our patients and clients. Occupational therapists use groupwork in different ways. We run activity groups which aim to teach task skills and encourage social interaction. We also take part in support groups where members share and explore their attitudes and feelings.

This chapter addresses three dimensions of groupwork. First, it outlines different types of occupational therapy groups and discusses the value and limitations of groupwork in general. Second, it offers practical guidelines for planning groupwork. It analyses the factors involved in preparing a session and setting up a longer-term group.

Managing a group involves more than simply running a planned session, however. In order to manage a group, the therapist needs to understand what is happening in the group and why. The final theme, therefore, focuses on such understanding and explores some core theories of group dynamics and the evaluation process.

GROUPS IN OCCUPATIONAL THERAPY

Occupational therapists are involved in groups that span a wide range of activities from psychodrama to bingo. One occupational therapist might specialise in psychotherapy, while another employs a whole variety of practical and social group activities. What links such a diverse range of groups to occupational therapy? The answer lies within the use occupational therapists make of activities and their core concern to further the occupational performance of individual clients.

The aims of groupwork treatment are usually complex. A practical activity group, for example, will often have multiple aims, such as to teach skills, boost confidence and increase social interaction. However, within that group, specific treatment objectives for a particular individual may run counter to the overall group aims. As the first step towards understanding the roles of groups in occupational therapy, this section will first map out the range of groups available and then explore their value and their limitations.

Types of groups

Groups can be classified as being predominantly activity based, support based, or a mixture of the two (Fig. 14.1). This distinction seems to encompass the wide range of groups in which occupational therapists engage.

Activity groups (e.g. cookery) involve task and/or social elements. Task groups aim to develop skills and tend to be orientated towards an end product and the individual. Social groups, by contrast, are for recreation and aim to encourage social interaction.

Support groups (e.g. creative therapy) focus on communication and/or psychotherapy. These groups emphasise the group process rather than the end product. Communication groups aim for

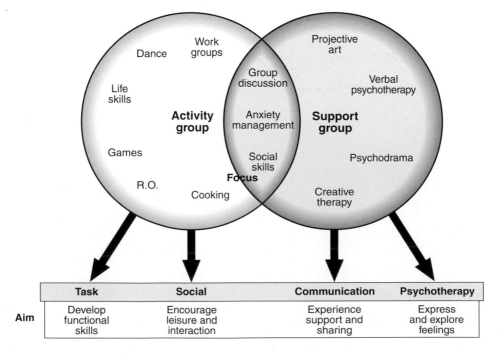

Figure 14.1   Classification of groups in occupational therapy.

group members to give each other support and share experiences, while psychotherapy groups aim to help participants gain insight and explore their feelings (Finlay 1993).

This classification of groups should not be interpreted rigidly. Any activity can be designed to fit along the continuum of task–social–communication–psychotherapy. In fact, all the elements may be on offer in any one group but shift according to what the group is doing and group members' responses. Thus, members might simultaneously share feelings (psychotherapy) and give each other support (communication), while having fun (social) and learning a new hobby (task). Further, it is important to recognise that different individuals may well react differently to the same activity. A role play, for instance, can be experienced as fun by one person, a practical way of learning a skill by another, and it may trigger all sorts of emotional reactions in a third person.

Approaches to groupwork

Occupational therapists utilise a variety of approaches to groupwork. To give some sense of the range involved, four different approaches (Finlay 1999) are described below. The first two approaches fall loosely under the banner of activity groups, while the last two are more in tune with the aims of support groups.

Skills-focused groups

A number of approaches to groupwork focus on developing individuals' skills. One example is the *directive group*, a highly structured approach to groupwork developed by Kaplan (1988) for lower functioning psychiatric patients who have performance difficulties. Here, the aim of the group is to improve members' self-care, task performance and basic interaction. The group meets daily and follows a set format using a range of activities (for instance, games, crafts or exercises). Applying these ideas to working with the elderly, Trace & Howell (1991) found the use of purposeful activity maximised their contact with their clients.

Taking a slightly different approach, Mosey (1986) recommended teaching skills in a developmental sequence. She outlined five stages of development of *group interaction skills*: parallel group, project group, egocentric cooperative group, cooperative group and mature group. Patients or clients are placed into the group environment (made up of activity, therapist and other members) that best suits their developmental level. Members are encouraged to interact and develop their skills progressively. For example, a patient operating at a parallel group level is given opportunities to work alongside others. In order to encourage interaction the therapist can limit the equipment available and direct the patient to share with one other person. Salo-Chydenius (1996) described a successful social skills training programme with patients with long-term mental illness where group activities designed to teach basic communication skills were structured to mirror this developmental sequence over the course of 12 sessions.

Occupational behaviour groups

Many occupational therapy groups explicitly aim to develop productive and satisfying occupational roles. Arising from Reilly's (1974) occupational behaviour model and Kielhofner's (1995) human occupation model, these types of groups utilise different work and leisure activities. Borg & Bruce (1991) described their *therapeutic activity group* where occupational therapists use activity to structure patients' participation, the goal being to enable them to make decisions and take responsibility, develop skills and gain validation. Similarly, Howe & Schwartzberg (1986) developed a *functional group* geared to enhancing the occupational behaviour of participants through work, play and self-maintenance tasks. Basic goals are to elicit purposeful, self-initiated and spontaneous group-centred actions.

Cognitive behavioural groups

Here, members are taught to understand the connection between their negative thoughts and their anxious or depressed behaviour. The range of groupwork commonly practised in this field encompasses social skills training, assertiveness training and anxiety management courses. Role play is used frequently to provide individuals with opportunities to rehearse new behaviours while other members act as role models. Homework assignments such as keeping a log of thoughts and behaviours also encourage group members to generalise their learning (Yakobina et al 1997).

A number of therapists have devised and evaluated the use of anxiety management groups (see, for instance, Prior 1998a, 1998b; Rosier et al 1998). These types of groups aim to increase group members' skills and confidence to manage their anxiety while group members give each other support.

Psychodynamic creative therapy groups

In their book *Occupational therapy: a communication process*, the Fidlers (1963) explored the role of the unconscious, interpersonal relationships and the symbolic potential of activities. Activities are offered to help individuals to express their thoughts and feelings. Interactions within the group offer the opportunity for sharing, ego strengthening and reality testing, and individuals are encouraged to develop social awareness and a sense of belonging.

This theory has underpinned many types of occupational therapy groups, spanning the use of art, drama, music, poetry and dance. Leary (1994) described a range of activities which can be used to develop self-awareness based on themes such as 'Who am I' or 'Caring about each other' or 'My problem is'. Atkinson & Wells (2000) look in detail at the application of psychodynamic creative therapy activities.

The value of groups

Special qualities of groups

A group is more than a collection of individuals. Members of a group are bonded together by their group identity and shared purposes which will only be realised by interacting and working together (Mosey 1973). Each group has a life and identity of its own. So what are the special qualities of a group that a therapist can tap?

- First, any group involves multiple relationships. A group member can draw on the therapeutic potential of having relationships with several people at once rather than working with just one therapist. Groups are sometimes conceptualised as a hall of mirrors where multiple transferences take place (Blair 1990).

- Second, groups provide a natural learning environment where individuals can interact, find role models and advise each other. Norms and pressures within a group shape attitudes and behaviours as members respond to others' expectations.

- Third, groups can be enormously supportive. Members gain strength from feeling connected to others and being accepted by them. Pleasures, hopes, uncertainties and pains can be shared. Often, emotions in a group become amplified as people react to and identify with each other. This in turn helps members to express and explore their feelings.

- Finally, groups are a dynamic source of ideas and creativity. People are invariably stimulated and energised by others as they bounce ideas off them.

Yalom (1975) offered an in-depth analysis of 11 curative factors of group therapy:

1. instillation of hope
2. universality
3. imparting information
4. altruism
5. the corrective recapitulation of the primary family group
6. development of socialising techniques
7. imitative behaviour
8. interpersonal learning
9. group cohesiveness
10. catharsis
11. existential factors.

Yalom's research has been adapted and replicated by many researchers. In particular Falk-Kessler et al (1991) explored the extent to which these factors are valued within occupational therapy groupwork. They found that both patients and therapists perceived group cohesiveness, hope and interpersonal learning as the most helpful. Emphasising the need to deliver services that are valued by clients, Lloyd & Maas (1997) note research findings which indicate clients also feel positive about the use of activities.

Value of different group formats

Occupational therapy literature is full of examples of the use and value of groups (see Tallant 1998 for a comprehensive review). A central and recurrent theme in this literature is that groups are a tool to promote change, teach skills and encourage social contact.

A number of occupational therapy researchers have investigated the value of activity groups over talking groups. Klyczek & Mann (1986) compared different treatment programmes at two psychiatric day centres. The programme offering more activity rather than psychotherapy was found to be significantly more effective for developing decision-making skills, use of leisure time, self-esteem and vocational adjustment. McDermott (1988) considered the effect of three group formats: task, activity-based verbal and verbal. She found that, while the task group resulted in more positive communications and more interactions between members, the verbal and activity-based verbal groups facilitated more discussion of feelings. All three groups were seen as beneficial for learning.

Crouch (1987) compared occupational therapists' assessments of psychiatric patients made during two types of groups (art and discussion groups) with assessments carried out by other team members over the course of a week. Her results suggest that occupational therapy groupwork can be a quick and effective means of assessing patients' functioning.

Group versus individual treatment

Groupwork and individual therapy are two different treatment tools which mental health therapists draw upon. Both have their value for particular people, times and situations. They are not mutually exclusive, and many patients and clients can benefit from involvement in both, either concurrently (Box 14.1) or by using one as a precursor to the other. Any discussion of when to use groupwork and/or individual treatment must necessarily relate to individual needs and aims of treatment, as well as to practical issues such as the availability of suitable groups, and the treatment context.

In general, if a person's mental health problems are either created by or result in interpersonal difficulties, then a group offers the more relevant context in which to explore such difficulties, gain support and learn how best to cope. Groupwork will be an appropriate choice of treatment if the patient or client:

- has the skills and awareness to interact and share with others in a group
- has problems related to social interaction and relationships
- feels isolated and is without others to offer support or constructive advice
- is threatened by the intensity or intimacy of one-to-one work.

Box 14.1   Example 1: concurrent individual and group therapy

J. H. Lacey (1984) developed a structured treatment programme for women suffering from bulimia nervosa which involves both individual and group treatment. Five clients meet on one half-day a week for 10 consecutive weeks. Each client starts by having a half-hour individual session with her therapist, then all five clients meet in a group session run by two therapists (one of whom is their individual therapist).

Lacey advocates an eclectic theoretical orientation combining psychodynamic, behavioural and cognitive approaches. The individual sessions initially employ behavioural and cognitive techniques where the client agrees to a contract to maintain a prescribed diet and to write a daily diary of food intake and the emotions/events surrounding it. The sessions develop into insight-directed supportive psychotherapy as the client identifies the emotions involved with her eating patterns.

The group sessions aim to provide mutual support in changing members' eating habits. They also provide a safe place to explore feelings. The groups tend to be fast-moving and have 'much expressed affect, sometimes to the extent that the therapist needs to prevent the group members from "bingeing" with emotions' (Lacey 1984).

Groupwork is contraindicated when the patient or client:

- is threatened by being in a group and is unable to relate to others
- is unmotivated to engage in groupwork
- is too self-absorbed to be aware of others' needs
- is too acutely ill, fragile or aggressive to concentrate and contain his own behaviour, so that the interactions would be destructive
- has problems which feel too intense and complicated to work through adequately in a group situation (as can be the case when someone has experienced sexual abuse or other trauma).

Therapists who enjoy and are skilled at groupwork may tend to opt for groupwork as their preferred treatment option. However, the wider treatment context also needs to be taken into account. Is there enough supervision available? Is there sufficient demand for a group? What are the practical constraints regarding timetabling and staff availability? Would the group fit in with treatments the other team members are offering? Will other team members be supportive? If the answers to these questions are in the negative, then setting up a group is ill advised.

Group treatments are often seen as an economic option, as we can treat several people simultaneously; however, cost-effectiveness only works if the treatment is effective as well. At times a patient or client's problem can be more simply and efficiently handled on an individual basis, for instance, in behavioural goal-setting. Furthermore, it can often take more time to manage a group for the following reasons:

- a group session will often last over one-and-a-half hours whereas an individual consultation may only last 30 minutes
- extra time needs to be set aside for group leader preparation, discussions and evaluation
- people still need to be seen individually to prepare them, and to evaluate and document their progress.

Running a group is rarely the easy option!

There are strengths and limitations to both formats. Ultimately, the question of which treatment to offer remains a matter for professional judgement. Whatever decision is made, it should be a joint one, taken in consultation with the patient or client and the treatment team.

PLANNING GROUPS

Planning a group, whether it is for a single session or setting up a longer-term group, is a complicated business. It is a time-consuming, challenging exercise in problem solving and creativity. This section will describe how, in order to prepare for a session, the therapist needs to think through the aims of treatment, choose activities and structure the session, arrange the environment, grade and adapt treatment, and then motivate the members to attend. Setting up a longer-term group involves making practical decisions about the group, marketing it and then preparing prospective members. (For an in-depth account of group leadership see Cole 1998.)

PREPARING A SESSION
Aims and objectives

The initial task when preparing a session is to formulate its aims and objectives. Aims can be viewed as the intended overall gain, objectives as the specific, measurable outcome targets.

Aims and objectives ensure that the group activity is purposeful. Knowing the point of the session gives group members goals to strive for and so increases their motivation. For leaders, knowing what has to be achieved gives clues about how to structure the session. The aims and objectives will also provide baseline criteria for evaluating both group and individual progress.

Activity groups and support groups have different aims and objectives. Activity groups aim 'to develop work skills' or 'to encourage leisure pursuits', and may well focus on an end product. Examples of group objectives relevant here are 'by the end of the session members will be able to centre the clay on the pottery wheel' or 'members will be able to explain confidently how to cook chicken korma'. In addition to group objectives, individuals may have their own personal objectives such as 'Paul will share tools/materials with another member during the craft session'.

Support groups aim 'to encourage members to explore feelings and give each other support'. Group interactions and relationships are usually seen as more important than the activity or end product. This focus on feelings and process may make formulating objectives difficult or even inappropriate. However, the therapist could have general objectives for a session such as 'by the end of the projective art group members will be able to describe at least one point they like and dislike about themselves'. Individuals may have their own objectives such as 'learn how to say "no" assertively'.

Choosing the activity

It has been said that 'The analysis of occupations and their prescription as therapy are the unique skills of the occupational therapist' (Hagedorn 1992). Indeed, it could be argued that the appropriate selection and systematic application of activity is the crucial pivot of most occupational therapy intervention.

The choice of type of group activity follows naturally from the aims. As Borg & Bruce (1991) stated: 'In order for activity to be therapeutic, it must successfully bond the goals of therapy with the nature of the activity itself'. An aim to improve skills, for instance, guides the therapist towards work on craft activities; whereas aiming to increase self-confidence in relationships points towards support group activities such as social skills training or creative therapy.

The primary factor guiding activity selection should be what is meaningful to the people concerned. The activity needs both to maintain a person's interest and to appeal to his personal and cultural values. Some individuals find group games childish and demeaning. A housewife may not value cooking. A person may perceive clay as dirty and dislike touching it. A man might prefer knitting to woodwork. Not all people will

wish to take part in Christmas festivities. Activities designed to promote independence may not be valued. In all these cases the interest and beliefs of the individuals must be respected and the therapist's own values temporarily suspended.

Kremer et al (1984) investigated the degree of meaning different activities held for chronic psychiatric patients. The activity of cooking was found to be significantly more meaningful than craft or sensory awareness groups. The authors suggested that possible reasons for this are that it is an age-appropriate, culturally meaningful, concrete, productive activity which offers oral stimulation.

The group members' level of functioning will then influence what activities are selected. Members may not have the skills to carry out certain tasks, or individuals could have some physical limitations such as mobility problems or sensory deficits. Alternatively, the group as a whole might not have enough trust and cohesion to allow self-disclosure.

Structuring the session

When the type and level of activity have been chosen, the next step involves creating and planning the full session. In order to do this the overall structure of the group session can be visualised as involving five different phases. These phases differ in quality and emphasis depending upon the type and level of group, but each phase needs to be considered to some degree:

1. *Introduction.* The members are first welcomed and introduced to each other, where necessary. Some groups may benefit from ice-breaking games such as throwing a bean bag and calling out each other's names. The group activity is also likely to need some initial explanation.

2. *Warm-up.* Longer warm-up periods are required for new or 'feelings-based' groups, while a familiar craft activity group will not require much warm-up time. Typical warm-ups include: physical exercise to energise a group; humorous activities to relax members; nonverbal games to prepare for a role-play.

3. *Action*. This phase is the main part of the session where the activity or activities selected to achieve the group aims are implemented. The action may involve carrying out a single task (for example, painting a group picture) or working through a series of exercises (such as in drama therapy). If there are to be several exercises, it may be useful to focus on some theme so that an idea or experience can be followed through.

4. *Wind-down*. Having a period to wind down is important for any group and may be fulfilled in different ways. A closure activity may be used to draw threads together or relax the group. Alternatively, clearing up may signal a transition period towards ending the group. Some verbal psychotherapy groups rely on the presence of a clock to allow members to prepare themselves when the time is coming to a close. At the very end of the group, the therapist might conclude with a few key comments and will try to acknowledge individuals' contributions.

5. *Post-group*. It is essential for the leader or leaders to have some time to evaluate the group and record what happened. Post-group discussions allow the leaders time both to reflect on the group and to gain support for themselves.

An example of planning a session is given in Box 14.2.

Organising the environment

When planning a group, as much attention should be paid to organising the environment as to devising the group activity. This involves attending to both practical/physical and more abstract/psychological considerations.

Practical planning needs to take into account furniture, equipment and physical safety. First, consideration should be given to what furniture is needed and how it should be positioned. These are important decisions as they not only have practical implications but can also affect group members' expectations – tables and chairs laid out in a formal style are likely to promote very different behaviours from those encouraged by having large floor cushions strewn around.

Second, equipment and materials need to be planned in advance to check their availability and condition. Third, physical safety must be ensured: this involves complying with health and safety regulations and considering the safe handling of materials, equipment and substances. There should also be adequate lighting, warmth, space and ventilation for comfort. While these last aspects may not be totally within the occupational therapist's control, there should at least be awareness of their potential positive and negative effects on the group. A lively game, for instance, would not be the best choice in a room which contains obstacles and is very warm.

On a more abstract level, the environment can communicate much about attitudes/expectations; it can set the scene by creating an atmosphere, and can promote emotional safety. Messages about expectations can be implicit in the choice of equipment and surroundings. For instance, having particularly artistic paintings on an art room wall can be potentially threatening to

---

Box 14.2 Example 2: a therapist's plan for a projective art group (adapted from Finlay 1993)

Introduction (10 minutes). (a) Introduce self, then ask each person to say his or her name. (b) Acknowledge newness of group/activity to all members. (c) Establish aim of not trying to paint 'pretty' pictures but to express self and gain support. (d) Describe typical format of painting then talking about picture. (e) Lay down group rule that there should be no interpretation of paintings except by the individual.

Warm-up (5 minutes). Painting to music consisting of different moods and tempos. Aim to have fun, relax the group, introduce notion of expressing self through painting. Members to offer brief feedback comments about how they experienced the activity.

Action (30 minutes). Paint (a) 'how I see myself – what is important to me in my present life'; (b) 'how I would like it to be'. Each painting to take approximately 15 minutes, including sharing and discussion time.

Wind-down (15 minutes). (a) Group picture using a large piece of paper; start by having a painting conversation with a neighbour; gradually try to have contact with other group members. (b) Feedback about the group. (c) Each member is invited to say 'one thing positive for me in today's session'.

Post-group (approximately half an hour) Write notes and give feedback to team.

members who perceive they are expected to be artistic. Or, to take an opposite example, supplying only thick paint brushes to an art group signals that accurate, detailed paintings are not required. Atmosphere is equally important and can be created. A work atmosphere, for example, is promoted by laying out the furniture in an appropriate manner and ensuring distractions are kept to a minimum. Also, rooms can carry atmospheres by their other functions and associations. Outpatients, for instance, sometime find it hard to return to a group held on the ward, as it provokes painful memories or a return to sick role behaviour. Linked with atmosphere is the need to promote emotional safety. Having some private space which is free from interruptions is a prerequisite for any group where feelings are being expressed and building trust is a key aim. Sometimes, a separate room is not a practical possibility, but there are other ways of establishing boundaries, such as by using room dividers.

Grading and adapting treatment

The ability of therapists to grade and adapt activities, in ways which transform occupation into therapy, is the fundamental process underlying occupational therapy intervention.

The demands of an activity and the amount of stimulation/pressure within the environment are graded in three main ways:

1. by gradually increasing the level of difficulty of the activity
2. by breaking down the activity into component parts
3. by increasing the type and number of roles a member is to play.

In a woodwork group, for example, the technical demands of the task can be increased, or a group member may be encouraged to begin to take on a teacher role, helping others.

Activities are adapted when they are altered to suit the background, ability and values of an individual and the circumstances of the situation. For example, a cooking activity might be switched after the discovery that the planned beefburgers would not suit a Hindu member of the group. Again, if a group seems bored or understimulated during an activity, the therapist would endeavour to make the session more interesting (perhaps by introducing an element of competition), or might even abandon the activity altogether.

Box 14.3 illustrates how an activity might be graded and adapted.

Box 14.3 Example 3: grading social interaction in a photography group

Sue became acutely anxious when required to interact with others. In order to work on these difficulties, she joined the photography group. She had always wanted to pursue photography as a hobby and was keen to develop her skills.

The occupational therapist and Sue negotiated the following hierarchy of goals where she was required to interact with others increasingly over the course of 10 sessions:

1. Be a nominal member of the group; work alone taking photographs; interact only with the therapist.
2. Work on an individual activity alongside a group activity.
3. Work with one other person in the group taking photographs outside.
4. Work with the same person in the group room and darkroom.

5. Work with another person in the group room and darkroom.
6. Join the group when they are being taught a technique; no particular interaction required.
7. Work with others in the group.
8. Join the group in an outing to photography museum.

By the third session, Sue managed goals 1–4 fairly easily. Her involvement with the photography tasks enabled her to handle the goals for interacting without too much anxiety. During the fourth session, however, Sue had a panic attack prior to going in the darkroom with a male member of the group. The planned darkroom activity was adapted to accommodate her difficulties. Sue had not anticipated her reaction to the more intimate contact with a man, and was able to explore this further in her individual psychotherapy sessions. With extra encouragement and support she achieved the rest of her goals.

Motivating members

One of the most common problems confronting workers in the mental health field is that of clients lacking motivation to engage in treatment. If a client does not want to join the group activity, then disentangling what is causing the lack of motivation becomes the first task.

Does the client lack drive as a product of his illness, institutionalisation or medication? If this is the case, care needs to be taken to make the group activities relevant, reasonably stimulating and enjoyable for the individual. A study by Polimeni-Walker et al (1992) demonstrated that patients frequently considered escape from hospital routine and relief of boredom as the most important reasons for participating in an occupational therapy group. While this calls into question whether they are deriving the optimal benefits of therapy, it should be recognised that they might have their own perceptions of what they are gaining.

Alternatively, can the client's reluctance to attend a group be put down to uncertainty, anxiety or confusion about the purpose of the group or treatment? In this case, careful explanation and preparation is needed, giving the clients time to air their questions or concerns.

If clients can see the purpose and value of treatment, invariably their motivation is correspondingly increased. It is the therapist's job to clarify how and why treatment might be relevant and to ensure the activities have meaning for individuals. Ideally, clients should be actively involved in planning their own treatment. This not only engages them in treatment; it also ensures they take some responsibility for future progress.

SETTING UP A LONGER-TERM GROUP

A longer-term group is one that continues and is set up to last for a fixed number of weeks or to run indefinitely. The decision to establish either type of group should be made in response to a clear demand which could come from professional colleagues who see an unmet need, or from the clients themselves. Whichever is the case, therapists have an ethical and professional responsibility to provide appropriate treatment which meets needs and not simply one they themselves would like to carry out!

There are three main stages involved in setting up a longer-term group (Fig. 14.2). First, there is a preliminary planning period when decisions about the type, level and aims of the group are made. Specific issues concerning leadership, group membership and the timing of the group need to be considered. The second stage of setting up a group involves marketing it to prospective members and referral agents. The third stage, of member preparation, may well involve several interviews to select, then prepare, the members.

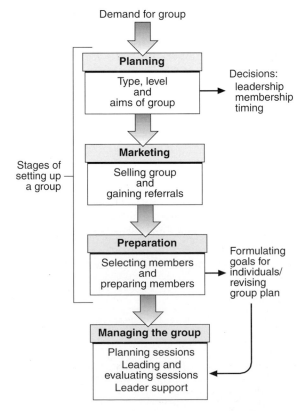

Figure 14.2 The stages involved in setting up a longer-term group.

Planning

Once the aims of the group have been established, several other decisions need to be taken. First, consideration is given to the number of leaders and their respective roles. For a longer-term group it is best to have more than one leader as it allows a division of labour. For instance, in a support group, one leader can take a more confronting role while the other supports. In a task group, one leader might work with individuals on an activity while the other leader oversees the group process. Having more than one leader enables them to give each other continuing support. There is also the advantage that the group can continue if one leader is absent.

Second, there are a number of group membership issues to be resolved:

Size of group. The optimum size for a psychotherapy group is usually considered to be six to nine people. Activity groups can run with more or fewer members, providing there are enough staff to attend to individuals.

Open versus closed groups. Support groups generally function best as closed groups, which allow group cohesion and trust to develop with continuing relationships. Activity groups are able to operate as open groups, although when a lot of interaction between members is necessary it is better to have a core of regular attenders.

Mix of members. Support groups operate best when members function at a similar level so they can identify with each other. They need to be different enough, however, to challenge each other and offer new ideas. Activity groups can often tolerate a greater degree of heterogeneity between members. Having members at different functioning levels may be useful. For example, a higher functioning member can assist another who is less able.

Third, in terms of decisions about timing, consideration should be given to:

- when and how often the group should take place
- the length of the session
- how many weeks or months the group should run for

- whether the group session should be time-limited or open-ended.

In general, support groups take place once a week or fortnight and last for an hour or an hour and a half. Usually, they are strictly time-limited as this predictability contributes to emotional safety. Activity groups, on the other hand, can take place more often, for longer periods, and may well allow open-ended attendance.

Marketing

After the preliminary planning, the next stage is to gain referrals. Initially, the referral procedure needs to be established and a relevant referral form designed. Then the group needs to be advertised and marketed in a way appropriate to the unit. Examples of marketing methods designed to give information about the group are: sending out letters to referral agencies, distributing leaflets around the ward, and putting up poster displays in outpatient departments and GP surgeries. It is important to remember that marketing a group also means marketing occupational therapy, and the more professional the letters and posters look, the more successful the group will be in the long term.

Member preparation

Once the members have been selected, they need to be actively prepared for, and engaged in, the group. This may be done, for instance, by having a couple of pre-group interviews with each member. Preparing members for a group is a crucial step and may well make a difference to whether or not the group is sustained.

The aims of a pre-group interview are:

1. *Relationship building*: to introduce the prospective member and therapist to each other.
2. *Information giving*: to give information about the group and clarify expectations.
3. *Information receiving*: to begin to get to know and understand the needs of the individual member.

4. *Support*: to acknowledge his or her anxieties and uncertainties.
5. *Assessment*: to establish the baseline assessment criteria.
6. *Treatment planning*: to negotiate the individual's treatment aims and objectives.

When the pre-group interviews have taken place and prospective members have made a positive commitment to attend the group, the therapist can concentrate on managing the group.

MANAGING THE GROUP

Managing a group involves much more than simply running a planned session. Groups invariably go in different directions from the plan, and activities have to be modified along the way. Problems can erupt, for example conflict may break out or members might resist an activity. The group therapist needs to understand what is occurring and why, and then to be able to handle these events. The therapist needs to be aware of, and continuously to evaluate, both individual processes and the group process.

In order to begin to explore how to manage a group, this section will consider some of the core elements of group dynamics theory and the evaluation process. Box 14.4 offers a sample analysis of one group's development over time and highlights some typical problems and some of the techniques used to manage a group.

Group dynamics

Group dynamics are the 'forces, social structures, behaviours, relationships and processes which occur within groups' (Finlay 1993). This section looks briefly at some of the phenomena which occur within groups, i.e. roles, relationships and group evolution. (See Cole 1998 for a further exploration of group dynamics in occupational therapy.)

Roles

Every group member will assume a number of group roles. Some roles are formally ascribed and involve an official position with associated status and responsibilities, such as 'chairperson'. Members also take on informal roles, for instance: 'the counsellor' or 'the stirrer'. Benne & Sheats (1978) outlined three kinds of group roles:

Box 14.4 Example 4: the 'next-step' group

The 'next-step' group is a support group which aims to help people who have recently lost important life roles to adjust to and cope with their new situation. Treatment methods employed include creative/expressive activities and discussion.

Group objectives
By the end of the 12-week course members will be able to:

1. describe the significance of different life roles for them
2. analyse different ways members relate to each other and how some behaviour can be unhelpful or destructive
3. list ways of replacing lost roles
4. demonstrate at least one new behaviour or coping strategy.

Members
Sarah is the group therapist.

Peter (aged 40) is a single parent of two sons who have recently left home. He feels dissatisfied and stressed but he denies any feelings of loss and remains aloof and critical in the group.

Dave (aged 30) needs to find a new role and identity as an ex-drinker. He lost a good job and relationship through drinking. He has now found a new job and is well motivated to change his behaviour.

Alison (aged 21) is shortly due to complete her university course. She is anxious about exams, confused about her future options and fears losing her independence on returning home to her parents with whom she has a poor relationship.

Pam (aged 38) has recently been through a difficult divorce and she is trying (unsuccessfully) to withdraw from benzodiazepines which she has taken for a number of years. She is tense, vulnerable and lonely.

Ian (aged 53) has recently been made redundant from his job in industry and is unlikely to get another. Having a work role is important to him and he is both bitter and depressed.

Box 14.4   cont'd

EVOLUTION OF GROUP

Session	Activity and focus	Comments on group process/development
1	Art: 'paint self now/before'	'Forming' stage. Members anxious and dependent on Sarah who tried to pull out common links. Members experienced tension and discomfort with new and unfamiliar activity.
2	Collage: 'aspects of self: inside/outside'	Members resistant to activity; once engaged, some self-disclosure. Members began to recognise similar pains beneath able exteriors and trust began. Peter denied having feelings, which annoyed the others.
3	Drama 'buttons: life story and important events'	'Norming' stage. Norm established of doing trigger activity then each member 'tells their story'. Interaction minimal so Sarah pointed out common areas. Some anger towards Sarah for not solving problems; she in turn challenged the group to assume more responsibility.
4	Art: 'feelings: one aspect of myself I don't like/one I do like'	Group cohesion increased as three members expressed deeper feelings. Pam, Ian, Dave each became tearful and supported each other. Peter remained critical and aloof from the group.
5	Drama: 'family sculpts: now/ideal'	'Storming' stage. Open conflict occurred between Alison and Peter as they appeared to project family roles onto each other. Peter was scapegoated by Alison, Dave and Pam who formed a subgroup. Sarah asked Peter and Alison to sculpt their problem family situations in turn (an unplanned activity).
6	Role-play: Alison practised being assertive with her parents	'Performing' stage. Conflict was reduced. Members pulled together to help Alison successfully 'handle' parents. Peter played a parent, was constructively helpful and received positive feedback. Sarah remained fairly active/directive.
7	Drama: 'trading qualities: what I need to cope better in future'	Exercise led by Sarah encouraged members to recognise positive aspects in everyone. Self-esteem and group cohesion boosted.
8	Role-play: Peter tried a psychodrama and talked to his absent sons	Peter felt safe enough to try a psychodrama and learn new ways of relating to his children. Alison and Dave took on the children's roles. The session was deeply painful for Peter as he came to terms with some home truths about his relationships. The group was supportive of him.
9	Flipcharts: 'Roles and daily activities: what they are/what needs to change'	Prior to the group activity, Ian said he wanted to leave the group as he was not finding it of benefit. Sarah wondered if the previous week's emotional session was to blame. The group members persuaded Ian to stay for their sake. In the flipchart activity, members gave each other constructive suggestions and cohesion was high.
10	Role-play: Dave practised saying 'no' to an alcoholic drink	All members participated actively in the role plays and listened well to each other. Dave was successful in finding an assertion formula. Sarah directed the role play but otherwise her interventions were minimal.
11	Drama: 'Preferred scenarios: moving fantasy on to reality'	Preferred scenario exercise prompted members to express their wish for the group to continue. 'Storming' stage as members expressed anger towards Sarah who maintained the group has to end. Issues of loss, sadness and anger were raised.
12	Art: whole group painting, and Evaluation: 'one thing gained'	'Performing' stage. Acceptance of ending though members still expressed resistance. Generally cohesive group and positive feelings were expressed. Members recognised that work on their problems still needed to continue beyond the group.

- group task roles, such as information-giver and initiator, where members coordinate their effort towards problem solving and carrying out a task
- group-building and maintenance roles, which include 'followers' and 'harmonisers', among others
- individual roles which aim to satisfy individual's needs, for instance 'blocker' or 'recognition seeker'.

The roles adopted are determined by the contribution the individual wishes to make and by the demands of the group goals and other members' needs. For instance, a person who is characteristically a follower may well assume a leader role if one is needed to achieve a task and others do not oblige. Roles are typically functional in that they serve individual or group interests in some way. For example, the clown role can be unconsciously enacted to protect members by enabling the group to evade difficult issues.

If the therapist is to manage the group effectively, she needs to be aware of roles adopted by individuals and those which are required by the group; then the therapist needs to be able to enable positive and effective role behaviours to emerge. A prime concern is to facilitate members in taking on different roles. For instance, enabling an individual with low self-esteem to assume a leader mantle successfully will enhance his confidence. Or, a person might be encouraged to try out a new role behaviour, such as being assertive, in the safety of the group prior to adopting the role in real life.

Group therapists need to be aware of what roles the group needs in order to achieve its goals. A work group requires workers and technicians; social groups benefit from clowns and encouragers; communication groups need risk-takers and gate-keepers. Therapists might even select the members for a group with a view to such balance.

When problems arise within the group, the leader would do well to analyse roles played or required. An apathetic group may have been influenced by an apathetic controller; a silent group may need an initiator or facilitator; an angry group may need a spokesperson or a harmoniser; when conflict erupts between two members, this could signal competition for a leader role.

Finally, the therapist needs to be aware of her own roles and how they contribute to the group process. Consider the situation where members of a group are dependent and needy. Might this have arisen in response to an overly protective carer-therapist? In some situations, the group therapist may need to adopt a *laissez-faire* role to encourage others to be more active. In other circumstances, she may need to become more directive. The group therapist can also act as a model for members to follow, for example, when members emulate the 'free-child' leader.

Intragroup relationships

There is a vast pool of literature (e.g. Bales 1970) analysing interactions in groups. Some frequently reported findings are as follows:

- Individual participation is a function of group size, personality, status in group, knowledge and physical location within the group.
- High participators tend to give information/opinions and speak more to the group as a whole. Lower participators, on the other hand, tend to contribute more by expressing agreement or asking questions, and direct these more to individuals.
- Those who contribute more receive more messages from others and those who contribute little are likely to be ignored.
- As members feel safer with each other, they spend more time expressing feelings and can tolerate disagreement more without an increase in anxiety.

Argyle (1967) described interactions in groups in terms of task and sociable activities (Table 14.1). Members interact both to achieve the group task and to attend to social and emotional needs. Quieter members may still be actively

Table 14.1 Task versus sociable activities and interactions (Argyle 1967)

	Task	Sociable
Verbal	Information and discussion related to the task	Gossip and chat, jokes and games, discussion of personal problems
Nonverbal	Task performance, helpful nonverbal comments on performance, nonverbal signals conveying information	Communicating interpersonal attitudes, emotions, self-presentation

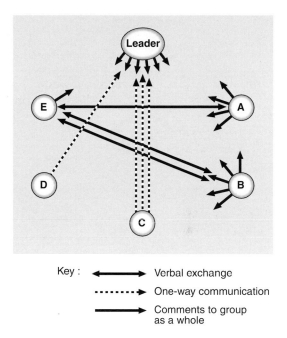

Key :
- ⟷ Verbal exchange
- ┅┅➤ One-way communication
- ➤ Comments to group as a whole

Figure 14.4 Verbal communications occurring in a group.

involved at a nonverbal level, supporting the group.

Moreno (1953) made a special contribution to understanding relationships between group members. His analytical tool, the sociogram, has been widely used to represent visually the underlying social structure of groups.

The sociogram in Figure 14.3 plots the relationships in one group. It highlights a core subgroup or clique. F is an outsider who wishes to become a member; D and E have some connection to the main clique through E's relationship with C; G remains isolated. The sociogram in Figure 14.4 represents the amount and direction of verbal communication in another group where

C and D are notably directing all their comments to the leader, whereas A, B and E interact as a group.

Beyond simply describing such relationships, further analysis is necessary to explore their quality and impact. For instance, in the case of Figure 14.3, is the core subgroup advantageous and a source of strength and support? Or is it potentially destructive, as allegiance to the wider group is diminished, impairing full group cooperation? In Figure 14.4, are C and D somehow dependent on the leader? Do they find interacting with others difficult in some way?

Once the group therapist has begun to understand what is occurring in the group, she can develop the interactions. Therapists can facilitate interaction by using themselves and the activity as treatment tools and ensuring the environment is supportive (Fig. 14.5).

Evolution of a group

Groups which come together regularly over a period of time usually evolve through

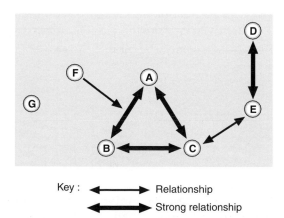

Key :
- ⟷ Relationship
- ⟺ Strong relationship
- ⟵ One-way relationship

Figure 14.3 A relationship sociogram representing subgroupings.

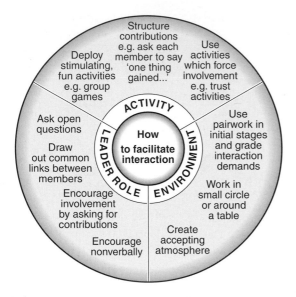

Figure 14.5   How to facilitate interaction.

a number of stages where members experience distinct sets of feelings, preoccupations and behaviours. These stages overlap and are not necessarily sequential, nor will all stages necessarily be experienced by every group. The key point is that every group faces certain developmental issues as part of its ongoing dynamics.

Tuckman (1965) encapsulated the stages experienced by groups using the terms: forming, storming, norming and performing. In the forming stage, members ask questions about what is expected of them and the purpose of the group. It is a period of orientation, dependence, testing and anxiety about fitting in. The storming stage involves intragroup conflict. Members feel resistant to the group task and may express hostility to the leader for not solving their problems. The norming stage is a time for cohesion; a strong group culture emerges and pressure is exerted to conform to group norms. In the performing stage the group works effectively; trust is high and members focus on achieving the task at hand.

Group leaders need to understand these stages in order to identify the needs of individuals and ensure they have appropriate expect-

ations of the group. The therapist also has a key role to play in facilitating some resolution of each stage. In the early stages of a group, the therapist will want to clarify aims and encourage members to take part actively. When the group experiences conflict, she will encourage supportive relationships and honest communication while keeping the group safe. As the group becomes more cohesive and productive the therapist might step back or encourage greater risk taking. In the ending stages the group will need help to acknowledge feelings of impending loss and tie up unfinished business. Box 14.4 gives an account of a leader helping a group to move through these stages.

Evaluation

Occupational therapists have a professional responsibility to evaluate their work. Evaluation is necessary to establish whether patients or clients are benefiting from the therapy and to measure any progress. Evaluation is also essential to clarify what needs to be achieved in future sessions, and can be used to develop the therapist's group skills and interventions.

Methods

A range of evaluation methods, both objective and subjective, is available to therapists (Fig. 14.6).

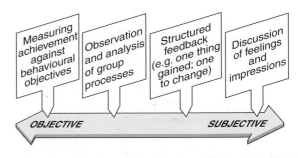

Figure 14.6   Continuum of subjective–objective evaluation methods.

On the whole, evaluation methods towards the subjective end of the spectrum tend to be more suitable for support groups, while activity groups require more objective outcome measures. Thus, in a psychotherapy group members will be regularly invited to express their feelings about the group and its progress, while in task-orientated groups progress is more appropriately assessed in terms of individual performance and skills (Table 14.2).

In practice, several evaluation methods are likely to be employed for each group: for instance, feedback from group members, observations and analysis of the group processes and measurement of progress using behavioural outcome measures.

Recording group progress

It is difficult to document what has occurred in a group in a succinct fashion, as the record needs to capture both individual behaviour and the complex group processes involved. Some therapists write a brief summary of group events/themes (see Box 14.4) and record individual progress separately (see Table 14.2).

Alternatively, visual means of recording, such as sociograms or chronograms, can be helpful for representing complex group dynamics. Cox's (1973) group therapy interaction chronogram (Fig. 14.7) offers a succinct way of recording events that occur in the initial, middle and end stages of a group, as well as any positive and negative responses between members.

Supervision

Finally, as part of the evaluation process, every therapist needs support and opportunity to reflect on experiences and develop skills. Supervision offers this. Before starting any group it is important to arrange supervision, whatever the basis (for example weekly one to one sessions or monthly peer-group support). Supervision should offer a safe forum in which to:

- evaluate what occurred in the group
- consider different ways of handling the group
- explore co-leadership issues and tensions.

Table 14.2 Evaluation of an individual's behaviour in an activity group

	Session			
	1	2	3	4
Task performance Concentration Instructions Problem solving	2 had to work with him individually	2	1 concentration improved	0
Social interaction Awareness of others Verbal interaction Sharing	2	2	1 awareness and sharing prompted	1
General behaviour Presentation Orientation Activity level	2 hypoactive	2	0 medication changed	0

0 = no problem; 1 = some problem; 2 = severe problem.

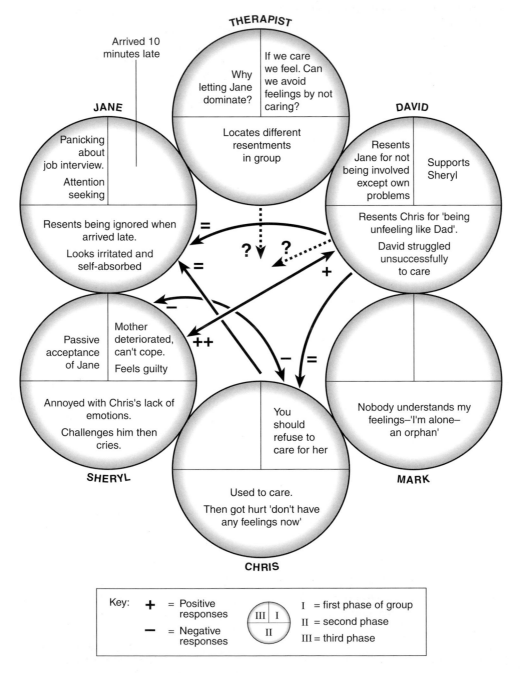

Figure 14.7 Example of Cox's chronogram.

Arguably, those therapists running support groups should have supervision more often in order to explore their feelings and any counter-transferences. But feelings can be aroused in activity groups too, so these should not be ignored.

SUMMARY

This chapter has sought to explore the use of groupwork in occupational therapy. First, it considered different types of groups and their value. Practical guidelines were offered for how to prepare a session and set up a longer-term group. The final section focused on group dynamics theory and evaluation methods. It stressed the need to understand group processes in order to manage them.

Occupational therapists exploit the learning opportunities within a variety of group situations. However, the curative potential of groupwork is neither random nor inevitable. Group experiences are powerful and can be destructive as well as beneficial. For occupational therapy groups to be effective, individuals must be enabled actively to participate in the group process. Therapists need to guide and support patients or clients through their group experiences. As group therapists, success depends on our capacity to unfold and manage sensitively the complex dynamics involved when interdependent people relate to each other.

Groupwork is always a challenge and, as such, it is always a learning experience for the therapist too.

REFERENCES

Argyle M 1967 The psychology of interpersonal behaviour. Penguin, Oxford

Atkinson K and Wells C (2000) Creative therapies: a psychodynamic approach within occupational therapy. Stanley Thornes, Cheltenham

Bales R F 1970 Personality and interpersonal behaviour. Holt, Rhinehart and Winston, New York

Benne K, Sheats P 1978 Functional roles of group members. Journal of Social Issues 4: 41–49

Blair S 1990 Occupational therapy and group psychotherapy. In: Creek J (ed) Occupational therapy and mental health, 1st edn. Churchill Livingstone, Edinburgh

Borg B, Bruce M 1991 The group system – the therapeutic activity group in occupational therapy. Slack, Thorofare, New Jersey

Cole M B 1998 Group dynamics in occupational therapy: the theoretical basis and practice application of group treatment, 2nd edn. Slack, Thorofare, New Jersey

Cox M 1973 The group therapy interaction chronogram. British Journal of Social Work 3(2): 223–256

Crouch R 1987 A study of the effectiveness of certain occupational therapy group techniques in the assessment of the acutely disturbed adult psychiatric patient. British Journal of Occupational Therapy 50(3): 86–91

Falk-Kessler J, Momich C, Perel S 1991 Therapeutic factors in occupational therapy groups. American Journal of Occupational Therapy 45: 59–66

Fidler G S, Fidler J W 1963 Occupational therapy: a communication process in psychiatry. Macmillan, New York

Finlay L 1993 Groupwork in occupational therapy. Chapman and Hall, London

Finlay L (1999) When actions speak louder: Groupwork in occupational therapy. Groupwork: an Interdisciplinary Journal for Working with Groups. 11(3): 19–29

Hagedorn R 1992 Occupational therapy: foundations for practice models, frames of reference and core skills. Churchill Livingstone, Edinburgh

Howe M, Schwartzberg S 1986 A functional approach to group work in occupational therapy. J B Lippincott, Philadelphia

Kaplan K 1988 Directive group therapy. Slack, Thorofare, New Jersey

Kielhofner G (ed) 1995 A model of human occupation: theory and application. Williams and Wilkins, Baltimore

Klyczek J, Mann W 1986 Therapeutic modality comparisons in day treatment. American Journal of Occupational Therapy 40: 606–611

Kremer E R H, Nelson D, Duncombe L 1984 Effects of selected activities on affective meaning in psychiatric patients. American Journal of Occupational Therapy 38(8): 522–528

Lacey J H 1984 Time-limited individual and group treatment for bulimia. In: Garner D, Garfinkel P (eds) Handbook of psychotherapy for anorexia nervosa and bulimia. Guilford Press, New York

Leary S 1994 Activities for personal growth: a comprehensive handbook of activities for therapists. McLennan and Petty, Sydney

Lloyd C, Maas F 1997 Occupational therapy group work in psyciatric settings. British Journal of Occupational Therapy 60(5): 226–229

McDermott A 1988 The effect of three group formats on group interaction patterns. In: Gibson D (ed) Group process and structure in psycho-social occupational therapy. Haworth Press, New York

Moreno J 1953 Who shall survive? (revised edn). Beacon House, New York

Mosey A 1973 Activities therapy. Raven Press, New York

Mosey A 1986 Psychosocial components of occupational therapy. Raven Press, New York

Polimeni-Walker I, Wilson K, Jewens R 1992 Reasons for participating in occupational therapy groups: perceptions of adult psychiatric in-patients and occupational therapists. Canadian Journal of Occupational Therapy 59(5): 240–247

Prior S 1998a Determining the effectiveness of a short-term anxiety management course. British Journal of Occupational Therapy 61(5): 207–213

Prior S 1998b Anxiety management: results of a follow up study. British Journal of Occupational Therapy 61(6): 284–285

Reilly M 1974 Play as exploratory learning. Sage, Beverly Hills, CA

Rosier C, Williams H, Ryrie I 1998 Anxiety management groups in a community mental health team. British Journal of Occupational Therapy 61(6): 203–206

Salo-Chydenius S 1996 Changing helplessness to coping: an exploratory study of social skills training with individuals with long-term illness. Occupational Therapy International 3(3): 174–189

Tallant B 1998 Applying the group process to psychosocial occupational therapy. In: Stein F, Cutler S (eds) Psychosocial occupational therapy: a holistic approach. Singular Publishing, San Diego

Trace S, Howell T 1991 Occupational therapy in geriatric mental health. The American Journal of Occupational Therapy 45(9): 833–838

Tuckman B W 1965 Developmental sequences in small groups. Psychological Bulletin 63: 384–389

Yakobina S, Yakobina S, Tallant B 1997 I came, I thought, I conquered: cognitive behaviour approach applied in occupational therapy for the treatment of depressed (dysthymic) females. Occupational Therapy in Mental Health 13(4): 59–73

Yalom I D 1975 The theory and practice of group psychotherapy, 2nd edn. Basic Books, New York

15

Creative activities

Jennifer Creek

INTRODUCTION

Occupational therapists have access to a wide range of activities which can be used with their clients to achieve therapeutic ends. One group of activities, that has gone in and out of fashion over the years but which still has an important place in therapy today, is creative activities. Creative activities require the individual to incorporate something of himself into the production of an idea or end product, for example a poem or a piece of embroidery. They therefore have a very personal dimension. Occupational therapists use a full range of creative activities, selecting the most appropriate one to achieve the goals of particular clients.

This chapter will define creativity, describe the characteristics of creative people and outline the creative process. The therapeutic potential of creative activities will be discussed and some practical pointers given for organising creative therapy sessions. An occupational therapy theory of creativity will be described briefly. The chapter will end with an example of a creative activity used with women with enduring mental health problems.

First, it will be useful to consider what is meant by creative activity, or creativity.

WHAT IS CREATIVITY?

To create is to 'bring into existence, give rise to, originate'. To be creative is to have the ability to create, to be inventive or imaginative, to show imagination as well as routine skill (Sykes 1976). Stein (1974, p. 6) defined creativity as 'a process as a result of which novelty is achieved'. This novelty may be in form, appearance or relationship (Beeman 1990). True creativity is a process, taking place over a period of time, which is characterised by originality, has some value to the individual or to society, and is fully developed (MacKinnon 1962, quoted in Harrington 1990). Creative activity, therefore, is activity which involves imagination and has a novel, worthwhile product. The product may be concrete, such as a painting or piece of writing, or it may be an original idea or train of thought.

Creativity is an ability which can be developed, although some people seem to have more creative potential than others. Everyone has the ability to be creative to some extent, although not everyone will be capable of producing entirely original creative work. Stein (1974, p. 6) suggested that: 'Individuals vary in their ability to meet the requirements for the different stages of the creative process. Some individuals can fulfil all aspects of the creative process, but most seem to be able to handle certain aspects better than others.'

Characteristics of creative people

It might be expected that highly creative people are also highly intelligent but this is not necessarily the case.

Milgram (1990) described four types of intellectual ability:

1. *General intellectual ability.* This refers to the ability to think in abstractions and to solve problems in a logical and systematic way. This ability can be measured by IQ tests.
2. *Specific intellectual ability.* This is a distinct intellectual ability in a particular area, such as music or mathematics. Such abilities are usually reflected in achievement in particular subjects at school.
3. *General creative thinking.* This is the ability to 'generate ideas that are imaginative, clever, elegant or surprising' (p. 217) and to produce original solutions to problems.

4. *Specific creative talent.* This refers to the ability to produce socially valued, novel products in areas such as art, writing, science, music, business or politics. Such talents may be evident in children but are not normally fully developed until adulthood.

No correlation has been found between general or specific intellectual ability and general or specific creative ability. This means that a person with a low IQ or someone who has never attained academic qualifications may still be capable of thinking creatively and producing original, creative work. Conversely, a person with high academic achievements or in a very senior administrative job may not perform well in activities that demand creative ability.

Creative activity requires a certain amount of courage and independence (Beeman 1990). Human activities always have a social context, and truly original work may appear shocking to others at first. The creative thinker, artist or scientist must be prepared to face disapproval or ridicule before his or her work is accepted. This is not usually the case for most small acts of creation, but only for major original works that change the way we see the world. Most people's creativity is shaped by their social environment; very few people are able to shape others' perceptions of the world by their work.

Creativity is usually a synthesis or reformulation of existing ideas and experience (Beeman 1990), therefore a person needs to have experience and knowledge in order to create.

The creative process

The chapter so far has stressed that although creative activity frequently has an end product it is a process which takes place over time. Various researchers have described the creative process as consisting of a series of predictable stages (Poincare 1970, Weisberg 1986, Beeman 1990). These are:

1. *Preparation.* This is a period of time when information is taken in and the individual may be consciously trying to solve a problem or produce a piece of work without success.

2. *Incubation*. The work is put aside and not thought about consciously, but work is continuing unconsciously, sorting and evaluating the information and material that has been absorbed.
3. *Illumination*. If the incubation stage has been successful the individual will experience sudden illumination and a surge of energy to resume work.
4. *Verification*. This is when the solution to the problem is worked out in full, or the painting is completed, or the book written. The insights provided by the illumination stage are put into practice.

The next section looks at how creative ability can be used in therapy to assist people to overcome mental health problems.

CREATIVE ACTIVITIES AS THERAPY

When someone is facing difficulties due to illness or disability, a capacity for thinking and acting creatively will influence the way in which problems are approached and will enhance the ability to find solutions. To this extent, creativity is an important aspect of any occupational therapy intervention. There is also a range of interventions which specifically aim to tap into the client's own creative potential. These are often known as creative therapies and include such techniques as art, drama, dance, music, pottery and certain types of writing. Creative activities may be used with people of any age and with any type or level of dysfunction.

In this section we will first describe what is meant by creative activities, look at the value of creative activities as therapeutic media and consider how people's creative potential might be supported and expressed. An occupational therapy theory of creative ability that can be applied to any client group is then described.

What are creative activities?

It is possible to approach many of the activities of daily life creatively and use them as vehicles for self-expression. For example, cooking may be seen as a routine chore or it can be an opportunity for exploration and experimentation. Self-care can be nothing more than a regular habit, or it can be a chance to express personality and mood through clothes, make-up, hairstyle, grooming and personal style. Housework, that notoriously dull routine, can be given a creative dimension if the living environment is used as an extension of the personality and as a space for personal expression.

Other activities are valued as carrying a specific potential for creative expression. For example, sewing, knitting, DIY, painting and decorating, pottery, furniture restoration, upholstery, gardening, dancing, writing and cake decorating are all activities which people may engage in for the pleasure of creating as well as, in some cases, because of economic necessity. Adult education classes are often a forum for learning new creative skills or practising existing ones.

The range of creative activities available to the occupational therapist is vast. These may be carried out in hospital occupational therapy departments, on wards, in day centres or in day hospitals. Community facilities may be accessed, for example suggesting an evening class for a client recovering from depression or supporting a person with learning difficulties while he takes a college course in a creative skill.

Some of the creative activities that might be used as part of a therapeutic intervention are listed in Box 15.1.

The value of creative activities

Creativity has an evolutionary value for the human race in that it leads to finding original solutions to problems of survival and, further, contributes significantly to advances in human knowledge and understanding. It also has value for individuals, both for the pragmatic purpose of solving problems in daily life and for enhancing quality of life.

The ways in which creative activities can be of therapeutic value for individuals include the following:

Box 15.1 Creative activities that might be used in therapy	
painting	flower arranging
drawing	mosaics
collage	stained glass
découpage	photography
pottery	enamelling
papier mâché	candle making
marbling	singing
puppetry	dancing
embroidery	playing musical
patchwork	instruments
dressmaking	writing stories or poetry
knitting	tie-dye and batik
crochet	drama
calligraphy	conjuring
gardening	juggling
woodwork	decorating Easter eggs
weaving	making Christmas
macramé	decorations

• *Increasing motivation*. People find creative activities pleasurable and will actively seek opportunities to exercise their creative potential. 'Play generates energy because it is a pleasure in itself, an intrinsic end' (Gordon 1961, p. 119).

• *Enhancing learning*. Reilly (1974) highlighted the importance of a playful approach to learning new skills. She proposed a hierarchy of learning in which playful exploration is the first stage, leading on to practice to a level of competence and finishing with the application of newly learned skills to achieve personal goals.

• *Increasing satisfaction and self-esteem*. It is intrinsically satisfying to produce an original piece of work or an original idea, independent of the personal or social value of the product. Creative activity is therefore an important source of personal satisfaction and self-esteem.

• *Enabling self-expression*. People have a need to express their feelings, whether joyful or painful. Feelings which are not expressed may leak out in inappropriate actions or in overreaction to apparently trivial events. Creative activities are a socially acceptable and controllable medium for expressing strong feelings which may otherwise seem overwhelming.

• *Facilitating projection*. Hagedorn (1995) pointed out that in the field of mental health, creative activities are used projectively, 'to enable the individual to gain insights into his situation'. For example, the client might be invited to paint a picture of how he is feeling. Independently of the conscious use of imagery to express his feelings, he will also project unconscious material into his work which is then available for discussion and analysis.

• *Providing opportunities for sublimation*. The human drive to be creative is so strong that it can be used as an outlet for the feelings arising from frustration of other needs. For example, a client might be encouraged to write a poem about the experience of unrequited love.

Enhancing creativity

Although creativity is a natural process, and a pleasurable one, there are various factors which might inhibit its expression. Environmental influences, such as an improverished physical environment during childhood, or adults who discourage messy activities, might lead to an unwillingness to risk trying out new ways of thinking or behaving. Burke (1977) described how the intrinsic urge to act translates into a sense of personal causation – the initiation of action intended to have an effect on the environment. The development of personal causation can be blocked by lack of opportunities to make choices and by repeated experiences of failure. People with a weak sense of personal causation exhibit unwillingness to initiate action and may appear helpless and hopeless. Du Toit (1991) identified certain personal characteristics which inhibit the expression of creativity, including lack of adaptability, poor self-control, apathy and aloofness. Finally, survival needs take priority over other, higher needs (Maslow 1968), therefore creative expression may be inhibited by physiological need or by feelings of insecurity.

One of the greatest challenges to an occupational therapist is to find activities which tap into the client's creative potential and overcome these barriers. The following list gives some of the conditions which the therapist can provide in the therapeutic environment to facilitate creative expression:

• The environment should be stimulating, containing a variety of attractive objects to look at and handle. In an art room, for example, these might include prints of well-known paintings, found objects, dried flowers, interesting pots, fabrics, shells, stones and examples of work.

• For an activity which requires a theme or topic, such as creative writing, it may be helpful to brainstorm at the beginning of the session to stimulate the client's own ideas. For example, the group might be asked to suggest settings for a romantic short story, the more unlikely the better. They may then be asked to think of improbable ways in which the hero and heroine might meet. Introducing an element of absurdity or humour into the exercise demonstrates that it should not be taken too seriously and can help to stimulate creativity.

• Materials and equipment should be of good quality and readily available. For example, if the activity is pottery there should be a plentiful supply of clay ready to use, enough hand tools and turntables or boards for everyone, a water supply, overalls and cleaning cloths. Many materials are attractive and can be displayed advantageously to stimulate clients' interest, such as fabrics, beads, threads and yarns in a sewing room.

• Items which might be copied or which might be perceived to set an unachievably high standard should be removed. For example, if clients are having a free painting session, it is not a good idea to have postcards or photographs available to copy. These would focus undue attention on the end product rather than on the process of creativity.

• Participants in any creative activity should be given all the information and instruction they need to complete the activity successfully. For example, when leading a pottery session it is important to emphasise the careful preparation of clay so that air bubbles are removed and the work is not lost in the kiln. The level of ability of the client and his present mental state should always be taken into account in selecting a suitable method for teaching new skills or imparting information.

• The focus of the session should be on the creative process and not on the end product. The therapist should avoid praising a particular piece of work for its beauty or skilful execution if other clients might compare their own work unfavourably with it and become inhibited. Praise can be given for participation, effort and for finishing the activity.

• Enough time should be allowed for people to work at their own pace, without pressure. If work cannot be finished during one session, or if the client expresses a wish to continue to practise a new skill, there should be further opportunities to continue.

• The therapist should treat everyone's work with respect, irrespective of the quality of workmanship or stage of completion. This is partly a symbolic valuing of the client himself and partly modelling, so that the client learns to value his own efforts and productions. For example, all pieces of work should be kept unless the client expressly asks for a piece to be destroyed.

• The environment should be secure and free from casual interruptions. Clients may be inhibited by having other people wandering in and observing them at work. For example, if a small group of clients has been doing creative dancing together for a few weeks, they may have learned to be comfortable with each other but may be extremely embarrassed if an outsider sees them performing.

If people are anxious about trying creative activities it is helpful to provide more structure and a more concrete topic to start with. The amount of structure can be reduced as they become more confident in the activity. The structure may be inherent in the activity used, for example cross-stitch embroidery is a more structured activity than free painting, or it may be in the way the session is organised. For example, a first creative writing session could involve clients in writing a short description of a building they know or writing an imaginary conversation between two people they know. A later session might require them to describe feelings or pretend to be someone else and write in the first person. As the group gains confidence and skill they might progress to writing short stories on topics of their own choice.

An occupational therapy theory of creativity

De Witt (1992) demonstrated how the development of creative ability can be used as a framework for therapeutic intervention, drawing on the earlier work of du Toit, a South African occupational therapist. Du Toit (1970) called her model 'Creative ability' and described it as being concerned with the way in which people realise, define and extend themselves by expressing their potential through creative action. Creative ability denotes 'the combination of an inner volition or drive towards action, and the externalisation or expression of that volition in action' (du Toit 1974, p. 87).

Creative ability in an individual is manifested in his creation of a tangible or intangible product. The quality of his action (Doing) reflects the quality of the volitional component of his 'Being'. The level of his 'Doing' is characterised by the level of his ability to form relational contacts with materials, people and situations, by the measure of his anxiety control, by his manifestation of originative ability and by the quality of his preparedness to actualise himself through exercising effort in action which makes maximal demands on his potential. (du Toit 1970, p. 39)

Du Toit (1970) also described the following four aspects of creativity:

1. *Creative capacity* – the total creative potential of a particular individual
2. *Creative response* – the positive reaction which the individual displays towards any opportunity for activity
3. *Creative participation* – the process of being involved in all activities of life, not just in specific opportunities for creativity
4. *Creative act* – the end point of creative participation, the end product.

Creative action requires a positive attitude towards activity and a willingness to participate as well as basic creative potential. Creative ability, therefore, affects the degree and quality of the individual's activities in all areas of life: personal care, productivity, social relationships and leisure.

The development of creative activity is a lifelong process, starting at birth and continuing into old age. It is subject to the same influences and constraints as other aspects of human development (see Ch. 3). Three stages and six substages in the development of creative ability can be identified, as shown in Figure 15.1.

Creative ability is not a static characteristic but varies with the degree to which the individual feels secure and with the demands that are made on him. Psychiatric illness can interfere with creative ability, either temporarily or permanently. Box 15.2 shows the level of function that might be observed in clients operating at the different levels of creative ability.

COMPONENT	Volition	Action
DEFINITION	Inner condition of the organism that initiates or directs its behaviour towards a goal	Exertion of motivation into mental and physical effort resulting in the creation of a tangible or intangible end product
DEVELOPMENTAL STAGES		
I Preparation for constructive action	Tone Self-differentiation	Predestructive Destructive Incidental
II Behaviour and skill development for norm compliancy	Self-presentation Participation: Passive Imitative	Explorative Experimental Imitative
III Behaviour and skill development for self-actualisation	Participation: Active Competitive Contribution Competitive contribution	Original Product-centred Situation-centred Society-centred

Figure 15.1 The development of creative ability (adapted from de Witt 1992).

> **Box 15.2**   Levels of creative ability
>
> **Preparation for constructive action**
> Patients at this level are dependent, unable to provide for or care for themselves in any way. Activity is purposeless and they have little or no control over bodily functions. They lack awareness of the self as a separate being or awareness of others. Language is absent or very basic.
>
> **Behaviour and skill development for norm compliance**
> Patients at this level are exploring and learning about the self and the environment and developing a sense of self. They have many of the skills of independent living and are able to apply them if given support and encouragement. Awareness of others is developing. Conversational skills are improving although conversation may reflect the individual's psychopathology.
>
> **Behaviour and skill development for self-actualisation**
> People at this level are rarely seen as hospital in-patients. They are able to cope independently, to recognise when they have problems and to change their behaviour to meet personal needs. They are able to form consistent and lasting interpersonal relationships although there may be an element of selfishness. They may prefer not to take responsibility or initiate projects with other people. At the lower end of this level, people may have a wide range of interests but organisation of time for adequate relaxation may be a problem.

Creative ability has two components: volition and action. Volition governs action and action is the manifestation of volition, so if either component is deficient then creative ability will be impaired. The therapist assesses the client in terms of these two factors across all areas of daily life activity. Assessment is based on direct observation of the client's performance in a wide variety of situations.

Intervention is planned to stimulate the client's volition or to give a positive direction to actions. The types of activities used will depend on the developmental level of the client's creative ability (de Witt 1992). For example, clients operating at the first level, preparation for constructive action, might include people with profound learning difficulties or those with severe psychosis. At this level, the aims of intervention are to:

1. facilitate awareness of the self and of the therapist
2. encourage awareness of the environment

3. stimulate sensory and motor reflexes to promote biological tone.

Treatment sessions should be short. Alertness and concentration can be maintained through the presentation of stimuli, such as speaking the client's name, presenting objects from the environment to be touched and explored, and changing the client's position and posture. As the client demonstrates increasing receptivity to stimuli they can be gradually upgraded until the client is ready to move on to the next level.

Clients at the second level, behaviour and skill development for norm compliancy, will include many of the people the occupational therapist works with in a psychiatric setting. At this level, the aims of intervention are to:

1. encourage awareness and exploration of the self and of the physical and social environment
2. faciliate the development of personal and social skills to support community living
3. encourage awareness of and compliance with social and group norms.

This level covers a wide range of abilities so activities should be graded as the patient's abilities improve. The initial phase of treatment is therapist-directed, moving towards patient-directed activities as the patient develops skills and begins to show preferences. It is necessary for the therapist to be encouraging and supportive in the early stages of intervention in order to make the patient feel safe. The patient should be asked for opinions and ideas and given choices about activity. Activities should be varied and will include personal care, sport and recreational activities, group activities and tasks with a concrete end product, such as art or cooking. Emphasis is placed on the patient's interaction with materials and processes rather than on the end product.

The third level of creative ability, behaviour and skill development for self-actualisation, is not often seen in psychiatric patients since it represents an ability to function in all areas of life. The individual may have a problem but is able to try out new ways of behaving in order to find an acceptable solution.

ORGANISING CREATIVE ACTIVITIES

Creativity has already been defined as the ability to be inventive or imaginative. Creative activities are therefore those which offer opportunities for the client to produce original work. The skill of the therapist is in adapting or synthesising activities to make it possible for people to access their own creative potential. This section describes how a creative activity session might be organised, using tie-dying as an example.

Tie-dying as a creative group activity

This session is planned for a group of women with enduring mental health problems who have never done the activity before. They are attending a day centre on a sessional basis.

Planning and preparation

Half a day is set aside for the activity, allowing for a tea or coffee break while work is in the dye bath or drying. The group know beforehand what activity they will be doing so they can wear suitable clothing. A room is chosen which has good lighting, a sink, tables with washable surfaces, chairs and a washable floor covering. The room is prepared before the group arrive. Buckets, bowls, measuring jugs, kettles, spoons, cold water dyes, dye fixative and salt for preparing the dye are set out on one workbench against the wall. One container of dye may be already mixed for the demonstration. Drying racks, washing powder and an iron are available. Aprons or overalls are available to protect people's clothes. Tables are put together in a square so that everyone can sit together. Fabrics for dying, string, clothes pegs, dye samples, examples of tie-dying, books and any other materials are set out on the main work table.

Running the group

When the group arrive they are invited to sit at the table for a demonstration of the activity. If people arrive early, they may be offered a cup of tea or coffee on arrival and have the opportunity to look at books and samples before the group starts. The therapist tells them what they are going to make and shows examples of finished products. The group are then shown some examples of different tie-dye effects and told how these were obtained. The therapist demonstrates three or four simple methods of tying or clamping cloth to achieve different effects. She points out that there are other methods people can try if they feel confident. She puts her samples into the prepared dye bath and invites people to select their materials and choose a technique to start with. She suggests that they choose different textures and weights of material to see how this affects the finished result.

People are encouraged to work at their own pace on their own pieces of work. The therapist moves around the table, encouraging and offering advice if it is sought. If a piece of work looks as though it is too loosely tied she will suggest that a better effect may be obtained by tightening the ties. The therapist's manner of approach is important because she wants to ensure that people experience success but wishes to avoid sounding critical of their efforts. If anyone is having difficulty deciding what to do she goes through the alternatives with them again. When someone is ready to put work in the dye bath the therapist asks him to choose a colour and shows him how to mix the dye. Other people are invited to watch the process if they wish to.

When everyone has at least one piece of work in the dye bath, a tea break may be suggested. The session is planned so that everyone can be active throughout, while all working at their own pace. After a break, the first pieces of work should be ready to come out of the dye bath. They are rinsed thoroughly, washed and hung to dry. The drying rack should be near a heater so that the cloth dries as quickly as possible. Once the work is no longer dripping wet, the ties may be cut and the cloth ironed dry. Group members are encouraged to look at each other's work as it is finished.

Ending the session

At the end of the session, some work will still be in the dye bath. The therapist promises to finish the process and leave the work to dry so that people can collect it on another day. Finished work may be taken away.

SUMMARY

This chapter began by considering the nature of creativity as an aspect of human functioning and described the creative process. The therapeutic value of creativity was then discussed, both the value of being able to think of creative solutions to problems and the value of activities which are seen as especially creative, such as art, music and drama. Ways of structuring activity sessions to enhance the expression of creativity were discussed. An occupational therapy theory of creative activity was described briefly. This theory was developed by South African occupational therapists for application with any client group, not just people with mental health problems. The chapter ended with a description of how to set up and run a creative activity group, tie-dying.

REFERENCES

Beeman C A 1990 Just this side of madness: creativity and the drive to create. UCA Press

Burke J P 1977 A clinical perspective on motivation: pawn versus origin. American Journal of Occupational Therapy 31(4): 254–258

de Witt P A 1992 Creative ability – a model for psychiatric occupational therapy. In: Crouch R B (ed) Occupational therapy in psychiatry and mental health. Lifecare Group, Johannesburg

du Toit V 1970 Creative ability. In: Du Toit V, Patient volition and action in occupational therapy. Vona and Marie du Toit Foundation, Hillbrow, South Africa

du Toit V 1991 Initiative in occupational therapy. In: Du Toit V, Patient volition and action in occupational therapy Vona and Marie du Toit Foundation, Hillbrow, South Africa

Gordon W J J 1961 Synectics. Harper and Row, New York

Hagedorn R 1995 Occupational therapy: perspectives and processes. Churchill Livingstone, Edinburgh

Harrington D M 1990 The ecology of human creativity: a psychological perspective. In: Runco M A, Robert R S (eds) Theories of creativity. Sage, Newbury Park

Maslow A H 1968 Towards a psychology of being. Van Nostrand, New York

Milgram R M 1990 Creativity: an idea whose time has come and gone? In: Runco M A, Robert R S (eds) Theories of creativity. Sage, Newbury Park

Poincare H 1970 Mathematical creation. In: Vernon P E (ed) Creativity. Penguin, Harmondsworth

Reilly M (ed) 1974 Play as exploratory learning. Sage, Beverley Hills

Stein M 1974 Stimulating creativity. Volume 1. Individual procedures. Academic Press, New York

Sykes J B 1976 The concise Oxford dictionary. Oxford University Press, Oxford

Weisberg R 1986 Creativity, genius and other myths. Freeman, New York

16

Life and social skills training

Mary Roberts

INTRODUCTION

Onlookers watch with fascination as a lump of clay is transformed into a beautifully shaped pot by an experienced potter at the wheel. People cheer and extol the virtues of the winning competitor in a sport. In each case exceptional skills have been displayed, usually resulting from a combination of talent, practice and hard work. Everyday activities also require a vast repertoire of skills which are gained with effort as a person develops. Whether exciting or mundane, skills are an essential part of a human being's interaction with his environment.

Mental illness can cause disruption and deficit in an individual's skills. The processes which enable the growth of potential talents or skills may be inhibited. Abilities which are used daily and which are taken for granted can become impaired and deteriorated.

An occupational therapist aims to enable the client to function at his optimum level when mental health problems arise. This invariably means that the client will either be assisted to learn new skills or to reestablish old ones. The ability to apply skills training in the context of therapy is a skill in itself, and one that an occupational therapist has to acquire. This chapter will examine the occupational therapist's role and perspective in skills training.

WHAT ARE SKILLS?

Definition of skills

Skills enable people to operate as individuals and contribute to their functioning as part of the society in which they belong. Some skills are needed to help a person survive, for example being able to obtain and/or prepare food. There are also skills which help individuals to follow and develop a sense of self-identity, such as being a wage-earner or artist.

Skill, according to the Concise Oxford Dictionary (1976), is facility in an action or in doing. Skills are involved in achieving tasks and are dependent on abilities. Hence a skill is something we know how to do and feel comfortable with when putting it into action. Once learned, it often becomes automatic, for example applying the brakes when driving a car. Initially the driver will learn where the brake is in relation to the foot, how hard to press it and on what occasion to do this. With practice, the driver will learn to differentiate between, for example, slowing down in traffic and doing an emergency stop until he can stop, without hesitation, in a way which is appropriate to the situation. Skills have physical and mental components which link closely together – an ability to tie shoelaces is hindered not only if a person does not have the motor skill to manipulate the laces, but also if he feels too anxious to learn how to do so.

In occupational therapy, a skill is defined as a performance component which evolves with practice. Skills are grouped according to the emphasis of the occupational therapy approach used, for example psychosocial function or cognitive ability. They form the basis of performance, behaviour, cognition and social interaction. A description of these concepts will provide further clarification:

Performance

The concept of 'performance' is one used frequently in occupational therapy. In relation to skills, it is the process or manner of functioning, which incorporates what a person does and how it is done. Performance is the outward expression of skills.

It also includes the degree to which an individual is competent, that is, whether there is achievement or failure in doing an activity. A person's perception of competence can vary according to the demands of the situation and his view of himself.

Behaviour

Extensive studies in psychology have provided insights into behaviour which have enabled well established interventions, such as behavioural approaches. Behaviour is defined as acting or reacting in a specific way. This can be particular to the individual but there are also behaviours which are common to human beings in general.

Complex interactions within the human being produce behaviour, often in patterns. For example, walking into a room full of people in a meeting and being able to show the right amount of formality and confidence requires previous knowledge, an ability to judge a situation, appropriate body language and so on.

Behaviour includes the response of an individual based on attitudes and values, verbal and nonverbal communication. Sometimes it is innate, developing under the influence of heredity, and sometimes it is produced by environmental factors or a combination of both (Argyle 1978). Behaviour can be changed by reeducation, illness or trauma.

Cognition

Cognition involves the mechanisms of knowing and perceiving. It includes the skills of reasoning, mental processing, thinking, memory, planning and problem solving. Aspects of cognition are essential to the development of performance. Associated skills are restricted if there are problems in cognition. In psychology and occupational therapy literature, cognition is well documented (Ch. 13).

The use of cognitive skills in intervention can be effective in dealing with some mental health problems.

Social interaction

Social interaction is the process by which individuals communicate, react and behave with one another in society. Doble & Magill Evans (1992) describe it as the ability to receive and selectively attend to social information in the environment by which a person is able to interpret situations and adapt his response accordingly. The processes required for this are: receiving and interpreting social messages, planning social output, interactional style, and social enactment.

A person will use various combinations of verbal and nonverbal communication, assertiveness, negotiation and cooperation (Mosey 1986) in his interactions. His responses will partly depend on personal goals, that is what he is trying to accomplish in the interaction. They are also guided by cultural expectations – the rules of behaviour outlined by group norms (Franklin 1990). For example, in one culture it may be acceptable to greet someone by shaking hands but in another it may be considered offensive to touch another person in public.

These skills contribute to competent social behaviour, enabling the person to be comfortable in society. They also facilitate the making and sustaining of interpersonal relationships. Difficulties in social interaction are often one of the aspects of mental health problems and, as such, are commonly dealt with by occupational therapists.

Acquisition of skills

Theorists in social psychology, language and sociology identified stages of growth and development in the areas described above as they explored human development from birth to maturity. For example, physical motor, social language, activities of daily living and sociocultural skills were identified by Gesell, areas of psychosocial development were described by Erikson, while Grant and Freud developed psychodynamic theories. Needs were linked to motivation by Maslow, and Piaget explained cognition (Llorens 1991). Such theories form a basis of knowledge and understanding of how skills are aquired.

Early work in skills training emphasised social behaviour. The work was mainly done by social psychologists and included research into behaviour, verbal and nonverbal communication, behaviour modification and the ability to change. Jones (1967, in Argyle 1978) analysed social behaviour. Rogers (1967, in Gadza & Brooks 1985) researched social and life skills training which formed the basis of the first training model in social skills developed by Carkhuff (1969, in Gadza & Brooks 1985). Trowser and Argyle (1978) began to categorise what was described as social inadequacy and formulated social skills training programmes to deal with it.

Social skills training is well documented and described elsewhere (Argyle 1978, Franklin 1990). A plethora of social skills exercises are used by a number of different professions, including those working in prisons and the probation service, personnel and business management and education, as well as those working within mental health. The occupational therapist is advised to search psychology literature for specific topics required for study and ideas relating to particular interventions.

Evolution of skills concepts in occupational therapy

When we consider the contribution of occupational therapy to life and skills training it is interesting to explore how the profession's theories have come to complement and progress the concepts discussed above. The early work in both psychology and occupational therapy has been built on by others, such as Mosey and Kielhofner, to formulate models and approaches for practice. Ayres's work (Llorens 1991), which later became the 'Sensory intergation theory', described the function and dysfunction of the central nervous system relating to purposeful activity. Llorens (1976), also with an emphasis on activities, synthesised the developmental theories. Her work added to the understanding of the nature of the acquisition of skill for mastery, the role of trauma in disrupting the developmental cycle and the idea of using activities, tasks and interpersonal interactions to reinstate skills.

The use of purposeful activity

Activities are characteristic of, and necessary to, human existence (Cynkin & Robinson 1990). Knowledge about skills has developed within the context of the way occupational therapists use activities to achieve multiple and complex treatment aims (Creek 1996). The foundational knowledge of occupational therapy is in the meaning of occupation and purposeful activity (Gillette & Kielhofner 1979).

There is an ongoing debate about what the term purposeful activity should include (Breines 1984, AOTA 1993, Hong & Yates 1995, Pedretti 1996, Golledge 1998). The main points within the term are that the activity should be goal directed, will be part of everyday life and be determined by its context. It will have meaning and interest, unique to the individual, but will have different meanings at different times (Breines 1984, Hong & Yates 1995, Creek 1996).

Purposeful activity is an integrated part of therapy and is meaningful in its relation to the treatment goal (Golledge 1998). If the activities have no meaning to the client they do not have a therapeutic value (Creek 1996). Purposeful activity provides the incentive and opportunity for the individual to achieve mastery, thus gaining a sense of inner assurance and competence (Fidler 1981). The occupational therapist and client cooperate to produce change and development (Breines 1984, Dickerson 1995).

The learning and acquiring of skills is seen as integral to an individual's relationship with 'doing'. Fidler (Fidler & Fidler 1978) describes doing as purposeful activity (in contrast to random activity) which is a process of investigating, trying out and gaining evidence of one's capacities for experiencing, responding, managing, creating and controlling, in order to become a competent and contributing member of society. Doing provides the means to develop and integrate sensory, motor, cognitive and psychological systems. In a similar vein, Stewart (1994) states that doing allows an individual to experience reality, to achieve, to fail, to explore and to grow. The points that mind, body and social self are developed through what we do are endorsed by Creek (1996).

These ideas echo Reilly's (1974) concept that through 'doing' in play, a human being develops skills leading to mastery of the real world. She described play as part of a system of learning which, through imagination, uses symbols to represent reality. There are three stages in the play sub-system: exploration, competency and achievement.

- *Exploratory behaviour* tests the environment looking for rules, either during childhood or when an event is new. (This is inhibited if there is high pressure for need fulfillment or anxiety).
- *Competency* is dominated by a drive actively to influence the environment and be influenced by it through feedback mechanisms. Practice is essential for learning during this period.
- *Achievement* inherits the learning acquired in the previous two stages, focuses on excellence, and is linked with the person's expectations.

Skills are, therefore, attained through development, learning and practice with experience. There are inherent characteristics in these processes which affect the direction of skill acquisition. For instance, in order to ride a bicycle a child will need to develop the appropriate level of musculoskeletal size and strength, coordination and balance, and, later, the ability to appreciate safety measures. Incapacity in any of these areas will influence the acquisition of the skill.

A skill has to be internalised and this is done either through learning by copying someone else or by gaining a knowledge and understanding of the process required for the skill. Either way the process has to be experienced and practised regularly, repeating each stage until it is achieved. For example, when making a cake, repeated attempts to follow the same recipe, rectifying mistakes and acquiring knowledge on the way usually achieve a good result in the end.

Good results at each stage are important, both to increase understanding and to build up confidence. Poor results and a sense of failure can mean that attempts at learning the skill are abandoned. Success and achievement are important factors in supplying the incentives to learn a skill. These are closely followed by self-esteem and approval. All these contribute to motivation (see Ch. 7), which is the driving force behind occupational behaviour and therefore an essential element in acquiring skills. It prompts the individual to seek out and master new skills. It contributes to the 'urge to explore and master the environment, i.e. fitness and responsiveness to external demands and to personal drives for competence' (Kielhofner 1985).

The ability to learn is, therefore, an important element of skill acquisition and is facilitated by appropriate instruction and training. An understanding of the learning process and the difficulties experienced in this area by clients with mental health problems is essential for occupational therapists involved in any form of skills training.

Learning theory

Learning may be defined as a change in behaviour that occurs as the result of experience.

Learning theory offers an explanation of how individuals reach a particular level of competence in cognitive performance, rather than looking at patterns common to all. The overall level of competence achieved is seen as important, rather than the age at which skills are developed.

A major difference between cognitive developmental theory and learning theory is that, in the latter, skills are thought to be acquired through the individual's interaction with the environment and are not dependent on prior learning of more basic skills.

Learning theory presents a model of how skills are learned and also suggests ways in which learning can be facilitated. Learning is seen to take place through a variety of experiences, including:

- habituation
- conditioning
- transfer of learning.

Habituation

Habituation is learning not to react to stimuli that are constant or irrelevant, for example not to listen to the background hum of traffic noise. New sights and sounds attract immediate attention but, once the judgement is made that they are irrelevant, the individual learns to ignore them.

This has implications for the design of a therapeutic environment. Small changes, such as turning off the radio, can be used to reactivate a client's attention.

Conditioning

Conditioning is the acquisition of conditioned responses, or the making of new associations between elements in the environment. There are two types of conditioning: classical conditioning and operant conditioning. Both these techniques are extensively used to change people's behaviour, that is, to teach new skills. In classical conditioning, a behaviour normally produced in response to one stimulus is transferred to another stimulus, for example, a client with severe learning difficulty feels pleasure when he drinks coffee. By always giving him a cup of coffee at the end of a treatment session the therapist teaches him to associate therapy with coffee and he learns to feel pleasure when attending a treatment session.

Operant conditioning increases or decreases the likelihood of a behaviour being repeated by applying a positive or negative stimulus immediately after the behaviour. For example, if the therapist praises a client every time he performs a task, he is more likely to repeat it. If she ignores him when he shouts inappropriately, he is less likely to shout. Behaviour can be shaped towards a desired pattern by rewarding any operant behaviour that approximates to the desired behaviour.

Transfer of learning

Learning one skill often affects the learning of other skills, either by facilitating or by interfering with their acquisition. When earlier learning has a positive effect on later learning it is called transfer of learning; for example, learning to use a gas stove in the occupational therapy department will help a person to learn to use the gas cooker in their new flat. When the effect is negative it is called negative transfer; for example, learning how to use one type of computer in occupational therapy can make it difficult to get used to a different one at home. Negative transfer effects can slow down the learning process when new skills are being learned but they do not usually persist.

Transfer occurs because of similarity of content, the way in which the skill is learned, and the principle behind solving the problems, or a combination of these.

Simulated tasks give preliminary practice when dangerous skills are being learned or when the real situation is inaccessible. However, simulation is only useful if there is positive transfer from the simulated task to the real one and no negative transfer (Munn 1966). For example, an occupational therapist designed an activities of daily living (ADL) assessment unit for stroke victims in which all the fitments were adjustable so that the essential features of the home environment could be simulated. It was found that even confused clients responded automatically to familiarly positioned features, demonstrating that learning was transferred from the home environment to the unit. It could therefore be assumed that further learning would transfer from the unit to the home environment and this was found to be the case (Smith 1979).

Skill deficits caused by mental illness

The process of mental illness itself undermines the individual's performance, behaviour, cognition and social interaction. Secondary factors of illness may mean that skills in these areas have not been developed, for example a dysfunctional family background may have affected the learning process early in the person's life. Institutionalised methods of providing care instead of an enabling approach (whether in a hospital or community setting) can inhibit the

individual's development of skills in all these areas.

The occupational therapy approach is important because it helps to maintain an adequate level of skills and prevent deterioration. Certain skill deficits apparent in the major categories of mental illness are the focus of intervention. The following descriptions of such skill deficits are not definitive, as the problems in reality are complex, but some of the main areas of difficulty are indicated.

Psychotic disorders

During an acute onset of psychosis, when the symptoms such as hallucinations are florid, functional ability can be grossly impaired because of the effect of thought disorder. Perceptual difficulties will mean that the person is unable to interpret some aspects of reality. Action, learning and performance are therefore disrupted, sometimes in unexpected ways. For example, a patient may be unable to peel potatoes because they transform into snakes before his eyes. There may also be difficulty in filtering out irrelevant stimuli or information when doing a task. These problems result in poor acquisition of skills. There is some evidence to suggest that elements of sensory integration may be affected, such as coordination, balance, manual dexterity (King 1974), which will also influence physical performance.

A deterioration in skills may also be experienced if the illness emerges over a long period of time. This can be particularly true during the slow onset of negativism when symptoms take on a chronic form. The sufferer may have developed problems early in life and therefore school work and learning would be affected. Often, further education and career pursuits are interrupted and a work history will show a downward trend towards less skilful and demanding jobs. Behaviour may be bizarre and social and life skills may be lacking. Interests and hobbies are not pursued so that social and emotional withdrawal is increased. Alternatively, a person may have become excessively involved with an interest which has become part of his delusional system so that skills required for anything other than this interest, for example looking after himself, may not have been acquired. The general disorganisation caused by the symptoms affects the maintenance and growth of skills in cognition, performance, behaviour and social interaction.

Affective and neurotic disorders

The illnesses in this category are characterised in the acute phase by strong emotional responses such as anxiety, guilt, self-reproach, despair and, as a result, can also cause temporary deterioration in some existing abilities. Skills may be lacking initially for a number of reasons associated with the factors contributory to the illness. As a consequence, the individual may habitually respond to situations in a maladapted way, for example, by over-reacting or with learned helplessness.

Mood swings can interfere with a person's judgement. Abilities may be viewed in an unrealistic way, either under- or overestimating them. Similarly, the person may have no notion of his own potential to develop skills. Behaviour may be inconsistent as a result of mood swings. These difficulties affect the person's motivation to learn or cope with problems for which he needs new skills. The feeling of being controlled by emotional responses or irrational thought undermines confidence to increase skills. Physical discomfort, such as tiredness and lethargy, hinders the development and maintenance of some skills, therefore they deteriorate. Conversely, activity may be speeded up through agitation and mistakes and failures occur or things are left incomplete. These also lead to a loss of confidence and a sense of failure, often out of proportion to the event. This will mean that more courage is required to respond to the challenge of learning a new or different way of doing something. Apathy may consequently occur, resulting in a vicious cycle of few skills leading to less effort to attain skills therefore further reduction in skills (see Burke's theory of 'Pawns and origins', p. 130).

Preoccupation with worries can undermine learning, causing a lack of attention which prevents the absorption of information, thus interfering with memory (retention and recall). The application of skills is also hampered through lack of attention and concentration.

In chronic form these illnesses often have associated social and family problems making the person's situation unstable. Energy is used up coping with social and environmental problems and stressful situations with few resources left to accommodate change. This affects skill development and consolidation. Sometimes, there is a store of skills in the pre-morbid personality but, due to 'secondary gain', energy is devoted to maintaining the sick role.

There are other problems indirectly caused by the after-effects of illness which can interfere with skill training and acquisition. Often clients may be unable to apply themselves: they may have days when they are feeling particularly unwell or troubled; the side-effects of medication may produce difficulties such as tiredness or discomfort, or time-keeping can be erratic. Consequently, occupational therapy sessions are not attended regularly and this interferes with the learning process.

THE OCCUPATIONAL THERAPIST'S ROLE IN SKILLS TRAINING

The occupational therapist has several contributions to make in enabling people to acquire and re-acquire skills after mental illness. The focus of occupational therapy in this context is the skills the client needs to promote mental health and wellness. The emphasis is on how to improve the quality of life if there are permanent difficulties or how to draw out potential abilities. The therapist has a role as mediator, enabler, guide and teacher.

As a mediator, an occupational therapist will structure and organise the learning experience and provide feedback to the learner on his performance (Christiansen & Baum 1991). This has to be done in a way which will draw on the person's strengths, bearing in mind their vulnerability and insecurity. By facilitating the learning process the therapist acts as an enabler, empowering the client to gain and use skills. It is, therefore, important to understand any barriers to learning, such as the effect of the person's illness or previous learning problems. She can then help the learner to work through them and overcome them. The therapist directs the learning process, thus acting as a guide, providing and encouraging appropriate activities and creating an environment in which the individual, with his unique abilities and deficits, can learn. The ability to teach at an appropriate level and provide relevant instruction and materials is also essential.

It is necessary to apply a 'just right challenge' (Robinson 1977) in order to build a sense of achievement and restore confidence in skills.

Individual or group sessions are used to do this, depending on the needs of the clients or the resources available. For some, individual sessions with the therapist will remove the threat of comparison with others and provide the appropriate situation to build concentration and confidence. In other cases, using the group interactions and process will enhance learning by providing stimulation and social contact. Careful planning is required, not only to enable the person to learn or relearn a skill in a supportive environment, but also to take into account the needs of an individual affected by illness and, sometimes, a variety of difficult social circumstances. Some of these points are highlighted in the history of Mrs X, in Box 16.1.

Box 16.1 Case example 1

Mrs X was an outpatient aged 45. She was recovering from depression which recurred periodically. One of the contributory factors to her illness was chronic social problems. She also suffered from anxiety, especially when required to do something new, and became very negative about her own abilities. Her self-confidence and self-esteem were low.

Aims of intervention
To build confidence and increase self-esteem
To provide opportunity and support for doing something new
To improve her concentration and memory by following written instructions

Activity chosen: patchwork
Mrs X had previously attended anxiety management and enhancing self-esteem courses and had shown herself to be well motivated, but she needed to apply her knowledge in practical situations. She wanted to try patchwork because she had seen her friend make a quilt. Mrs X used sewing as a means of relaxing and managing stress. By attempting patchwork she was using skills already familiar to her in a challenging new way. Mrs X also wanted to improve her concentration and memory in order to resume her hobby of reading.

Approach of therapist
Care was taken to make the task manageable, ensuring successful stages, to reduce anxiety and anticipation of failure. Although Mrs X wanted to make a quilt, after discussion with the therapist it was agreed that a patchwork pattern on her nephew's cot cover would be easier to begin with. Support and encouragement were given initially to help her through hindrances to learning such as her negative over-reaction to difficulties.

The activity was also used to remind her of relevant issues she needed to practice from the previous courses.

Environment
This was arranged to avoid any possibilities of failure, because Mrs X was so nervous she could easily have been put off. There was sufficient space to cut out and sew. It had to be clean and dust free. The scissors had to be sharp; the needle and thimble were of a size which was comfortable and the same sewing cotton was available for each session. Seating was arranged to accommodate Mrs X's back problem and she was situated where there was good lighting. She was placed slightly apart from others, initially, because she was too shy to let them see her work. As her confidence grew she became more sociable and was able to allow others to see and comment on her work.

Teaching methods
Mrs X was shown each stage as she was ready for it by demonstration and verbal instructions. To reinforce these and to help her work independently she also had written instructions and pictures. The process was adapted when she took fright at the prospect of making her own templates. In order to avoid this becoming an obstruction to the whole learning process she was provided with one made by the therapist.

Progress
Gradually Mrs X was confident enough to work on her own, succeeded in making the patchwork and designed and completed the layout on the cot cover on her own at home. She was very pleased with the finished article. She subsequently made some draught excluders out of patchwork, on her own, and solved the problem of templates by deciding to buy plastic ones!

Facilitating change

Learning causes a change in behaviour (see p. 279 occupational therapy contributes to this by teaching new and adaptive skills to the client. Building confidence enables a person to respond to a situation in a new way. This produces different feedback and can stop the vicious cycle of failure, thus increasing self-esteem. An increasing awareness of abilities gives the individual new expectations of himself (Kanfer & Goldstein 1981) and this can affect the attitude to learning. By providing opportunities to develop skills and observe the results the therapist is enabling the client to become competent through doing, thus changing attitudes which affect behaviour.

There is also a need to be able to cope with the inability to change. Change may not occur for a number of reasons (for example the prognosis of the illness, failure of medical treatments, the client's fear of change), or because of social circumstances. Consequently, it is important to enable the client to have a quality of life within the limits of his difficulties, to make adjustments, and to be able to gain skills which provide a sense of satisfaction within his limitations.

SKILLS FROM THE PERSPECTIVE OF FOUR PRACTICE MODELS AND APPROACHES

As has been stated earlier, a goal of occupational therapy is to enable people to function at their optimum level, and there are a number of practice models which highlight ways to bring this about. Each model has its own perspective on how to develop and harness certain skills. More detailed information about the models is dealt with elsewhere (see Further Reading, p. 293), but certain aspects are relevant here. Generally, problems are explained in terms of dysfunction and maladaption. It is suggested that each model has its contribution to make in facilitating the acquisition or reestablishment of skills, depending on the individual's circumstances. A pragmatic and holistic approach in their use is therefore advised.

The model of human occupation

In this model (Kielhofner 1985), the outward manifestations of skills are evident in performance. These in turn are driven by volition and habituation.

Volition

Volition has three components which are personal causation, values and interests:

1. Personal causation is a person's self-perception of his effectiveness in the environment which will include his belief in his skills and his ability to exert control, including his anticipation of results.
2. Values are those principles or standards by which the person judges things or actions to be good, right and important.
3. Interest is the disposition to find occupations pleasurable. It is generated by action and the individual's personal experience of an activity. Some interests are preferred to others, and this is related to the degree of enjoyment and complexity in the activity and its appeal to the senses. If the experience of an activity is a good one, interest grows and the inclination for future action is increased. Interest, therefore, acts as an important factor in motivation. The development of an individual's interests has been formed by the values of family, peer groups, culture, and educational background. Interests are affected by a person's openness to new experiences, his developmental level and the available opportunities in the environment. Matsutsuyu (1969) stated that interests are influenced by early experience, stimulate positive and negative emotional responses, sustain action and are part of a person's self image. One study (Roberts 1994) reflected some of these points in that interest seemed to be associated with the inherent processes of an activity and how that activity was valued. Attaining achievement was also a significant factor since interest was increased as a successful end product or goal became a likely outcome of doing an activity. Clients were also strongly motivated to overcome difficulties by interest in their particular activity.

Habituation

Behaviours become habituated into roles (expectations of behaviours which accompany particular functions), habits and routines. These work in conjunction to produce skilled behaviour expressed outwardly as performance.

The components of performance are skills and skill constituents:

1. Skills in this context are defined as abilities which a person has which lead to accomplishment of a goal under variable environmental conditions. These include: perceptual motor skills, which are those of manipulating the self and objects; process skills, which are problem solving and planning abilities; and communication/interaction skills for cooperating and interacting with people.

2. Skills constituents are subcomponents of skills which are symbolic (images which guide performance), neurological (actions produced by the central nervous system) and musculoskeletal (the production of movement).

It can be seen, therefore, that when volition and habituation are affected by mental illness, performance in certain areas will also break down. This model gives some guidance as to which skills need to be 'repaired' or developed and what motivates the client in particular areas. A person's sense of effectiveness, belief in skills and routines are affected by mental illness. It is often the case that the person's roles and interests are also disrupted and the model can contribute towards making a profile of what the client is normally like and the potential areas of development.

Cognitive disabilities model

This model (Allen 1982) aims to describe cognitive limitations caused by chronic illness and identifies the remaining functional ability so that the expectations of the clients are realistic. There are six cognitive levels which are characterised by variations in relation to:

- attention
- apparent purpose

- experience
- behaviour
- duration and process of action.

Permanent impairment is assumed in persons with chronic psychiatric disorders and in some people with brain damage. The management of permanent residual limitations is the focus of the model, rather than improvement or alteration. There is a particular emphasis on task analysis so that the cognitive dimension of performance is known. This provides the means for a task to be adapted to match the maximum ability of the individual. Since an individual can then gain a sense of achievement, the distress caused by failure is reduced. For instance, a client functioning in the model's level four may be able to learn the process of chopping vegetables by copying and repetition. He can then make an acceptable contribution (with guidance) towards group cooking in a hostel but would not be expected to cook meals on his own.

The model differs from other approaches in psychiatry in its acceptance of residual disability. It therefore provides guidance for enabling clients in this position to function at their optimum without putting them under undue stress. The expected skills are laid out clearly in the model handbook (Allen et al 1992) and task-orientated activities are used for gaining achievement. It can be argued that if an individual is able to build and apply skills within his cognitive limitations it will also have a positive effect on his behaviour.

Mosey's adaptive skills approach (Mosey 1970)

Mosey's work is specific to psychiatry. It identifies, in depth, psychosocial functioning and the problems associated with lack of skills and learned maladaptive responses in this area. These are described as affecting task planning, performance, interactions and ability to identify and satisfy needs. The skills required are called performance components, of which there are four, as follows:

1. *Sensory integration.* This is defined as the process of receiving and utilising sensory stimuli

which includes tactile sub-systems, postural and bilateral interaction and praxia.

2. *Cognitive function.* This refers to the cortical processes which use information for thinking and problem solving. These include: attention, thought processes, levels of conceptualisation, intelligence, dealing with factual information, and ability to identify and follow through a plan to deal with problems.

3. *Psychological function.* This deals with the processing of information from past events plus that currently available in the environment in order to view self and others realistically. This is seen as a dynamic state which includes needs, emotions, values, interest and motivation.

4. *Social interaction.* This is seen as the ability to engage with others in casual and sustained relationships, the ability to interpret situations socially and to structure social interplay. Social skills are defined as the capacity to relate to others in a way which is satisfying to self and others. They include communication, dyadic and group interaction skills.

An individual uses the performance components in occupational performances which are described as 'organised patterns of behaviour through which an individual engages in and meets the demands of the environment' (Mosey 1986, p. 64). They are categorised as family interactions, activities of daily living, school/work, play/leisure/recreation and temporal adaptation. Role behaviour in relation to these is seen as dynamic because it is changeable and capable of being redefined.

From these concepts, Mosey developed three models for practice of which *recapitulation of ontogenesis* is the one particularly relevant to the acquisition of skills. The term itself means returning to an earlier stage of development to rectify maladaption. It is linked to cognitive and social learning theory and uses aspects of the developmental and humanistic frames of reference. Mosey identified six adaptive skills: perceptual motor, cognitive, dyadic and group interaction, self-identity and sexual identity. They are acquired sequentially, linked chronologically and evolve in complexity and adaptive

potential. They are subdivided into skill components which are the stages in which they are learned. Mosey advocated the use of experiential learning through activity (individually and in groups) to adapt responses and improve skills.

This approach provides a means of checking on which stages of skill acquisition have been missed or where the individual is stuck. It is then possible to place the person into a learning situation where skills can be extended by starting at a natural stage of development.

Model of adaptation through occupation

This model, developed by Reed & Sanderson (1984), centres on skills assessment, development and retraining, and this is seen as the main concern of occupational therapists. It is based on problem solving and emphasises autonomy, actualisation and accomplishment. Occupations are identified as natural vehicles for human normal development and adaptation for the primary learning of skills. Participation in occupation enables adaptive responses. Occupational performance results from developmental motivation and the learning of many skills. Component skills are integrated into patterns and are configured appropriately to the requirements of the situation, for example, particular roles. Skills in this context are:

- motor activities
- sensory and cognitive functioning
- psychological and emotional behaviour
- social awareness
- work adjustment
- avocational interests and leisure activities.

Occupational performance is influenced by environmental factors which are physical, biopsychological and sociocultural. The context and content of these may enhance or impede learning or performance. When a person has the occupational skills and is able to use them to fulfil needs and meet demands, he has achieved a state of adaptation and health.

A person may lack in motor, sensory, cognitive, intrapersonal or interpersonal skills and, in this model, the occupational therapist aims to:

develop
improve } skills in
reestablish } order to
maintain

prevent
remediate } dysfunctional
minimise } performance

The general focus on skills development makes the model suitable for use with psychiatric as well as physical conditions.

METHODS OF SKILLS TRAINING

ADAPTABLE TEACHING TECHNIQUES

There is little documentation about the planning, organisation, knowledge of teaching methods and care for detail which an occupational therapist needs in order to provide opportunities for clients to acquire appropriate skills. It is nevertheless a main function of the occupational therapist to do this. She has to be adaptable and flexible in the methods used bearing in mind the specific needs of the client. One of the core skills of an occupational therapist is to design a unique therapeutic programme of activities for the client (Hagedorn 1992), often including a means to enable the client to achieve or adapt specific skills. To do this, an occupational therapist has to attend to the approach used, the learning environment and the teaching methods.

The attitude and approach of the therapist

The therapist aims to build a sense of achievement and confidence in the client so that motivation is enhanced, learning takes place and skills are increased. The therapist's own attitude and approach are a crucial part of this process. There is collaboration between client and therapist so that information is not imposed on the client but a means is found to begin at a stage appropriate to the client learning needs.

Many aspects of being a therapist will also come into play in the skills training role. In particular, the therapist will draw from the conscious use of self as described by Mosey (1986), which means that the interactions with the client will be planned. Acknowledging the individuality of the learner, the therapist will reflect carefully on her approach and it will depend on the situation. It may not be possible to take the same approach with the client in every session. The client's moods and condition are unpredictable and so the therapist has to be accommodating and well prepared, having considered a number of options of how to teach particular aspects of a skill.

Consideration has to be given to how facts and concepts are communicated. It is important to instruct the learner at a level which will make understanding easy, using words and concepts which are familiar to him and working at his pace. This is done in a way that is non-patronising, protecting the client's dignity, acknowledging his inherent capacity but bearing in mind the possible cognitive difficulties brought about by illness.

It is necessary to allow the learner freedom to learn by avoiding criticism and embarrassment. The therapist offers the learner respect, acceptance and a sense of security by being patient and non-judgemental. The aim is to alleviate fear and to provide reassurance and encouragement. The client needs support as he tries out new skills, experimenting with abilities which do not yet feel comfortable. The support is withdrawn at an appropriate time when he becomes competent. In fact, it is appropriate in the latter stages to provide or seek out opportunities which challenge the learner to increase the new skill.

The therapist's manner should be relaxed so that the learner feels free to make mistakes without feeling as though it is a disaster. Equally, it is important to give sufficient guidance so that the learner avoids making so many mistakes that he becomes disheartened and learning does not take place. To avoid pressurising the learner the therapist remains objective about his progress, keeping expectations balanced and realistic. The therapist also has to have knowledge of the skills to be acquired or provide an appropriate instructor. If support workers or instructors are involved in the situation mutual cooperation is important to ensure consistency of approach.

The learning environment

The occupational therapist not only has to design a unique programme to incorporate suitable intervention procedures in a therapeutic sense for each individual, but also a specific learning environment has to be created to facilitate the person's optimum ability to learn while handicapped by illness or residual dysfunction. The intention is to eliminate as many external barriers to learning as possible. The following should, therefore, be arranged with care:

- Attention to the details of basic comfort – such as appropriate heating, lighting, ventilation, room layout and seating arrangements – is essential for all learning. This will help to alleviate some of the general problems already discussed (pp. 280, 281) such as lack of concentration, preoccupations, anxiety and fatigue.
- Particular consideration is also given to the atmosphere. Is the atmosphere conducive to thinking and reflection? Is the encouragement of conversation and discussion desirable? What things will distract the learner? Certain distractions will negate the learning process, for example, observers, people wandering in and out, too much extraneous stimuli. How much noise is acceptable? For some, a hub of conversation, music or background noise may be comforting. For others, silence and a sense of calm will be necessary. Willson (1987) advises 'selective stimulation' with clients who cannot filter out stimuli. This means that the environment is organised so that it only contains those things which will enhance the learning process.
- Space is also a relevant issue. The close proximity of others, including the therapist, may make the client feel tense. Therefore, in order to learn, he may need to be provided with sufficient body space as well as work space around him. There are also occasions when a place for 'time out' is important so that the learner can take a break when fatigued or experiencing difficulty.

- Consideration has to be given to which place is the best setting to achieve learning goals. If the skill to be acquired is a practical activity, there has to be available an adequate area, suitable and functioning equipment, choice of, and relevant, materials to enhance motivation, reduce frustration and ensure achievement. The traditional occupational therapy department has a role in providing the client with the safe environment, equipment and support in which to initiate some skills. In some cases learning is more likely to take place when the learner is actively involved in a situation which is not in a department or unit. The community setting obviously has potential for giving the client opportunities to practice in real situations. (As the community services develop and the larger psychiatric hospitals close this is an issue that the profession needs to address.)

A number of the points in the above sections are summed up in the requirement for careful preparation, both in the therapist's approach and in the organising of the environment. Careful preparation is also necessary in the application of teaching techniques.

Teaching methods

The methods employed to convey information are of paramount importance because, if chosen appropriately, they will increase the client's chances to learn and acquire skills. Each person learns in his own individual way. Since this process is impeded by mental health problems, the occupational therapist teaching skills will use teaching techniques which take into account the presenting problems of the client. She will also need to know what the client's premorbid personality was like, and about aspects of his educational background and previous learning capacity. This will be evident in part from his school, work history and interests, but also in his on-going response to activities and the learning process. This information is used to devise teaching techniques individualised for the client's learning needs. The method will allow for the client's fluctuating condition and be readily adapted when required, as illustrated in the case example in Box 16.2.

In order to provide personalised learning situations for the client it is advantageous to be aware of various teaching techniques. There are techniques which enhance the learner's own learning strategies, increasing the sense of achievement and confidence, as summarised in Box 16.3.

There are also teaching strategies which are particularly useful when dealing with the implications of mental illness and its effect on learning. Some of these are described below:

- *Clear verbal instructions and repetition.* These techniques allow the learner time to absorb what is being said. Make short comments which describe the procedure or concept succinctly, avoiding lengthy explanations. Check if the learner has understood what has been said. Repeat the points when necessary.
- *One concept at a time.* Break a process down into stages so that the learner is shown one concept and masters that before going on to the next stage. In this way learning is split into achievable tasks. The challenge for the learner, therefore, is not so great that he gives up and he is able to feel in control (see Box 16.4).

Box 16.2   Case example 2

Mr Y is in hospital having his medication adjusted. He suffers from hallucinations which are causing him intense distress at present. At times, when he concentrates hard, he is able to do an activity despite them. He and the occupational therapist agree that an interesting activity would help alleviate some of his distress. He begins to learn how to do marquetry (which he could continue at home and develop as a hobby). There are times when he is able to follow verbal instructions and can be left to work alone. On other occasions he finds this difficult and, until his condition is more settled, the therapist will sit next to him and work with him, helping him to do one small section at a time.

Box 16.3   Helpful teaching techniques (paraphrased from Christiansen & Baum 1991)

Learning strategies can influence successful acquisition of performance skills by teaching techniques that help learners to:

- use self-motivation and reinforcement to sustain interest in what is being learned
- focus attention and concentration on relevant and important information (and ignore irrelevant and distracting information)
- acquire, organise and interpret new information
- enhance memory
- use rational principles and problem solving to make their own decisions (for helping themselves)

Box 16.4   Breaking down a process to teach a task

Example: Using a wood plane correctly (when the user is right-handed)

METHOD	KEY POINTS
Take a firm stance, facing the bench with your feet slightly apart. This enables you to swing the weight of your body from one side to the other.	Always keep the cutting edge of the plane sharp.
Hold the handle of the plane in the right hand and the knob in the left hand.	
Start the stroke with your weight on the right foot, then, keeping an even pressure on the knob, follow the body through, finishing with the weight on the left foot.	Always plane with the grain, not against it, or the wood will split.
When planing the ends of a piece of wood work inwards to the centre from one end and repeat the process for the other end. If you plane straight across from one end the edges will splinter.	Avoid letting the plane slip from the horizontal, either at the beginning or the end of the stroke, or the ends of the work will become rounded.
Give the movement smoothness and rhythm and do not force the plane.	

- *Key points*. It may sometimes be necessary to state the obvious and draw attention to main points because this will reinforce learning. This will also help to clarify a process and enable the learner to progress.

- *Instant feedback*. Feedback should be positive and constructive and as immediate as possible to guide the learner where he is succeeding and what errors he is making. It is preferable to deal with errors by first pointing out what has been done well and then suggesting improvements. This is especially necessary when a practical task is being attempted, for example in the use of tools.

- *Reinforcement*. It is essential to provide or find a means of making opportunities to practice newly learned skills. This is important, not only to reinforce what has been learned until the learner is competent but also to overcome the inhibiting factors of illness. Poor motivation and lack of confidence make practising techniques difficult. Tasks which are set for clients to reinforce learning are sometimes best negotiated with the client so that they become achievable. Again, feedback and discussion on the results should be a part of the process to encourage a continuous progression.

- *Demonstration*. Showing the learner how to do something is often an advantage because it enables the learner to understand a process more clearly than if it is just explained. If a demonstration takes place it may bypass some of the cognitive difficulties inherent in the illnesses such as a poor attention span. By using this technique the therapist can also spend time with the learner providing encouragement and support.

- *Experiential learning*. This will provide the learner with an experience which enhances the learning process. Examples of this are the therapist going with the client to practice using a library, or doing a role play. Often a client with mental health problems may not have the motivation or courage to initiate a situation on his own, such as going to an adult literacy course. It is important for the therapist to facilitate secure situations where the learner can gain the experiences that he needs.

- *Duration of session*. Timing is an essential element in the learning process. It is important to arrange sessions so that they are not so long as to overwhelm the learner in terms of length of time, fatigue and attention span. It also has to allow learners to reach a point of clarity in learning so that they do not leave a session feeling confused, thus impairing the process of acquiring a skill.

- *The individual within a group context*. Teaching techniques will be required which suit the individual as he learns a skill, whether he is alone or in a group. When the occupational therapist runs a group, whether it is practical or not, she will take into account the learning needs of each group member. The group will be planned so that the clients in the group are compatible and the size is comfortable. It is necessary to meet clients' emotional and learning needs in order to facilitate the development of skills. The group process and the activity are used to achieve these ends (Mosey 1973). Consequently there will be learning goals for each individual as well as the group as a whole.

Some of these points are highlighted in Box 16.5 where the teaching techniques for two people are compared. One person has no mental illness and the other has suffered a psychosis.

Emotional skills

Strategies which make it easier to teach 'emotional' skills such as anxiety or anger management or building self-esteem are also worth contemplating.

Much of the material available for the average person – such as handbooks, leaflets and tapes about acquiring skills – usually has plenty of information relating to a subject, often more than is required in order to add interest. Methods of teaching which convey very detailed information pose difficulties for some people with mental health problems. In the same way that clients cannot cope with too much sensory stimuli in the environment they can also find too much information clouds an issue for them and they cannot select what they need. Simpler information, if it is available, is often childish and can undermine

Box 16.5	Teaching techniques for making a coil pot, adapted to clients with different needs

A client of average ability and not affected by illness	**A client of similar ability recovering from a psychotic episode**
Ensure that the environment has adequate light and is comfortable, and have enough appropriate tools to hand.	Add to these points the need to organise the environment to be quiet, not over-stimulating. Seat client on his own to reduce distractions.
Give clear, concise instructions.	In addition to this, be calm, supportive and encouraging, but do not fuss, and give the client his required space.
First, demonstrate hand wedging.	Demonstrate hand wedging and show pictures of this (and next stages), thus reinforcing the information.
Second, show how to roll out coils of clay, prepare base and pinch coils into place.	Expect to work through one stage at a time, depending on the degree of tolerance, attention and preoccupation observed in the client.
Third, advise on care of clay by covering with a damp cloth to prevent cracking.	Repeat the relevant movements of each process if necessary and give as much guidance as is required to ensure success.
The client may finish these processes in one or two sessions, depending on size of pot and time available.	Allow for a lower standard than may be assumed for the age and expected ability of the client. If the client is able to tolerate it, move on to the next stage, but end with a complete stage to ensure achievement.

the client's self-respect. It is better, therefore, to design information which will suit the occasion. In this way a balance between easily understood information and a respect for the client's adulthood can be attained.

For those clients who require it, some of the following points can be helpful:

In some cases, when the client may have one main issue to deal with more than any other, it is advisable to use the previously mentioned technique of one concept at a time and break down ideas into individual elements. For example, a client may need to learn how to breathe slowly so that he can deal with panic but be unable to cope with exploring all the facts relating to the fight and flight mechanism, which must be held back until a later date. Simplify written information and have handouts which summarise the main points. These will then serve as an easy reminder when required.

Some clients have reached a stage psychologically when they are ready to assimilate information regarding their emotional needs. They are able to utilise cognitive techniques to enhance their insight and motivate themselves to using coping strategies. Other clients, especially those with enduring mental health problems, may have a vicious cycle of response or experience strong symptoms that make them feel helpless. In this case, particular help is needed in raising awareness of how to isolate the problem and deal with it. This process can be facilitated by use of symbolism (Reilly 1974) conveyed by visual aids, games, aspects of creative therapies such as use of paints and clay.

Alternatively, the situation may need to be depersonalised in order to gain a perspective on it that will enable the client to progress. Story telling is a good way of accomplishing this, for example a story about how a fictional person achieved his aim by setting goals. Another means is to provide opportunities to discuss real-life events by, for example, showing a video. Sometimes discussion is inappropriate because the person needs the experience of a technique being successful before they can move forward. The best teaching technique therefore is to provide an opportunity for active participation.

USE OF ACTIVITIES TO TEACH SKILLS

As indicated above and in the section on models and approaches, activities and the process of doing are a natural part of daily life and therefore a dynamic means by which skills can be taught. Reilly (1974) viewed activity as an intrinsic part of the learning process and Fidler (Fidler & Fidler 1978, Fidler 1981) advocated 'doing' for the development of performance skills. Doing is seen as an integral part of self-expression and becoming 'I'. The human being's interaction with objects in the environment provides him with the opportunities to experiment and gain feedback. Doing is defined as 'enabling the development and integration of the sensory, motor, cognitive and psychological systems; serving as a socialising agent, and verifying one's efficacy as a competent, contributing member of one's society' (Fidler & Fidler 1978). Understanding the nature and relevance of 'doing' to human adaptation can enhance the teaching strategies of an occupational therapist. There are many ways in which an occupational therapist will apply the process of doing in order to develop a client's skills. Task-orientated activities and parallel groups are two useful examples.

Task-orientated activities

Traditionally, in occupational therapy, task-orientated activities are associated with the concept of doing, be it a practical, functional or creative activity. A task is a constituent part of an activity. Young & Quinn (1991) stated that a sequence of tasks combine to form an activity. It is through the precise analysis of activities broken down into tasks that the learning process in occupational therapy is often facilitated. The therapist will therefore encourage the client to do a task as part of the skill acquisition process whether it is participation in a craft group or role playing a job interview. Mosey (1973) identified task skills which serve as a guide to what is normally expected and how the therapist can enable their development. They are:

- a comparable rate of performance
- appropriate use of tools
- willingness to engage in tasks
- sustained interest
- following instructions (verbal, written or demonstration)

- acceptable tidiness
- appropriate attention to detail
- solving and organisational abilities related to the task.

Parallel groups

The process of doing tasks can also serve as a stepping stone towards the development of group interaction skills. A way of achieving this is to use the parallel group concept.

The participant in a parallel group works at a task in the presence of other group members (Mosey 1986). There is a small amount of interaction with other members of the group in that tools are shared. The therapist will provide support to the clients in the group and will be a strong leader. The activities are well within the client's ability and assistance is given when required. Two or more doing the same activity is encouraged because this increases interaction.

Parallel groups are a useful means of skills training because they provide a secure forum for doing tasks, giving opportunities for guidance and support while the client is doing the task and learning to interact. Also, the environment and therefore the degree of stimulation can be controlled. For clients with enduring mental health problems parallel groups can be a starting point for developing both the task and interaction skills that they need.

SUMMARY

Skills are an essential part of the human being's interaction with the environment and form the basis of performance, behaviour, cognition and social interaction. Skills are acquired by development, learning and practice. Mental illness affects a person's skills in varying degrees, causing deficits or difficulties in relation to them. Occupational therapy has a role in enabling the person to recover, adapt or acquire skills. The occupational therapist facilitates the learning process by a combination of enabling, guiding, teaching and mediating.

Practice models argue for the necessity to develop skills in order to be able to function and highlight different perspectives on how to achieve this.

Occupational therapists use particular methods of teaching to facilitate skills training. They are adaptable and flexible, taking into account the individual needs of the client while affected by illness and providing a suitable level of challenge. The approach of the therapist, the learning environment and the use of activities are important factors in this process.

REFERENCES

Allen C K 1982 Independence through activity: the practice of occupational therapy (psychiatry). American Journal of Occupational Therapy 36(11): 731–739

Allen C K, Earhart C A, Blue T 1992 Occupational therapy treatment goals for the physically and cognitively disabled. American Occupational Therapy Association, Rockville

American Occupational Therapy Association 1993 Position paper: purposeful activity. Americal Journal of Occupational Therapy 47(12): 1081–1082

Argyle M 1978 The psychology of interpersonal behaviour. Cox and Wyman, London

Breines E 1984 The issue is: an attempt to define purposeful activity. American Journal of Occupational Therapy 38(8): 543–544

Christiansen C, Baum C (eds) 1991 Occupational therapy: overcoming human deficits. Slack, Thorofare, New Jersey

Concise Oxford Dictionary 1976 Clarendon Press, Oxford

Creek J 1996 Making a cup of tea as an honours degree subject. British Journal of Occupational Therapy 59(3): 128–130

Cynkin S, Robinson A M 1990 Occupational therapy and activities health: towards health through activities. Little Brown, London

Dickerson A E 1995 Action identification may explain why the doing of activities in occupational therapy effects positive changes in clients. British Journal of Occupational Therapy 58(11): 461–464

Doble S E, Magill Evans J 1992 A model of social interaction to guide occupational therapy practice. Canadian Journal of Occupational Therapy 59(3): 141–150

Fidler G S 1981 From crafts to competence. American Journal of Occupational Therapy 35(9): 567–573

Fidler G, Fidler J 1978 Doing and becoming: purposeful action and self-actualisation. American Journal of Occupational Therapy 32(5): 305–310

Franklin L 1990 Social skills training. In: Creek J (ed) Occupational therapy in mental health: principles and practice. Churchill Livingstone, Edinburgh

Gadza G M, Brooks D K 1985 The development of the social/life skills training movement. Journal of Group Psychotherapy, Psychodrama and Sociometry 38(Spring): 1–10

Gillette N, Kielhofner G 1979 The impact of specialization on the professionalization and survival of occupational therapy. American Journal of Occupational Therapy 33: 30

Golledge J 1998 Distinguishing between occupation, purposeful activity and activity. Part 1. Review and explanation. British Journal of Occupational Therapy 61(3): 100–105

Hagedorn R 1992 Occupational therapy: foundations for practice, models, frames of reference and core skills. Croom Helm, London

Hong C S, Yates P 1995 Purposeful activities? What are they? British Journal of Occupational Therapy 58(2): 75–76

Kanfer F H, Goldstein A P 1981 Helping people change. Pergamon Press, Oxford

Kielhofner G (ed) 1985 A model of human occupation, theory and application. Williams and Wilkins, Baltimore

King L J 1974 Sensory integrative approach to schizophrenia. American Journal of Occupational Therapy 28: 529–536

Llorens L A 1991 Performance tasks and roles throughout the lifespan. In: Christiansen C, Baum C (eds) 1991 Occupational therapy: overcoming human deficits. Slack, Thorofare, New Jersey

Matsutsuyu J S 1969 The interest checklist. American Journal of Occupational Therapy 23(4): 323–328

Mosey A C 1970 Three frames of reference for mental health. Slack, Thorofare, New Jersey

Mosey A C 1973 Activities therapy. Raven Press, New York

Mosey A C 1986 Psychosocial components of occupational therapy. Raven Press, New York

Munn N L 1966 Psychology: the fundamentals of human adjustment, 5th edn. Houghton Mifflin, Boston

Pedretti L W 1996 Occupational therapy: practice skills for physical dysfunction, 4th edn. Mosby, St Louis

Reed K L, Sanderson S N 1984 Concepts of occupational therapy. Williams and Wilkins, Baltimore

Reilly M (ed) 1974 Play as exploratory learning. Sage Publications, London

Roberts M E 1994 Doing a task orientated therapeutic activity – the client's response. Unpublished MSc dissertation, University of Exeter

Robinson A 1977 Play: the arena for acquisition of rules for competent behavior. American Journal of Occupational Therapy 31: 248–253. Cited in: Yerxa E J 1993 Occupational science: a new source of power for participants in occupational therapy. Journal of Occupational Science 1(1): 3–8

Smith M E 1979 Familiar daily living activities as a measure of neurological deficit after stroke. Unpublished fellowship thesis, College of Occupational Therapists, London

Stewart A 1994 Empowerment and enablement: occupational therapy 2001. British Journal of Occupational Therapy 57(7): 248–254

Willson M 1987 Occupational therapy in long term psychiatry, 2nd edn. Churchill Livingstone, London

Young M, Quinn E 1991 Theories and practice of occupational therapy. Churchill Livingstone, Edinburgh

FURTHER READING

Bruce M A, Borg B 1987 Frames of reference in psychosocial occupational therapy. Slack, Thorofare, New Jersey

Fidler G S 1969 The task orientated group as a context for treatment. American Journal of Occupational Therapy 23(1): 43–48

Hayes R L, Halford K W, Varghese F N 1991 Generalization of the effects of activity therapy and social skills training on the social behavior of low functioning schizophrenic patients. Occupational Therapy in Mental Health 11(4): 3–20

Hopkins H L, Smith H D (eds) 1993 Willard and Spackman's Occupational therapy, 8th edn. Lippincott, Philadelphia

Kielhofner G 1992 Conceptual foundations of occupational therapy. F A Davis, Philadelphia

Rose N 1989 Essential psychiatry. Blackwell Scientific Publications, London

Yerxa E J 1967 Eleanor Clarke Sagle lecture 1966. Authentic occupational therapy. American Journal of Occupational Therapy 21(1): 1–9

Yerxa E J 1980 Audacious values: the energy source for occupational therapy practice. Cited in: Kielhofner G 1983 Health through occupational theory and practice in occupational therapy. F A Davis, Philadelphia

17

Therapeutic play

Lily I. H. Jeffrey

INTRODUCTION

In the 20th century, child analysts and later child psychologists and child psychiatrists focused their skills on devising treatment interventions to help emotionally disturbed children. Occupational therapists working in multidisciplinary teams in the field of child and adolescent mental health have contributed their own specific approach to enhance the therapeutic milieu created by these teams. The role of the occupational therapist in the field of child and adolescent mental health is described in a later chapter in this book (Ch. 22). This current chapter describes how occupational therapists use therapeutic play in the assessment and treatment of emotionally disturbed children.

Young children are unable to express their emotional needs and conflicts since they lack the verbal ability of adults, who often use intricate thought concepts and sophisticated language. Childhood has a language of its own – play. For occupational therapists wanting to understand and help emotionally and behaviourally disturbed children, it is essential to learn their 'play language' in all its developmental aspects so that the child can communicate freely with the adult. The child is constantly communicating through play. The occupational therapist needs to be skilled at tuning into and interpreting this complex language of childhood.

PLAY

From the first persistent attempts to reach and grasp his rattle to the sophisticated computer games of infinite variety and complexity, the years of childhood, for the normal healthy child, are filled with a rich diversity of experiences as he engages in play activity of one kind or another throughout most of his waking hours. The study of play illustrates the complex nature of this activity (Miller 1973, Bruner et al 1976), and focusing on the purpose of play in childhood has produced numerous theories (Ellis 1973).

The therapeutic value of ordinary play

Play assists and enhances all aspects of development: physical, emotional, social, cognitive, perceptual, sensory integration and language. It is a medium for forming and sharing relationships, either the mother–child or parent–child relationships, extending to siblings and other family members then peers and other adults. Play time provides the child with his own 'space' to work out his own problems, often at an unconscious level, for example repeating certain play themes over and over again and so mastering his anxiety. As he symbolically expresses his fears and fantasies, he becomes the ruler of his play world and so works through his inner turmoil. Through play he is able to express (and so become aware of) his own feelings, especially towards safe inanimate objects that do not retaliate. He becomes aware of his potentials and limitations in regard to different play materials. He has his own likes and dislikes, he forms his own self-awareness and identity. He receives praise and recognition from the various skills he acquires. This builds up his confidence in his own abilities, establishes a positive self-image and develops his self-esteem.

Play as a medium for therapy

Play has many purposes in the therapy session. It is used to establish a therapeutic relationship with a child by providing a neutral shared experience. The inanimate play object provides a link between therapist and child without, at this stage, feelings being revealed. The play assists the assessment processes, that is, diagnostic, behavioural, developmental and continuous assessment. The child, through different play activities, can regress and use play symbolically to release tension and aggression. He can enact his unconscious and conscious needs and conflicts with the play materials, as well as expressing fears and fantasies. By interpreting all these activities the therapist helps the child to gain insight. The child can alter his attitudes, improve his way of relating to adults and peers, and practise these new ways of behaving in the social setting of play-group therapy. The child develops new skills and uses his creativity, which can sublimate basic needs in a socially acceptable way, and he receives praise and recognition so that his confidence and self-image are improved.

THERAPEUTIC PLAY: AN INTRODUCTION

The use of play as a therapeutic medium to help emotionally and behaviourally disturbed children is a complex area of work. The field ranges from using therapeutic play as a method of communicating effectively with a child to the use of play therapy within the context of a transference relationship, which promotes emotional growth. Many children with a multitude of disorders benefit from these types of intervention. Different types of play therapy are practiced by many professions. It is one of the many therapeutic strategies used in the field of child psychiatry and needs to be complementary to other forms of treatment.

Children who need therapeutic play

Every child experiences stress of some kind in his life. This is normally worked through by the child himself, with help from his parents and extended family, his peers, teachers at school, or other significant adults that he meets in the community. These children usually have access to rich play environments and supportive relationships. The child needs to play out upsetting experiences, with the support of a trusted adult, just as an adult would need to talk about such events with colleagues, friends or relatives.

Some children, for a variety of reasons, develop distressing psychological symptomatology and need to be referred to the multidisciplinary team in a child mental health service. Occupational therapy is one form of treatment available in this setting.

The psychological disorders of childhood and adolescence

The list below is adapted from the World Health Organization's *ICD 10 Classification of Mental and Behavioural Disorders* (WHO 1992):

- neurotic disorders, such as anxiety states, phobias, obsessions, compulsions, hysterical disorders, hypochondriasis, school refusal
- attachment disorders
- developmental disorders, including learning disorders, speech and language delay, perceptual problems, abnormal clumsiness
- hyperkinetic disorder/attention deficit disorder
- affective disorders
- epilepsy
- enuresis
- encopresis
- psychoses, including infantile autism, schizophrenia, disintegrative psychoses, *folie à deux*
- psychosomatic disorders such as asthma, eczema, ulcerative colitis
- anorexia nervosa, bulimia, obesity
- conduct disorders
- non-accidental injury
- sexual abuse
- elective mutism
- post traumatic stress disorder
- stammering
- tics
- Gilles de la Tourette syndrome.

Therapeutic play for children under stress

Therapeutic play can help any child who is under stress, such as the child who is admitted to hospital, perhaps as an emergency or with an illness that requires prolonged or painful treatment. Therapeutic play in its various forms can help by allowing the child to express his fears. Through preparation play, staff can explain the complicated procedures necessary in treatment.

Therapeutic play helps the chronically sick child and the child with a permanent physical handicap to make the necessary emotional adjustments to cope with life with a handicap, by allowing expression of frustrations and exploring methods of deriving satisfaction from alternative activities. Child therapists have also described their work with dying children.

Children coping with difficult family situations, including separated or divorced parents, and looked after children need to communicate their anxieties, fears and frustrations at these situations. Within the context of a therapeutic relationship with a trusted adult, therapeutic play provides a means of communication so that these children can express their feelings of despair that the parental situation cannot be altered. It also provides a situation where the child can be helped to adapt to these circumstances, for example the child can be prepared for the necessary adjustments needed for a successful looked after situation or adoption, and also provides support in the months after this event to ensure that a smooth transition is made. The neutral adult (child therapist) provides the support and opportunity for expression of frustrated feelings, which the child is unable to express in the new parental situation.

Children who are physically or sexually abused need this type of help to work through all the feelings associated with this traumatic experience, which, if left unheeded, would scar them emotionally for the rest of their lives. The child in a bereaved family needs help with his adjustment to the tragic event yet often his needs are overlooked by the grieving adults around him.

The multidisciplinary team

The multifactorial aetiology of the psychological disorders of childhood needs to be investigated by a team of professionals. Traditionally, diagnosis and formulation of problems were carried out by a tripartite group composed of child psychiatrist, child psychologist and psychiatric social worker. With the development of day and in-patient units, teams expanded to include nurses, teachers and occupational therapists. As the complexities of the child's disturbance emerged, speech and language therapists, EEG staff, child psychotherapists, community psychiatric nurses, dietitians, nursery nurses and so on have all contributed to the team approach.

In today's community centred health environment, with the great demands on scarce resources, the Health Advisory Service has outlined a tier approach to identify service delivery at different levels (NHS Health Advisory Service 1995). Liaison with other health professionals and support for staff in other agencies, such as education, social services and the legal system, are complex areas of the work.

Interventions for the disturbed child and his family

How are children with emotional and behavioural problems and their families helped? As the causes of these disturbances are numerous and variable, so the types of treatment available are many.

Beginning with the child himself, he may have individual or group therapy or it may be necessary to seek a new accepting environment in a residential unit, so that relief is given to both child and parents and the destructive emotional climate is not perpetuated in the home. The child may need specific remedial and educational help, and attendance at the unit school, either as an in-patient or on a daily basis in a day unit, may be essential. Some units focus on behavioural problems and use a variety of behavioural/cognitive techniques to reduce or eliminate these problems. The use of pharmacotherapy in child psychiatry has increased in recent years.

Parents, too, need help. This could be in the form of supportive psychotherapy on an individual or group basis, or perhaps specific marital help is required. Often the approach is to treat the whole family in family therapy, using a variety of models.

The occupational therapist providing individual and/or group therapy is indeed the voice of the child in the multidisciplinary team, and can present problems solely from the child's point of view. This cannot be done without communicating effectively with the child in the play setting and observing the child's mental state, behaviour and level of emotional functioning. Occupational therapy provides a method for the child to solve his own psychosocial and developmental problems.

Occupational therapy and therapeutic play

The therapeutic use of selected and graded activities is one of the core skills of the occupational therapy profession. This is based on the occupational science philosophy that every person, from birth to death, is an occupational being. Occupations range from personal care and domestic daily living skills to work or its substitutes, and to the multitude of leisure activities in which the individual participates. The key occupation of childhood is play.

Throughout its history, the profession, in the field of mental health, has undertaken activity analysis to understand the therapeutic use of purposeful activity and the intrinsic qualities that give the activity its therapeutic value.

In the middle of the 20th century, occupational therapists in the USA developed an eclectic approach to object relations theory. The object relations frame of reference has been defined as 'the theoretical approach which views persons, media and activities as objects invested with psychic energy. Interaction with these objects is necessary to satisfy personal needs and promote psychosocial growth and ultimately leads to self actualization' (Bruce & Borg 1987). These therapists concentrated on the core skills of the profession by examining the psychodynamics of activities and the therapeutic relationship. They encouraged activity analysis in the light of the unconcious symbolic significance of the objects used (Fidler & Fidler 1963).

The theory of the psychodynamics of activities and the therapeutic relationship, which are key components of occupational therapy in the field of mental health, are evident in relation to developmental play therapy, described in a later section of this chapter (p. 300).

THEORETICAL FRAMEWORKS FOR CHILD THERAPY

When reviewing the literature on the effectiveness of child psychotherapy, Kazdin (1988) listed 235 different types of interventions, many using therapeutic play. These therapies are provided by therapists from different professional backgrounds – child psychiatrists, clinical psychologists, child psychotherapists, social workers, occupational therapists, nurses and play specialists or play leaders using play on paediatric wards or in paediatric clinics. The following sections of this chapter describe some of the major approaches to child therapy which use play as a therapeutic medium.

TYPES OF CHILD THERAPY

The major types of child therapy include the following:

- psychoanalytic psychotherapy
- relationship therapy
- nondirective (client-centred) therapy
- developmental play therapy
- directed play therapy
- group play therapy
- family therapy.

Psychoanalytic psychotherapy

Child psychotherapists practicing psychoanalytic psychotherapy have extensive training provided by establishments recognised by the Association of Child Psychotherapists. During this training, at least 4 years in length, students undergo a personal psychoanalysis (Clarkson & Pokorny 1994).

Courses at the different training schools are based on various analytical approaches: Kleinian, post-Kleinian, Anna Freud, Margaret Lowenfield and Jungian.

The focus of therapy is the child's unconscious, that is, his 'inner world'. The therapist is dealing with the child's unconscious anxieties and defences. These are clearly demonstrated in the transference relationship that develops between the child and the therapist. In this relationship the child experiences unconscious needs that were unmet and unconscious conflicts that were unresolved with significant figures (parents) in his early life. The transference relationship reflects the emotional level that the child has reached and is fixated at. The aim of therapy is to resolve these past conflicts and unmet needs and to help the child to progress from the fixated level, through the normal phases of emotional development until he attains the appropriate emotional level for his chronological age.

Through the accepting transference relationship, the child displays and experiences his needs as he is no longer required to repress them in his daily life. This experience brings awareness, with interpretation insight is gained and, within the relationship, he is helped to mature. Klein (1932) indicated that in the analysis of children the free play of the child is a direct substitute for the verbal free association of the adult in psychoanalysis. The child produces unconscious material in his symbolic play and reveals his inner world. The acceptance of this material by the therapist, and her interpretation, helps the child to gain insight into his fears, frustrations, conflicts, needs, anxieties and fantasies and helps him work through and integrate his feelings.

Often, the child participates in role reversal with the therapist, in a symbolic way. The child becomes a significant adult figure in his life and the therapist is directed to take on the role of the child. The child then masters his fears and conflicts in the real relationship by acting out the adult's role as he sees it. Freud (1920) described how, in play, the child no longer accepts the inevitable control of his life by adults but takes control of his own play world and reconstructs disturbing situations with the play material, where he directs the course of action and so masters his anxieties.

The repetition of a particular play theme illustrates the child's unconscious anxiety about a particular situation and the therapist, by interpreting the anxieties, helps them to diminish. The repetition helps the child to integrate his feelings and anxieties into his general experience.

Relationship therapy

Relationship therapy, based on the work of Otto Rank (Menaker 1982), emphasises the therapeutic relationship between child and therapist. The focus of sessions is on the 'here and now' relationship. Therapy begins at the presenting level of emotional development of the child and the feelings expressed in the therapy sessions towards the therapist form the basis of the maturational experience.

This type of therapy is suitable for any age range but for younger children a play experience is added for communication purposes.

Nondirective (client-centred) therapy

This is probably the most common form of play therapy used in the UK and North America. It was devised for children by Virginia Axline (Axline 1947) from the therapeutic work of Carl Rogers with adults, that is, client-centred therapy (Rogers 1967).

Axline's work is based on her theory that the child's innate drive to achieve maturity must be given the optimum facilitating environment to reach that goal. She suggests that this can be done:

- by providing an 'ideal' play environment so that the child can play out all his bewildering feelings and, in so doing, become aware of them, acknowledge them, and eventually direct and control them
- by providing an adult who accepts and understands all these feelings completely, reflecting

back the feelings so that they are clarified for the child.

The therapist does not direct the child's play in any way, limit setting is minimal, and the therapist presents a concerned, consistent approach, aware of all that the child is communicating in his play and ensuring that the child realises that he is accepted, whatever feelings he displays. She allows the child to be himself. This increases his confidence and self-esteem. The child is completely free to realise his potentialities and so he matures. By learning to understand and accept himself, he learns to understand and accept others.

The nature of the therapeutic relationship

Practitioners new to the field often query the differences between relationship therapy and nondirective therapy. The difference lies in the nature of the therapeutic relationship. In nondirective therapy, the therapist has a quiescent approach, using reflection of feelings as the main form of communication, whereas relationship therapy uses the 'here and now' feelings of the child for the therapist to explore the child's level of emotional functioning. In relationship therapy the accepting therapist allows the child to express these feelings and actively explains (interprets) their significance in the relationship and so helps the child to mature.

Developmental play therapy

Developmental play therapy is based on developmental theories, that is, Hellersberg's psychophysical theory of development and Freud and Peller's psychosexual theories of development (Peller 1952, Hall, 1954, Hellersberg 1955) (Table 17.1). These theories explain the complex play patterns which the child presents in play therapy sessions. Jeffrey (1984) has outlined how a knowledge of these three theories in relation to the child's play in therapy provides the therapist with a sound theoretical rationale for providing an initial assessment that gives a baseline of the child's emotional state and subsequently, as therapy proceeds, provides a method of measuring

Table 17.1   Developmental play therapy. (Adapted from Jeffrey 1984, with kind permission from the British Journal of Occupational Therapy.)

Phases of therapy	Psychophysical (Hellersberg)	Psychoanalytical (Freud)	Psychosexual (Peller)
Phase 1	Sensory/tactile	Oral	Narcissistic
Phase 2	Motor	Anal	Pre-oedipal
Phase 3	Representational	Phallic	Oedipal
Phase 4	Constructive	Latency	Post-oedipal

progress. For this to be achieved, the play takes place in the context of relationship therapy using nondirective play.

The aim of this therapy is to allow the child, within the context of the therapeutic relationship and with the use of appropriate play activities, to achieve his appropriate level of emotional development for his chronological age. This method of therapy is based on developmental theories that suggest that, for healthy personality development to occur, the child needs to progress through each stage of emotional development successfully before tackling a further phase. If the child's needs at one stage are not satisfied, he is fixated at that particular level, he does not mature and does not become a well-integrated adult who can cope with the ordinary stresses and strains of life.

It is essential, therefore, that the therapeutic experience provides a good therapeutic relationship that permits the child to relate to the therapist and play out the particular level of emotional development he has reached. The child is free to choose whatever activities he wishes to participate in. He is not expected to achieve, as he would be in the school situation, nor is he expected to conform to a particular standard of behaviour. In this atmosphere of therapeutic freedom, he is enabled to demonstrate his particular problems. The therapist empathetically accepts, explores and clarifies his feelings and interprets the type of relationship he forms with her and also the behaviour he produces. However, more importantly, in this type of therapy it is by allowing the child to use the play material as he wishes, reflecting his stage of emotional development, that this phase is worked through. This is because the child's

needs are satisfied both by the type of relationship he is experiencing and by the type of therapeutic play he can indulge in. The child, by this biopsychosocial approach, re-experiences his early development, makes up the deficiencies and hence achieves emotional maturity.

Directed play therapy

Directed play therapy is used when the therapist decides to use the play medium for a specific therapeutic aim and directs the use of play materials by the child so that, if possible, the objective is achieved. Often this involves contriving, through play, the re-enactment of past, present or future disturbing events in the child's life, for example using therapy dolls to help express her guilt and fear about being sexually abused by her father, or helping the child express feelings about separation from a loved parent when parents have just divorced, or rehearsing feelings about particular painful procedures if the child is about to be admitted to hospital, explaining the need for the procedures and exactly what is to be done.

Directed play techniques have been used for over 60 years with a multitude of aims and objectives. An early paper on the subject (Levy 1939) described how, in imaginative play, the normal child copes with anxiety. Levy harnessed this in 'release therapy'. With older children he encouraged them to re-enact a situation that had particularly troubled them and was a precipitating factor in their particular symptomatology. For younger children he did not explore actual events but allowed them to indulge in play of a primitive nature, for example messy sand, water and clay, which the child used in a variety of ways. This expression of basic aggressive feelings and accompanying regressive play released the child from the controls of a too-strict upbringing, when too high expectations and demands were made of him.

A wealth of directed techniques exists for different types of psychological disorders in childhood:

- Theraplay (Jernberg 1979) was devised for children who, for a variety of reasons, have either missed or not responded to normal sensory motor play in the first 2 years of life.
- Gardner (1971) has used his 'mutual storytelling technique' to help children with all types of psychological problems. He uses both audiotapes and videotapes of the child and recommends the use of these items of equipment rather than toy props, as the child enjoys participating in the adult world of communication, and is not distracted by fantasy material, and so produces his own imaginative creations in verbal form.
- Gardner has also devised the 'talking, feeling and doing' game specifically for children who find it difficult, even with his story technique, to express their needs and conflicts (Gardner 1975).
- O'Connor (1982) has also suggested that the older child needs to verbalise, rather than just play out, feelings and has devised the 'colour your life technique', so that feelings are expressed verbally through the use of significant colours.
- A useful source of directed techniques is found in *Counselling Children* (Geldard & Geldard 1997). The authors, an occupational therapist and a psychologist, present a wide range of play and therapeutic activity, with the therapeutic objectives of each technique clearly illustrated.

Group play therapy

Group therapy for emotionally disturbed children in the form of 'activity group therapy' was first introduced by Slavson (Slavson & Schiffer 1975). His colleague Schiffer (1971) introduced this form of therapy for the younger age group, naming it 'therapeutic play groups'.

Group therapy can never be a substitute for individual therapy. Group therapy has different aims and objectives and, although it is a very useful adjunct to individual therapy, it cannot replace the one-to-one therapeutic relationship, if that is what the disturbed child requires for his particular disorder. It is also essential that children placed in groups must have a potential for social development and social play, whatever their chronological age, and that they are not fixated at an earlier level of development.

The group, with the adult therapist or therapists and the peer group of children, reflects the family situation with parents and siblings or reflects the school situation with teachers and classmates. From an assessment point of view, the child interacts in this new 'family' or new 'school' set-up as he has done in the previous settings. The child plays one adult against another, as he does at home. His sibling rivalry difficulties are reflected in the new 'family' setting. Within the warm, empathetic atmosphere of the group, his difficulties are displayed and accepted. In the group, adults do not repeat emotionally charged parental interaction and peers are encouraged to understand the child's difficulties, just as their own difficulties are being accepted and tolerated. So, in this therapeutic situation, the child can try out new ways of behaving and relating. As the child feels more accepted, a positive self-image develops, he accepts more responsibility for his behaviour, becomes more independent and matures.

Certain children do not benefit from group therapy, for example severely deprived children, autistic children, severely neurotic children and some psychotic and brain-damaged children. The child with a learning disability should not be placed in a therapeutic group of this nature as he is scapegoated.

Occupational therapists use groups for a variety of therapeutic objectives. Forward (1965) illustrated how they could be used for children from different diagnostic and behavioural categories, for example encopretic children, aggressive children. Trafford (Silveira & Trafford 1988) described how throughout their young lives children need to function in groups. She outlined a variety of directed techniques to facilitate interaction.

Family therapy

When considering different models for family therapy, it is important to remember the young child in this setting. Some family therapists make provision for the child by having play materials available. However, it is also important to understand how the young child is affected by the family dynamics within the group, hence the importance of having a child therapist present who can organise play materials that allow the child to communicate at his correct maturational age and emotional developmental level. The child does not have the verbal abilities of the adults present, but he will communicate through his play. The child therapist's role in this setting is to draw the attention of the family and family therapist to the communication of the young child. She must also help the child by clarifying the adults' communication at a level he can understand.

Therapists have derived different approaches to including children in this setting, for example, conjoint play therapy for the young child and his parent (Safer 1965) and the specific participation of the child in family therapy (Villeneuve 1979).

PRACTICAL GUIDELINES FOR USING THERAPEUTIC PLAY

The child, having been assessed by the multidisciplinary team, is referred for occupational therapy. To ensure a successful outcome of treatment, many practical considerations need to be examined at this stage. These include the roles of the participants, the child himself, the parents, the therapist and the play environment. Therapy needs careful introduction, skilful handling throughout the course of treatment and successful termination.

THE ROLE OF THE PARENTS

It is vital initially that the parents or carers understand the child's need for therapy. It is also important to gain their cooperation and commitment to bringing the child for regular sessions.

Parental commitment

Children who are in-patients or day patients in a unit with an occupational therapist can easily attend for sessions. This is not so with out-patients. Often, parents or carers find the weekly commitment of bringing the child to the unit a considerable drain on their time. It helps if it can be arranged that the parent sees medical and social work staff at the same time as the child is having therapy and so are having their own needs attended to.

Some units have devised imaginative programmes, with occupational therapists providing individual or group sessions for the children and having activity groups, for example for depressed young mothers who are isolated from close and extended family. Supportive coffee and chat groups with another member of staff, when practical handling problems can be discussed, are an alternative.

Introducing child therapy to parents

It is useful to give an information leaflet to the parents explaining the general principles of therapy. This can be discussed with the parents to clarify any difficulties prior to beginning treatment. The parents' consent for treatment should be gained and recorded in the notes.

The information leaflet should explain how playing out problems for the child is a substitute for the talking out of problems by the adult, and that the child needs a therapeutic relationship with the occupational therapist, a neutral figure, away from his ordinary daily living activities. The length of treatment (difficult to predict but often long) must be indicated and it must be stressed that the parents' commitment is vital, especially in relation to bringing the child regularly.

From a practical point of view, it is important to emphasise to parents that all types of activities are used, including messy paint and clay, and that they can help by allowing the child to come to the unit in clothing suitable for these activities.

THE ROLE OF THE OCCUPATIONAL THERAPIST

Therapists planning treatment for children will be influenced by their education and training, knowledge, skills and experience. It is essential for therapists to focus on the difficulties that the individual child is having at home or at school. Therapists must provide a play environment that enables the child to communicate his views of the problem.

Assessment

The initial phase of the intervention has several purposes:

- It is therapeutic, allowing the child to build up a relationship with the therapist in a permissive, trusting atmosphere.
- In this accepting situation, the child reveals his problems as he sees them. Again, self-revelation accompanied by ventilation of feelings is therapeutic.
- The child's mental state is noted.
- The child's maturational level is assessed.
- The child's behaviour in the setting is noted.
- The emotional stage that the child has reached is determined by the type of play he uses in a nondirective setting and the type of relationship he forms with the therapist.

This essential information must then be conveyed to the multidisciplinary team by the therapist, so that future treatment and management can be planned.

Treatment

Once the therapist is aware of the child's emotional developmental level and has the knowledge of the child's specific problems, therapy sessions can now take place in the context of a therapeutic play environment using one of the theoretical frameworks previously outlined in this chapter.

Education and training

The occupational therapy profession recognised the need for postgraduate clinical courses in the field of child and adolescent mental health in the middle of the 20th century. A 2-year course in play diagnosis and play therapy, developed at the Institute of Family Therapy in Ipswich, was approved by the College of Occupational Therapists (College of Occupational Therapists 1990). A 1-year generic course for nurses, teachers and occupational therapists was developed at the Fleming Nuffield Unit in Newcastle (Jeffrey et al 1979).

In addition to child psychotherapy training approved by the Association of Child Psychotherapists, the British Association of Play Therapists has in recent years recognised courses in psychodynamic play therapy.

Occupational therapists in the field of child and adolescent mental health may wish to extend their therapeutic skills by attending courses such as these.

Supervision

Hawkins & Shohet (1989) described good supervision in terms of the 'therapeutic triad', that is, the supervisor supporting and 'holding' the feelings of the therapist and child to allow therapy to progress.

All who practise therapy of this nature should have regular weekly supervision with a senior colleague where all children in therapy can be discussed. Children requiring these forms of treatment have had fearful, anxious, painful, depriving experiences. The therapist needs to contain these feelings for the child and, in turn, requires help to do this.

A skilful supervisor will be experienced in the field and will be able to help the therapist with planning therapy, making necessary adjustments to her approach, managing the acting out behaviour of the child and exploring progress in the context of developmental theories.

Supervising is a skilled task and training and experience in this role is essential, as well as being able to devote time to staff who require this support.

Recording sessions

Play sessions should be accurately recorded in detail. Piaget (Richmond 1970) suggested that, for the child, to play is to think. It is therefore essential to record the sequences of play within the session to understand the child's thought processes. Often, seemingly trivial themes in the child's play in the first few sessions only become recognised as significant after many sessions, when the child plays out a particular theme again and again.

Details to be noted are:

- What does the child choose to play with?
- How does he play with the toy – aggressively, secretly, not allowing the therapist to see and so on?
- Does the child include the therapist in his play?
- What is the nature of the interaction?
- What type of relationship is formed?
- How does the therapist feel towards the child?
- What limits need to be set?
- What type of behaviour is exhibited?
- What verbal communication accompanies the play?

These notes should be written during the session, if this is acceptable to the child, or immediately after the session for accuracy. This material is invaluable in supervision as it enables therapist and supervisor to explore the therapeutic process.

THE ROLE OF THE CHILD

Often a child's introduction to a child psychiatry unit is surrounded by anger and guilt, both for the parents and the child. The child's behaviour has become intolerable and help is needed. The parents feel they have failed in their upbringing of the child. The child may have been threatened with all sorts of dire consequences if his behaviour does not improve, so it is very important when meeting him to begin immediately to clarify the role of the unit and the therapy to be provided.

Introducing the child to therapy

At the introductory visit it is important for both child and parent to meet the occupational thera-

pist and see the play room. It should be acknowledged that the therapist knows that the child has been having some difficulties and his life has not been happy (there is no need to discuss the problems in detail) and that the therapist is there to help him. The procedure for attending sessions should be explained, for example, the parent will be seeing the social worker, or member of the medical staff while the child comes for his 45-minute session with the therapist. The therapist will collect him from the waiting room and they will return there at the end of the session.

The initial phase

The first session may be clouded with separation difficulties for both parent and child, and this must be worked through. Sometimes this can take several sessions and occasionally the child finds the situation so threatening that the parent needs to remain in the room. It is best, at this point, just to use the time to introduce the child to all the play materials available and allow him to enjoy himself and be at ease, rather than focus on the therapy when the parent is present.

For the child who can separate, the therapist indicates that she knows the child has been having problems; again there is no need to elaborate. The child will communicate his view of the problems in his own time. The therapist must explain that coming for regular sessions to play in this room with her will help. The child is then introduced to the play materials and given permission to play with anything he likes. Children vary in the time they take to settle into the play situation, usually depending on their previous separation experiences and degree of anxiety, but the therapist conveying her interest and approval in what they are doing gives the secure framework necessary.

Often in the first few sessions the child (usually depending on his age) will become anxious after a time. This is partly normal separation anxiety, but sometimes children have been threatened that they will be sent away, and feel that they will not be taken back to their parents at the end of the session. If a child becomes very anxious, it is best to terminate the session at this point and take him back to his parents.

Setting limits

Even in nondirective play therapy, some limits are essential. First, the therapist must be in control of the play situation. If she is not, the child finds this a very threatening experience. Many disturbed children have not had consistent experiences in their lives. The variations in the same adult's reactions to single facets of their behaviour has left them confused, with no idea of which behaviour is approved and which is not. The limits within the therapy situation provide this consistent approach by the therapist, and so order can be given to the child's life during the play session. Later this generalises to the rest of his life.

Limits also demonstrate the concern that the therapist has for the child. They are there for the child's well-being; for example, he must not harm the fabric of the room, the therapist, the other children or himself, and he must not destroy the toys. If the child does break these limits, he is out of control, the situation is frightening for him and later he experiences considerable guilt. The limit is set at the appropriate time when this deviant behaviour is displayed.

Sometimes the child wishes to take the play materials home with him. This expresses a need to take the play situation home. This must be interpreted to the child in terms of a simple explanation, that the work of therapy takes place in the session and is not repeated in other situations. Some therapists suggest that the very young child needs a toy to take home as a 'transitional object' to remind the small child that the play experience is there and will return.

Some therapists do not display paintings and other projective work and do not allow it to be removed from the playroom. Again, remember that this is not ordinary play, but therapy, and children need to know that the feelings expressed in the play room are confidential and are contained there by the therapist, that is, the therapist takes care of the child's work which is stored in his own drawer.

Testing out the therapist

The child also tests out the therapist by using certain types of behaviour, for example running out of the room, deliberately flooding the sand tray, putting the lights on and off, painting the floor, walls or furniture, throwing toys at the therapist or deliberately hurting another child.

Careful management techniques need to be worked out to handle this acting out. As well as interpreting the child's need to use this behaviour, realistic explanations should be given as to why he cannot carry it out and limits firmly set.

Terminating therapy

The child, having worked through his problems, must be given ample warning that therapy will end. He needs time to work through leaving what has been an intense relationship with the therapist. The child is helped in this process by reviewing his original reason for referral, indicating how he has progressed and helping him with plans for the future. The child may produce symptoms again in an attempt to retain the therapy situation but, by careful preparation, he will be ready for the discharge date. Sometimes children in a residential unit continue to attend the unit for outpatient therapy while they settle into their new surroundings or return to their original home and school. Again, termination must be judged with care, when the child no longer needs the support offered.

THE PLAY ENVIRONMENT

The entire aim of creating the child-centred play environment is to allow the child to communicate. Through the play medium, with toys and other play activities, he obtains the therapeutic experience he requires to develop or to restore his emotional well-being.

A CHILD-CENTRED ENVIRONMENT

A room should preferably be specifically designed for play and reserved solely for this purpose. The child needs to feel free to be himself in that room and does not want the atmosphere clouded with previous memories and associations, for example a classroom, a medical room in the school, or a room previously used when parents have been interviewed.

The room must be completely child-centred, with child-sized furniture of various heights. The therapist's office should preferably be elsewhere as a desk, telephone, filing cabinets and notes do not enhance the play atmosphere.

A useful arrangement is a partly carpeted area so that both child and therapist can sit on the floor, with the rest of the room having a vinyl covering for sand, water, paint, clay and other messy activities. An easy chair is an asset, as therapists who use 'reading therapy' will find that the story atmosphere created in this setting is very useful. The room must convey a sense of privacy, for example windows should be of frosted glass to a certain height if there is the likelihood of the sessions being observed from outside. It is important that the child feels he can trust the play environment. If the therapist wishes to use one-way screens, sound recording or videotape equipment, this must always be fully explained to the child.

Display and storage of toys

Display of toys, other play materials and books must always be considered carefully. Open shelving is required for the display of toys, all readily accessible to the child. In some instances, there is a need to restrict certain play materials and there should be lockable storage cupboards, so that the therapist can control the play environment.

Some therapists like to exhibit the children's pictures and other products of play sessions on pinboards or in display cabinets. This really should be the child's decision; remember that he is revealing his inner emotions through these media and may not want them to be displayed for all to see. In contrast, other children may need recognition for their efforts.

Safety

Tools must be kept in a lockable cupboard with shadowboards for easy identification and check-

ing at the end of the session. Paint, glue and so on should be stored in a lockable metal cupboard.

The therapist must be able to control the water and electricity supply to the room. Enclosed strip lighting should be installed for safety purposes.

Sand and water play

When planning the 'messy' play area, careful thought is needed about the site of the sand tray, or trays, in relation to the sink. It is important that they should not be constantly flooded as this impedes the play of other children attending that day. Ideally, three types of sand in separated trays should be available:

1. dry sand for pouring
2. damp ordinary sand for modelling
3. very messy wet sand.

A useful arrangement, if it is not possible to have three sand trays or if space is scarce, is to have one sand tray stand, with one tray in place, and underneath two stackable trays with the other types of sand available and exchanged when necessary. Two lids are also useful to cover the sand tray and the top container, to control the use of this material. Some therapists prefer a sandpit at floor level. A play sink (child height), so that the child can indulge in water play without being restricted to a small handbasin, is an essential feature. It is useful if this sink is at a height for comfortable sitting for child and therapist, that is, knee room must be available.

Space is very important and a cluttered atmosphere confuses the child. A playroom with restricted materials is often far more effective than one where the child is overwhelmed by too much to choose from. Remember the room is designed to facilitate communication and if a good therapeutic relationship is established the child will convey his needs with the limited materials available.

Toys and play materials

The toys and play materials used are all available to allow the child to communicate and express his feelings. They are also needed to assess the child's emotional development level and to allow him to fixate, regress and eventually mature emotionally through the relationship experience and participation in the play activity.

Different types of play therapy require different play materials, but the following selection, based on the developmental play therapy model (Peller 1952, Hall 1954, Hellersberg 1955), should cater for most children's needs. (See the section on Developmental play therapy, p. 300.)

General equipment

- overalls, or plastic aprons
- sponges for quick mopping up
- dustpan, brush
- squeezy mop
- paper towels, wastepaper bins.

Phase 1: Sensory/tactile/oral/narcissistic

- Materials for bubble blowing: a suitable container for a mixture of washing-up liquid and water. Bubble masters, as these give instant success.
- Food activity of some sort (Fig. 17.1), for example simple sweet-making with instant

icing, or introducing food into the session, for example orange juice and biscuits.

- Tea-party toys for dolls and small children: cups, saucers, spoons, teapot, milk jug.
- For the older child, still fixated at this stage, food preparation at a more sophisticated level and using the department's kitchen, if this is appropriate.
- Musical instruments and singing activities. It is useful to have a suitable selection of tapes.
- Dry sand for pouring, sand tray and toys for sand play.
- A variety of toys for object-related play, for example a post box, and inset trays.

Phase 2: Motor/anal/pre-oedipal

- If available, an outside adventure playground is ideal for this type of play, or visits to the local adventure playground.
- Indoors, a gym is also ideal. However, even in a restricted space, movement games can be devised, for example a play tunnel.
- Hammer toys and simple woodwork activity also provide suitable movement activities.
- Water play in the sink is important at this stage, with suitable water-play toys for pouring waterwheel, boats and so on.

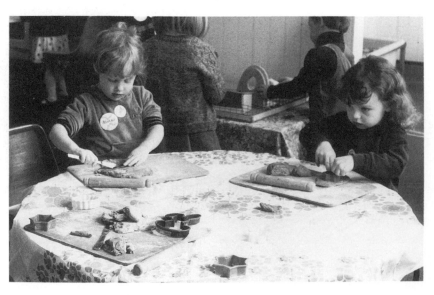

Figure 17.1 Phase 1: sensory/tactile. Children baking.

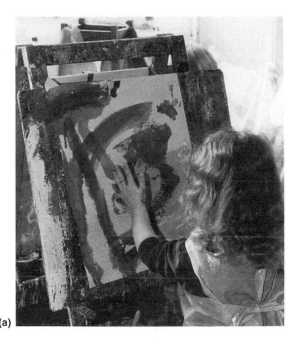

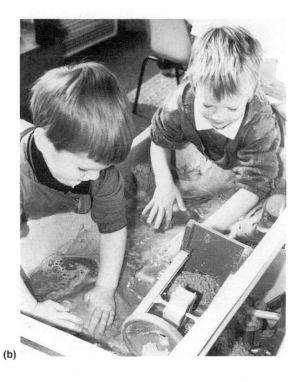

Figure 17.2 Phase 2: motor. (**a**) Finger painting. (**b**) Wet, soggy sand.

(a)

(b)

- Clay should be available for smearing at this stage. Finger painting, with water paste and liquid paint is ideal (Fig. 17.2a).
- Play dough (home-made) is excellent, with boards, rolling pins and cutters.
- Dolls, with cot, clothes, feeding bottles (real size), bath, potty, and so on.
- A sand tray and toys for wet, messy sand play (Fig. 17.2b).

Phase 3: Representational/phallic/oedipal

- A selection of fairy stories, with the text on one page and illustration on the opposite page.
- A dolls' house, dolls and furniture.
- A farm and layout (Fig. 17.3). Domestic animal families.
- Wild model animals. Fantasy animals, such as dragons.
- A play mat with a garage and transport toys, police cars, ambulance, aeroplanes, motorbikes, cars, helicopters, a fire brigade, a train set and so on.

- Miniature figures: policemen, firemen, ambulance driver, for instance.
- Domestic play equipment and play dough.

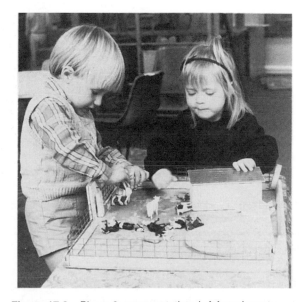

Figure 17.3 Phase 3: representational. A farm layout.

- A Wendy house, cot, doll bed, chairs, table, cooker, doll family.
- Dressing up clothes and other props for imaginative play. A toy telephone.
- Puppets and a puppet theatre.
- A miniature hospital and miniature hospital figures.
- Drawing materials: paper, pencils, crayons, felt-tip pens, brushes, liquid paint and palettes.

Phase 4: Constructive/latency/post-oedipal

A selection of constructive and creative activities for use in a group, as follows:

- Construction toys: Duplo, Lego, Helter-Skelter (Fig. 17.4a).
- Table games: picture lotto, picture dominoes (Fig. 17.4b).
- Clay or plasticine for modelling.
- Materials for collage: glue, paint, paper and bits to stick on.

To equip a new play therapy room, a selection of toys should be made from each of these phases.

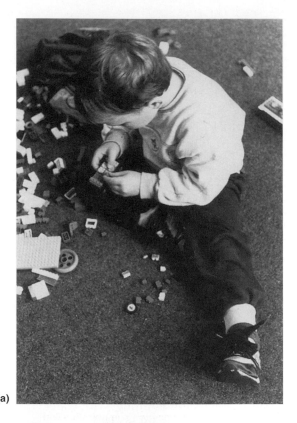

(a)

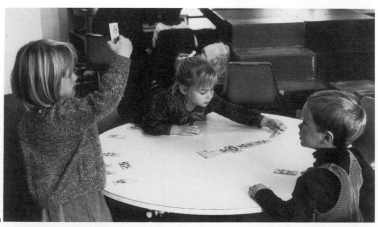

(b)

Figure 17.4   Phase 4: constructive. (**a**) Lego. (**b**) Picture dominoes.

SUMMARY

The many pressures of modern life are manifesting in various ways in today's society. Children may be either directly or indirectly affected by homelessness, unemployment, divorce, reconstituted families, drug or alcohol abuse and other life events.

Children who are suffering from a chronic or terminal illness, those who are looked after or adopted, children suffering from non-accidental injury or sexual abuse, suffer from excessive stress and unhappiness.

More and more adults under stress seek help in the form of counselling, therapy or self-help groups. It is essential that children under stress can receive appropriate help too. Therapeutic play is one form of help. Occupational therapists must contribute their knowledge of children and of their problems to the multi-disciplinary team. In that setting the occupational therapist is indeed the voice of the child.

REFERENCES

Axline V M 1947 Play therapy. Ballantine Books, New York

Bruce M A, Borg B 1987 Frames of reference in psychosocial occupational therapy. Slack, New Jersey

Bruner J S et al 1976 Play: its role in development and evolution. Penguin, Harmondsworth

Clarkson P, Pokorny M 1994 The handbook of psychotherapy. Routledge, London

College of Occupational Therapists 1990 Occupational therapy reference book 1990. Parke Sutton, Norwich

Ellis M J 1973 Why people play. Prentice Hall, New Jersey

Fidler G S, Fidler J W 1963 Occupational therapy: a communication process in psychiatry. MacMillan, London

Forward G E 1965 Group therapy for the emotionally disturbed child. Occupational Therapy 28 (9, 10, 11)

Freud S 1920 Beyond the pleasure principle. In: On metapsychology, vol. 2, 1984. Pelican Freud Library. Penguin, Harmondsworth

Gardner R A 1971 Therapeutic communication with children: the mutual story telling technique. Jason Aronson, New York

Gardner R A 1975 Psychotherapeutic approaches to the resistant child: the talking, feeling and doing game. Jason Aronson, New York

Geldard K, Geldard D 1997 Counselling children. Sage, London

Hall C S 1954 A primer of Freudian psychology. World Publishing Company, New York

Hawkins P, Shohet R 1989 Supervision in the helping professions. Open University Press, Buckingham

Hellersberg E F 1955 Child growth in play therapy. American Journal of Psychotherapy 9: 484–502

Jeffrey L I H 1979 Generic training in the psychological management of children and adolescents. Journal of Workers for Maladjusted Children 7(1): 32–41

Jeffrey L I H 1982a Occupational therapy in child and adolescent psychiatry: the future. British Journal of Occupational Therapy 45(10): 330–334

Jeffrey L I H 1982b Exploration of the use of therapeutic play in the rehabilitation of psychologically disturbed children. Fellowship thesis. Available from the British Library and the College of Occupational Therapists, London

Jeffrey L I H 1984 Developmental play therapy: an assessment and therapeutic technique in child psychiatry. British Journal of Occupational Therapy 47(3): 70–74

Jernberg A 1979 Theraplay. Jossey-Bass, San Francisco

Kaplan C, Telford R 1998 The butterfly children. Churchill Livingstone, Edinburgh

Kazdin A E 1988 Child psychotherapy. Pergamon Press, Oxford

Klein M 1932 The psychoanalysis of children. Hogarth Press, London

Levy D 1939 Release therapy. American Journal of Orthopsychiatry 9: 713–736

Menaker E 1982 Otto Rank: a rediscovered legacy. Columbia University Press, New York

Miller S 1973 The advisory psychology of play. Penguin, Harmondsworth

NHS Health Advisory Service 1995 A thematic review of child and adolescent mental health services – together we stand. HMSO, London

O'Connor K J 1982 The color your life technique. In: Schaefer C, O'Connor K J (eds) Handbook of play therapy. Wiley, New York

Peller L E 1952 Models of children's play. Mental Hygiene 36: 66–83

Richmond P G 1970 An introduction to Piaget. Routledge and Kegan Paul, London

Rogers C R 1967 On becoming a person. Constable, London

Safer A 1965 Conjoint play therapy for the young child and his parent. Archives of General Psychiatry 13: 320–326

Schiffer M 1971 The therapeutic play group. Allen and Unwin, London

Silveira W R, Trafford G 1988 Children need groups. Aberdeen University Press, Aberdeen

Slavson S R, Schiffer M 1975 Group psychotherapies for children. International Universities Press, New York

Villeneuve C 1979 The specific participation of the child in family therapy. American Academy of Child Psychiatry 44–53

World Health Organization 1992 The ICD 10 classification of mental and behaviour disorders. WHO, Geneva

FURTHER READING

Overviews of the field

Dodds J B 1967 A child psychotherapy primer. Human Sciences Press, New York

Haworth M R 1964 Child psychotherapy practice and theory. Basic Books, New York

Jeffrey L I H 1982a Occupational therapy in child and adolescent psychiatry: the future. British Journal of Occupational Therapy 45(10): 330–334

Jeffrey L I H 1982b Exploration of the use of therapeutic play in the rehabilitation of psychologically disturbed children. Fellowship thesis: available from the British Library and the College of Occupational Therapists, London

Oaklander V 1978 Windows to our children. Real People Press, Utah

Schaefer C 1976 Therapeutic use of child's play. Aronson, New York

Schaefer C, O'Connor K (eds) 1962 Handbook of play therapy. Wiley, New York

Recent publications, 1990–2000

Carroll J 1998 Introduction to therapeutic play. Blackwell Science, Oxford

Cattenach A 1992 Play therapy with abused children. Jessica Kingsley, London

Cattenach A 1994 Play therapy: where the sky meets the underworld. Jessica Kingsley, London

Cattenach A 1997 Children's stories in play therapy. Jessica Kingsley, London

Copley B, Forryan B 1987 Therapeutic work with children and young people. Robert Royce, London

Geldard K, Geldard D 1997 Counselling children. Sage Publications, London

Gil E 1991 The healing power of play. Guilford Press, London

Jennings S 1994 Play therapy. Blackwell Scientific, Oxford

Jennings S 1997 Introduction to developmental play therapy. Jessica Kingsley, London

Kaplan C, Telford R 1998 The butterfly children. Churchill Livingstone, Edinburgh

McMahon L 1992 The handbook of play therapy. Tavistock/Routledge, London

Ryan V, Wilson K 1996 Case studies in nondirective play therapy. Baillière Tindall, London

Varma V P (ed) 1992 The secret life of vulnerable children. Routledge, London

Webb N B 1991 Play therapy with children in crisis. Guilford Press, London

West J 1992 Child centred play therapy. Edward Arnold, London

Wilson K, Kendrick P, Ryan V 1992 Play therapy – a non-directive approach for children. Ballière Tindall, London

Psychoanalytic psychotherapy

Boston M, Szur R 1983 Psychotherapy with severely deprived children. Routledge and Kegan Paul, London

Bettelheim B 1978 The uses of enchantment. Penguin, Harmondsworth

Copley B, Forryan C 1987 Therapeutic work with children and young people. Robert Royce, London

Daws D, Boston M 1977 The child psychotherapist and problems of young people. Wildwood House, London

Freud A 1966 Normality and pathology in childhood. Hogarth Press, London

Freud S 1909 Analysis of a phobia in a five year old boy. In: Case Histories, vol. 10, 1977. Pelican Freud Library. Penguin, Harmondsworth

Freud S 1920 Beyond the pleasure principle. In: On metapsychology, vol 11, 1984. Pelican Freud Library. Penguin, Harmondsworth

Klein M Reprinted 1975 The psychoanalysis of children. Hogarth Press, London

Lowenfield M 1968 Play in childhood. Cedric Chivers, London

Winnicot D W 1971 Therapeutic consultations in child psychiatry. Hogarth, London

Winnicot D W 1980 The piggle. Penguin, Harmondsworth

Nondirective play therapy

Axline V M 1969 Play therapy. Ballantine Books, New York

Axline V M 1971 Dibs: in search of self. Penguin Books, Harmondsworth

Kaplan C, Telford R 1998 The butterfly children. Churchill Livingstone, Edinburgh

Relationship therapy

Allen F H 1942 Psychotherapy with children. Norton, New York

Menaker E 1982 Otto Rank: a rediscovered legacy. Columbia University Press, New York

Moustakas C E 1973 Children in play therapy. Aronson, New York

Moustakas C E 1979 Psychotherapy with children. Harper and Row, New York

Rank O 1978 Truth and reality. Norton, New York

Rank O 1978 Will therapy. Norton, New York

Taft J 1933 The dynamics of therapy in a controlled relationship. Macmillan, New York

Developmental play therapy

Hall C S 1954 A primer of Freudian psychology. World Publishing, New York

Hellersberg E F 1955 Child growth in play therapy. American Journal of Psychotherapy 9: 484–502

Jeffrey L I H 1984 Developmental play therapy: an assessment and therapeutic technique in child psychiatry. British Journal of Occupational Therapy 47(3): 70–74

Peller L E 1952 Models of children's play. Mental Hygiene 36: 66–83

Peller L E 1954 Libidinal phases, ego development and play. Psychoanalytical Study of the Child 9: 178–198

Directed play therapy

Gardner R A 1971 Therapeutic communication with children: the mutual story telling technique. Aronson, New York

Jernberg A 1979 Theraplay. Jossey-Bass, San Francisco

Levy D 1939 Release therapy. Journal of Orthopsychiatry 9: 713–736

Nickerson E, O'Laoughlin K (eds) 1982 Action orientated therapies. Human Resource Development Press, Amherst

O'Connor K J 1982 The color your life technique. In: Schaefer C, O'Connor K J (eds) Handbook of play therapy. Wiley, New York

Schaefer C, Reid S (eds) 1986 Game play: therapeutic use of childhood games. Wiley, New York

Group play therapy

Forward G E 1965 Group therapy for the emotionally disturbed child. Occupational Therapy 28(9, 10, 11)

Ginott H G 1961 Group psychotherapy with children. McGraw-Hill, New York

Schiffer M 1971 The therapeutic play group. Allen and Unwin, London

Silveira W R, Trafford G 1988 Children need groups. Aberdeen University Press, Aberdeen

Slavson S R 1945 An introduction to group therapy. International Universities Press, New York

Slavson S R, Schiffer M 1975 Group psychotherapies for children. International Universities Press, New York

Family therapy

Safer A 1965 Conjoint play therapy for the young child and his parent. Archives of General Psychiatry 13: 320–326

Villeneuve C 1979 The specific participation of the child in family therapy. American Academy of Child Psychiatry 44–53

Client groups

18

Acute psychiatry

Lynn Yarwood   Valerie Johnstone

INTRODUCTION

Acute mental health problems are those which are serious and which include a high degree of risk of harm to self or others. The acute episode may occur as a relapse of an enduring mental health problem, as a reaction to significant life events or as the first presentation of an illness. Occupational therapists work with clients with acute mental health problems in a variety of settings. These include:

- acute admission in-patient units
- day hospitals
- community services
- specialised units for people suffering from a specific disorder, for example eating disorders
- a combination of the above (e.g. partial hospitalisation programmes).

Local policies and resources, along with client need, determine the treatment setting for the client. Community care means that many clients receive treatment in their home environment; however, hospital admission may be necessary, particularly if there is risk of harm to self or to others, self-neglect or medication issues. Clients who are admitted to an acute psychiatric in-patient unit are usually severely ill and have experienced deterioration in their ability adequately to fulfil their normal daily roles. A period of hospitalisation means loss of contact with familiar daily activities. Having to cope with the strange physical environment, abnormal sociocultural surroundings and unfamiliar pattern of activities may intensify feelings of stress, anxiety and role dysfunction.

The main purposes of admission are to:

- provide a thorough assessment
- initiate treatment
- reduce symptoms
- provide a place of safety
- plan discharge and reintegration into the community.

Other chapters outline the various community settings in which the occupational therapist may work. The acute inpatient unit setting will be described here.

THE ACUTE IN-PATIENT UNIT SETTING

These units, which may be single-sex or mixed and have a bed occupancy of up to 30, are commonly placed within either a psychiatric or a general hospital. Some units only admit clients with a particular illness, while in others, clients with a wide variety of diagnoses may be found. Communal sitting and dining are the norm, with the old dormitory-style wards of the past rapidly being replaced with single and sometimes *en suite* bedrooms. However, the importance of increasing the client's right to privacy can create problems when clients need close observation for their own safety. Careful consideration has to be given to the design of the accommodation to minimise potential risks and allow discreet observation of the occupant by staff.

Many clients are unable to leave the ward for various reasons during periods of the admission therefore an area of the ward needs to be available for those who wish to participate in a range of recreational, social and therapeutic activities. Facilities for clients to participate in activities off the unit are also essential as this can help reduce feelings of frustration and containment. In addition, provision should be made for clients, if they so desire, to carry on with some of their normal daily routines. For example kitchen facilities may be available on the ward to enable patients to prepare simple meals, and laundry facilities for washing and ironing.

Informal and formal admissions

The majority of clients are admitted to hospital on an informal basis which means that they come into hospital voluntarily. However, some clients who are suffering from a mental illness may be detained formally under a section of either the Mental Health Act 1983 (DoH 1983) or the Mental Health (Scotland) Act 1984 for assessment or treatment. These Acts are utilised where there are concerns regarding the health and safety of the client and/or there is a need to protect others.

The multidisciplinary team

A typical multidisciplinary team (MDT) on an acute in-patient unit may include nurses, medical staff, psychologists, social workers, physiotherapists, art therapists and occupational therapists. In order to plan effective services for the aftercare of clients, community staff, such as community psychiatric nurses, social workers and community-based occupational therapists, should also be recognised as vital members.

Due to the often volatile nature of acute units and the need for interventions to be specific and intensive, effective communication within the team is essential. The role of each member needs to be clearly identified and agreed by the team to ensure that interventions are effective and carried out efficiently and safely. In order to do this, the occupational therapist must develop assertiveness skills that can be used to negotiate and define role expectations and ensure that the team and the client have a clear understanding of the role of occupational therapy including referral systems, assessment procedures and interventions used. It is also essential to have a knowledge of risk issues and of the individual client's mental health status – which can change within hours – according to the Mental Health Act 1983 or the Mental Health (Scotland) Act 1984. Daily contact with other team members and the use of multidisciplinary notes can greatly enhance this communication process. (See Ch. 10 for further information about the multidisciplinary team.)

Current issues within acute in-patient psychiatry

The nature of acute wards has changed, particularly over the past two decades. Clients who are admitted have more acute symptoms than in the past but tend to spend less time on the unit (Moore 1998). This preference for short-term admissions emerged in the early 1970s as a result of the rising costs of hospital care and the increasing effectiveness and availability of medication (Crory et al 1974). However, a new problem has arisen. Figures issued by the Department of Health (1995) showed that admissions in recent years have risen by 50%, with some units consistently having a bed occupancy rate of over 100%. This has increased the pressure on beds and led to even shorter admissions.

Moore (1998) discussed the findings of the Acute Care Inpatient Study (ACIS), a 3-year nationwide study which highlighted the effect that patients being admitted with more acute symptoms and the decreased length of stay has on the role of therapeutic interventions and activity. It found that, although acute units are fairly successful at reducing clients' symptoms and catering for basic physical needs, wider, long-term needs are not being adequately met.

The emphasis on symptom reduction and short-term admission has implications for the occupational therapist. The validity of the role of occupational therapy in this setting and the value of working with clients who are acutely ill is sometimes questioned, particularly when resources are scarce. Among the problems that may be encountered by occupational therapists are job dissatisfaction and frustration from rarely seeing clients' goals being met, the inability to address long-term functional problems adequately and emotional strain resulting from working with clients in a state of acute distress.

Nevertheless, occupational therapists have a key role in meeting some of the wider needs identified in the acute care in-patient study and must be confident that the interventions they provide are appropriate to the in-patient setting and effective in meeting both the short- and long-term functional needs of clients. The problems related to shorter admission can be overcome with the development of a clearly defined theoretical framework which allows the occupational therapist to provide effective interventions which meet the client's needs within the short period of available time.

Readmission and relapse

In an acute psychiatric setting, it is not uncommon to meet some of the clients on more than one occasion. This may be because of a period of relapse in their mental state, frequent episodes of crisis, or a combination of the two. The term 'revolving door syndrome' is frequently used to describe this group of clients as they are regularly readmitted to hospital. It is essential that all members of the team, including the occupational therapist, are aware of any attitudes of scepticism or a sense of failure in both themselves and the client on such occasions. The factors which contribute to readmission and relapse are certainly worth examining while withholding judgement and bias. It may be that the client functions at his best with regular periods of hospitalisation, almost 'topping up' his skills and strategies to cope with daily life. The fact that the client has survived in the community since the last admission to hospital can be considered a success rather than a failure. Whatever the reasons for readmission, each individual client is worthy of reassessment and subsequent intervention.

OCCUPATIONAL THERAPY IN THE ACUTE SETTING

Attitudes, principles and core beliefs

Many texts exist which identify and examine the core values of occupational therapy and related disciplines (Mocellin 1988, Cynkin & Robinson 1990, Kielhofner 1992, Hopkins & Smith 1993, Hagedorn 1995, Yerxa 1998). Although the aim of this chapter is not to reiterate or summarise this wealth of information, it does seem relevant to highlight the values which are most pertinent to acute psychiatry. Thus, the practice of occupational therapy in acute psychiatry can be considered within a philosophical context and with an understanding of core values, assumptions and beliefs.

The uniqueness of occupational therapy lies in its focus on occupation as central in promoting and maintaining health and well-being (Law et al 1998). When an individual experiences an acute psychiatric illness, whether in hospital or not, it is likely that his ability to engage in the meaningful daily activities that support a range of occupations has diminished. In this situation, medical models can dominate as a reductionist approach is utilised and the search is on to identify symptoms and alleviate illness. If the individual is admitted to hospital, he will also experience a significant and relatively sudden environmental change which lessens his chances of maintaining any degree of normal daily life and routine. At this time the occupational therapist has an essential role to play in the promotion of independent and meaningful occupations and activities.

A sound understanding of illness allows the occupational therapist to appreciate the client's situation and work in parallel with the multidisciplinary team. However, the occupational therapist must also understand occupational therapy concepts of health to be able to offer a unique contribution to intervention that is grounded in the philosophical basis of the profession.

Occupational therapy theory

Occupational science is an emerging discipline that aims to study systematically all aspects of the relationship between humans and occupation (Wilcock 1991, Yerxa 1993). It searches for evidence that can be used to justify the historical assumptions and beliefs of the occupational therapy profession. Such evidence can be used to inform the practice of occupational therapy. Furthermore, there seems to be increasing emphasis on the idea that health is not just the

absence of illness, but is a state which reflects quality of life and experiences of well-being (Wilcock 1998, Yerxa 1998).

When someone is suffering from an acute psychiatric illness, attention is commonly focused on symptom reduction, medical treatment and protection of the client within a safe, caring and supportive environment. This practice is essential and extremely effective, however, the occupational needs of individuals are also paramount at this time. Since occupational scientists suggest that occupational deprivation can be detrimental to health (Wilcock 1991), it would seem that alleviation of symptomatology and illness in isolation is insufficient for a healthy recovery.

An area of study which is of particular interest to occupational therapists is that of flow theory. Emerson (1998) reviewed the related literature, making particular reference to the work of Csikszentmihalyi, who has explored flow theory in depth, and suggests that flow is a subjective psychological state that exists when an individual is totally involved in an activity. To achieve flow, individuals must be engaged in the 'just right' challenge; the essential skill of the occupational therapist is, therefore, to find activities which can engage people in the acute stage of an illness. During an acute illness, clients can become immersed in symptoms and distress. It can be argued, however, that to reach some level of flow state can not only reduce symptoms but also promote a healthier state of mind. Although the symptoms and worries of clients do not disappear, some quality time out can ease their distress and allow them to feel more able to cope with their situation.

Motivation and change

Motivation theory has been widely researched, particularly in the field of psychology (Bernstein et al 1988). The word motivation comes from *movere*, the Latin word meaning 'to move'. It can be further defined as the influences that account for initiation, direction, intensity and persistence of behaviour (Geen et al 1984). The study of motivation focuses on the internal and external influences that might drive a person to act.

Motivation is a key focus in acute psychiatry. Understanding what it is that motivates each individual is essential for treatment to be effective. All aspects of motivation should be considered, from basic instincts and drives through to the need to maximise one's potential. These motives are clearly defined in Maslow's hierarchy of needs which indicates that basic physiological and safety needs must be at least partly satisfied before needs for belongingness and love, esteem and self-actualisation can influence an individual's behaviour (Maslow 1968).

It is not unusual in the field of psychiatry to hear the term 'resistance' being used when an individual does not seem to be complying with treatment. Although this idea of resistance can be understood from a variety of theoretical frameworks, De Shazer (1988) questioned this concept when he talked of the 'death of resistance' within the field of brief psychotherapies. He believes that such a phenomenon simply indicates that the client's and the professional's goals are different.

Sociologists have explored ideas that include the sick role and the patient career. In practice these are often referred to when it is thought an individual has a preference for living in a hospital setting and seemingly enjoying the benefits of illness. This is a crucial time to revisit concepts of motivation and, with the client, explore patterns and stages of change.

Prochaska & Di Clemente (1983) developed a model of change which is particularly useful to consider when the client is thought to have some degree of control over his behaviour. Stages of change identified in this model include pre-contemplation, contemplation, action and maintenance. Intervention will typically vary depending on the stage the client is at. Examples may include motivational interviewing during pre-contemplation, or support to develop coping strategies during maintenance.

The main treatment tool used by occupational therapists is that of meaningful activity which meets client's goals. However, the context and the nature of the activity must be carefully considered, agreed and planned in collaboration with the client. Failure to do so could result in 'resistance' since the goals are wrong, the motives are not important or the stage of change has been misjudged. For example, a young male client may tell the occupational therapist he likes to play pool with his friends. The occupational therapist then assumes that pool would be a useful activity to use to help develop a therapeutic relationship with the client. However, the client disagrees or simply does not want to play. This may be because the motives – which could include social contact with friends, time away from parents or the consumption of alcohol and banter while playing – are missing. It can therefore be seen that the context of activity must be considered to achieve therapeutic outcomes.

DIAGNOSIS

Occupational therapists are not primarily concerned with diagnosis or the application of a medical model but do work within medical settings where their role is to analyse the relationship between health, illness and the effects on occupational functioning. It is essential that a sound understanding of illness, disability and concepts of health exist in the profession. Mental illness usually develops as a result of a combination of biological, psychological and social influences. The occupational therapist, therefore, has to examine the relationship between clinical presentation and function within a biopsychosocial perspective.

The range of disorders encountered in an acute psychiatric setting is diverse. Although similarities exist between diagnostic groups, each client will differ in presentation. For example, no two clients suffering from schizophrenia are the same or have the same needs. During the acute phase, two clients may both hear voices, but for one this symptom may result in high levels of distress and agitation while the other may withdraw from daily life and spend most of the time in bed.

The art of occupational therapy is to collaborate with the client to examine effects on function and to define associated needs. It is therefore inappropriate for an occupational therapist to treat each client according to diagnosis. Instead, every client should be approached as an individual, with emphasis placed on how their symptoms affect their ability to function in daily occupations.

The following section will briefly introduce the main categories of diagnosis followed by a general appraisal of the effects of illness on function.

SCHIZOPHRENIA

Schizophrenia can occur at any age with peak onset in late adolescence or early adulthood. There are a number of possible causes for this illness including biological, psychological and social factors. Prognosis is influenced by the nature of the initial presentation with acute onset usually indicating a good prognosis and slow, insidious onset indicating poor long-term outcomes. Furthermore, because the prodromal changes often start to appear in adolescence or early adulthood, the normal psychological, social and emotional milestones of development can be interrupted. The illness can have a devastating effect on both the individual concerned and their family.

Clinical features

The symptoms that have been considered as diagnostic of the condition have been termed 'first rank' symptoms by the German psychiatrist Kurt Schneider (Kendell & Zealley 1988), and consist of:

- *Auditory hallucinations.* The patient hears voices speaking his thoughts out loud and/or he hears voices having a conversation about him or commenting on his actions.
- *Thought withdrawal/insertion.* This is the sensation of thoughts being put in or being taken away from the patient's mind.
- *Thought broadcasting.* The sensation of thoughts being broadcast to others.
- *External control of emotions.* The client feels controlled by an external influence.
- *Delusions.* These are strong beliefs that the client holds in the face of logical argument.

- *Somatic passivity.* The patient experiences bodily sensations imposed by some external agency.

Other features may include visual, tactile or olfactory hallucinations.

The chronic illness may have a similar presentation but is primarily characterised by thought disorder and negative symptoms such as:

- Reduced levels of activity
- Lack of motivation
- Flattened affect
- Social withdrawal.

Treatment

As the causes of this illness are complex, so is the treatment, which includes:

- *Medication.* The use of antipsychotic drugs is common although there are often undesirable side-effects. These drugs are effective in treating the first rank symptoms. In recent years increasing emphasis has been placed on the treatment of negative symptoms which define the chronic illness.
- *Psychosocial interventions.* These include psychoeducation, family interventions, cognitive therapy, interventions which address social functioning.

AFFECTIVE (MOOD) DISORDERS

The term affective (mood) disorder is applied to conditions where the primary manifestation is a disturbance of affect, either depression or elation. The possible causes of these disorders include genetic and biochemical factors along with early life experiences and stressful life events. These disorders are commonly categorised as:

- *Unipolar,* where the presentation is either of mania alone or, more commonly, depression alone
- *Bipolar,* where episodes of both mania and depression are experienced.

Clinical features

The clinical features of the affective disorders depend on the presenting phase of the illness.

The terms endogenous and reactive are used to classify depression. Reactive depression usually follows some life crisis such as bereavement or the loss of a job, and endogenous is so named if the depression appears unrelated to external events and there is evidence of diurnal variation of mood with accompanying sleep disturbance. However, it is often difficult to distinguish between the two types and their presentation is similar. The term hypomania is used to describe a less severe episode of mania. See Table 18.1 for the clinical features of affective disorders.

Treatment of mania

- *Medication*. In the acute phase, medication, including antipsychotic drugs, is used to reduce elation, overactivity and delusional ideas. Mood stabilisers are often added to the regime at this stage or a later stage with the aim of preventing future relapse.
- *Support and environment*. It is essential that the client experiencing mania be supported in a protected environment which avoids overstimulation. Failure to do so could result in the client acting on their beliefs, which could have devastating consequences following recovery.

Treatment of depression

- *Medication*. A variety of antidepressants is available.
- *Electroconvulsive therapy (ECT)*. This is used when a rapid response to treatment is required to avoid a serious risk to health. However, it must be used cautiously when treating the depressive phase of a bipolar illness since it can elevate mood, resulting in mania.
- *Provision of basic needs*. Acutely depressed clients can require assistance to meet their nutritional, sleep and self-care needs.
- *Psychological*. Supportive counselling, cognitive therapy and the psychotherapies can all be effective in the treatment of depression.

PERSONALITY DISORDERS

Personality disorders are described as common and difficult to treat by Waldinger (1990) who

Table 18.1 Clinical features of affective (mood) disorders

	Mania	Depression
Mood	Characterised by elevated mood, excessive cheerfulness and optimism and irritability	Depressed, miserable, sad with diurnal variation
Activity	There is a marked increase in activity levels with evidence of restlessness, distractability and disinhibition	Energy levels are reduced, with evidence of psychomotor retardation and poverty of movement. Apathy and agitation can exist along with a deterioration of cognitive functioning (i.e. concentration and memory)
Speech	Speech is fast and pressured, flitting from topic to topic (flight of ideas). Associations are casual and often triggered by rhymes or puns	Speech is impoverished, monotonous and slow; in severe cases clients can become mute
Ideation	Ideas and beliefs are commonly grandiose in nature with excessive self-confidence. Delusions can exist in relation to religion, persecution, wealth and power	Feelings, ideas or delusions of guilt, unworthiness and hopelessness with hypochondriasis and suicidal ideation
Physical	Disturbances of sleep and appetite are common features of mania. If symptoms are not treated, clients can suffer from exhaustion, rapid weight loss, malnutrition and dehydration	Sleep disturbance, appetite and weight loss, loss of libido, fatigue and general aches and pains

explores this diagnostic category in detail. The question is asked, when do personality traits become personality disorders? Acknowledgement is given to the paucity of knowledge which exists about the causes of specific personality disorders, although some assumptions and theories refer to deprived or traumatic childhood experiences, hereditary character traits and other biological, environmental, social and psychological factors. Generally speaking, the personality disorders are characterised by:

- inflexible and maladaptive responses to stress
- nearly all areas of a person's life are affected
- the individual is seemingly untroubled by the illness and does not see himself as others see him
- the individual feels the problem is external and blames the environment
- the individual's unacceptable behaviour commonly results in rejection by others
- further complications, including psychotic episodes, suicide, self-harm, depression, antisocial behaviour and substance misuse
- difficulty in sustaining stable relationships
- difficulty learning from past experiences.

There are many recognised types of personality disorder, which range from dependent, schizoid and obsessive-compulsive to borderline and psychopathic personality disorders.

Treatment

Treatment is considered difficult since, in the field of acute psychiatry, people diagnosed with personality disorder often present with accompanying complications such as depressive or psychotic symptoms. These symptoms can be treated and the treatment of the personality disorder itself can vary from psychodynamic psychotherapy, to address early life trauma, to cognitive behavioural therapy or social skills training.

CONFUSIONAL STATES

A client may be admitted to hospital in an acute confusional state. This can be a feature of several psychiatric disorders, although possible physical causes must also be considered. The team has an important role in assessing the cause of the confusion before treatment can begin and the following must also be considered:

Acute (toxic) confusional states

These occur in physical illnesses such as infection, intoxication and vitamin B deficiencies, and are usually of a short duration. They have a rapid onset characterised by:

- clouding of consciousness: disturbance of awareness of the environment, lack of attention and concentration
- disorientation for time and place
- hallucinations.

Treatment will depend on the underlying physical cause of the confusion.

Chronic organic states

Dementia

This is a progressive state of permanent intellectual impairment characterised by:

- clouding of consciousness
- memory impairment
- disintegration of personality
- cognitive impairment
- disorientation for time, place and/or person
- emotional lability
- hallucinations
- behavioural changes.

The treatment of dementia is described in Chapter 21.

SUBSTANCE MISUSE

Abuse of alcohol or drugs and other substances is generally characterised by a maladaptive pattern of alcohol or substance use leading to significant impairment or distress, as manifested by the following clinical features (the presentation will depend largely on the type of alcohol or drug use, the social environment and the personality of the individual):

- *Psychological*. Disorientation, delirium, disinhibition, irritability, aggressiveness, depression, paranoid ideas, jealousy, suspiciousness, hallucinations, memory impairment.
- *Social*. Neglect of family, work and social obligations, financial difficulties, conflict with law and society, housing problems, loss of interest in social activities.
- *Physical*. Deterioration of self-care, loss of appetite, ataxia, tremors, gastric problems, hepatitis.

Treatment

Detoxification. The client must be detoxified before meaningful therapy can begin. Usually, this can be done as an outpatient; however, some clients will be admitted to specialised units or general acute units for detoxification, particularly if there has been failure of outpatient withdrawal, insufficient psychosocial supports, there is severe impairment, or the living situation encourages continued substance misuse.

Psychosocial. This will focus on confronting denial, fostering an identification as a recovering person, recognising the negative consequences of the misuse, avoiding situational cues that stimulate craving and formulating support plans and lifestyle changes.

Psychotherapy. This is useful when it focuses on the reasons for the client's substance misuse.

Behaviour therapy. Teaching the user ways to reduce anxiety, relaxation techniques, assertiveness skills, self-control skills and new strategies to master the environment.

ANXIETY AND STRESS RELATED DISORDERS

Anxiety states may form part of any psychiatric disorder or may occur on their own. Although anxiety is a normal response in certain situations, it becomes pathological when it occurs:

- for no apparent reason
- as a result of an actual event, but its duration and intensity are out of proportion
- as a specific fear of objects or situations, for example a fear of open spaces.

The anxiety and stress disorders include:

- phobic anxiety disorders
- panic disorder
- generalised anxiety disorder
- obsessive-compulsive disorder
- post traumatic stress disorder.

Clinical features

Physical symptoms include dry mouth, diarrhoea, nausea, tightness of chest, hyperventilation, palpitations, increased frequency of micturition, blurred vision, dizziness, headache, sleep disturbance, fatigue, restlessness and muscle tension.

Behavioural symptoms include social withdrawal, the use of maladaptive coping strategies such as alcohol misuse, avoidance of anxiety provoking situations and panic behaviour which results in leaving the difficult situation abruptly.

Psychological symptoms include apprehension, feeling of dread, irritability, poor concentration, distractibility, thinking errors, sensitivity to noise and poor memory.

Treatment

Before treatment for anxiety commences, it is essential to consider a differential diagnosis, as there may be an underlying physical cause for the symptoms. Treatment may include:

- *Physical symptoms*: medication, relaxation therapy
- *Behavioural symptoms*: systematic desensitisation, flooding
- *Psychological symptoms*: cognitive therapy, counselling, psychotherapy.

EATING DISORDERS

The eating disorders have been described as a widespread clinical problem. The onset of these disorders is typically during adolescence, with a high prevalence among women. A variety of causative factors have been considered, including genetic and hormonal factors, psychological disturbance, familial relationships and social factors.

Anorexia nervosa

Anorexia nervosa is a syndrome of self-starvation with criteria for diagnosis including a below standard body weight, a profound wish to be thin, an intense fear of obesity, deliberate weight loss and amenorrhoea. The main features include:

- a distorted body image and sense of body size
- vomiting and purging
- excessive exercise
- decreased libido
- particular avoidance of carbohydrates in the diet
- extremely rigid rules about food and eating.

There are many physical complications which are consequential of the illness and, at worst, extremely low body weight with symptoms of malnutrition can result in danger to life.

Bulimia nervosa

Bulimia nervosa is a disorder characterised by frequent episodes of binge eating with self-induced vomiting and laxative and diuretic misuse. In contrast to anorexia nervosa, individuals suffering from bulimia are generally aware that their eating patterns are abnormal but feel unable to stop or change their eating behaviour. The body weight of the individual usually fluctuates and depression is common following binges. There are a number of associated physical complications, which are a result of frequent vomiting.

Treatment

This may occur in a variety of settings depending on the client's needs and resources available. Intervention includes physical treatments, medication and the behavioural, cognitive and psychotherapies. Where there is significant risk to health due to weight loss, the priority of treatment is to increase body weight and satisfy nutritional needs before psychological treatment can commence.

THE OCCUPATIONAL THERAPY PROCESS

The occupational therapist working in an acute in-patient unit needs to develop specific skills in rapid assessment of needs, goal setting, prioritising key problems, providing effective short-term interventions and discharge planning which takes into consideration the long-term functional needs of the client.

Referral

Some units may operate a system of blanket referral whereby all clients admitted are assessed by the occupational therapist. More commonly, clients are referred according to individual needs following discussion with the multidisciplinary team. The preferred system will depend on a number of factors including staffing, resources, unit capacity and service philosophy. On receipt of the referral, the occupational therapist must first consider the level of priority of the needs of the client. This is essential when the demand for occupational therapy outweighs the resources available. Box 18.1 lists priority criteria within an acute in-patient occupational therapy service.

Consent to treatment

Central to occupational therapy philosophy is the importance of working closely with clients to determine treatment goals and outcomes. This collaborative relationship can be influenced in an acute psychiatric setting by:

- an individual refusing treatment or not being able to participate in the process
- the medical model
- client need as perceived by the team versus the client's personal wishes.

These are areas that must be addressed by the multidisciplinary team. Whatever decisions are made regarding treatment the occupational

Box 18.1 Priorities within as acute in-patient occupational therapy service

High priority
- There are concerns regarding health and safety at home
- The mental health problem has had a significant impact on the client's ability to perform daily tasks and essential life roles
- There is evidence of poor pre-morbid functioning which has contributed to the admission
- Poor support systems exist
- Functioning has significantly altered with poor indication of reasons why
- There is a clear relationship between stress, vulnerability and occupational balance
- Occupational deprivation has a significant impact on health

Low priority
- Need for direction in activity but no difficulty initiating or carrying these out
- Primary reason for referral is a medical programme (e.g. detox, medication review)
- Extracontractual referrals (ECRs) where rapid move on is expected

therapist must ensure that they are well justified and ethical.

Therapeutic relationships

The term therapeutic relationship is one used commonly in the treatment setting. It is, however, much more than a simple term. It is a rich, complex phenomenon which provides the basis for all therapeutic intervention. It is a relationship between therapist and client which respects the differences between personal and therapeutic boundaries and follows a process from establishing initial rapport to the development of trust, respect and collaboration. In the acute psychiatric setting, the occupational therapist needs to assess and treat individuals quickly and effectively. It is therefore essential for the occupational therapist to become an expert in therapeutic relationships and develop the ability to:

- establish rapport
- respect the wishes of the client
- use honesty and strive to develop a collaborative approach
- adapt to communicate effectively with all kinds of people.

Safety and risk issues

Whether occupational therapists are working with clients on a ward, in the community or in a client's home they must constantly be aware of clients' and their own safety and ensure that measures are in place to minimise risk.

The following must be carefully considered and decisions discussed and documented prior to contact with any client who has an acute mental health problem:

- policies and procedures regarding safety and risk (e.g. observation policy)
- outcomes of risk assessment
- views of the multidisciplinary team
- location of meeting place
- action plan in case of emergency
- informing someone of whereabouts and expected time of return
- alarm systems
- access to equipment or tools
- client history of violence
- content of hallucinations or delusional beliefs
- history of substance misuse
- risk of suicide.

Assessment

Once the referral has been discussed and agreed, the process of assessment is initiated. Information about a client's needs must be gathered and analysed within a short time by the occupational therapist working in the acute in-patient setting. Occupational therapists can utilise a variety of assessment tools. The method chosen will be influenced by:

- the reason for admission
- the client's mental state
- areas of need identified by the team
- areas of need identified by the client
- the preferred theoretical framework of the occupational therapy service and the team.

Assessment tools

The methods used may include:

- brief, regular contact with the client
- observation

Box 18.2	A typical week for a basic grade occupational therapist working in an acute in-patient unit				
	Monday	Tuesday	Wednesday	Thursday	Friday
8.30	Weekly planning meeting with OT team	Preparation for meeting	Supervision with senior OT	Clinical supervision with TI	Planning for sessions
9.30	Planning and preparation for sessions	Multidisciplinary team meeting	Preparation for sessions	Multidisciplinary team meeting	CPD forum/Basic grade support meeting
10.30	Relaxation group		Lunch group		Individual session
11.00		Initial interview		Initial interview	
11.30	Meeting with nurse to discuss client				Individual session
12.00	Notes	Treatment planning		Treatment planning	
12.30			Lunch		
1.00	Preparation for group	Preparation for group	Preparation for group	Preparation for home visit	Attend handover on the ward
1.30	Lifestyles group with senior OT	Pottery group with TI (technical instructor)	Activity group with senior OT and TI	Pre-discharge home visit to carry out community and daily living skills assessment	
2.00					Handover of a client to community OT
2.30.	Feedback from group and notes				
3.00		Feedback from group and notes	Feedback from group and notes		Notes and administration
3.30	Trust occupational therapy monthly staff meeting		Review with client	Writing report	
4.00		General administration (e.g. phone calls)			

- interview
- use of activity
- standardised assessment
- specific assessment (e.g. assessment of domestic skills).

Further information about methods of assessment can be found in Chapter 6.

Throughout the assessment, the occupational therapist gathers information about the client's:

- normal daily routine
- productivity, self-care and leisure roles
- perceptions of the factors which influence his function and occupations
- hopes, aspirations and goals
- strengths, abilities and achievements.

The occupational therapist works with the client to determine what is reasonable to accomplish in a short time, ensuring that goals are specific and realistic and using the initial and ongoing findings to form a plan of intervention.

Intervention

Occupational therapy intervention is subject to the same influences as those outlined in the assessment section, above. In addition to this, the resources available, skills of staff and the therapist's caseload will determine the nature of therapy.

Interventions used in this area are wide and varied and it is difficult to describe and justify every possibility. This section on intervention will therefore attempt to provide the reader with

an insight into one way that an occupational therapist and occupational therapy service may operate within an acute in-patient setting (see Boxes 18.2 and 18.3).

The two case studies in Boxes 18.4–18.7 attempt to consolidate the chapter content while considering the diversity of factors which may influence clinical reasoning and therapeutic outcomes in practice.

Evaluation

It is vital that occupational therapists examine both the processes and outcomes of their interventions in order to provide clients with a high

---

Box 18.3   An example of an occupational therapy group programme

	Monday	Tuesday	Wednesday	Thursday	Friday
AM	Relaxation	DIY group	Relaxation	Self-image	Anxiety management with nurse
	Gardening	Computer	Lunch (ladies)	Lunch (men's)	Mini-activity (arts and crafts)
PM	Lifestyles	Pottery	Activity group (Arts & crafts)	Fishing group	Creative writing
	Woodwork		Younger person's group	Pre-discharge	Woodwork

Box 18.4   Case example 1

Fiona is a 28-year-old woman who lives with her partner and two children, aged 5 and 2. She is well known to psychiatric services having been under the care of a consultant psychiatrist and CPN for over 9 years. She has been admitted to hospital on several occasions with a number of formal admissions when she has been detained under the Mental Health Act for assessment and treatment. Fiona's diagnosis is borderline personality disorder, which is complicated by frequent depressive episodes, alcohol and drug misuse, deliberate self-harm and a number of serious suicide attempts. It is believed that her mental health problems stem from a traumatic childhood when she was sexually, physically and emotionally abused. Surprisingly, Fiona has developed and sustained a reasonable relationship with her partner and with the support of her GP and health visitor has managed to care for her children appropriately. On this occasion Fiona was admitted to hospital informally following escalation in her depressive symptoms and considerable risk issues related to her alcohol

consumption and self-harm, with evidence of increased suicidal intent. Shortly after admission Fiona was discussed at the weekly multidisciplinary meeting. The team showed scepticism and believed that the main role of admission was to provide a safe environment and alleviate the crisis and considered Fiona a low priority for occupational therapy intervention. However, at the meeting the occupational therapist asked questions about Fiona's daily occupations, which seemed to have diminished with the deterioration in her mental health. It was agreed that the occupational therapist should assess Fiona on the basis that her occupational needs should be considered immediately, rather than waiting for her mental state to improve. The occupational therapist made explicit her beliefs about occupation and that improved occupational functioning might have a role to play in Fiona' recovery. However, she was also aware that her input would depend on Fiona's readiness to change and motivation to improve her lifestyle and therefore her state of health.

Box 18.5 Case example 1, part 2

Occupational therapist's thoughts and findings

Is this client a priority? Yes, there is evidence of the mental health problem having had a significant impact on ability to perform in daily tasks and essential life roles, poor pre-morbid functioning contributing to the admission, and occupational deprivation having an impact on health.

Need to familiarise self with Fiona quickly and decide the most appropriate form of assessment. Important to offer choice and respect wishes. Honesty and collaboration important to establish initial trust and start to develop therapeutic relationship.

It is essential to acknowledge and validate Fiona's situation without focusing totally on negatives; try to elicit details of strengths, competencies and exceptions to the problem.

A key motivating factor for Fiona is her children.

Need to assess Fiona's commitment and ability to plan for the future. Achievable goal setting is very important to both esteem and confidence while avoiding failure. Short-term goals are more successful when they are planned within the context of a longer-term outcome. If this is difficult for Fiona, the goals have to be smaller until she is able to think about her future.

There is evidence of feelings of low self-esteem affecting Fiona's occupational performance. The use of solution orientated techniques has begun to identify competencies. Her negative thoughts are affecting her daily activity and she has increasingly felt unable to cope. This has resulted in her ceasing many of her daily activities. Through the application of a cognitive behavioural approach Fiona can begin to recognise and appreciate improvement through successful participation in activity. This will reinforce changes in behaviour resulting from changes in thinking.

Due to the concerns of the team about the suicidal ideas that Fiona has been expressing, the kitchen environment must be safe and close supervision in place.

Fiona has been able to set herself some goals, which would help her achieve 'flow' and engage in problem-free time. We now need to think about steps towards achieving these.

The regular use of COPM (Canadian Occupational Performance Measure) will positively reinforce successful achievement as it considers the client's satisfaction with performance. Fiona will be provided with evidence of her abilities, which in turn will increase her self-esteem. The tool will assist Fiona to decide what she wants, needs and is expected to do in her daily life.

Actions

Brief introduction to Fiona to arrange further assessment. Honesty used when explaining reasons for occupational therapy referral.

Initial interview with Fiona took place in an interview room, at Fiona's request. Further explanation of occupational therapy and purpose of the interview (i.e. to gather information re occupations and functioning). Mutual decision not to discuss current problems in detail but for Fiona to be aware of occupational therapist's knowledge about her situation.

Fiona described feeling hopeless and helpless with very little opportunity for achievement and positive regard. She was able to recognise that there were times when she was less distressed, which was when she was busy helping her children. When asked what happens on the days that she feels she has been a good mother she describes spending time playing games and drawing with them. She also feels it is important that the children are well fed and she enjoys cooking for them and her husband.

Fiona was able to make a relationship between meaningful occupation and her state of health. She became more animated and expressive when talking about her abilities and important life roles. Fiona was asked to imagine herself in the future and think about a 'miracle'. The aim was to invite Fiona to think creatively about what she would like to be doing that would indicate a more satisfying life. The occupational therapist gathered information which described her miracle day, which included cooking for the family, wearing comfortable clothes and helping old people in a part time job.

Fiona was asked to think about a scale of 1–10, where 10 indicates her goals have been met. When asked to place herself on the scale Fiona put herself at a 2. She felt that simply planning her goals merited a notch on the scale. To get to a 3 on the scale she stated that she needed to do some cooking.

The occupational therapist suggested to Fiona that perhaps she would she like to bake some cakes for them to eat when they next visit. Fiona agreed but expressed anxieties about how she would manage. They explored what needed to happen for her to be successful and at the same time feel safe in the kitchen, and developed a plan based on this.

Fiona had a successful kitchen session with the occupational therapist and enjoyed seeing the children's faces when they visited later that day.

A week later, during an OT review, Fiona agreed to complete the COPM and through this identified her long-term goals. Scaling questions continued to be used.

Box 18.6 Case example 2

Alistair is a 54-year-old divorced man who lives alone and has little contact with his ex-wife and two adult children. His neighbour, with whom he has a good relationship, became concerned about him as he noticed a deterioration in his self-care and expressed his concerns to Alistair's GP. The GP referred Alistair to the community mental health team and a community psychiatric nurse carried out a home visit. This was followed by a joint visit with the consultant psychiatrist. They noted that Alistair displayed poverty of speech, appeared cowering and anxious, he was half dressed and his home was in a generally dirty and unkempt state with evidence of urinary and faecal incontinence. He was also disorientated in time, place and person. Alistair agreed to go into hospital informally.

Treatment during the first few days of admission consisted of basic nursing care as follows:

1. Building him up nutritionally
2. Addressing his self-care needs
3. Providing a safe environment
4. Assessment.

As his nutritional needs were met Alistair became less confused, however, it was noticed that the content of his speech was depressive, with ideas of guilt and unworthiness, and his sleep pattern was poor, as was his appetite. At the multidisciplinary meeting it was decided to commence antidepressant medication and the occupational therapist was asked to see him with the aim of:

- contributing to the ongoing assessment
- assessing daily living skills
- identifying his post discharge needs.

quality service, and with up-to-date, effective interventions. Finlay (1997) suggested that evaluation of what we do is fundamental to our integrity and confidence as therapists. Occupational therapists working in an acute psychiatric setting must ensure that interventions are evidence based and effective in meeting the needs of their client in a short period of time. Evaluation should take into account the following:

- evaluation of self through reflection and supervision
- regular evaluation with the client through the use of, for example, outcome measures, questionnaires
- Evaluation of the service by clinical audit, consumer surveys, outcome measures, views of the multidisciplinary team.

It is essential that any occupational therapy programme is flexible and is regularly reviewed and evaluated to ensure that the needs of the client group at any time are being met.

Discharge planning

Planning for discharge should begin at the time of admission and should involve all members of the multidisciplinary team, including community based staff (Canton 1984). In order to contribute effectively to this process, the occupational ther-

apist needs to have a good knowledge of community resources and ensure that clients are safe to return home and adequately prepared to cope with their normal environment. One of the frustrations often encountered by occupational therapists working in acute in-patient settings is that clients are discharged before successful completion of occupational therapy interventions. To alleviate this problem, short-term care must be viewed as part of the total spectrum of services. Managers should plan services that allow for cross-boundary working and flexibility in service provision with the in-patient occupational therapist being able to offer short-term follow-up or refer the client on to community based occupational therapists for longer-term intervention.

SUMMARY

This chapter has described the role of occupational therapy in acute psychiatry. The multidisciplinary team and current influences in this field have been introduced while inviting the reader to consider attitudes, principles and core beliefs which define practice. The types of illness experienced by clients have been briefly outlined and the effects on occupational functioning highlighted. The occupational therapy process within this setting has been demonstrated through practical examples.

Box 18.7 Case example 2, part 2

The occupational therapist's thinking and findings	Actions taken
I need to make an initial contact with this client.	Initial contact made on the ward. The occupational therapist found Alistair sitting in the dining room drinking a cup of tea on his own. The occupational therapist introduced herself to Alistair and asked him if he would mind having a chat with her, and asked where he would prefer to meet. Alistair chose a small sitting area. The occupational therapist briefly explained the role of occupational therapy and the reasons for the meeting. She told him that she was aware of the difficulties he was having at home prior to admission and asked if he would be willing to work with her to address some of the difficulties. She reassured him that his goals are important and that they could work together to achieve them. He agreed to meet with her again.
From the information I have gathered from the team, the initial contact needs to be brief and informal due to Alistair's anxieties, his withdrawn state, his difficulties in expressing himself and limited tolerance of people. The initial contact needs to be in a place familiar and comfortable for him.	
I need to begin to develop a therapeutic relationship with Alistair to gain his trust. Perhaps some problem-free talk would be useful to find out his competencies, desires, hopes and stage of change. His basic needs are partly being satisfied – is it possible to begin to look at the next stage? I will meet with him tomorrow and suggest that he make a cup of tea for us to drink while we talk. This is a cultural norm and will provide an appropriate environment for problem free talk. I can also begin to assess his ADL skills through the activity.	The occupational therapist talked to Alistair about his home life, his likes and dislikes, his hobbies and interests and his habits over a cup of tea, which the client made successfully. During this conversation Alistair mentioned that he used to enjoy art. The occupational therapist explored this further and found that Alistair became more animated as they talked and brighter at the occupational therapist's suggestion that he visit the occupational therapy department to look at the art materials available.
Competencies have been identified through the process of problem-free talk. Participation in art will provide a forum for assessment. This links with the belief of the relationship between occupation and health.	
When engaged in an activity that gives him pleasure and at which he is competent, objectively Alistair appears to reach a flow state. He can concentrate for periods of up to 1 hour, is animated and expressive, makes decisions and relates to others.	Alistair initially had 1–1 art sessions with the occupational therapist then agreed to join a mini-activity group and continued to attend regularly. After 2 weeks the occupational therapist and Alistair sat down to review progress and started to consider longer-term needs. At this review Alistair and the occupational therapist agreed what needed to happen for him to be able to return home.
Safety, skills and ability to manage at home independently need to be assessed. Alistair also needs to regain his confidences in his abilities.	Alistair engaged in four 1–1 sessions in the kitchen with the occupational therapist. He continued with his art session and started to do this independently outwith the art groups.
When a session is organised, Alistair can successfully and safely prepare himself a nutritious meal, his mental state has improved and discharge is imminent. However, can he maintain this independently in the community? His budgeting, meal planning and shopping skills still need to be assessed.	The occupational therapist and CPN carried out a home visit with Alistair to assess and identify continuing needs following discharge. Referral was made to community based occupational therapist to continue working with Alistair in the community and enable him to make a successful transition from hospital to community.

Occupational therapy services need to respond to a number of significant factors which may include:

- short admissions, pressure on beds and rapid turnover of clients
- poor role definition and role blurring
- dominance of the medical model
- lack of resources
- limited evidence base for practice
- flexible and weekend working.

Within the ever changing climate of health care, the future and success of occupational therapy in acute in-patient psychiatry is also dependent on efficient service delivery which is evidence based and responds to current trends. This challenge is paramount.

REFERENCES

Bernstein D A, Roy A, Srull T K, Wickens C D 1988 Psychology. Houghton Mifflin, Boston

Canton C L M 1984 The impact of discharge planning on chronic schizophrenic patients. Hospital and Community Psychiatry 35(3): 225–262

Crory S, Sebastian V, Mosey A C 1974 Acute short-term treatment in psychiatry. American Journal of Occupational Therapy 28: 401–406

Cynkin S, Robinson A M 1990 Occupational therapy and activities health: towards health through activities. Little Brown, Boston

Department of Health 1983 Mental Health Act 1983. HMSO, London

Department of Health 1995 Mental health in England. Statistical Bulletin. HMSO, London

De Shazer S 1988 Clues: investigating solution in brief therapy. Norton, New York

Emerson H 1998 Flow and occupation: a review of the literature. Canadian Journal of Occupational Therapy 65(1): 37–44

Finlay L 1997 The practice of psychosocial occupational therapy. Stanley Thornes, Cheltenham

Geen R G, Beatty W W, Arkin R M 1984 Human motivation: physiological, behavioural and social approaches. Allyn and Bacon, Boston

Hagedorn R 1995 Occupational therapy: perspectives and processes. Churchill Livingstone, Edinburgh

Hopkins H, Smith H (eds) 1993 Willard and Spackman's Occupational therapy, 8th edn. Lippincott, Philadelphia

Kendell R E, Zealley A K (eds) 1988 Companion to psychiatric studies. Churchill Livingstone, Edinburgh

Kielhofner G 1992 Conceptual foundations of occupational therapy. F A Davis, Philadelphia

Law M, Steinwender S, Leclair L 1998 Occupation health and wellbeing. Canadian Journal of Occupational Therapy 65(2): 81–91

Maslow A 1968 Towards a psychology of being. Van Nostrand, New York

Mocellin G 1988 A perspective on the principles and practice of occupational therapy. British Journal of Occupational Therapy 51(1): 4–7

Moore C 1998 Acute in-patient care could do better, says survey. Nursing Times 94(3): 54–56

Prochaska J O, DiClemente C C 1984 The transtheoretical approach – crossing traditional boundaries of therapy. Dow Jones Irwin, Illinois

Sainsbury Centre 1998 Acute problems: a survey of the quality of care in acute psychiatric wards. Sainsbury Centre, London

Waldinger R J 1990 Psychiatry for medical students, 2nd edn. American Psychiatric Press, Washington DC

Wilcock A A 1991 Occupational science. British Journal of Occupational Therapy 54(8): 297–300

Wilcock A A 1998 Occupation for health. British Journal of Occupational Therapy 61(8): 340–345

Yerxa E J 1993 Occupational science: a new source of power for participants in occupational therapy. Occupational Science: Australia 1(1): 3–10

Yerxa E J 1998 Health and the spirit of human occupation. American Journal of Occupational Therapy 52(6): 412–418

19

Long-term illness

Kath Snowden   Gary Molden
Sheila Dudley

INTRODUCTION

Increasing client independence and autonomy is the keystone of the rehabilitation process and should underpin all actions and planning in working with clients. While such a principle can apply to all circumstances regardless of the nature of the setting, whether this is an institution or the community, there are certain issues more particular to institutional practices. This chapter explores the multiple and complex issues which influence treatment within long-stay settings and also those which transcend setting and are fundamental to successful professional practice.

The most significant issue relating to the effect of particular settings upon the lives of clients is that of living in an institution. In such settings the system and organisation may seem to be of a rigid and begrudging nature. Opportunities for a client to practise or initiate skills, to change and grow as a person or to be independent and autonomous can be made difficult by institutional practices and routines, although these may be necessary in part to maintain certain levels of safety and competence in care and treatment.

It is often within these or similar boundaries that occupational therapists find themselves, either as students or as qualified professionals, eager to make a difference to another person's life. Success in this area lies ultimately in the ability to appreciate, understand and act on the multiple factors which affect the learning and uptake of skills. Equally, it lies in the ability to view individuals as important, not only in their own right, but also as people in a reciprocal and dynamic social structure which has shaped, and will continue to shape, their lives, and will also be shaped by their actions upon it. Accordingly, in this chapter information is provided on serious mental illness and medication. One major current model of schizophrenia which is particularly useful in informing approaches to the occupational therapy process is described and related to that process.

The effects of institutionalisation upon autonomy are examined with reference to the role of the therapist and the importance of therapeutic relationships in ameliorating them. Case examples are provided as illustrations of links between the clinical, ethical and professional factors involved in successful treatment outcomes. Finally, attention is drawn to relevant government legislation on the care of individuals with serious mental illness which, it is suggested, is equally relevant to care within institutions as in the community.

It is the study of such principles as a true understanding of the nature of serious mental illnesses, the complexity of factors which affect learning and the importance of context that informs the content of this chapter.

CLIENT DISORDERS

The disorders the occupational therapist will encounter in the long-stay environment are those that, by their very nature, have a significant and enduring impact on the individual's social and psychological functioning. The impairments that the illness cause are exacerbated by secondary handicaps and disabilities which necessitate the need for long-term supportive care.

Multiple problems

Most of the long-stay population suffer from chronic psychiatric illnesses, with about 80% suffering from schizophrenia. However, disproportionately high levels of other disabilities, such as learning difficulties, physical disabilities, epilepsy and sensory deficits, are also found in the long-stay population. These secondary disabilities often indicate individuals whose pre-morbid functioning was at a significantly lower level than the norm, and this has implications for personal and social functioning both prior to and, especially, following the onset of psychiatric illness.

Behavioural problems may also be encountered within the long-stay population and these may be a management problem, especially when they are aggressive, sexual or self-destructive in nature. There may also be behavioural problems associated with the nature of the institution.

What we see, therefore, is not just individuals with primary psychiatric disabilities but individuals who may be multiply handicapped and presenting with multiple problems. Some of them have been within 'the system' for many years.

Schizophrenia

Schizophrenia is the major mental illness encountered in the long-stay setting, therefore a description is necessary. It is a psychotic disorder characterised by a constellation of symptoms which affect the individual in the areas of thought, perception, affect and motor activity.

The diagnosis of schizophrenia has been a difficult one. However, since Schneider's (1959) identification of first and second rank symptoms, much research has been done in order to provide a standardised system for the reliable diagnosis of schizophrenia. These diagnostic systems include the PSE-CATEGO system (Wing et al 1974) developed in the UK, and DSM-IV (American Psychiatric Association 1995) in the USA.

Both these systems identify 'core symptoms' which correspond to Schneider's first rank symptoms and, as such, are used to make a diagnosis of schizophrenia. These can be categorised as follows:

1. *Auditory hallucinations*

- Hearing voice(s) commenting on one's thoughts or actions. These voices speak about the subject and refer to him in the third person.

- Hearing voices talking to each other about the subject (third party auditory hallucinations).

2. *Delusions of influence*

- Delusions of control; the subject feels that he is under the control of some force other than himself or, conversely, the subject may feel that he is able to control other people's will, mood or behaviour.
- Somatic passivity; the subject believes that external alien forces are penetrating his mind and body and interfering with bodily functions. These forces can be alien thoughts, radio waves, X-rays or microwaves.

3. *Thought disorders*

- Thought insertion; the subject experiences thoughts that are not recognised as his own.
- Thought broadcast; the subject hears his thoughts spoken out loud or believes that the thoughts are broadcast so that others can hear them.
- Thought block/withdrawal; the subject experiences sudden stopping of his thoughts. In the absence of any other explanation, the subject may feel someone has taken thoughts from out of his head.

Although these symptoms are identified for diagnostic purposes as core symptoms, they are not the only ones experienced. Individuals may have visual, tactile or olfactory hallucinations; they may have delusions that events or colours have special meanings, for example that people with grey hair can read the individual's mind. Emotional incongruity may also be a difficulty, whereby the individual's emotions may be inappropriate for the circumstances, for example laughing when talking about committing suicide.

The above symptoms are generally referred to as *positive symptoms*, as they are generally excesses and pathological in nature. However, schizophrenia can also lead to a large range of deficits which are termed *negative symptoms*. These tend to be deficits in functioning and include:

- flatness of affect and emotional blunting
- apathy and lack of motivation
- reduced activity levels
- psychomotor retardation
- attentional problems; poor concentration, distractibility
- reduced social awareness.

One of the long-term effects of schizophrenia can be a syndrome described by Wing (1978) as 'clinical poverty syndrome' which is characterised by a large number of the above negative symptoms. These symptoms can occur at the same time as positive symptoms but most often persist long after the positive symptoms have subsided. They are mostly resistant to neuroleptic treatment and present, when compounded by the secondary disabilities mentioned earlier, a great challenge to those working in the long-stay environment.

The stress–vulnerability model of schizophrenia

Current research is investigating a number of areas which may be indicated in the aetiology of schizophrenia. At present it is thought that individuals have a predisposition to developing schizophrenia and that this predisposition is an enduring vulnerability trait. The potential causes of this vulnerability are:

- genetic factors
- pathological brain changes
- birth trauma/defects
- environmental factors, such as diet or infection.

However, by themselves these factors do not account for or explain the symptomatic flare-ups or relapses that are the nature of the schizophrenic experience. What the stress–vulnerability model proposes is that schizophrenia is a result of environmental stressors reacting with this underlying vulnerability.

Both positive and negative symptoms can be seen as a function of the interaction between an individual's problem-solving and coping skills, his support networks and the amount of life stresses that impinge on the individual. This type of interactional process is shown diagrammatically in Figure 19.1.

A number of interesting features can be drawn from this model. First, the model suggests that chronicity is a function of repeated relapse and, second, that relapse or an increase in psychotic symptoms can be triggered in one of two ways, either by an increase in stressful events (either personal or environmental) or, conversely, by a decrease in social problem-solving skills or a reduction in support networks. Thus, it strongly supports the case for intervention and for a philosophy of care that is aimed at preventing relapse, reducing personal and environmental stress, improving social, problem-solving and coping skills, and strengthening support networks.

The stress–vulnerability model and the occupational therapist's role

For most of our working lives we may strive to offer treatment which can readily be identified as the occupational therapy approach. We usually see this approach as our discrete professional contribution to a package of care. All too often, however, these discrete contributions lead to narrow or prescriptive professional parameters and role boundaries. The almost inevitable result of role defensiveness is professional boundary disputes, which may divert some of our daily effort from client care.

As a model, stress–vulnerability can be seen to have the attributes of all good models in that it can

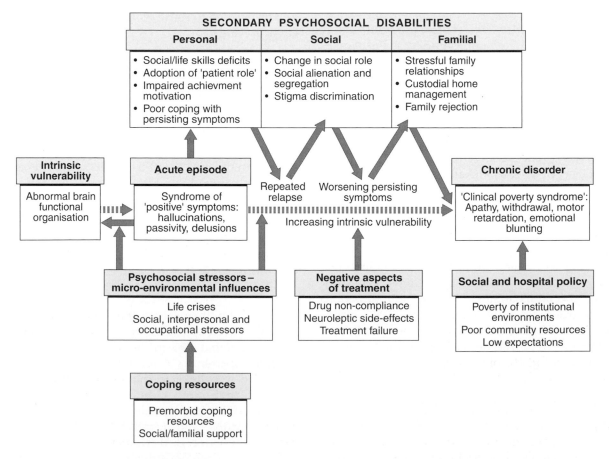

Figure 19.1 A vulnerability–interactionist model (referred to in this chapter as stress–vulnerability). (From Birchwood M J, Hallett S E, Preston M C 1989 Schizophrenia: an integrated approach to research and treatment. Reproduced by kind permission of the Longman Group UK Ltd.)

'provide an explanation of clinical phenomena and suggest the type of intervention the therapist should make. It is the link between theory and practice' (Creek & Feaver 1993). What it does not do, however, is specify the nature of the professional who should carry out these interventions. It is not limited to one profession for its application and there is no reason why it should be.

The validity of the stress–vulnerability model continues to be strengthened as clinical evidence is amassed to support its explanation of the phenomenon of schizophrenia. This has potentially groundbreaking implications for the development of professional roles as it offers all professions the opportunity to operate to a unifying and relevant model of schizophrenia. In other words, we can share a starting point with each other – a common understanding of the nature of the illness we wish to treat.

The implications for all professions are immense. Areas once considered to be the sole province of one particular profession are now contained within one unifying model. Social function, for example, cannot be teased out as a separate clinical entity but is co-dependent on all the other variables contained in the model (Birchwood et al 1989). How then can the occupational therapist claim social skills training as a distinct professional responsibility? How do we move forward as professionals when the basis on which we have traditionally built our roles is open to question? There are no easy answers and these challenges are shared by all professions working with schizophrenia in the National Health Service today. The main concern, perhaps, has to be that we remain open minded and seek opportunities to develop as a profession within this framework. It is difficult to say, at the present time, how our practice will differ in 20 years time, but the point is that at least some aspects of it should.

Other psychiatric problems

As mentioned above, schizophrenia is found in 80% of the long-stay population. Other psychiatric problems include: bipolar affective disorders, chronic personality disorders, such as schizo-affective disorder, chronic substance abuse, chronic neuroses, and a growing number of early onset dementias. There may also be a small percentage of people with behavioural problems which have no formal diagnosis.

Effects of institutionalisation

Another factor which may have an effect on the individual is that of the institution itself. Institutionalisation is a recognised concept and much has been written on the subject. (For a full discussion, see Goffman (1961) or Barton (1959).)

Briefly, it can be argued that individuals become dependent on the institution. Their self-esteem and decision-making capacity reduces; they may become apathetic, passive and lack initiative; they may lose interest in anything outside the institution. When we examine these manifestations of institutionalisation we see that they are similar to the negative symptoms identified in schizophrenia. Barton (1959) identified a number of features of institutions that contribute to this condition. These include:

- enforced idleness
- staff attitudes, for example brutality, bossiness and teasing
- loss of friends and personal possessions
- loss of contact with the outside world
- ward atmosphere.

All these factors make the institutional environment one of the major areas for potential change for the benefit of the long-stay population.

What the occupational therapist working in this environment will need to bear in mind is, first, how these problems of institutionalisation may magnify and compound the negative symptoms experienced by the individual and, second, how the institution and the nature of the organisation influence and shape both the behaviour of the individual and also that of the staff working in that environment.

CARE AND TREATMENT

Much has been published over the past few years, both as legislation and guidelines, regarding the care of those with serious or long-term mental illness, including the Care Programme Approach (DoH 1990b), *Guidelines on the Implementation of Supervision Registers* (DoH 1994c), *Health of the Nation* (DoH 1992) and *Working in Partnership* (DoH 1994a). Reports on a number of incidents (DoH 1994b) have added to the wealth of literature concerning this client group.

Resource issues aside, these initiatives have been invaluable in highlighting the nature and extent of care, along with the professional skills and range of services, needed to ensure that appropriate interventions, safety measures and long-term monitoring take place. This, combined with recent clinical research findings as described in this chapter, has brought this hitherto neglected client group to the forefront of mental health provision.

It is unfortunate that, apart from the general move towards community resettlement from long-stay insitutions, the main emphasis has been on care and support for clients fortunate enough to be placed in community settings. Staff working in long-stay ward environments need to be as acutely aware of the need to improve overall packages of care for those clients who may not, in the foreseeable future, be discharged from hospital. Keeping abreast of research and legislation will assist this process and should help to promote staff motivation in this very demanding area of work.

Medication

As detailed in this chapter, interventions aimed at ameliorating personal and environmental stress and enhancing coping skills play a major role in preventing relapse and improving prognosis. However, medication continues to play an important part in the overall treatment of clients with severe mental illness.

The introduction of neuroleptic drugs in the 1950s had a huge impact on the management and treatment of clients with psychotic illness. This led directly to more opportunities for clients whose positive symptoms and resultant behaviours had previously necessitated hospitalisation. The range of drugs now available in both oral and injectable form is used widely as part of an overall treatment package. Indications for use include:

- acute and chronic schizophrenia
- schizo-affective disorder, often in combination with antidepressants or other drugs
- acute manic states
- challenging behaviours.

While the obvious benefits of medication in relieving positive symptoms are evident in a high proportion of clients, 5–10% do not respond. Furthermore, neuroleptics (major tranquillisers) continue to have substantial drawbacks. The negative symptoms which often persist after an acute episode are largely unresponsive to neuroleptic drugs and approximately 40% of clients on long-term maintenance doses do relapse. Methods of predicting which clients will benefit are unreliable, however, and in the absence of more effective medical treatment many clients in long-term institutions, in particular those suffering from schizophrenia, receive maintenance doses of neuroleptics. In all cases those clients in receipt of major tranquillisers should be given the minimum effective dose, not least because of the many severe and often irreversible side-effects.

On a positive note, recent years have seen the introduction of atypical neuroleptics such as olanzapine. These new drugs have shown promising effects for many clients and may help to ensure compliance with medication due to a reduction of negative side-effects.

Effects of neuroleptics

Neuroleptic drugs usually take effect over a period of 2–6 weeks. There is a reduction in delusions and hallucinations, thought disorder and paranoid thinking.

These drugs also have a sedative effect on agitation and restlessness. Following reduction in acute symptoms, a maintenance dose is generally prescribed to prevent recurrence of acute symptoms. Medication may be given intramuscularly or orally, the latter having the specific advantage of the ability to adjust dosage, for example in the case of a fluctuating mental state or in response to the emergence of side-effects. Intramuscular injection is often prescribed for clients who are acutely agitated, or as a long-term measure to ensure compliance.

Side-effects

In common with individual responses of positive symptom reduction, vulnerability towards developing side-effects varies from client to client. All neuroleptics, however, have at least some of the following side-effects:

1. extrapyramidal: parkinsonian type rigidity, tremor and dyskinesia; acute dystonias, akathesia and tardive dyskinesia (spontaneous movements of mouth and tongue)
2. Anticholinergic: dry mouth, blurred vision, difficulty in micturition and drowsiness
3. hormonal: gynaecomastia, sexual dysfunction, menstrual disturbances
4. cardiovascular: hypotension
5. allergic reactions: jaundice, photosensitivity
6. haematological disorder: although rare, includes agranulocytosis and haemolytic anaemia
7. others:
   — weight gain
   — agitation
   — insomnia
   — neuroleptic malignant syndrome.

Examples of neuroleptic drugs

1. phenothiazines: chlorpromazine, thioridazine, fluphenazine
2. butyrophenones: haloperidol, droperidol
3. thioxanthenes: flupenthixol
4. dibenzoxazepines: loxapine, clozapine (used in the treatment of resistant cases. There is a high risk of agranulocytosis, so there must be regular blood tests and monitoring).

Other drugs commonly used include:

- lithium carbonate
- antidepressants
- benzodiazepines, e.g. Valium.

It is, unfortunately, common practice for clients in long-stay institutions to be maintained on regular and high doses of medication. While medication will continue to play an important role in the client's overall care management, the impetus must always be that of reducing dosage or of discontinuation, particularly so where positive symptoms are less distressing than the actual side-effects of medication. The occupational therapist and other professionals involved can play a crucial role in monitoring these effects and thus contribute to ensuring that the safest minimum dose is given. Emphasis on environmental factors will help this process.

Environmental factors

The move to close many of our existing long-stay wards for the mentally ill, and the ways in which treatment and support are now developing, open up new opportunities and possibilities for those clients who would previously have been destined to life as an in-patient. Unquestionably, good quality, well-resourced community care packages are a preferred option for care. However, the principles that underpin care, as outlined in this chapter, should be pursued regardless of setting. Conversely, poor institutional practice can be as evident in a community-based group home, or indeed in the client's own home, as in the institution itself.

While efforts can be made to improve substantially the actual physical environment of the ward, relationships, professional practices and the quality of individual care plans will have a greater impact on outcome and general satisfaction for clients.

Avoiding a generalised approach to care is particularly problematic within in-patient settings, although not peculiar to them. Wherever possible, interventions and skills training should take place in environments relevant to the problem experienced. This demands that the therapist think creatively of ways in which to achieve this, and requires cooperation from ward managers and others involved in the client's overall care. The use of available resources in ways that promote client choice can often pose a threat to established practice within a ward setting. Goffman (1961) highlighted the tendency for institutional practice to meet the needs of service providers rather than those of clients.

This poses a considerable challenge to all professionals working in institutional settings, but person-centred practice should nevertheless be promoted, through education and determination and by focusing on the client's strengths and skills as opposed to the constraints set down by the service setting. Many examples of effective client-centred services are widely available, though good practices are not common nationally.

The need for consistency

The nature of long-term mental illnesses, and of the institutional setting, leads to many long-stay clients suffering from disintegration of thought or actions. Given this disintegration, it is essential that the input to these clients is specific and consistent in nature. However, it is not unusual for the occupational therapist to find herself based in a department separate from the environment in which she is to work. If a common direction and philosophy is to be ensured, this will involve considerable effort from all parties to communicate effectively and develop a clear understanding of their respective roles.

Integration does not necessarily demand that all professionals share the same office or staff room. What matters is that component parts of the service work well together as a whole and that useful and meaningful links are made between professionals and departments to assist this. In practice this means that the occupational therapist, often a minority in the multidisciplinary team, needs to ensure that she communicates effectively with the team in order to develop and maintain a consistent approach.

The therapeutic relationship

The needs of any client extend beyond skills acquisition or the competence of the therapist in reaching this. We all share fundamental human needs for love, warmth, support, trust and security – some of the foundations of healthy relationships. The question is therefore posed: is it the strength of a supportive and healing relationship which forms the cornerstone of successful intervention or the sophisticated techniques learned in colleges and universities?

The inadequacy of our intervention techniques is often experienced by students or newly qualified therapists entering the field of long-stay psychiatry. The complex needs of the client, and the rate at which an individual's mental state or motivation levels can change, mean that the novice cannot always rely on the presence of comforting routines. However, the therapist starts to note that despite these disturbances and influences on practice, progress is still made. Thus, the question arises: is there another factor at work?

Time, when embraced as a therapeutic opportunity, gives the therapist the chance to form trusting, warm and secure relationships, elements particularly identified as crucial to clients with schizophrenia. Any relationship based on trust and a feeling of security provides a foundation for the client to reach out and to be able to risk failing, because there is a secure place to return to. Clients will risk learning new skills when they know that they can trust us to support them in all their endeavours. Goering & Stylianos (1988) identified the therapeutic relationship as a third crucial element, interactive with two other facets of rehabilitative treatment, that is, the development of competence and support systems.

Maggie and Jordon Paul (Paul and Paul 1988) emphasised the relevance of a strong relationship to the promotion of client autonomy: 'The stronger and more secure we become, the more willing we are to be ourselves whilst encouraging our loved ones to do the same.' In other words, healthy relationships, which are not based on deep power or control needs of the professional are a fundamental underpinning of achievement of autonomy by the client.

To reach this level of personal and professional maturity is the result of lifelong development and self-exploration. Regrettably, such levels of insight do not automatically arrive with our degrees at graduation. Personal growth requires constant attention and active self-intervention. If we are secure and comfortable with ourselves, we will not have the desire to change or dictate a way of being to another. We will possess the maturity to practise within rehabilitation precisely because we are able to encourage our clients to become themselves, to act their own way, to set their own goals (Box 19.1).

Case management

The introduction of the Community Care Act (DoH 1990a) and the Care Programme Approach for people with a mental illness (DoH 1990b) has led to a need for services to set up case-management systems to support clients with severe mental illness in the community. The main features of an effective care programme approach system are:

- assessment (multidisciplinary)
- allocation of a care coordinator (to take overall responsibility for the coordination of care)
- care planning
- review/revision (at least 6-monthly)
- information technology
- quality standards.

It should follow that the above features are relevant in a long-stay ward environment. For example, a client had been referred to community services for resettlement after a period of 40 years in hospital. On discharge the client was registered with a local general practitioner and, in line with good care management practice,

---

Box 19.1 Case example 1

Rose was 56 and had been in hospital since her early twenties. She suffered with schizophrenia, although her symptoms were well controlled and she was a humorous and popular individual. Her daily activities were based on visiting other areas, both in the hospital and nearby town, and she returned to the ward only to eat or sleep.

Rose did not engage with ward or occupational therapy staff, nor did she participate in life or activities on the ward/department. There were no opportunities to assess her needs or skills, therefore the options for progress were seen to be as follows:

1. to design a programme using known reinforcers to encourage attendance at ward/department sessions, or
2. to get to know Rose; use assessment carefully and thoroughly.

The therapeutic issues involved in selecting either option 1 or 2 were held to be that, while option 1 might produce some involvement with ward/department activities, it would be perhaps at the expense of trust and client opinion. Option 2 was held to acknowledge the effects of memories of locked wards or oppressive practice upon behaviour, acknowledge time as an ally, accept that current behaviour might reflect a need to avoid stressful situations in order to reduce arousal levels, and finally, acknowledge the independence shown in mind, spirit and actions as positive manifestations despite years of incarceration in an institution.

Initially, option 1 was tried by the team without success. The reasons, on evaluation, were held to be a failure to acknowledge the factors outlined above in option 2. The team then set up a treatment plan which involved building a relationship with Rose and building up new, positive experiences when on the ward. Staff joined her on her travels and welcomed her on her return, spending quality time with Rose on her terms. After 5 months, Rose chose to spend more time on the ward and asked to join in activities. In other words she had begun to trust again and was available for therapeutic interventions. In essence, the second approach succeeded because it:

- acknowledged the power of warm and trusting relationships
- maximised and recognised the power of intrinsic motivation
- placed staff in a position to begin a true and joint assessment of need
- maintained Rose's current coping skills in controlling arousal levels and did not attempt to replace them on her behalf
- used time to help unravel the many complex reasons the original behaviours had arisen
- was based on the client's strengths, not on ward needs.

Essentially, Rose had made contact again with the world in which she lived, the only true starting point for treatment.

received a general health assessment. While in hospital she had frequently complained of abdominal pain and constipation and was prescribed a laxative to remedy this. It was discovered, once she was discharged into the community, that she was in fact in the later stages of cervical cancer and she died 12 months later. Had her care while in hospital included regular holistic assessment and review of her care, this tragedy might not have happened.

It is important, then, that each client is allocated a worker who will draw together all the relevant and regularly reviewed information from other professionals involved. This role could be taken on by a ward occupational therapist, nurse, psychologist or other professional, and assessment might include the following categories (Tameside and Glossop Community and Priority Services NHS Trust 1996):

- the caring network (e.g. relatives, friends)
- leisure and social network
- emotional support
- medication
- symptoms/causes of illness
- employment/vocation
- self-care
- housekeeping
- accommodation needs
- financial difficulties
- personal health
- safety.

It is all too easy to assume that, because a client has been known for many years, he does not require regular assessment and review. By adopting some of the approaches aimed at effective community care, this extensive risk of denying inpatients fundamental general health and mental health care can be avoided.

Autonomy and independence

The important words 'autonomy' and 'independence' are frequently and often interchangeably used by therapists throughout their professional career, yet this ease of reference belies complexities of meaning and of the issues involved. If we give insufficient consideration to the meanings of these words, thus limiting their definition, so too will the scope and emphasis of our practice be limited.

There is a danger in viewing autonomy and independence as personal attributes, skills to be acquired or personal goals to be attained. This view divorces the individual from the world he lives in, the life context which affects and is affected by his existence and interactions with it. Once this road has been taken, responsibility for success weighs too heavily with the client. Equally the therapist may begin to rely on techniques or batteries of assessment and checklists which show, in great detail, how many skills or subskills are still required by the client in the professional-led search for client success. If, as a profession, we acknowledge the importance of independence and autonomy, we need to investigate their meanings in order to ensure breadth and relevance of practice.

Broadly speaking, autonomy is held to be personal freedom, self-government or freedom of the will. At a personal level, it can include freedom of thought, intent or action (Gillon 1985) but, as already indicated, personal freedom or rights exist in a context, for example that of a large institution or long-stay ward in a general hospital (O'Neill 1984). Independence may be usefully defined as the position of not being dependent on authority or, alternatively, not relying on others for one's opinions or behaviours. Crucially, these definitions do not separate the individual from the context of his life, rather they place him relative to it in a reciprocal relationship. At the simplest level a client may learn how to make a cup of tea for himself in the occupational therapy department. However, on return to the ward, opportunities to carry out this skill or to use it autonomously may not exist. At this point the client may indeed be independent in the skill yet not autonomous in the true sense, due to the limitations the system or organisation places upon the chance for autonomous practice.

The crucial issue about independence, especially within the framework of serious mental illness and clinical competence, is its fundamental relationship with its apparent opposite, dependency. Dependency is always a matter of degree.

Support is welcome when any individual is ill or suffering a life crisis. The problems arise when either support is withdrawn prematurely or not even offered, or continues to be provided when the need for support has diminished. Unless we judge dependency needs correctly (Box 19.2), we actively deny the client the opportunity to be independent and autonomous at any level, a result opposite to that which our interventions are meant to achieve.

What are the characteristics of a system or organisation which is autonomous in nature? They include intent to be responsive and dynamic in nature and practice, and having built into their service design, routes and forums where ideas and issues can be channelled in order to adapt the system to meet the changing needs of the individuals within it (Rosenheck 1988). Thus, autonomy is not simply the province of the client, nor even the province of the organisation alone. Autonomy can only be truly considered when both the person and the system are evaluated and understood relative to each other in a dynamic and reciprocal relationship (Benner 1984).

The role of the therapist within the autonomy framework

How is the role and breadth of occupational therapy practice affected by this understanding? Again, using the analogy of a client who has attained the skill of making a cup of tea in the

---

Box 19.2 Case example 2

Jimmy was in his mid-forties and had schizophrenia. He had been in hospital since his early twenties and was in a small, independent area of a long-stay ward. He suffered with severe thought disorder and delusional systems and chose to remain isolated, although he informed staff that he was lonely. Time was spent by staff in getting to know and assess Jimmy. His isolation and active avoidance of staff were acknowledged, and many months were allocated to gaining rapport and a fuller picture.

The main areas indicated by assessment were that: self-care and household skills were good; shopping provided a limited but reasonable range of goods; cooking was sporadic, ranging from one, cold item to a small, hot meal; and isolation was both a coping skill to reduce arousal and a problem as it led to loneliness.

At this stage, there was sufficient evidence to draw up goal plans around shopping, cooking and social skills, but not enough information to determine whether these problems were due to lack of skills or were symptomatic of more complex factors. Thus, a further period of assessment was organised around social isolation and cooking/nutrition. To achieve this, staff approached Jimmy several times each day and offered to spend a short time with him if he wished. Also, for a period of one month, staff recorded details of every meal Jimmy made. After the assessment period, the information was analysed and the results correlated with mental state entries in the nursing Kardex. The results showed that more than 70% of the meals were cold and required little or no preparation, the balance were mostly simple, hot snacks and a tiny proportion were a two- or three-item hot meal. A crucial piece of information emerged from this exploration of Jimmy's eating patterns and habits. The pattern correlated with strong, daily fluctuations in mental state, indeed one was a precise indicator of the other. Cold, simple meals were evident when Jimmy's mental state was worse.

As mental state fluctuations dictated how well Jimmy ate, rather than a skills deficit per se, a goal plan was drawn up in support of this. At every meal staff offered a range of support in order to maximise his skills, either 100% staff help, some support as required, or none. Jimmy chose the levels he required at each meal:

- As a result of receiving support, Jimmy was able to cook hot meals much more frequently, and his diet improved accordingly. Also, due to the reduction in his stress levels associated with eating he began to tolerate social interaction and began, after some months, to actively seek this. His loneliness decreased.
- It is clear that if cooking skills/sessions had been targeted initially, not only would the interventions have added to stress/arousal levels but the opportunities to use any skills eventually learned in this fashion would always be limited by mental state fluctuations.
- Jimmy's increased tolerance of relationships and staff involvement opened the door to long-term, useful joint assessment of need so that other areas, such as shopping, improvement in cooking range/repertoire and development of personal interests, could be achieved.

Ultimately, the flexibility of the approach acknowledged the devastating effects of a serious and fluctuating mental illness. As already stated, independence and dependence are fundamentally linked. By offering Jimmy the opportunity to dictate support levels, independence became feasible, as he was able to match support with his own, self-determined needs.

department, the role of the therapist would extend to addressing, in some way, the system affecting practice on the ward. This is not to say that the system or any organisation is intentionally rigid or unforgiving, nor that occupational therapy departments are in any way exempt from these issues. All practice can be traced back to a particular event or rationale which shaped regulations and beliefs at that time: the issue may well be that unlimited tea-making cannot happen on a ward because of financial restrictions or because someone was once badly scalded.

The crucial point is whether or not the system is open to influence or reexamination of issues and practice in light of new information brought to bear. This is a necessary process if the individuals working within an organisation are to be able to convert clients' changing clinical and personal needs into practices which support development, growth and independence.

The role of the therapist therefore includes attending meetings, working cooperatively and with an open mind with other professionals and being involved in multidisciplinary forums whose activities include organisational planning. It is here that all professionals can make an impact on the system and can contribute to adapting the nature of the organisation, to meet the changing needs of the client. Thus, time spent in clinical activities is only one of the ways in which client autonomy and independence is addressed. Many professionals fear that the amount of time apparently spent in nonclinical activities fuels the idea that somehow one is not being a 'real' occupational therapist. On the contrary, if autonomy is an issue of context as well as individual need, then practice must reflect this.

Professional growth and development

Working in long-stay psychiatry can provide the occupational therapist with important opportunities. Serious and enduring mental illnesses, by their very nature, continue to affect an individual for the course of his or her life and the successful therapist will harness this nature and welcome time as an ally to get to know the person and their unique circumstances. Equally, the long-

stay environment exposes the therapist to opportunities which are necessary for the growth of the professional self: a development intrinsically bound to successful outcomes in treatment.

This latter issue has been coherently and sensitively explored by Gail Fidler (1966), who examined the relationship between professionals and learning as a growth process. The parallels between the issues she raised and the experiences which characterise long-stay psychiatry can be appreciated by applying the principles she described, first to oneself as a student or professional and second, to an imaginary client.

Fidler (1966) suggested that skills, facts and knowledge are indeed necessary tools of independence but it is how and why these are implemented which measures, clarifies and promotes professional autonomy and growth. It is crucial that students are allowed time, opportunity, security and support to integrate ideas and actions with their emotional, psychological, social and intellectual selves. Equally, they must have the opportunity to experience the stress and frustrations of this dynamic process whilst they continually embrace concepts, or even discard facts previously held dear, to form an integrative whole. This process promotes true learning for the individual; that which has been learned is all the more useful because each aspect has been so thoroughly experienced and explored (Fisher & Noble 1960). If we are able to acknowledge that the growth process is valuable for ourselves, then our next step is to acknowledge that it is equally valid for our clients. The learning and human needs of our clients and ourselves are one and the same.

The successful implementation of this process for our clients is thus heavily reliant on the strength of our professional self. This involves a lifetime commitment to developing the deep personal and professional maturity required not to impress our own values, experiences and processes upon another, but to allow them to embark on the same valuable journey. True learning involves stress associated with the drive to create order from the chaos of constantly changing ideas and reference points in our lives. Our clients deserve the same consideration when learning to live as we are granted during our professional training: the permission to struggle, and support while doing so.

THE OCCUPATIONAL THERAPY PROCESS

One of the cornerstones of occupational therapy is the belief in the therapeutic use of purposeful activity. In the long-stay environment, the term 'purposeful' can be qualified as activities which are intended to address two main areas:

- to enable the individual to attain his optimum level of independence within the constraints of the nature and severity of his illness and the nature of the institution
- to prevent relapse and reduce chronicity.

This second strand of care is often neglected by concentrating on the first.

Assessment and treatment are often based on a mixture of behavioural, cognitive and humanistic techniques. While these are important parts of the occupational therapy process, there are two major factors that need to be borne in mind when assessing and treating long-stay clients:

1. *Knowing the illness*: positive and negative symptoms, thought disorders, attentional and cognitive deficits, secondary handicaps and disabilities will all influence treatment.

2. *Knowing the effects of the illness on the individual*: what the attentional and cognitive problems may be and how they may influence the treatment plan.

Hemsley (1978) saw the behaviours present in schizophrenia as an attempt to adapt to or cope with the chronic cognitive impairments that occur in schizophrenia. These cognitive deficits may include cognitive distortions, difficulties processing and responding to external stimuli, thought disorders, information overload and psychophysiological arousal. Hemsley also stated that treatment without understanding of the client's basic impairment may either fail or actually result in making symptoms worse.

The stress–vulnerability model argues a positive correlation between stress and arousal, whereby increased stress increases arousal leading to psychological disorganisation which contributes to attentional and cognitive dysfunctions (Neuchterlein & Dawson 1984). This suggests interventions aimed at reducing arousal levels, which should therefore help reduce psychological deficits which in turn should facilitate personal development.

Assessment

No treatment or rehabilitation regime can be implemented without full knowledge of the nature and extent of the person's illness, and therefore, before treatment occurs, we need to make an assessment of how illness affects function. This assessment is an integral part of the occupational therapy process.

Assessment has a number of aims which are discussed elsewhere in this book, but in the long-stay environment assessment is informed by a number of issues, including validity and reliability.

Validity and reliability of assessment

Whether assessments are valid is a concern for all members of the multidisciplinary team within the long-stay institution and this concern has a number of aspects.

Firstly, there is the context of the assessment, that is, whether assessment occurs 'in vivo' or in a role play/simulated environment. Assessments that mirror the 'real' situation as much as possible have much greater validity, but this raises the issue of the trade-off between reliability and validity (Levy 1973). In essence, the more realistic the assessment situation, the more likely it is to be valid; the more structured and artificial the situation, the more variables can be controlled and the more reliable the results will be, but the assessment is then less likely to be valid. This trade-off needs to be considered by the occupational therapist when working with individuals, especially when attempting to recreate normal experiences at the same time as controlling the environment in order to encourage or reproduce behaviour.

Another concern relating to the validity of both assessment and treatment is that of the context of the institution. As occupational therapists, we pride ourselves on the purposeful use of activity to increase independence; however, do we consider the influence of the organisation on the individual's independence? Case example 3 (Box 19.3) highlights this dilemma.

By not giving due regard to the influence of the setting on the individual, occupational therapists may be in danger of becoming 'activity-focused' and not 'system-focused'. This may lead to excellent skills in planning and task analysis to the detriment of relevance to the individual in terms of his personal development.

In conclusion, there is a need to alter the type of institutional care the individual receives, both to promote the individual's quality of life and also to ameliorate the negative effects of the institution. These changes can occur in two main ways:

1. through changes in the philosophy of approach and interactions that occur within the institution, and
2. through changes in the structure and organisation of the institution, so that autonomy and normalisation are fostered.

Treatment

When designing treatment programmes for individuals with long-term mental health problems there are many issues that should inform treatment. These include the nature of the illness (Box 19.4), the primary and secondary handicaps that it causes, the individual's adaptation to the illness, and the potentially deleterious effect that the institution may have.

All the above need to be considered if the needs of the individual are to be understood, and treatment programmes designed that are effective in preventing relapse and increasing independence. In the mainstream long-stay institutions occupational therapy has tended to concentrate on the 'bread and butter' areas of:

- daily living skills
- physical and social activities
- creative and industrial therapies and social skills training.

While these are valuable areas of work for the occupational therapist in the long-stay setting, there are a number of strategies that have been identified from the stress–vulnerability model which may be useful for further study.

Box 19.3   Case example 3

Mr B had been on a long-stay ward for the last 20 years. He was referred to the occupational therapy department where it was identified that he lacked basic activities of daily living skills. A treatment plan was drawn up to teach him these basic skills.

For 3 months Mr B attended the occupational therapy department twice weekly and at the end of the period was able to manage to make tea and toast successfully. However, ward regulations and routines did not allow patients to make their own tea or toast on the ward.

In this case we might ask: Is Mr B any more independent? Is the treatment programme valid? Are the activities 'purposeful' within the context of the institution?

Box 19.4   Case example 4

An individual with chronic schizophrenia will still have acute episodes of positive symptoms which are preceded by prodromal stages which may be identified. Intervention at the prodromal stage may actually prevent acute psychosis beginning (Birchwood & Tarrier 1992).

Jim was a 64-year-old man who had been on a long-stay ward for 23 years. He left the ward most mornings and wandered into the local village and to the local bookies where he was well known. At certain times he would return complaining that dog(s) had attacked him and he would be quite shaken. This would be followed by periods where Jim would isolate himself and his paranoia would increase; he would be certain that these dogs 'knew' about him and that some force was setting the dogs on him. This would generalise to other residents and eventually staff who were 'out to get him'. An assessment plan was set up to monitor the frequency of these psychotic episodes and possible trigger factors. After 9 months' assessment, the multidisciplinary team concluded that Jim's mentioning of dogs attacking him was a prodromal sign and should therefore be taken seriously by the team who increased input at these vulnerable times to prevent relapse.

Reducing cognitive and attentional deficits

Some 50% of people with long-term schizophrenia will suffer from attentional dysfunction, that is, difficulties in determining, selecting, filtering and producing clarity of thought and also in suppressing irrelevant thoughts and ideas. Spaulding et al (1986) highlighted three possible strategies for reducing cognitive and attentional deficits:

1. Raising the level at which psychophysiological arousal causes psychological disorganisation. This is generally thought to be neurophysiological in basis and therefore changes in medication may raise the individual's threshold for disorganisation (Falloon & Liberman 1983).

2. Regulation of arousal. If arousal leads to disorganisation, which is linked with relapse, then ways of lowering levels of arousal can only be beneficial for individuals. Occupational therapists frequently use stress reduction techniques in the field of acute mental health, and there is now evidence to show that these stress reduction techniques can be modified for people with chronic mental health problems (Zeisset 1968, Smith 1980, Lukoff et al 1986).

Lukoff et al (1986) used a number of stress-management techniques, including daily yoga exercises, stress education sessions, sessions to encourage acceptance of psychotic symptoms, and sessions to increase self-esteem, along with a token economy for a group of patients with schizophrenia. They compared this group with a control group who received social skills training. They found that the stress-management group showed at least as great, if not greater, improvement on measures of psychopathology, while the social skills group showed greater improvement in social functioning.

3. Interventions which help the individual organise cognitive functioning: This strategy is aimed at reducing the confusion that illness causes.

Box 19.5 illustrates how both the treatment and the environment may be adapted to alleviate attentional deficits. The occupational therapist will use most of these strategies in any treatment setting; however, in the long-stay setting they become essential components of treatment and, in some cases, may well become the treatment themselves.

Duration and frequency of activities

The individual in long-term psychiatric care can often suffer from poor social skills and social

---

Box 19.5 Occupational therapy strategies for planning treatment for clients with attentional deficits

External factors
- The setting may be noisy and busy, or what may seem quiet to the therapist may seem overstimulating to the distracted or aroused client. Even the actions of the therapist can contribute to this overstimulation. Strategies here would include minimising external noises or interruptions, maintaining a clean, uncluttered work area and reducing unnecessary actions by the therapist.
- If a client experiences difficulties in distinguishing between relevant information present in the environment, the therapist needs to promote clarity about the task in hand by giving immediate and relevant feedback in order to maximise learning.

Internal factors
- There may be difficulties in maintaining attention due to intrusive thoughts and hallucinations. Where these are particularly problematic, joint identification of coping strategies may be necessary and may

include: thought stopping techniques, self-instruction, and identification and reduction of stressors which may increase arousal.
- There may be difficulties in maintaining attention due to problems with internal information filtering processes. This may result in problems with short-term memory and completing complex tasks. Useful coping strategies here would include:
  — helping the client by using simple language
  — using task analysis to break activities down into easy steps
  — ensuring prompts and reinforcement are frequent and relevant
  — keeping sessions short when the client is especially aroused
  — repeating sessions frequently in order for learning to occur.

For a fuller discussion of cognitive remediation see Green (1993), Lieberman & Corrigan (1993) and Spaulding et al (1986).

withdrawal and it is these social skills and situations that depend so much on both cognitive and attentional skills. As many of the training efforts that occupational therapists use will also depend upon cognition and attention, we need to give careful consideration to the duration and frequency of activity. Occupational therapy programmes are often designed with the activity dictating the duration and frequency of sessions. If it is accepted that attentional problems affect learning skills, and therefore the ability to generalise skills, then sessions will have to be of shorter duration but of greater frequency.

The service should aim to provide flexible levels of intervention as this will match the fluctuating needs of care of the client group.

Focusing on the individual

Occupational therapists in the long-stay environment may be put under pressure to provide therapy for large numbers of ward patients on the pretext that it may be the only therapy they receive. This ethos must be questioned very closely by the occupational therapist. If the individual's constellation of deficits is unique, then we can rule out a 'cookbook' approach to treatment, and therefore individualised assessment and treatment regimes may always be necessary.

However, occupational therapists do carry out group activities, especially in the areas mentioned previously, and small groupwork in these areas can be valuable if consideration is given both to the varying levels of need and also the varying amount of stress and demand put on individuals within sessions.

Evaluation

Evaluation of treatment in the long-stay setting is as important as in any other setting. It has often been erroneously assumed that long-stay clients do not change over time and, therefore, meaningful work cannot be carried out with these chronic patients. Both these stereotypes are untrue and, in order that they are refuted, it becomes vitally important for the team to gather

and share accurate information about the client as any change may occur very slowly.

Involving carers

In considering the most appropriate treatment approaches, it is vital to involve the client's carers or relatives in establishing previous abilities, interests, dislikes, etc. The damaging effects of the illness itself, combined with secondary deficits, often cloud our ability to establish what were the previous norms.

It is important to identify the current perceptions held by the carer if he is to contribute in a meaningful way to the overall care of the client. Lack of education concerning illness, and more specific education on how the illness may affect the carer on an individual basis, are vital areas to be addressed. There is now much evidence as to the value of providing education for families of clients living at home. This approach must also be ensured for those carers who visit clients on the long-stay ward. In institutions where retraction of long-stay wards is planned, this important area of involvement must not be missed if any subsequent resettlement of clients back to their district of origin is to have optimum effectiveness.

CONCLUSION

Whether the therapist is working in an institution or any long-stay setting, the principles which guide and underpin practice remain the same. A real understanding of the nature of serious mental illness should drive our practice and generate and support our philosophical debates. This understanding should also be used positively to review our traditional roles as occupational therapists working with the seriously mentally ill. There will be new opportunities to expand our practice if we take advantage of emerging knowledge about serious mental illness as guided by the stress–vulnerability model. Equally, given that consistency of approach among all professionals has been identified as crucial to treatment success, the therapist owes the client a move towards integrated practice methods in order to secure this outcome.

It is not uncommon for occupational therapists to evaluate activities. It is, however, more uncommon to evaluate them in relation to both a contextual framework, the organisation, and the issues of autonomy. It is feasible to create a ward or department programme filled with apparent structure and daily activity where clients are busy all day, as too are the satisfied therapists who have implemented this. However, if the activities bear no relation to true client needs, the meaning of their lives and how they interact with their world, the programme has merely achieved activity without purpose or true autonomous intent.

Rehabilitation is, by nature, an issue of autonomy. The care of clients who are moved into the community is currently a more likely area to be influenced by new approaches and government legislation, yet these are transferable to different settings. The problems of institutionalisation, however, are not necessarily solved by moving clients out; the attitude of staff is a crucial factor in deinstitutionalising practice.

Where clients live in any institutional setting, the therapist faces the danger of not recognising that autonomy is as much an issue for herself as for the client, together with the concomitant responsibility for addressing the organisation's capacity to change. Unless staff address the issues of institutionalisation, as our part of the bargain, we will still be writing about this problem in a further 50 years. If that is the case, we are not practising successful rehabilitation and are failing as therapists to address the true clinical and philosophical issues concerning our responsibilities of client autonomy and true rehabilitation.

SUMMARY

In this chapter we looked at the disorders that are encountered in the long-stay setting, and in particular the stress–vulnerability model of schizophrenia was described. The effects of institutionalisation were discussed.

Issues of client-centred care and treatment by occupational therapists, as members of multidisciplinary teams, were covered, including medication, the need for consistency and the importance of the therapeutic relationship. Autonomy and independence, both as regards clients and the professional growth of the occupational therapist, were considered.

The process of occupational therapy in the long-stay setting was discussed, including aspects of assessment, evaluation and the involvement of carers, and finally, the broader professional responsibilities of occupational therapists in this area were considered.

REFERENCES

American Psychiatric Association 1995 Diagnostic and statistical manual, 4th edn. American Psychiatric Association, Washington

Barton W 1959 Institutional neurosis. J Wright, Bristol, Washington

Benner P E 1984 Stress and satisfaction on the job (work meanings and coping of mid-career men). Prager, New York

Birchwood M J, Tarrier N 1992 Innovations in the psychological management of schizophrenia. Wiley, Chichester

Birchwood M J, Hallett S E, Preston M C 1989 Schizophrenia: an integrated approach to research and treatment. Longman, London

Creek J 1993 Feaver, models for practice in occupational therapy: part 1. Defining terms. British Journal of Occupational Therapy 56(1): 4

Department of Health 1990a Community Care Act. HMSO, London

Department of Health 1990b Care Programme Approach for people with a mental illness referred to specialist psychiatric services. HMSO, London

Department of Health 1992 Health of the nation: a strategy for health in England. HMSO, London

Department of Health 1994a Working in partnership: report of the mental health nursing review team. HMSO, London

Department of Health 1994b The report of the enquiry into the care and treatment of Christopher Clunis. HMSO, London

Department of Health 1994c Guidelines on the implementation of supervision registers. HMSO, London

Falloon I, Liberman R P 1983 Interactions between drug and psychosocial therapy in schizophrenia. Schizophrenia Bulletin 9: 543–554

Fidler G S 1966 Learning as a growth process: a conceptual framework for professional education. American Journal of Occupational Therapy 20: 1–8

Fisher M B, Noble J L 1960 College education as personal development. Prentice Hall, New York

Gillon R 1985 Autonomy and the principle of respect for autonomy. British Medical Journal 290: 51–53

Goering P N, Stylianos S K 1988 Exploring the helping relationship between the schizophrenic client and rehabilitation therapist. American Orthopsychiatric Association 58(2): 271–280

Goffman E 1961 Asylums: essays on the social situation of mental patients and other inmates. Doubleday, New York

Green M F 1993 Cognitive remediation in schizophrenia: is it time yet? American Journal of Psychiatry 150: 178–187

Hemsley D R 1978 Limitations of operant procedures in the modification of schizophrenic functioning: the possible relevance of studies of cognitive disturbance. Behaviour Analysis and Modification 2: 165–173

Levy P 1973 On the relation between test theory and psychology. In: Kline P (ed) New approaches in psychological measurement. John Wiley, London

Lieberman R P, Corrigan P W 1993 Designing new psychosocial treatments for schizophrenia. Psychiatry 56: 238–249

Lukoff D, Wallace C J, Lieberman R P, Burke K 1986 A holistic program for chronic schizophrenic patients. Schizophrenia Bulletin 12: 274–282

Neuchterlein K, Dawson M 1984 A heuristic vulnerability/stress model of schizophrenic episodes. Schizophrenia Bulletin 10: 300–312

O'Neill O 1984 Paternalism and partial autonomy. Journal of Medical Ethics 10: 173–178

Paul J, Paul M 1988 Do I have to give up me to be loved by you? Thorson, London

Rosenheck R 1988 System dynamics in complex psychiatric treatment organisations. Journal of Psychiatry 51: 211–219

Schneider K 1959 Clinical psychopathology, trans. M W Hamilton. Grune and Stratton, New York

Silverstone T, Turner P 1988 Drug treatment in psychiatry, 4th edn. Routledge, London

Smith R 1980 Development of an integrated coping response through cognitive-affective stress management training. In: Sarason I, Spielberger C (eds) Stress and anxiety, vol. 7. Hemisphere, Washington DC

Spaulding W D, Storms L, Goodrich V, Sullivan M 1986 Applications of experimental psychopathology in psychiatric rehabilitation. Schizophrenia Bulletin 12: 560–577

Tameside and Glossop Community and Priority Services NHS Trust 1996 Care programme approach system. Tameside and Glossop Mental Health Service, Ashton-under-Lyne

Wing J K (ed) 1978 Schizophrenia: towards a new synthesis. Academic Press, London

Wing J K, Cooper J E, Sartorius N 1974 Measurement and classification of psychiatric symptoms: an instructional manual for the PSE and Catego Program. Cambridge University Press, Cambridge

Zeisset R 1968 Desensitisation and relaxation in the modification of psychiatric patients' interview behaviour. Journal of Abnormal Psychology 73: 18–24

20

Rehabilitation

Clephane A. Hume   Anne Joice

INTRODUCTION

Rehabilitation in the context of mental health had its beginnings in the 19th-centruy programmes which encouraged patients to participate in work activities within the hospital, for their general welfare. With the introduction of phenothiazine medication in the 1960s, the rehabilitation and discharge of many long-term patients became a realistic possibility and an accepted area of work in psychiatric hospitals. Thus, preparation of clients for discharge became an important aspect of occupational therapy intervention.

In recent years, hospital closures and reduction in bed numbers and community care policies and legislation have led to a major focus on rehabilitation in the context of the community.

However, despite many changes in terminology and location of treatment, patients' needs remain constant and this chapter provides an introduction to rehabilitation as used in the field of mental health. Theoretical concepts are outlined, the context of practice is described, and areas that will be most relevant to occupational therapy are discussed. No treatment plan can be devised in isolation and therefore relationships with colleagues and significant others are also considered.

Needs and opportunities for education are considered and, last but not least, attention is given to some of the problems and constraints that concern the rehabilitation team.

WHAT IS REHABILITATION?

What do we mean by rehabilitation? Definitions are usually phrased in terms such as the following: enabling the individual to reach the maximum level of independence in the psychological, physical, social, spiritual and economic spheres of life.

Clark (1984) reminded us that rehabilitation is not about protecting clients, rather it is enabling them to have an experience of success and thus generating motivation to aim towards greater things.

One of the UK government's targets for mental health is to secure significant improvement in the health and social functioning of mentally ill people. This means that quality of life should be a key concern in any service. The need for effective rehabilitation services is obvious.

The World Health Organization (World Health 1984) described the rehabilitation process as 'all means aimed at reducing the impact of disabling and handicapping conditions in individuals and enabling them to achieve maximum integration into the community.' Although this statement was made in the context of rehabilitation assistants working with people with physical disability, it is a philosophy with which occupational therapists can identify. Hagedorn (1992) described the rehabilitation model of treatment as being problem based and focused on dysfunction. Varied activities, techniques and methods are used to enable the client to develop competence in the skills necessary for leading as full a life as possible. Rehabilitation thus involves helping the client to compensate for any disabilities and learn coping strategies. It is not appropriate to define general standards of independent function since the needs of individuals vary greatly. What is a realistic aim for one person may be totally unattainable for the next.

It is necessary to consider rehabilitation in the context of psychiatric illness and consequent disability and handicap. Caplan (1961) suggested that handicap associated with mental illness is superimposed on the actual illness and is both treatable and preventable.

Disability does not mean that the person is handicapped. Someone who suffers from hallucinations may be able to adjust to hearing voices and learn to carry on living an effective life so that he is not handicapped in his day-to-day existence.

Active intervention is required if the handicapping effects of, for example, a schizophrenic illness are to be minimised. In this instance the balance between stimulation and overstimulation of the individual is a fine one, which cannot be clearly defined. Too much pressure creates stress and precipitates retreat into psychotic behaviour.

Wing & Morris (1981) described three factors that contribute to handicap:

1. psychiatric disabilities arising from the symptoms and illness process
2. social disadvantages, such as poverty or unemployment
3. adverse personal reaction to illness.

To these can be added the complexity of problems with which people are confronted when these three factors are combined. Various approaches to treatment may be used within the rehabilitation process, for example the cognitive-behavioural approach for social skills training and the humanistic approach to develop self-esteem. Models of treatment may include the model of human occupation or the occupational performance model.

Although the focus of intervention is the individual, it is essential to remember that family, friends, neighbours, employers, fellow clients and staff all play a significant part in the treatment process and in the degree of handicap experienced. Both hospital and community resources may be involved. Increasingly the focus is on working with clients in the community, without recourse to admission.

The rehabilitation process will consist of different stages, according to the needs of the individual:

- identification of problems
- possible intervention
- follow-up support as required.

For the person leaving hospital, additional points should be considered:

- preparation for resettlement
- actual resettlement in the community
- follow-up support as required by the individual.

It should be recognised that progress in rehabilitation may be slow, often over a period of years, and will represent much hard work on the part of both clients and staff.

The differences between rehabilitation and long-term care

Many long-term care facilities are described as using a rehabilitative approach and this may indeed be the case. However, it is not helpful for units to claim to be rehabilitation units when they are in fact, providing continuing care. Euphemistic labelling helps neither staff nor clients and leads to false expectations. Consequently, there may be a feeling of failure when unrealistic goals are not achieved.

The long-term care unit, be it in the hospital or community, aims to provide continuing care, very often lifelong, for clients with severe handicap. Such people may have an ongoing illness, such as schizophrenia, or a chronic condition such as Korsakoff's psychosis, and require shelter (asylum) from the demands of everyday community life. The focus is on support through fluctuating periods of illness.

In a ward or community house providing continuing care aimed at improving, or at least maintaining, clients' quality of life, staff can still use a rehabilitative approach. The aim of rehabilitation in this situation is to enable the person to gain a higher level of personal independence in the hope that he may eventually move to an environment that allows him to be more independent.

Much of the difference lies in the team's attitude and approach to clients and this will be discussed later. Differences will also be evident in the physical environment and the daily routine of the unit.

The rehabilitative approach places more responsibility on the client. For example, if a client is going out somewhere, he will be expected to tell staff where he is going and when he is likely to return, whereas in the long-term unit he will be told to come back at a specific time. This difference in emphasis is subtle, but nevertheless significant and may be quite threatening to people moving from one unit to another with a less structured approach.

The long-term care ward in a hospital can seem to be an under-resourced area, with consequent poor morale among staff. It is useful to bear in mind some of the positive social contacts, the facilities and the supportive structure that a hospital provides.

Wing (Wing & Brown 1971) said that even the most intractable client retains the power to surprise the persistent therapist and, over a long period of time, clients may move from a long-term unit to a rehabilitation facility. Providing a high standard of care for chronic clients is in itself a laudable aim that should be encouraged and not neglected, be it in the context of a hospital or the community.

PRINCIPLES OF REHABILITATION

General guidelines

What are some of the principles by which staff should be guided in planning treatment programmes? Hume (Hume & Pullen 1994) considers them to be as follows:

- Listen to the client.
- Know the community.
- Pay attention to detail.
- Remember how the world has changed.

Using these principles as a general guideline, it is possible to devise individual programmes.

Listen to the client

All therapists listen to their clients but it may take a considerable amount of time to unravel the problems. Clients may be unaware of what their real difficulties are and it becomes a shared process of discovery to identify the principal problems. The therapist must know the individual and be sensitive to verbal and non-verbal cues. It is also desirable to involve other people, for example, the family, who know the client well and can therefore identify problems that the individual himself may not recognise.

Know the community

The therapist must also be aware of what resources and facilities the community in which the client is living has to offer. It is simply not possible to prepare a client adequately for discharge if the therapist is unacquainted with the area to which he is going. Likewise, it is necessary to know what the cultural norms are so that clients can be given appropriate advice or social skills training if required. The occupational therapist does not need to know everything herself. Knowing where to obtain the information is the crucial factor.

Pay attention to detail

It is easy to overlook apparently trivial factors that may prove to be enormous obstacles for a particular individual. Inability to cope with what seems an easy, everyday task may produce feelings of inadequacy and incompetence. Attempts to compensate for deficiencies may exacerbate any social stigma that the person is experiencing.

Another potential pitfall is to assume that skills will generalise, that is be transferred to another similar behaviour. Ability in some aspect of activities of daily living, for example, does not imply competence in others. It is necessary to be comprehensive but not over-zealous in carrying out relevant assessments.

Remember how the world has changed

Awareness of changes that have occurred in a community is obviously of more significance for long-term hospital residents but this does not mean that others will not come across unexpected differences. Even a brief stay in hospital can inspire a feeling of being a stranger in your own home, let alone the wider community. Clients who are moving from one culture to another will obviously need considerable help in learning about their new locality (Ch. 26).

Other principles

Further principles, for example: some of which are very familiar to the occupational therapist – can also be incorporated into the rehabilitation process.

- The need for graded programmes, with staged treatment goals that enable the client to build up to the ultimate goal. This is closely linked to activity analysis.
- Clients may need to be taught skills that they have never had the opportunity to learn, or they may need to improve on skills that have not been used much during a period of hospitalisation. This includes an element of reorientation to the everyday world.
- The therapist must bear in mind the proposed ultimate goal for each client. If someone is to move to a hostel where all meals are provided it is less important to focus on meal preparation than it would be for someone who will need to be self-sufficient.

Attitudes and approach

Attitudes are of paramount importance in carrying out rehabilitation programmes. In an environment in which staff change frequently, extra demands may be placed on clients to establish temporary relationships with their carers and continuity is lacking. Clients have a need for a consistent approach from staff. Rigid imposition of rules one day cannot be followed by a casual approach the next if clients – or staff – are to have any sense of security.

Clients require an approach that can be compared to good parenting, that is, one that allows them to feel it is safe and natural to fail. We all learn from our mistakes and subsequent encouragement to try again. Sometimes, of course, people need to fail to learn the extent of their limitations.

The client's attitudes must also be taken into consideration. What are his hopes and expectations? How realistic are these? How do his ambitions relate to the ideas of his family and friends? Are they at variance?

Another important factor is attitude towards medication. This is not the prime concern of the occupational therapist but it is worthy of consideration. Clients may want to discuss their feelings about the need to take medication on a long-term basis, often a contentious issue. Some clients may learn to adjust their own medication according to changes in symptoms but, if unexplained changes in behaviour occur, it is worth enquiring whether the person is failing to take medication as prescribed. It is easy to forget to take pills, especially when you do not feel ill. The use of long-acting depot preparations may help, as they are given by injection every 2–3 weeks. There is therefore no need to remember to take tablets other than to counteract side-effects.

Bridging the gap between hospital and community

Many people will not have been admitted to hospital. For those who have, much of the rehabilitation process can be seen to be geared towards educating and re-educating people for life outside hospital. Clients need to have information about local resources and support services, an important part of the preparation required before moving from hospital into the community.

Rehabilitation, as Caplan (1964) indicated, does not end with discharge, and people require continuing support to enable them to integrate successfully into the community. Adequate ways of providing such support are problematic but services in the UK are being developed following the NHS and Community Care Act of 1993 (DoH 1990).

Ways in which community integration may be achieved will vary considerably according to the skills of the individual and the support services existing in a particular locality. Each rehabilitation team must devise its own system for ensuring that clients are not lost after discharge. Some teams operate a key worker system which facilitates coordination of the people and resources involved. Where care is transferred to a voluntary organisation, medical supervision may be provided by the parent hospital or primary care team.

Whatever the system, one important consideration is to prepare the ground for the individual at the point of discharge. Are community support services ready to become involved? Have workers made contact with the client already? This is highly desirable, although sometimes impracticable, so that a known and trusted person can reduce the stress of change involved in moving to a new environment.

Is the individual familiar with the locality? With all good intentions, despite all the team's efforts, this may not be the case if accommodation suddenly becomes available.

Community support

When the person is engaged in a rehabilitation programme in the community (without being admitted to hospital), it is obviously necessary to ensure that all services are provided and coordinated in an efficient way.

There may be a community mental health team with particular commitment to rehabilitation or it may be that one particular member of the team has an interest in this aspect of work. Local authority services may be available and there may be liaison with voluntary organisations. The system is perhaps less important than ensuring that care is provided. Many people escape or get lost, particularly those with more chronic problems who do not keep appointments or attend day care and require a more assertive outreach service.

CONTINUED SUPPORT

Within recent years there has been a development of community mental health teams targeting people suffering from severe and enduring mental health problems. As indicated above, the rehabilitation team should have decided how support should be provided. In the case of someone leaving hospital it may be necessary to retain a monitoring role for a period of time, to ensure that the stress of community living does not precipitate any relapse. This may be achieved by providing support to the organisation in which the client is living, or maintaining contact with the individual so that prompt intervention can take place if required. Liaison between hospital and community services is essential and should occur well before discharge occurs.

Increasingly, the community mental health team will provide ongoing support and each individual may have a key worker responsible for ensuring that appropriate services are in place for long-term support. It may be part of the occupational therapist's job to be a key worker within the team. In the absence of community mental health teams, the individual may require contact with the hospital as a day patient or referral to a day centre. For others, follow-up outpatient appointments or attendance at a medication clinic may be all that is necessary.

Liaison with outside agencies

Rehabilitation cannot take place solely within the confines of the hospital or home. Knowledge of community resources has already been emphasised as essential for members of the rehabilitation team. Every attempt should be made to initiate contact with agencies which can contribute to the rehabilitation process. Such agencies are many and varied, although they are most evident in urban areas. Local councils of voluntary organisations or coordinating groups for services for the disabled will be able to provide information about local resources, as will social work information officers and local mental health associations. These bodies may be most concerned with special resources for people with particular needs (e.g. alcohol abuse). Self-help groups may focus on the needs of sufferers, carers or both and liaison with these groups is a valuable aspect of rehabilitation.

Contact with self-help groups serves to provide clients with information about potential sources of help. Occasionally, staff might be invited to attend such a group for the purpose of giving information. Voluntary organisations, such as the National Schizophrenia Fellowship, usually welcome contact from mental health workers and this is mutually beneficial.

Other agencies provide services for the community as a whole, for example church lunch clubs or community centres, and clients can be encouraged to become involved in these during transitional phases of their rehabilitation programme. Occasional consultative visits from staff are generally appreciated by these groups and provide the opportunity for discussion of various mutual concerns.

Education, leisure and employment resources should also be considered although staff will have to be selective, or liaison can become a full time job! No one member of the team can possibly be aware of everything, but if each member establishes contact with agencies most relevant to his work and interests, the result will be a wide ranging body of knowledge which should be recorded in a place accessible to all.

CONTEXT

The theoretical principles of rehabilitation can be applied in any setting, including the client's own home. 'Rehabilitation begins with diagnosis' (Caplan 1961). From the occupational therapist's point of view this does not necessarily mean a medical label, although this does indicate some of the common symptoms and problems that may be anticipated. The therapist should base her identification of the individual's difficulties on her own assessment of the functional problems consequent on the illness.

However, there are general considerations which should be observed according to the location of treatment, some of which will be described here.

Acute admission ward

It may not be possible to transfer a client out of an admission ward once the acute phase of illness is over. Beds in slower moving wards will not always be available. The nature of the acute ward means that there are difficulties in attempting to introduce a rehabilitation approach for appropriate clients. Staff must focus their attention on those whose immediate needs are most urgent. The person who is independent and not at risk will inevitably take second place and may not receive the support he requires to make further progress. Staff must be aware of this as a potential problem.

Admission to hospital provides support in that the person is relieved of the responsibility of everyday tasks. It is, nevertheless, desirable to prevent people becoming institutionalised by preserving as high a degree of personal independence as is consistent with their illness.

Often, those who are well enough are encouraged to spend time away from hospital, carrying on their usual activities as far as they are able. While it is important not to keep the person away from the realities of everyday life for any longer than necessary, it is important to establish a programme which meets the needs of the individual. If an admission is of only a few days' duration it is important to draw up specific goals as soon as possible so that these can be continued after discharge.

If the person is to be transferred to a rehabilitation facility, staff on the acute ward can ensure that he becomes independent in everyday matters, such as personal hygiene and clothes care, and takes responsibility for his bedroom and routine chores around the ward. This can facilitate the move to a unit where he will be expected to be independent in particular tasks. Liaison between units is essential in ensuring that both understand the philosophy and approach of the respective services.

Rehabilitation unit/transitional care

As the name suggests, this is a facility targeted at rehabilitation. The entire programme will be geared towards promoting independence and the environment should also be structured towards this end (Hume & Pullen 1994).

Although the difference in emphasis may be subtle, it represents a definite, potentially threatening change in personal responsibility for clients. From having been given 'safe' boundaries within which to operate, the client now finds that he has a greater degree of freedom and is expected to set his own limits, even though initially this is in relation to simple, undemanding tasks.

The unit may be part of a transitional care system in which, depending upon local resources, there may be a gradual progression from the unit to a half way house, hostel or ward in the community, or discharge to a group home. The client is thus prepared for living in a small group context prior to discharge.

As the person becomes more capable of handling responsibilities for himself, supervision is gradually reduced.

Hostel/ward in the community

Hostels provide an environment in which clients can live with minimal supervision. The term 'ward in the community' has come into use to describe the role of units in which long-term clients are cared for in houses in ordinary residential areas. Such units may also be run by voluntary organisations or local authorities. The two terms tend to be used synonymously, actual use being determined by local preference, although the term 'hostel' usually implies a greater degree of independence. For convenience, hostel will be used here.

Staff may only be present during the day, night cover being on an on-call basis. On the other hand, much valuable work can be done by night staff during the late evenings, when clients who are out during the day are on the premises.

As in any hostel, residents assume a high level of personal responsibility, for instance individuals may have front door keys. Personal differences are sorted out by the residents with minimal staff intervention and any domestic matters, such as chore rotas, are also tackled by the group. Clients have responsibility for their own decision making and the organisation of their day. Preparation of meals may not be required of clients in a hospital hostel and, as suggested above, this should be balanced according to the ultimate proposed accommodation for the majority. If most clients will eventually move on to hostels run by outside organisations, where the meals are provided, it is not essential for them to be able to cook for themselves. In such cases, clients can develop their skills on an individual basis rather than as a group. Services such as laundry and cleaning may be arranged on an individual or joint basis.

The occupational therapist may be based in specialised local authority or health service teams targeting the mentally ill living in hostels where her role may be assertive outreach to clients who have become 'homeless'. Her role in a hostel may be more of a consultative one, with specific group sessions, rather than that of a permanent staff member, especially if clients are in work placements during the day.

Where hospital based occupational therapists are responsible for community psychiatric services, the therapist will extend this consultative role to community hostels for discharged clients.

INDEPENDENT ORGANISATIONS

With a decrease in the number of long-term beds available in hospitals, there has been an increase in the number of independent and voluntary organisations offering 'Homes for Life'. The Scottish Association for Mental Health, Penumbra, and the Richmond Fellowship are examples of organisations that offer people accommodation that maintains the maximum level of function possible for an individual within a community environment.

Group homes

These are the community side of transitional care. They are small houses or flats obtained through a variety of sources, ranging from district housing authorities and local mental health associations to individual enterprises.

At the stage of moving out of hospital and into the community, clients obviously cease to be in-patients, and this is the time to help them to adjust to their roles as ordinary members of society.

Group homes will be supervised in a variety of ways according to local custom and practice. Community psychiatric nurses or social workers may visit, or care workers and home care staff. If the home is one among many organised by a large body, there may be a warden in overall charge. Often, volunteers or befrienders may be involved.

The role of the occupational therapist may be minimal or she may be a key worker for a group of residents. Community based therapists may be highly involved in giving follow-up support for group home residents or this may be provided on a day care basis.

Whichever system operates in an area, it is essential to remember that, however good the pre-discharge preparation programme has been, difficulties will always arise as a consequence of moving to a new environment. There is a great difference between a hospital half-way house and a real home in the community, even if the physical surroundings seem comparable.

Assertive community treatment teams

As already mentioned, patients with severe and enduring mental health problems can be difficult to engage in services and can easily be lost to follow-up. Assertive community treatment teams are a clinically effective approach to managing the care of people with severe mental illness in the community (Marshall & Lockwood 1998). It is a team based approach rather than one based on key workers. Team members share responsibility for the clients and attempt to provide all the psychiatric and social care themselves rather than using other agencies. This could involve carrying out interventions that are not normally the traditional role of a mental health worker but are not unfamiliar to an occupational therapist, such as assisting a client to change a light bulb or complete a disability living allowance application form. The client:staff ratio is low, from 10:1 to 15:1, and the team is able to continue contact and offer services to reluctant or uncooperative people.

OCCUPATIONAL THERAPY IN REHABILITATION

Realistic goals

Wherever the therapist is working, be it in a community mental health team, hospital or other location, setting realistic goals within the context of rehabilitation may be a frustrating process. Scarcity of resources may preclude desired aims, although lack of resources should never be an excuse for omitting particular targets. Constraints may nevertheless operate and it is important that clients learn to cope with the realities.

As already indicated, the expectations of clients and relatives may not be realistic and the therapist must also beware of projecting her own hopes onto the client. An objective approach is essential.

AREAS OF INTERVENTION

Assessment of need will identify the priorities of the individual and, from these, treatment programmes can be devised. The increase in

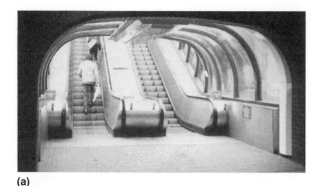

(a)

Figure 20.1 Personal independence can be promoted by familiarising clients with different aspects of life in the community. **(a)** Using escalators.

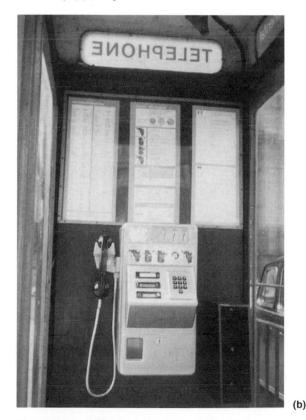

(b)

Figure 20.1 **(b)** Using a payphone and promoting appropriate social skills.

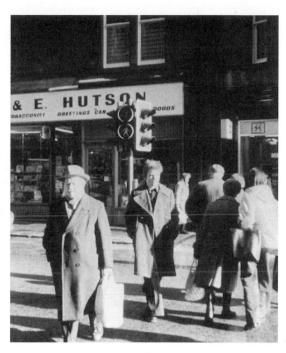

(c)

Figure 20.1 **(c)** Traffic signals and general road safety.

assessed using standardised assessment schedules or checklists (see Ch. 6), although units may devise their own forms.

Designing programmes relevant to the individual encompasses many aspects of the client's life and it is impossible to separate out any one aspect in practice. The main focus is likely to be on activities of daily living (ADL) but, for the sake of simplicity, aspects of care are here divided into four main areas:

- personal independence and social skills
- domestic and community living skills
- leisure
- work.

Personal independence and social skills

Included under this heading are self-care, interpersonal relationships and the social skills related to competence in both these areas. Decision making, day-to-day personal organisation and management of time (temporal adaptation) are also relevant (Fig. 20.1).

the numbers of standardised assessments has enabled occupational therapists to formalise the assessment process and measure outcomes in rehabilitation. Ideally, each aspect should be

Self-care, in the sense of personal hygiene, will probably be largely the responsibility of nursing staff but there are opportunities for the occupational therapist to reinforce socially acceptable levels of hygiene. Use of make-up, facial care (for both men and women), hair and hand care can all be included in self-care groups. The importance of other aspects of self-care, such as use of deodorants, menstrual hygiene and foot care, should not be overlooked. Safe sex and contraception, which may have been neglected elsewhere, can be incorporated naturally into self-care groups. Selection of clothes to enhance personal appearance may also need attention and can lead to lively group discussion!

In the context of rehabilitation, personal care often includes taking medication. This is largely the domain of nursing staff but it may sometimes be relevant to check that necessary medication is being taken. The occupational therapist may find that clients want to discuss this aspect of care along with other personal matters. It is essential that clients learn to administer their own pills. For those who are to attend a medication clinic it may be necessary to organise a visit to the clinic prior to discharge to establish contact.

Social skills

Competence in personal relationships must be considered and this is an area where social skills training may be required. Very basic skills may need rehearsal and clients who are withdrawn should practise asking for information and making their needs known to others. Non-verbal skills may be deficient and correct identification of emotional expression may require attention.

More sophisticated social skills might include dating skills and appropriate sexual behaviour, interview skills and assertive behaviour. The latter is a common area of difficulty, especially for those who have been in hospital for long periods or who tend to be self-effacing. Others may be inclined to aggressive outbursts and require to learn the difference between aggressive, assertive and passive behaviour in order to gain confidence and self-control.

Social skills training should always be integrated with practice, for example sharing a meal with a group of clients may provide a realistic opportunity to assess and improve interactive and hostess skills. Such refinements as passing salt and pepper may be lacking and conversation totally absent!

Any individual deficiencies in social skills, or problem areas related to specific conditions, should be dealt with as relevant. For example, someone who has alcohol-related problems may need to learn and practise how to refuse a drink that has already been poured and is being handed to him, before encountering the real situation.

Domestic skills

Teaching skills for coping with the practicalities of daily life is often seen as one of the occupational therapist's major contributions to rehabilitation. Certainly, domestic skills, including cooking and household management, are crucial in any programme. Without competence in these areas of life, survival in the community is likely to be problematic. Clothes care and awareness of general safety and security should also be part of any programme. It is tempting to try to cover all aspects of domestic skills, sometimes to a degree of competence well above that of the average citizen. Not all of us can change a fuse, replace a zip or repair broken glasses, but we know where to obtain the necessary assistance.

Wherever possible, treatment should take place in the person's own home, since a strange kitchen immediately puts someone at a disadvantage. In the context of long-term care, the ideal for someone being discharged from hospital is to practise household skills in the context of an assessment flat, where the client has a weekly allowance and learns to budget for food, heating and lighting.

Goals must be geared to the future. If the individual will eventually be using a launderette, then learning to use the washing machine in the occupational therapy department or the ward is not necessarily helpful. Instead, the occupational therapist can focus on ironing and discuss the meaning of some of the more obscure laundry labels so that 'dry clean only' clothes do not find their way into the wash.

Cooking may be a matter of refining existing skills in supportive surroundings, learning how to use relevant modern gadgets, such as microwave ovens, or it may necessitate covering the whole range of menu planning, budgeting and shopping, meal preparation and cleaning up. Hygiene and safety can readily be incorporated into kitchen activities as can nutritional education.

It is worth stressing that, although one kitchen assessment will demonstrate the individual's ability to produce a meal on that occasion, it does not ensure the motivation to do so in future nor the ability to cope with day-by-day economic menu planning.

For someone new to independent living, the rest of the home must be remembered, perhaps by shopping for bed linen, furniture or any other necessities for setting up home. Advertisers would have us believe that we require numerous gadgets and substances for efficient living so the realities need to be discussed.

Finally, remember that most rehabilitation units have an ever-open door and clients will need to consider security, keys and answering the door bell when there is no member of staff to do so. Practice of these latter skills is particularly important before people move into their own accommodation as well as subsequently.

Leisure

The value of leisure in maintaining a balanced and healthy lifestyle is often overlooked and discussion about the benefits of leisure may be required. Hospital life often provides a structured day of work and, to a greater or lesser extent, a range of leisure activities. For many clients, unstructured evenings and weekends may be a time of boredom and apathy and one of the important aims of the rehabilitation programme is to encourage them to plan how to use their free time. People need to learn to pursue their own interests rather than to rely on things

being organised for them because this will be their own responsibility once they leave hospital. Again, remember normality. We do not have to follow a hectic round of social activities to have a satisfying life. Watching television is an important activity for the majority of the population in the UK.

For many people in the community, a balance between relaxation and activity needs to be learned. A social network map may usefully indicate existing areas of contact and the use of a leisure inventory such as the interest check list (Matsutsuyu 1969), can be a useful way of introducing ideas, discovering preference and fostering time structuring habits. Identification of community resources for recreation and hobbies can also make clients aware of the range of opportunities available.

Sharing information about individual interests between clients may serve as an introduction to pursuits that may be continued on a long-term basis. Those clients who wish to do so can be encouraged to use special social resources within the locality, such as clubs run by local mental health associations. Support from a member of staff, a volunteer or another client may be necessary during the first visit. It is important that clients understand that other people will be sizing them up and that their welcome may not be all they had hoped for on the first occasion.

The cost of leisure activities is something that most people see as a potential barrier. Discovering resources that are free, or offer reduced rates to those on pensions or unemployment benefit, is part of the activity identification process. Assisting clients to build supportive social networks is essential to minimise the risk of readmission to a hospital as a result of isolation (Schoenfeld et al 1986).

For most of us, visiting or entertaining friends is a key leisure activity and one which may be denied to clients who have lost contact with family or friends. Volunteers may help by befriending individuals, inviting clients to their homes or arranging outings. Clients in hospital can be encouraged to return hospitality, thereby developing hostess skills for the time when they may be able to entertain others in their own home. Teaching social skills for dealing with unwanted visitors might also be contemplated.

Physical health may be promoted through sports and more energetic pursuits. Current research indicates the psychological benefits of such activity (see Ch. 12).

Work

In the current economic climate, what is the role of the occupational therapist in work rehabilitation? This question has been widely considered in the field of psychiatric rehabilitation. Monteath (1983) stressed that assessment and preparation for work are key functions of occupational therapy and this includes work in the widest sense, paid or unpaid. On the other hand, recognition that clients may require preparation for unemployment has to be accepted as a reality. As the proportion of the general public that is unemployed rises, so the stigma for clients who cannot find a job falls, but this does not negate the value of work programmes as a useful aspect of rehabilitation (Dyer 1993, Ekdawi & Conning 1994).

Recently, work hardening, preparing people to tolerate the rigours and demands of full-time work, has attracted considerable attention (Jacobs 1985). This is similar to the industrial units of the 1960s and 1970s.

Work may mean different things to different people, so it is helpful to establish a definition of work, whether full or part-time, paid, voluntary, sheltered or open employment or housework, so that a relevant programme can be devised for the individual. The therapist should have contact with statutory services (Department of Employment PACT teams) and be aware of local resources and training opportunities. Knowledge of local schemes designed to meet the needs of those seeking alternatives to remunerative employment should also be acquired.

For those who are able to return to an existing job or similar work, development of general work skills is an obvious requirement and a full-time simulated work programme may be indicated in order to develop work tolerance.

Most clients who experience difficulties at work do so because of social withdrawal rather than the actual job. Assessment of associated social skills should therefore encompass not only working relationships at different levels but also informal conversational situations, such as coffee breaks.

Pre-work groups, such as those described by Kramer (1984), are an excellent way of sharing knowledge, practising job-seeking skills and providing support to those undergoing interviews, particularly those which are unsuccessful. The opportunity to discuss the 'Do I tell them I've had psychiatric treatment?' dilemma gives people a chance to make up their own minds about how to tackle this issue for themselves.

Pre-vocational assessment may be carried out if an individual wishes to try out various types of work prior to determining priorities for job choice. If a change of job is indicated, further training may be organised. The possibility of gaining work experience through placement with local employers can also be investigated.

Liaison with voluntary agencies may provide work opportunities and the possibility of a reference for future job applications. Attitudes towards volunteers should be assessed, as the expectations of the agency may not match those of the worker in terms of commitment or task allocations.

It is possible that the occupational therapist may play a key role in the establishment and running of alternative work schemes or skill training projects. Imagination is required in devising such schemes, particularly to meet the needs of people with long-term illness.

The UK government's 'New Deal' initiative brought about the setting up of agencies run by local authorities, such as Job Coaching or Job Works, that seek out jobs then train and support people with mental health problems to remain in them. As with voluntary organisations, such schemes are often subject to temporary sources of funding.

PERSONNEL

One of the myths of rehabilitation is that it is an area in which high levels of staffing are not required. In fact, in order to carry out the necessary activities on an individual or small group basis, the reverse is true, whatever the location of treatment. In a study of rehabilitation resources in Scotland, McCreadie and colleagues (1985) investigated staffing in long-term wards, rehabilitation units and day care facilities. They reported that occupational therapy helpers devoted more time to long-term wards than any other staff group, while qualified therapists tended to work in specific rehabilitation units or day units. (The study did not include students.) Since the time of this research, many occupational therapy helpers in the UK have undertaken Scotvec/NVQ modular programmes and are eminently well qualified to take on this work. Although few in number, occupational therapy staff seem to be the most committed to hospital based rehabilitation services.

The multidisciplinary team

The multidisciplinary team in the rehabilitation setting will have the same membership as in any other hospital unit, depending upon local availability of staff. In addition to the core team is the extended team and the community team. The composition of the three teams will vary, but may be as follows:

Core team

- medical staff
- nurses
- occupational therapist
- social worker
- clinical psychologist

Extended team

- administrators
- chaplain
- catering staff
- ancillary staff
- volunteers

Community team

- community psychiatric nurses
- occupational therapists
- primary health care staff
- social services staff
- community workers
- voluntary organisations.

Membership of community care teams may be the same as that of the core team. This will vary according to the base, be it local authority social work services or a voluntary organisation. It should be remembered that much community care and support is provided by self-help groups and carers' groups.

Staff training

Inevitably, members of the team are educated according to the philosophies of their own professions. Individuals may have experience in a rehabilitation context during their initial professional education or not until postgraduate study, as is often the case with medical staff. Current debate about skill mix and patient focused care may alter this situation in future.

In order for a care team to have a cohesive approach, there is a need for in-service education. This may be done partly on an informal basis, with individuals explaining their treatment objectives to the team and the contribution they feel they can best make. Such sharing may help to iron out interprofessional differences and will also highlight individual areas of expertise. Staff can discuss attitudes and approaches, for example the difficulties of one professional standpoint being different from another or medical and social models of treatment resulting in conflicting aims. Alternatively, one team member may be concerned about the demands being placed on an individual client and wish to discuss this concern with other team members.

Formal training exists for professional groups, ranging from rehabilitation nursing courses to study days on a multidisciplinary basis. Organisations such as the World Association for Psychosocial Rehabilitation (WAPR) can extend contacts on a wider basis through study days and international conferences. Although this cannot strictly be regarded as training, the education component and exchange of ideas are valuable.

Staff in rehabilitation units have a responsibility to educate their colleagues in other areas. This is partly public relations but it also leads to more realistic referrals and expectations.

Staff support and supervision

An important aspect of any job should be provision of a structure for supervision and support. This is sometimes regarded as a sign of inadequacy rather than professional maturity, although there is growing recognition of the need for support, particularly in situations where a mix of skills is the norm.

In a situation where results may be slow, and setbacks not infrequent, it is essential that there is an arena for discussing the feelings of frustration or failure which may occur. A fresh, neutral opinion may inject alternative ideas or reinforce efforts to continue in the face of perceived difficulties.

Everyone needs affirmation for the task they are doing and rehabilitation staff are no exception.

The role of relatives

Often, particularly in the case of people with chronic illness, there is no known next of kin because of estrangement or death. Where relatives and significant others are involved, their contribution is crucial to the rehabilitation process. They may have their own specific needs for support in the situation.

Assuming that the client is in agreement, relatives will have contact with staff during visits to hospital or may arrange to be present when someone visits the home. Contact may be with a key worker, or with someone with particular expertise, according to need. The occupational therapist should play a part in such contact.

Carers may seek reassurance about the nature of the illness and possible outcomes. Although this should have been given at an earlier stage of the illness, initial worries may inhibit understanding therefore opportunities for further discussion should be offered.

Treatment planning requires the involvement of key people as soon as is practicable. Parents, spouse, employers and friends all have a part to play. Those most significant for the individual should be invited to discuss goals and aims. Their support and cooperation is vital; it may be impossible to achieve particular aims without it.

Joint interviews may be arranged to deal with emotionally loaded topics such as possible separation or desirable changes in behaviour patterns. Interviews may also focus on situations where conflicts in parental behaviour are creating problems for the client.

The work of Vaughn and Leff (Leff 1991) on emotional expression has made it possible to assess family groups in order to identify levels of emotional interaction. Patterns of interaction such as high incidence of critical comments or other emotionally demanding statements are referred to as 'high expressed emotion'. Once identified, such patterns of behaviour may be modified as families are taught how to respond differently. Relatives can be helped to understand that the client's experience is real for him and that they should not dismiss bizarre statements as nonsense. Reinforcing the content of delusional ideas by agreeing with the person's statements is not helpful in promoting contact with shared reality. Changing the subject, or some other diversionary tactic may serve to defuse a potentially difficult situation and families can gain much by the use of such strategies (Falloon & Pederson 1985).

Learning to set limits on unacceptable behaviour will not necessarily be easy. Families for whom the client's illness is a source of long-term stress may be supported through relatives' groups. Sharing practical information and coping strategies, or ventilating the stress of dealing with difficult behaviour, may relieve some of the feelings of anxiety or guilt.

In describing a needs based approach to the management of schizophrenia, Howe (1995) proposed a model of damage limitation. In order to change from a concept of crisis intervention to one of crisis prevention, she highlighted the need to implement improved education and training for service providers as well as support and information for the family. This model includes helping sufferers to keep well by understanding their own illness and highlights the need for liaison between all those involved in order to recognise early warning signs and minimise the chances of relapse.

Problems and constraints

The complaint is frequently made that resources are inadequate and money is not available to alter the situation. This should not become an excuse for lack of activity. What are other difficulties which the rehabilitation team has to face? A selection will illustrate some issues.

Role conflicts

One of the biggest problems for individual staff lies in the fact that the occupational therapist works in a multidisciplinary team rather than in a professional group. The classes of skills provided by any mental health worker have been defined by Joice & Coia (1989) as:

- statutory skills required by legislation
- professional skills restricted as a result of obtaining a professional qualification
- core skills not restricted to a discipline but expected of one more than another
- Basic shared skills common to all disciplines
- specialist skills obtained as result of an individual's special interest and enthusiasm.

Differentiating between the different classes of skills can be problematic and role blurring may lead to professional identity crises. Teams have to be specific about the skills that are expected of each discipline. Compiling a team operational policy can provide the mechanism for the multidisciplinary team to clarify each discipline's role. The sole representative of a profession can feel very isolated within the team, hence the need for support and supervision already mentioned.

Many health workers have been trained to care for clients rather than to let them do things for

themselves. This is not the occupational therapy ethos and standing back can cause conflicts at both a personal and interpersonal level.

Risk taking

Some of the tasks required within the rehabilitation process carry with them an element of risk taking behaviour, which can create tension and anxiety for the staff who feel, and are, responsible for their clients. Climbing stepladders or using potentially dangerous electrical appliances may be necessary skills they need to master and staff should be able to discuss their apprehensions in a supportive context. Real living does entail risks!

Motivation and interest

In many instances, staff are allocated to particular units rather than being able to choose where they work. This can mean that people may be sent to work in wards or areas which are not their principal interest. Rehabilitation is no exception to this and the subject must be dealt with openly to prevent undercurrents and dissatisfaction.

Applicants for posts, particularly for new projects, can be selected for enthusiasm as well as other qualities, and it is important that staff are supported during the planning stages, initial problems and in maintaining momentum after the implementation phase is over (Hume & Pullen 1994).

External constraints

Not all difficulties originate within the unit itself, although there may be a knock-on effect. After several months' work with an individual destined to move into sheltered accommodation, there may be no suitable place available at the time when he is ready to move and it is difficult to maintain momentum in such circumstances. Equally, sudden availability of accommodation may lead to a precipitate move and feelings of incomplete preparation, which raise anxieties.

An ongoing problem, shared by all working in the field of mental health, is that of stigma.

This may be aggravated by media reports of dramatic and unusual events which arouse prejudice and fears of the general public, thus making the achievement of clients' goals more difficult. Much education of the general public can be achieved during the process of establishing housing projects, resource centres or day care projects, so that everyone understands the problems and needs, and has a realistic understanding.

Burnout

A final difficulty, which is not peculiar to the rehabilitation team, is that of burnout. Working with the same clients, over long periods of time, with minimal progress can lead to feelings of disillusionment and rigidity in attitudes. Greater awareness of this has prompted investigation and preventive measures can now be identified and implemented (Pollock 1986).

Innovation should be encouraged rather than rejected and attempts can be made to avoid becoming static. Equally, the demands of recent reorganisation within health care necessitate understanding that change can be difficult and may be felt to be negating the value of current programmes.

Fidler (1984) outlined ways in which changes can be implemented to facilitate maximum acceptance of the new ideas by those who will be responsible for implementing them. A feeling of involvement and ownership is of paramount importance so that people (clients and staff) can make their views known and do not feel that change is being thrust upon them.

SUMMARY

The occupational therapist has the responsibility for continually evaluating treatment and for introducing techniques and methods appropriate to the current needs of patients and society. The work is anything but static and further research and evaluation are much needed.

The scope of rehabilitation is unlimited and it can be one of the most exciting areas of psychiatric practice. The location of work may change, but the needs of clients remain.

This chapter has considered the following points:

- what rehabilitation is
- the principles of rehabilitation
- transition from hospital to community
- community care
- the role of the occupational therapist in rehabilitation
- personal independence and social skills
- domestic skills
- leisure
- work and occupation
- the multidisciplinary team
- staffing
- role of the family in rehabilitation
- liaison with other bodies
- problems encountered in rehabilitation.

REFERENCES

Caplan G 1961 An approach to community mental health. Tavistock, London
Caplan G 1964 Principles of preventive psychiatry. Basic Books, New York
Clark D H 1984 The development of a psychiatric rehabilitation service. Lancet 2: 625–627
Department of Health 1990 NHS and Community Care Act. HMSO, London
Dyer J 1993 Rehabilitation and community care. In: Kendell R, Zealley A (eds) Companion to psychiatric studies, 5th edn. Churchill Livingstone, Edinburgh, ch 42
Ekdawi M, Conning A 1994 Psychiatric rehabilitation: a practical guide. Chapman and Hall, London

Falloon I, Pederson J 1985 Family management in the prevention of morbidity of schizophrenia: the adjustment of the family unit. British Journal of Psychiatry 147: 156–163
Fidler G S 1984 Design of rehabilitation services in psychiatric hospital settings. RAMSCO, Maryland
Hagedorn R 1992 Occupational therapy: foundations for practice. Churchill Livingstone, Edinburgh, ch 3
Howe G 1995 Working with schizophrenia: a needs based approach. Jessica Kingsley, London, ch 13
Hume C, Pullen I (eds) 1994 Rehabilitation for mental health problems. Churchill Livingstone, Edinburgh, chs 1, 7

Jacobs K 1985 Occupational therapy: work-related programs and assessment. Little Brown, Boston

Joice A, Coia D 1989 Skills of the occupational therapist working within the multidisciplinary team. British Journal of Occupational Therapy 52: 12: 466–468

Kramer L 1984 SCORE: solving community obstacles and restoring employment. Haworth Press, New York

Leff J 1991 Schizophrenia: social influences on onset and relapse. In: Bennett D, Freeman H (eds) Community psychiatry. Churchill Livingstone, Edinburgh, ch 6

McCreadie R, Affleck J, Robinson A 1985 The Scottish survey of psychiatric rehabilitation and support services. British Journal of Psychiatry 147: 289–294

Marshall, Lockwood 1998 Assertive community treatment for people with severe mental disorders. Cochrane Library

Matsutsuyu J S 1969 The interest check list. American Journal of Occupational Therapy 23(4): 323–328

Monteath H G 1983 Work rehabilitation in the current economic climate. British Journal of Occupational Therapy 46: 8

Pollock L 1986 The multidisciplinary team. In: Hume C, Pullen I Rehabilitation in psychiatry. Churchill Livingstone, Edinburgh, ch 6

Schoenfeld P, Halevy J, Hemley E, Ruhf L 1986 Long-term outcome of network therapy. Hospital and Community Psychiatry 37(4)

Wing J K, Brown G W 1971 Institutionalism and schizophrenia. Cambridge University Press, Cambridge

Wing J K, Morris B (eds) 1981 Handbook of psychiatric rehabilitation. Oxford University Press, Oxford

World Health 1984 (Leading article.) Policies. World Health (May): 5

21

Older people

Jackie Pool

INTRODUCTION

Ageing is a continuing part of lifespan development. Life expectancy, that is the length of time a person can expect to live, as predicted at the moment of birth, alters according to factors such as health, social circumstances and social trends. These must be favourable if life expectancy is to be achieved. The study of demographic trends shows that people are living longer as the barriers to achieving life expectancy are removed.

The 1991 census of Great Britain showed that people of pensionable age (65 years and over for men and 60 years and over for women) made up 18.7% of the population, an increase of 0.8% since 1981 (Government Statistical Service 1992). It is predicted that this trend will continue and that by 2026 the number of people aged 65 years and over will increase by 30%. The greatest increase will be in the number of very old people, that is those aged 85 years and over. In the population of England and Wales this figure will increase by 66% (Table 21.1).

The majority of older people live independently but these demographic trends do indicate an overall increased incidence of problems related to old age. Well-being depends on a balance of physical and mental health and social support. A breakdown of any one of these factors can lead to a breakdown of all three, therefore a holistic approach to working with older people is essential. Occupational therapists, with their wide range of knowledge and skills, are well equipped to work in this field.

Table 21.1 Projected change in population 1989–2026, England and Wales.(Source: Office of Population, Census and Surveys 1991.)

Age group	1989	2026	Absolute change, millions	Percentage change, %
0–4	3.3	3.4	0.1	3
5–14	6.1	6.7	0.6	10
15–24	7.7	6.7	−1.0	−13
25–44	14.6	13.9	−0.7	−5
45–64	10.9	13.6	2.7	25
65–74	4.5	5.5	1.0	23
75–84	2.8	3.7	0.9	33
85+	0.8	1.3	0.5	66
All ages	50.6	54.8	4.2	8

There is a commonly held belief that old age is a time of mental decline, but, as Twining observed in 1988, 80% of those who live to be 80 years or more show no sign of dementia. Indeed, only a small percentage of older people consult general practitioners about their mental health problems in comparison with other conditions such as circulatory or respiratory diseases (Fig. 21.1).

Occupational therapists working in the mental health field can offer a range of services to older people. This may be within the National Health Service, in specialist in-patient units for assessment and treatment purposes, or in day hospitals. There may be a respite care service offered and this is often coupled with the use of counselling skills to support the relatives and carers of this patient group. The implementation of the Care in the Community Act (DoH 1990) in 1993 has expanded the role of occupational therapists working with their clients living in the community. Older people who do not present themselves for treatment from the National Health Service may receive an occupational therapy

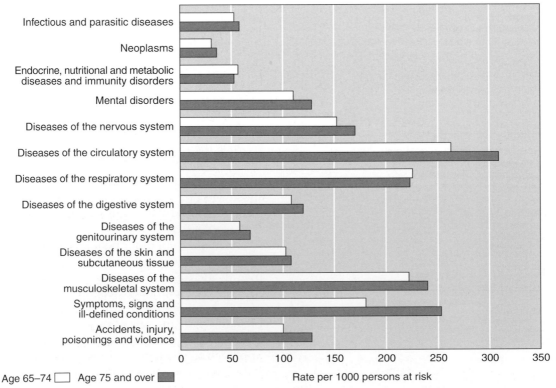

Age 65–74 ☐   Age 75 and over ▉   Rate per 1000 persons at risk

Figure 21.1 Causes of general practitioner consultations among people 65 years and over. (OPCS 1983 Morbidity statistics from general practice, 1981–1982.)

service from social service employed therapists. This may be achieved by direct referral and, in some cases, the general practitioner may be involved initially. This is often the case when relatives and carers seek professional help directly from their social services department. As the Care in the Community Act becomes more widely implemented there is also an increasing opportunity for occupational therapists to tender their services in a freelance capacity. Whatever the employment status of the occupational therapist, this diversity of career opportunities enables the needs of older people with mental disorders to be met in a variety of ways.

This chapter is set out in three sections. The first section looks at the ageing process. It promotes the concept of ageing as a positive experience and discusses theories of normal ageing, including biological theories, disengagement theory and activity theory. The social–psychological effects of ageing, cultural patterns and the multipathology of old age are also explored. The next section looks at mental disorders of old age, setting out the epidemiology, aetiology, pathology and clinical features of each. The final section explores ways of working with older people with mental disorders. Values and principles of practice are discussed. Then the occupational therapy process of assessment, treatment and care planning, implementation and evaluation is applied to this client group. In summary, the chapter looks at the challenge of working with older people with mental disorders in terms of changing attitudes, ensuring quality care and the need for ongoing research in this field.

THE AGEING PROCESS

Attitudes towards ageing

An understanding of normal ageing is essential if we are to understand mental disorders in old age. The mental capacity of older people is often underestimated. Provided they escape dementia and other brain diseases, healthy old people retain the ability to make their own decisions and to run their own lives. Old age can and

should be a positive experience, with more time available to engage in enjoyable activities, to spend with the family and to reflect. Unfortunately, some old people accept the belief that old age is a time of decline and this then becomes self-fulfilling. For example, there is a belief that all old people are incontinent, therefore an old person may accept incontinence as inevitable when there is probably a physiological cause which **can** be treated. This is just one example of how **atti**tudes to old age affect old people's self-attitudes so that they accept the avoidable as the inevitable, and thus contribute to the negative stereotype of old age.

This negative attitude to old age is not only held by older people, but reflects the attitude of society generally. We have inherited ageist attitudes and dogmas from our history and are applying them to today's society. However, Professor Eric Midwinter (1993), former director of the Centre for Policy on Ageing, suggested we should be adopting a completely revised concept of old age. Midwinter suggested that the construct of stages rather than ages is more useful and proposed three: childhood and socialisation, child-rearing and paid work, and the third stage in which people retire from one or both of these tasks.

WHAT IS AGEING?

Physiological ageing

An ageing process is any process in the individual which increases the likelihood of death in a given time interval. Ageing starts when physiological maturation stops. The ageing of individual organs depends on their type and cellular structure. For example, the heart wall becomes more rigid and the elasticity of large arteries is reduced. Lung capacity remains unchanged but vital capacity falls and there is a reduction in the elasticity of tissue. Muscle bulk and innervation is also reduced, causing myopathy and reduced muscle power. Muscle bulk can be increased by exercise but not the muscular cell count. There is, on average, a 1% reduction in physical function per year from the age of 30 years.

Reliable information about the structure of the normal brain in old age is difficult to find; many brains examined at post-mortem are likely to show the abnormalities of disease as well as normal ageing changes. These age-related changes may include reduced weight and volume of the brain, enlarged sulci and ventricles, thickening and hardening of blood vessels and the meninges, fewer neurones in some areas, and reduced amounts of neurotransmitters (Roberts 1989).

Psychological effects of ageing

Observations of healthy older people reveal evidence that there are only slight changes in memory function. Short-term memory is affected more than long-term but these effects are more apparent for recall than for recognition. If older people are given choices or cues their performance improves.

Learning tends to be slower but this is sometimes due to a tendency to persist with poor strategies. Slower learning does not necessarily mean that the final level of skill will be less, just that the older person may take a little longer to get there.

Some thought processes are more affected by old age than others. The most noticeable change is in the speed of reacting to something unfamiliar. Crystallised intellect (wisdom) changes less than fluid thinking (lateral thinking/problem solving).

These changes are not enough to affect everyday functioning but may be influential if the older person is under any type of stress, including physiological. Continuity characterises the personality in old age, with patterns emerging from maturity onwards. Therefore, marked personality changes are a sign of illness and not of ageing.

Old people are not all the same but there are differences between young and old people due to differences in background and upbringing. These are known as cohort differences.

Cultural patterns of ageing

Social conditions have had the greatest effect on the transition from a young to an ageing population in the UK. This country was the first to make the transition because it was the first to have an industrial revolution which led to improved living conditions. Whereas in developed countries the demographic transition has evolved, in developing countries the ageing population has been achieved artificially, by reducing the birth rate and improving the mortality rate, even among adverse social and environmental conditions. In some developing countries, even though poor social conditions still exist, the mortality rate from disease has fallen because of an increase in the availability of vaccinations and treatment. In some countries women have chosen to reduce their birth rates by being sterilised. This practice is encouraged by medical practitioners who receive fees for carrying out this service.

Attitudes to old age in the West can be seen as discriminatory, with older people being viewed as a financial drain on society: unproductive, dependent and in need of costly health care. In the East there is a tradition of viewing older people with respect and valuing their wisdom and experience. Unfortunately, this is now changing as the ageing population increases. In Japan, for example, it has been estimated that by the year 2020 one in four citizens will be over 65 years of age. The Japanese have become so worried about the cost of supporting their ageing population that they are considering 'exporting' it. Retirement cities in low-cost countries have been built as a way of moving large groups of old people out of Japan.

In the West there is a noticeable absence of positive images of old age in the media and an increasing obsession with methods of avoiding old age through diet, exercise, use of chemicals and surgery. When older people are used in advertising they usually support the negative stereotype rather than reflect the reality.

THEORIES OF AGEING

Theories that explain the processes involved in ageing have been produced by psychologists, biologists and sociologists. Aspects of these theories should be incorporated into the knowledge base of occupational therapy to increase therapists' understanding of the functioning of their older clients and to enhance clinical judgement, effective treatment and informed prognosis.

Developmental theories

Human development has fascinated men of literature and science throughout the centuries. The various developmental theories are dealt with in more depth in other books, such as Lewis's *The Mature Years* (Lewis 1969). Human development follows a sequence which may be viewed as occurring in stages. Arrival at each stage depends on many factors, including the maturity of the individual, gender, culture, class and the experiences they have encountered. Although the sequence of development is orderly, some individuals will reach these stages ahead of others. There are several theories of stages of development. Two which are particularly helpful when working with people with dementia are cognitive development and social development. Developmental theory is widely used in occupational therapy practice (Zemke & Gratz 1982) and forms the basis of such therapeutic techniques as reminiscence and validation. These can be used, for example, to help resolve the final developmental crisis of old age: the search for meaning in one's life in order to achieve integrity (Erikson 1959).

Biological theories

While a deep understanding of genetic and cellular structure is not essential for an occupational therapist, an awareness of biological changes and associated psychological factors is important for individual assessment. Equally important is a recognition of the sociopsychological impact that biological ageing can have. Relationships and status can alter as people begin to interact differently with the visibly ageing individual, sometimes to the extent that the psychological well-being of the older person is affected. This phenomenon is even more evident when the ageing individual is also displaying signs of a dementing illness. This will be discussed further in the section on working with older people with mental disorders.

Genetic theories

There are three hypotheses about the genetic factors which may cause ageing:

1. *Error accumulation* describes the formation of abnormal proteins which cause abnormal enzymes to rise to critical levels, leading eventually to death.
2. *Mutation* describes a more spontaneous change which, again, causes abnormalities to reach a critical level and leads to death.
3. *Programmed ageing* suggests that all individuals have a biological clock which is set at the moment of conception to run for a given length of time.

Cross-linkage

This theory suggests that abnormal bonds formed in collagen fibres lose their elasticity and eventually cause the organ to cease functioning.

Free radical

Oxygen molecules have pairs of orbiting electrons. Sometimes abnormal molecules are produced which have one electron missing. The remaining free electron acts like a magnet, attracting an electron from a neighbouring molecule. This sets off a sequence of cells changing their molecular structure and, as a result, body tissue becomes altered. The effect may be of ageing or of disease, such as cancer. The theory proposes that certain substances, including some linked to smoking, may increase the production of abnormal oxygen molecules and that others, such as vitamin E, may reduce them.

Social disengagement theory

This theory proposes that there is a mutual withdrawal of society from the individual (due to compulsory retirement, children growing up and leaving home, and so on) and of the individual from society (reduced social activities and a more solitary life). It is mainly based on a 5-year study of 275 people aged 50–90 in Kansas City (Cumming & Henry 1961). However, the theory came under criticism because it assumes that withdrawal from society is an inherent part of ageing. A follow-up study, including 55% of the original 275, showed that, although increasing age is accompanied by increasing disengagement, the most socially engaged people were the most happy (Havighurst et al 1968).

Disengagement may be cohort-specific, that is, it may have been adaptive to withdraw from an ageist society in the 1950s when the original study was carried out, but withdrawal may not be necessary now. Many of the social conditions which forced older people into restricted environments in the past have changed so that more active and socially engaged lifestyles are now possible (Turner & Helms 1989).

However, some older people do prefer to disengage and activity can decline without adversely affecting morale. A more leisurely lifestyle with fewer responsibilities can be seen as one of the rewarding aspects of old age.

Activity theory

This is the major alternative to social disengagement theory and is sometimes called reengagement theory. It asserts that the natural tendency of most older people is to associate with others, particularly in group and community affairs (Maddox 1963, Lemon et al 1972). By becoming more socially active, older people engage more in leisure activities. The achievement of leisure goals serves to sustain the older person's self-esteem and morale.

Social exchange theory

This theory criticises both disengagement and activity theories for not taking into account the physical and economic factors which may limit an individual's choice of how he ages. On retirement, an older person enters into an unwritten contract with society, exchanging the role of an economically active member of society for increased leisure and less responsibility (Hayslip & Panek 1989).

The hypothesis underpinning this theory is that the contract is achieved through mutual consent. In reality, retirement from paid work is artificially set by legislation which does not account for the disparate abilities and aspirations of older people. At the same time, although this exchange of leisure and work enables a society to utilise the work potential of younger people, unfortunately it does not encourage younger people to value their elders.

An evaluation of all of these theories suggests that each may refer to a legitimate process by which some individuals come to terms with the changes which accompany ageing. Therefore, each theory may be seen as an option and it will very much depend on the personality of the individual as to which option is chosen.

MENTAL DISORDERS IN OLD AGE

Altered patterns of disease in old age

As a person ages, there is an altered physiology which often only becomes apparent when an individual organ becomes stressed and has a diminished reserve of function with which to cope. Homeostatic mechanisms also become defective with ageing so that, although they may function adequately under normal conditions, they lose their reserve under stress. For example, temperature regulation is impaired and the facility for shivering is diminished; the thirst sensation is reduced, which may cause an older person to be liable to dehydrate. Together, reduced physiological reserves and impaired homeostatic mechanisms, when confronted with a stress factor, can contribute to tipping the balance into failure of the system.

In an older person this can cause the presentation and pattern of disease, and the reaction to it, to be different from the experiences of a younger person. In many cases the disease will present less dramatically, with vague, non-specific symptoms such as falling or collapse. Thus, information which conflicts with conventional medical ideology may lead to an inaccurate diagnosis.

The symptoms which most often lead to hospital admission are instability, incontinence and intellectual failure. These can be caused by a range of conditions, both physical and mental, and are often a combination of several. The occurrence of several different pathological processes together is common in old age and is called multiple pathology. The diseases may be related or can be totally separate.

Older people are susceptible to the same range of mental disorders as younger people, although they may present in a different way. These include: personality disorders, neuroses, psychoses and organic conditions. For many old people there may not be a clear disorder, but a breakdown of their physical health and/or social network can cause them to be vulnerable to mental ill health. For example, deafness combined with arthritis leads to social withdrawal which causes loneliness and a state of ill-being.

With all mental disorders in old age, the important point to consider is the wide range of potential differential diagnoses and the altered patterns of presentation. It is essential to work with each person as an individual and to carry out a comprehensive assessment. The specialist needs of this client group require the special skills of experienced multidisciplinary team members who embrace supervision and continued learning to keep abreast of current trends and research opportunities.

The most common organic and functional disorders affecting older people are described below.

ORGANIC DISORDERS

Organic disorders are disorders resulting from damage to, or changes in, the brain.

Dementia, or mental deterioration, is caused by disease of the brain, usually of a chronic or progressive nature, leading to multiple disturbances of higher cortical function, including impairment of memory, thinking, orientation, comprehension, learning ability, language and judgement. These changes occur in clear consciousness which assists in differentiating between dementia and acute confusional states.

The term 'dementia syndrome' is used to describe the clearly evident progressive decline of these cortical functions over at least a 6-month period. There is a group of organic disorders with similar signs and symptoms but with many different causes (Table 21.2) and pathology and prognosis will vary according to the cause. However, the concept of a single cause is no longer viable and mixed pathologies are common, especially in later onset dementia syndrome.

Alzheimer's disease

Epidemiology. The most common cause of dementia is Alzheimer's disease (AD), which affects approximately 5% of people over 65 and 20% of those over 80 (Alzheimer's Society 1999), and probably accounts for around 55% of all dementia cases.

Aetiology. Despite major advances in the study of Alzheimer's disease, the cause is not known. Epidemiological studies have confirmed that old age, a family history of AD, and the presence of Down syndrome are all risk factors (Henderson 1988). As with many diseases, it seems that the aetiology of AD is multifactorial. Genetic influences, in combination with environmental factors, lead to the development of the disease.

Pathology. A concrete diagnosis of Alzheimer's disease can only be achieved at post-mortem when generalised cerebral atrophy is evident along with shrunken gyri and widened sulci. Under microscopic examination, neuronal cell loss, plaques and tangles can be seen. The plaques are extracellular and consist of swollen, degenerating nerve structures with a central core of protein called amyloid. This protein is bound to aluminium silicate, hence the research into aluminium as a possible causal factor. The tangles are intracellular and consist of bundles of abnormal fibres. Plaques and tangles occur throughout the cortex but are particularly abundant in the temporal and parietal lobes, thus affecting memory and cognitive function.

Table 21.2 Causes of dementia (Tobiansky R 1993 Understanding dementia – Alzheimer's disease. Journal of Dementia Care 1(1): 26–29)

Primary cerebral degeneration	Inflammatory systemic diseases
Alzheimer's disease	Multiple sclerosis
Pick's disease	Systemic lupus erythematosus
Parkinson's disease	
Dementia of the Lewy body type	Cerebrovascular disease
Huntington's disease	Multi-infarct dementia
Progressive supranuclear palsy	Binswanger's disease
Wilson's disease	Lacunar infarcts
Spinocerebellar degeneration	
	Trauma and anoxia
Space-occupying lesions	
Tumours e.g. meningiomas, gliomas	Toxic causes
Cerebral (metastatic) carcinoma	Alcohol
Subdural haematomas	Drugs
Giant aneurysms	Poisons and heavy metals
Hydrocephalus	
	Metabolic causes
Cerebral infections	Hypothyroidism
Neurosyphilis	Hyper- and hypocalcaemia
Encephalitis/meningitis	Hypoglycaemia
AIDS	Hyper- and hyponatraemia
Cerebral abscess	Chronic hepatic encephalopathy
	Chronic uraemia
Prion diseases	Porphyria
Creutzfeldt–Jakob disease	
Gerstman–Straussler disease	Nutritional causes
Kuru	B_{12} deficiency
	Pellagra (niacin deficiency)
Storage diseases	Malabsorption
Metachromatic leucodystrophy	Thiamine deficiency
Adrenoleucodystrophy	
Cerebral lipidoses	

Clinical features. A particular feature of Alzheimer's disease is a steady decline of intellect and function as the disease progresses. The onset of the disease is marked by loss of recent memory, affecting the individual's ability to carry out intellectual tasks of daily living, such as planning, financing and shopping. As with other types of dementia the disease can manifest in a variety of ways depending on the area of the brain which has been affected (Table 21.3). The final outcome for people with Alzheimer's disease is death within 2–20 years from the onset of the illness. This large variation in prognosis may be due to the effect of psychosocial factors.

Dementia with Lewy bodies

Epidemiology. This type of dementia, which occurs in association with Parkinsonian features, was thought to be very rare until recent studies of the pathology of people with dementia at postmortem revealed that it is the second most common type of dementia, being roughly twice as common as vascular dementia (Perry et al 1989).

Pathology. There is a degeneration of the substantia nigra in the midbrain region. Normally, the substantia nigra is populated by nerve cells which contain a dark brown pigment. In Lewy body dementia these cells die and so the substantia nigra appears abnormally pale. Remaining nerve cells contain abnormal eosinophilic (pink staining) structures called Lewy bodies. These spread in the brain stem and in the cortical areas. As with Alzheimer's disease, there is some loss of neurones and plaques are present. However, neurofibrillary tangles are relatively sparse.

Clinical features. With this condition there is a development of dementia with features

Table 21.3 Lesion sites and neuropsychological deficits

Lobe	Dominant hemisphere	Nondominant hemisphere
Frontal	Expressive aphasia Agraphia Verbal apraxia Motor apraxia	Motor amusia Motor apraxia
Temporal	Sensory amusia Receptive aphasia Auditory agnosia Alexia Agraphia	Sensory amusia Metamorphosia Constructional apraxia
Occipital	Right hemianopia Alexia Colour agnosia Receptive dysphasia Constructional apraxia Dyscalculia Visual object agnosia Simultanognosia	Prosopagnosia Alexia Colour agnosia Dysgraphia Topographical disorientation Dressing apraxia Visual object agnosia Left hemianopia
Parietal	Tactile agnosia Constructional apraxia Visual object agnosia Visual spatial agnosia Agraphia Acalculia Right/left discrimination Finger agnosia Gerstmann's syndrome Somatognosia Asymbolia Ideomotor apraxia Ideational apraxia Simultanognosia	Tactile agnosia Constructional apraxia Visual object agnosia Visual spatial agnosia Agraphia (possibly) Acalculia (possibly) Right/left discrimination (possibly) Apractognosia Amorphosynthesis Unilateral neglect Dressing apraxia Prosopagnosia Topographical disorientation Anosognosia Alexia (possibly) Spatial relations syndrome

overlapping with those of Alzheimer's disease. The person with dementia with Lewy bodies will have a mild form of Parkinsonism with rigid limbs, tremor, bradykinesia and shuffling gait. Memory function may be less impaired than in Alzheimer's disease, but psychiatric symptoms, including visual and auditory hallucinations, are common. There is a sensitivity to antipsychotic medication. The main feature differentiating dementia with Lewy bodies from Alzheimer's disease and from vascular dementia is the variability of the symptoms, both at onset and as the disease continues.

Vascular dementia

Epidemiology. This type of dementia, which may be either a result of multi-infarcts or of vascular failure, accounts for about 15% of dementia cases.

Aetiology and pathology. Multi-infarct dementia is caused by cerebral arteriosclerosis disrupting the blood supply to the brain, causing the death of brain cells in the affected areas. Vascular disease may also be a result of the ageing process which leads to cerebrovascular failure and, subsequently, a decay of white brain matter. Both these causes of vascular dementia are most common in people who have general vascular problems and may be preventable. Unfortunately, as with other dementias, once the symptoms of this dementia have occurred they are not reversible.

Clinical features. Multi-infarct dementia caused by cerebral arteriosclerosis often has a rapid onset and a stepwise progression as further vascular accidents occur. Cerebrovascular failure is likely to have a more insidious onset and a smoother progression. The features of vascular dementia will vary according to the site of brain damage.

A comprehensive comparison of the further features of vascular dementia with Alzheimer's disease can be found in a good psychiatric textbook, for example *An Introduction To The Psychiatry Of Old Age* (Pitt 1982).

New variant Creutzfeldt–Jakob disease (CJD)

Epidemiology. The total number of suspect cases referred to the National CJD Surveillance Unit at 2 April 2001 was 1330. At this date the number of deaths of definite and probable cases of new variant CJD is 97.

Aetiology and pathology. This dementia is caused by prions, which are small infective agents made of proteins. Infection can occur between humans, for example following an injection of growth hormone from human pituitary glands which are contaminated with prions, or during neurosurgery. Infection can also occur through ingestion of infected food. In sheep, prions cause scrapie, and, in cows, bovine spongiform encephalitis (BSE), commonly known as mad cow disease. The disease is known to pass to cows when they graze on pasture infected by sheep. There is understandable concern that BSE is being contracted by humans, in the form of new variant CJD, if they eat infected neural matter from cows. There is evidence to support this, but other theories are also being investigated. Once a person has been infected with prions it may be decades before the onset of dementia, but when the symptoms

of dementia and ataxia develop, the process of the disease is usually very rapid (Livingston 1994).

Neuropathologically there is spongiform change, neuronal loss and astrocytic gliosis which is most evident in the basal ganglia and thalamus. The most striking pathological feature is amyloid plaque formation extensively distributed throughout the cerebrum and the cerebellum.

Clinical features. There is an early age of onset or death, the average being 27.6 years with a range of 18–41 years. The average duration of the illness is 13.1 months, with a range of 7.5–24 months. There is a predominantly psychiatric presentation, including anxiety, depression, social withdrawal and behaviour changes. Nearly all patients are referred to a psychiatrist early in the clinical course. After a period of weeks or months there is a development of cerebellar syndrome with gait and limb ataxia. Forgetfulness and memory disturbance develop later in the clinical course, progressing to severe cognitive impairment and a state of akinetic mutism. Myoclonus develops in the majority of patients and, in some, this is preceded by choreiform movements.

HIV-associated dementia

The ability of the retrovirus known as HIV to attack the brain directly was first reported in 1987 by Price and Navia of Cornell University. The virus infects the central nervous system and causes a brain disorder which slows the individual's thought processes and affects the ability to remember and to concentrate. This is one of the major complications of HIV infection, affecting most AIDS patients.

There are also motor features with leg weakness, loss of balance and unsteady gait. The individual becomes apathetic and socially withdrawn. If untreated, the infection progresses quickly and the patient will survive for only 6 months or less. However, there has been a dramatic decline of at least 50% in the incidence of HIV-associated dementia, as there has been in the incidence of all AIDS-related illnesses, since the introduction in 1996 of highly active anti-retroviral therapy (HAART).

HIV-associated dementia tends, by its nature, to affect a younger age group than the other dementias.

Other organic disorders

A variety of pathologies accounts for the remaining 5% of dementia cases including: space-occupying lesions; hydrocephalus; neurosyphilis; systemic disorders, such as hypothyroidism and drug toxicity, and Korsakoff's syndrome. The last is not strictly a dementia as it does not have a global cortical effect. It is caused by alcohol abuse resulting in a lack of thiamine and leading to memory impairment.

FUNCTIONAL DISORDERS

In functional disorders there is no evidence of damage or disturbance to the brain. As research adds to our knowledge and understanding of the process of these disorders it may be found that what was once termed a functional disorder is actually an organic one. For example, damage due to chemical changes may be discovered.

Older people may experience the same functional disorders as younger people, but they may manifest in different ways or, as with certain physical problems, may be dismissed as a natural part of the ageing process. The functional disorders which particularly affect older people are set out here.

Reactive depression

Reactive depression, sometimes termed neurotic or exogenous depression, is associated with major life events, especially those involving loss. Older people may experience many losses, including the loss of spouse, friends, financial security, physical health, sensory acuity, cognitive powers, social independence or work status. Surgery, acute illness or being institutionalised may also be significant, as studies have shown that older people are less able to tolerate acute stress than they are chronic stress (Fogel 1991).

Estimates of the prevalence of reactive depression in people over 65 vary widely, but depression may be more common in older people as it is this age group that experiences the most negative life events. Interestingly, as old people age further their coping strategies improve and they have lower rates of depression than younger old people.

Psychotic depression

The most significant difference between psychotic depression – also termed endogenous or unipolar depression – and reactive depression is the presence of delusions which may, for example, be of persecution, disease, sin, death or poverty.

Older people with a psychotic depression are likely to have had previous experience of it at a younger age. They often show a history of psychiatric illness and, possibly because of this, may also show signs of institutionalisation.

Diagnosing depression in an old person can be difficult because it often presents an atypical picture. It may be necessary to establish that there has been a change from the individual's usual mood and behaviour, which may perhaps have occurred years ago if the depression is of long standing. The fact that functional illnesses are treatable makes this thorough assessment worthwhile, particularly if there are signs of depression or if the old person displays insight, for example, reporting that they cannot remember rather than simply giving a wrong answer. If care is not taken, depression may be wrongly diagnosed as dementia because there are similarities between the two conditions (Table 21.4).

Paraphrenia

This condition, which is usually treatable, is characterised by delusions of persecution which are often accompanied by auditory hallucinations. The older person with paraphrenia will present as preoccupied, suspicious and sometimes aggressive. Unfortunately, the stereotype of old age as having these very characteristics may cause this condition to be accepted as

Table 21.4 Similarities between depression and dementia (Macdonald 1980)

	Depression	Dementia
Decline in mental functioning	Can't make effort to think or remember. Only remembers bad things: preoccupied with past misdeeds or regrets; ruminates about failure or death. Does not attend to surroundings. May have mental slowing.	Unable to connect similar ideas or to absorb new ones.
Withdrawal	Feels isolated and sometimes deservedly rejected. Can't make effort to join in social activities. May have retardation, physical and mental. Apathetic, hopeless, or despising themselves.	Thought processes too disordered for communication. Shallow, transient feelings, or feelings reduced generally.
Inappropriate social actions	May have persecutory ideas, may hear accusing voices. May have impulses to abase themselves. Early morning wakening with maximum depression of mood leads to wandering and suicide attempts.	Stereotyped (purposeless, repetitive) movements and behaviour. Disorientation in time leading to nocturnal activity.
Wandering	Searching (grief). Restlessness, agitation, anxiety, compelling thoughts. Early morning wakening or general poor sleep.	Disorientation as to place. Misrecognition of unfamiliar places and people.
Poor memory	Mental slowing, or too agitated and preoccupied with gloomy thoughts. Can't make effort, gives up easily.	Direct effect of underlying physical brain deterioration. Wrong replies given readily
Others	Crying. Incontinence. Weight loss. Angry outbursts.	

normal and go untreated. Alternatively, the older person may be labelled as having this condition when the problem is due to hearing loss.

WORKING WITH OLDER PEOPLE WITH MENTAL DISORDERS

The multidisciplinary team

Working with older people requires a holistic approach in a multidisciplinary team, in order to make a complete assessment and meet the possibly complex needs of this client group. The membership of the multidisciplinary team will vary according to the needs of the individual and the service setting. Commonly, a health service team would include a consultant in the psychiatry of old age, nurses, occupational therapists and social workers. A social services team may consist of social workers, home carers and occupational therapists. There is often an overlap between the two services, therefore good communication channels are essential. Increasingly,

multidisciplinary teams are also including service providers from the voluntary and independent sectors, if they are involved in an individual's care. The older person is the central figure in the team and, as such, he, or an advocate, should be consulted and informed about the care package.

When working with older people, team members should agree on common principles which meet their clients' basic needs and uphold their fundamental rights.

Values and principles of practice

Older people have the same basic rights to dignity, privacy, choice, independence and fulfilment as people of any other age group. When an older person experiences a mental health disorder these fundamental rights may easily be undermined by those giving care. Until recently there were few theories of care-giving and most work with older people was based on clinical experience. However, a theory of personhood and well-being has now been developed, in response to the particular needs of older people with dementia (Kitwood & Bredin 1992). This theory emphasises the primary importance of a socio-psychological approach to care-giving. It explains how the prevailing social psychology, which depersonalises the person with dementia, results in care which is well intentioned but lacking in insight and understanding and contributes to the dementing process. Personhood is essentially social and refers to the human being in relation to others, having status and being worthy of respect. When the individual is not accorded appropriate social interaction, well-being will suffer.

The theory proposes that a dementing illness is not necessarily a process of inevitable deterioration. Some people with dementia will score low on cognitive tests but will still function well as people, whereas others whose cognitive impairment is less severe will fare far less well. A dementing condition tends to be compounded by depression, anxiety, apathy or discouragement. Therefore a person with dementia may be in a state of well- or ill-being regardless of the degree of cognitive impairment. Kitwood proposed that there are four states of well-being: self-esteem, or a global feeling of personal worth; agency, that is, the ability to control personal life in a meaningful way and to produce and achieve; social confidence, or being at ease with others; and a fourth state of hope, or the retention of confidence that security will remain, and of optimism. There are twelve indicators that the person with dementia is experiencing one of these states:

1. the assertion of desire or will
2. the ability to experience and express a range of emotions
3. initiation of social contact
4. affectional warmth
5. social sensitivity
6. self-respect
7. acceptance of other dementia sufferers
8. humour
9. creativity and self-expression
10. showing evident pleasure
11. helpfulness
12. relaxation.

If social psychology which views the person with dementia as a problem and not a person to be related to can contribute to the dementing process, it follows that human interaction can bring about some return of mental function. The indicators of well-being enable care-givers to evaluate the quality and effectiveness of their interventions within a theoretical framework.

The occupational therapy process

The fundamental principles, philosophy and process of occupational therapy are the same when working with older people as with other age groups. However, practice draws on a broad range of theories, including physiological, behavioural, psychodynamic and cognitive concepts, and reflects the complexity of the physical, intellectual, emotional and social needs of older people. With this broad theoretical base, a variety of approaches may be used when working with older people with mental disorders. The key to successful intervention is to apply the occupational therapy process of assessment, treatment planning, implementation and evaluation in order to select the most appropriate approach and ensure a quality service.

ASSESSMENT

In order to assist the older person to become as independent as possible, it is first necessary to assess the individual's abilities, problems, wishes and interests. A problem-orientated assessment alone is too narrow, focusing on difficulties, whereas the treatment plan should also incorporate the person's abilities in order to use and maintain them. It is possible to motivate clients to be involved in therapy by building the programme of intervention on their wishes and interests.

A range of assessment methods may be used, including interviews, observation techniques and standardised tests.

Interviews

Interviewing an older person can be a lengthy process if a full history is to be obtained. When communication skills have been affected by mental disorder it may be tempting to interview the client's relatives or carers, but if the therapist utilises all her communication skills it is possible to achieve an informative interview with even the most dysphasic person.

The therapist should pay attention to the older person's non-verbal responses, including reactions, expressions, posture and tone of voice. The therapist also needs to use simple language and to ask closed questions when interviewing a person with dementia. The client must always be given time to respond. Possible sensory deficits should always be considered; it should be standard practice to allow for hearing or visual impairment. Making sure that a client is wearing his hearing aid, and that it is switched on and working, could prevent or correct a misdiagnosis of depression or dementia.

Observation

Observing the older person carrying out everyday functional tasks can reveal not only the person's level of ability in achieving an end result but also the presence of specific deficits for which treatment can then be planned. A functional assessment may be carried out in an occupational therapy department or in the familiarity of the person's own home.

The therapist uses skills in task analysis and activity analysis to select or design an appropriate assessment task. For example, making a cup of tea is an activity which tests the person's orientation, sequencing, memory, safety, perception and visuo-spatial skills.

Standardised tests

These are tools used to detect impairment and should therefore be used in addition to interview and observation in order to gain a full picture of the client. As the name indicates, the tests are designed to measure the client against set standards. They can be useful for determining the older person's baseline function and can then be reapplied after intervention to measure any changes. Not all standardised tests have been validated, but three which are well documented as valuable and reliable are the Allen Cognitive Level Screen (Allen et al 1992), the Dementia Rating Scale (Mattis 1998) and the Middlesex Elderly Assessment of Mental State (MEAMS; Golding 1989).

The Allen Cognitive Level Screen. The Allen Cognitive Level Screen (ACLS) uses a simple functional task as a screening assessment to analyse the level of cognitive disability. The cognitive disability model proposes that there are six cognitive levels, each of which can be described in terms of limitations associated with the medical condition and remaining abilities, as seen in patterns of behaviour in everyday tasks (Allen et al 1992). The levels range from level 6, where functioning is normal and no intervention is required, to level 1, where the person is profoundly impaired. An analysis of the results aids understanding of the patient's behaviour when carrying out everyday tasks. Optimum environmental stimulation and support can then be planned and implemented to decrease confusion, maximise functional capacities and help the person retain a sense of competence despite impairment.

Dementia Rating Scale. The Dementia Rating Scale (DRS) is a rapid but comprehensive measure of cognitive status for adults between the ages of 65 and 81 who have cortical impairment (Mattis 1988). It provides an accurate assessment of the progression and level of the person's behavioural, neuropathological and cognitive competence and can be used to plan programmes to maximise quality of life and to enhance intact abilities.

Middlesex Elderly Assessment of Mental State. The Middlesex Elderly Assessment of Mental State (MEAMS) is a screening test used to detect impairment of specific cognitive skills in older people and is designed to assist professionals working with older people to differentiate between functional and organic conditions (Golding 1989). The MEAMS requires the subject to perform a number of simple tasks, each sensitive to the functioning of a different area of the brain. It is therefore useful in treatment planning and as an indicator for further investigations.

Occupational therapy assessment in the multidisciplinary team

Assessment is a complex process requiring contributions from different members of the multidisciplinary team in order to obtain as accurate a picture as possible. The occupational therapist may be the first person to note a particular deficit which indicates that a specific area of the brain has been affected. Alternatively, the therapist may already have received a pathology report from colleagues, detailing the areas affected. She can then assess the implications of these findings on the person's functional ability.

The occupational therapist is often asked to provide information about a person's basic living skills, for example stating whether or not a person is safe to live at home alone or whether they require the assistance of a home carer, but can make a much wider contribution to the overall assessment of the client's abilities and needs. For example, the therapist may offer guidance to carers on how to help the old person to carry out tasks to their maximum potential. The occupational therapist will be able to advise not only whether the help of a home carer is required, but also how that help should be given (Box 21.1).

TREATMENT AND CARE PLANNING

When information about the older person's abilities, needs, wishes and interests has been gathered through the assessment process it can be used to formulate a plan of treatment. This is called a treatment or care plan. Where possible, the client should be involved in the treatment planning process, since understanding the aims of the programme will increase motivation to participate.

The treatment plan should follow the same format as for any other client group, with goals and objectives clearly defined so that all members of the team, including the client and his family or carers, are fully informed (see Ch. 7).

Traditionally, leisure activities have been the main treatment medium for older people. However, the key point when planning treatment is that the activity should be purposeful, both in achieving the goals of therapy and in the meaning it has for the individual. A basic living task may be just as effective in achieving therapeutic goals as a leisure activity, and it may be more appropriate for the older person who has never had time to participate in leisure activities and may feel uncomfortable being involved in them. A light domestic task, such as dusting, watering plants or cleaning shoes, may be as

---

Box 21.1 Case example 1

Mr Scott lived in a long stay hospital unit for people with dementia. He had been diagnosed as having Alzheimer's disease, and CT scans had shown lesions in the temporal and parietal lobes of the left hemisphere. Nurses were having difficulty helping Mr Scott to carry out many everyday tasks, although physically he was able to function well. Staff described him as lazy and deaf since he did not respond to repeated instructions from his carers and he was becoming increasingly withdrawn.

The occupational therapist carried out an assessment with Mr Scott by observing him getting dressed and watering the unit's plants. She found that Mr Scott was not deaf and responded to a calm, reassuring tone of voice by making eye contact and

smiling. It was evident that Mr Scott had a receptive aphasia and was therefore unable to follow the verbal instructions of his carers. In addition, the therapist observed that Mr Scott would start to get dressed but would abruptly stop and remain holding a sock as if unsure of his next move. Given the site of his brain damage this indicated the possibility of an ideational apraxia. She advised the carers to remain with Mr Scott while he dressed and to give him physical, rather than verbal, prompts when he was seen to falter, but to allow him to physically carry out the task himself. She also suggested that appropriate praise should be used to reinforce his achievements. In this way, Mr Scott was able to get dressed as independently as he was able, his self-confidence improved and he became less withdrawn.

effective as a leisure activity and the older person may feel more in control by engaging in a familiar activity.

Media for older people should be age-specific in order to increase motivation to participate. For example, when games are used, such as bowls or skittles, they should be played with adult equipment and not children's versions bought from toy shops.

Taking risks

Older people may be so protected by their carers that they are prevented from achieving fulfilment in their lives. There can be a temptation to stop someone attempting anything which may result in harm, particularly when they have a mental illness such as dementia. The relatives of the older person often wish for this protection, mistakenly believing that their father or mother is at risk of injury through carrying out certain activities. If the relatives are involved in the treatment planning process then they have the opportunity to discuss the use of any activities which involve an element of risk. Through discussion, agreement or compromise may be reached.

Appropriate risk taking is a normal part of everyday life and adds quality to the subjective experience. When we take a risk we usually consider the advantages and disadvantages and only act if, on balance, the reason for taking the action is worth the element of risk. The older person's right to take appropriate risks should be considered and appropriate opportunities built into the treatment plan. An older person with a mental disorder has the same legal and civil rights as anyone else. Restraining someone from carrying out an activity may constitute abuse. Protecting an older person from taking appropriate risks may do them more harm than enabling them to do so; this is the balance which needs to be considered (Box 21.2).

TREATMENT IMPLEMENTATION

A variety of media and methods is covered comprehensively in Section 4 of this book. In addition, there are many relevant publications, some of which are recommended for further reading, at the end of this chapter.

Some techniques

This section will consider some of the techniques which are frequently used with older people with mental disorders. Each of these approaches employs effective communication as its vehicle. Without good communication, treating the older person with respect for his dignity and individuality, all these approaches fail. It may be the process of these therapies, rather than the outcome, that is important because if the basic values underpinning good practice with older people are carried out then their personhood and well-being will be assured.

Anxiety management

Older people may experience anxiety, which affects their ability to function, in the same way as people of other age groups. The cause of this disorder in an older person may be a reaction to loss, or to the onset of disease, or it may be a

---

Box 21.2 Case example 2

Mrs Jones lived in a residential home for older people. She was diagnosed as having a dementia and was ataxic. Mrs Jones had a walking frame but constantly forgot to use it and was having frequent falls. The manager of the home applied to the occupational therapist for a chair from which Mrs Jones would find it difficult to rise, thus preventing her from walking about and protecting her from falling.

The occupational therapist worked with the staff and manager of the home, helping them to recognise Mrs Jones's right to get up and move around and the importance of mobility to her physical health. The therapist then assisted the staff to plan Mrs Jones's care so that they reduced her risk of injury from falling by assisting her to walk at planned times and prompting her to use her frame at others. To compensate for times when staff were not available, another resident, who was a friend of Mrs Jones, was encouraged to prompt her to use the frame.

In this way, Mrs Jones's care was planned so that appropriate risk taking was built in, but the element of risk was reduced to a minimum.

disorder which has carried on from a younger age. Anxiety management and relaxation techniques can be used to assist older people, even those with dementia, to take control of their own feelings in the same way as they are used to assist younger people.

Reminiscence

Reminiscing was once thought to be an indication of mental deterioration but it is now viewed as a positive experience which should be encouraged. Reminiscence has many values: as a way of preserving one's identity, searching for meaning and relevance in one's life, or reviewing past experiences of solving problems in order to solve current ones. Reminiscence can therefore be therapeutic and can be utilised by occupational therapists to assist clients to resolve conflicts or maintain self-esteem by preserving a sense of identity, as well as being a social or recreational activity.

A vast selection of media can be used to trigger reminiscence, including material published for this purpose in the form of videos, audio tapes, photographs and pictures. Libraries, museums and community groups are also useful sources of archive material.

The use of a life story book can help an older person to piece together his past in order to preserve a sense of identity. The information can also be shared with others, for example as a living history project with schoolchildren, or simply with carers. Appreciating the history of the older person promotes his self-esteem and enables others to be empathetic.

Reality orientation

Reality orientation (RO) is a treatment method which aims to stimulate people to relearn basic facts about themselves and their environment by systematically presenting and reinforcing relevant information. It is therefore only appropriate to use this method with people who are able to learn and it is not suitable for a person with dementia who has lost this cognitive skill. Rimmer (1988) offered a useful assessment tool which uses interview to assess the older person's level of orientation and to determine if RO is appropriate. RO is traditionally used with people with a dementia but it is also helpful for others who are disorientated, perhaps because of living in a long stay unit and being institutionalised.

Reality orientation can be practised in two ways. The 24-hour approach involves all members of the treatment team consistently reinforcing information which helps the older person orientate himself. The person is always addressed by his preferred name, and cues, such as clocks, calendars and notice boards, are also used. Individuals who are severely cognitively impaired, and who may have become so disorientated that they are not self-aware, may respond to direct sensory stimulation which aims to increase awareness of self.

Group RO is a selective approach used with a small group of people of a similar level of ability. The group meets regularly and each meeting lasts for about half an hour. The aim of group RO is to stimulate each of the participant's senses selectively in order to assist them to become more aware of their surroundings and themselves. The occupational therapist should identify the people most likely to benefit from this approach.

Validation therapy

This approach was developed to give validity and dignity to the feelings expressed by disorientated older people who can no longer benefit from reality orientation. The concept of validation may be used with a wide group of people and may also be seen as an issue of good practice. However, validation can be used as a therapy to assist the client to begin to resolve past conflicts by expressing their feelings to someone who empathises. It is thus possible to reduce problem behaviours which are symptomatic of internal conflicts.

Sensory stimulation

It is commonly accepted that sensory stimulation is necessary for physical and mental health. The concept of sensory deprivation relies on the theory that environmental stimulation leads to an appropriate response. Without this stimulation, no response will be forthcoming. This theory has been explored in relation to people with dementia and taken further to propose that sensory deprivation may add to, or even cause, dementia; and that it is possible to use sensory stimulation to reverse, or at least slow down, the disease process. Sensory stimulation can be achieved in many ways. At a simplistic level, the opportunity for sensory engagement with the environment can be enhanced by presenting everyday features to individuals. These environmental features may include objects such as ornaments, fabrics, plants, flowers or animals. Food is particularly valuable because it can be multisensory, incorporating opportunities for visual, olfactory, tactile, auditory and gustatory stimulation. Occupational therapists who recognise this can bring the environment to the person and ensure that the full value of the experience is derived by encouraging exploration.

In addition to using everyday environmental features, it is possible to use special environments and objects which aim to elicit specific responses. Originally developed as a leisure experience for people with severe learning difficulties and sensory disabilities, Snoezelen is a facility which is now used on a much wider scale. It is a non-directive approach which presents items of sensory equipment for exploration and development. Whole rooms can be dedicated to the arrangement of Snoezelen equipment, but small portable items can be presented to individuals in their own homes. The use of Snoezelen with people with dementia is relatively new, but positive therapeutic outcomes have been described (Pinkney & Barker 1994). In addition to stimulating and maintaining the body's ability to receive information through all of the sensory modalities, and thus stimulating neurological responses, Snoezelen promotes the development of a therapeutic relationship between the person with dementia and his care giver. In fact the relationship becomes a partnership in which the caring role is exchanged for one of equality and both participants are engaged in exploring and enjoying the environment.

Music is a medium which has therapeutic benefits going far beyond the immediate one of auditory stimulation. While language deterioration is a feature of cognitive disability, musical abilities can still be preserved. This may be because the fundamentals of music are not based in the lexical and semantic functions of naming and reference but in tone and rhythm (Aldridge & Brandt 1991). Music has a history as a means of communication, and varying tones and rhythms elicit primitive responses in mood and basic physiological functions such as heart and respiration rates. These are sub-cortical responses which can be stimulated even in people who have severe cortical damage but whose sub-cortex remains intact.

Behavioural therapy

This systematic approach may be used to reduce problem behaviours associated with dementia, such as aggression, inappropriate urinating, undressing or shouting. An assessment is carried out to determine the nature, frequency, triggers and consequences of the problem behaviour. This information is then used to plan a staged intervention until the desired new behaviour is elicited and the undesirable behaviour removed. More information about behavioural methods of assessment and treatment can be found in Chapter 13.

Group versus individual treatment

The decision to use an individual or a group approach should depend on the needs of the older person. Groups may be appropriate for some activities, particularly those which aim to promote social skills and verbal interaction, but the group must be carefully selected for size and composition. If the group is too large, or has members of varying levels of ability, it can be frustrating for participants. Large group outings can also be counter-productive as they may not promote a positive image of older people but rather contribute to negative stereotypes of old age. Often, an individual approach for a short length of time will be more beneficial, and will enhance the client's personhood and well-being more, than a longer period in a group.

Using volunteers

Group, rather than individual, treatment or care is sometimes selected in an attempt to provide a service for a larger number of old people. Lack of staff may mean that the needs of the individual cannot always be met. If this is the case, it is worth considering the use of volunteers. When a treatment or care plan has been formulated with clear objectives the volunteer can be guided to help the old person to achieve these. The volunteer will also find it beneficial to work to a plan and will appreciate being given direction. Most volunteers tend to give up because of having too little, rather than too much, to do.

Environmental adaptation

In addition to using the treatment techniques described, occupational therapists have a role to play in adapting the older person's environment to promote function at the optimum level. This may require the provision of equipment, to enable the person to overcome a physical problem. For example, large-handle cutlery may be provided for someone with arthritis, or a raised garden constructed for someone in a wheelchair.

Alternatively, the adaptation may meet the psychological need of the person. The design of residential or day units for people with dementia can affect their orientation, mood or thought processes. The occupational therapist can advise on the use of colour, plants or ornaments to act as environmental clues. The occupational therapist may also apply her knowledge or perceptual deficits when advising about décor. For example, functional problems arising from an inability to discriminate between a figure and its background can be overcome by the careful use of colour and lighting. The provision of quiet areas and areas which are stimulating to the senses will affect the user's mood and, in the case of people with dementia, their levels of expressed emotion.

EVALUATION

The occupational therapist must continuously monitor the outcomes of her intervention with clients to determine the effectiveness of the treatment or care plan. The evaluation should include a reassessment using the standardised tests which were used to establish the client's baseline of function. It will then be possible to make a comparison between the client's level of function before and after therapeutic intervention.

In this way the therapist can evaluate the effectiveness of her treatment. If the evaluation shows that occupational therapy is not effective, then the programme may need to be modified. This may involve the deletion of unattainable goals or the modification of goals partly achieved. It is also important to modify the programme of intervention when evaluation shows that therapy is being effective, as new goals will need to be added as progress is made.

Consultation with the client is also important to determine his level of satisfaction with his treatment or care. Although in cases of chronic dementia a cure will not be possible, it is possible to promote a positive outlook in the client by involving him in the evaluation process and reinforcing when goals have been achieved.

SUMMARY

This chapter has focused on the positive aspects of old age and on the rights of older people to be treated in the same way as other client groups. Part of the challenge of working with older people is to change the attitudes of others, and of old people themselves, by disproving the myths and negative stereotypes of old age.

The impact that mental disorders in old age can have on physiological and social well-being should not be overlooked. Multipathology calls for skilled care and treatment by experienced occupational therapists and requires application of the occupational therapy process within a framework of appropriate theories.

The field of work with older people with mental disorders is becoming increasingly stimulating as levels of knowledge about conditions and methods of intervention improve. Occupational therapists have a role to play in clinical practice and have much to contribute to research in this area. Demographic trends have led to older people constituting an increasingly large number of occupational therapists' clients. An opportunity therefore exists to test out hypotheses about intervention, to evaluate new techniques and to document and publish findings.

Finally, the role of occupational therapists in educating others working with older people is clear. Apart from providing education about the wider role of occupational therapy there is also scope for educating others, including colleagues, relatives and carers, about the potential of older people for functioning independently and the techniques which can be used to achieve this.

REFERENCES

Aldridge D, Brandt G 1991 Music therapy and Alzheimer's disease. British Journal of Music Therapy 5: 28–36

Allen C K, Earhart C A, Blue T 1992 Occupational therapy treatment goals for the physically and cognitively disabled. American Occupational Therapy Association, Rockville, MD

Alzheimer's Society 1999 Fighting dementia for two decades. Annual Review 1998/99, 1 Alzheimer's Society, London

Cumming E, Henry W E 1961 Growing old: the process of disengagement. Basic, New York

Department of Health 1990 NHS and Care in the Community Act. HMSO, London

Erikson E H 1959 Identity and the life cycle: selected papers. Psychological issues (monograph). International Universities Press, New York

Fogel B S 1991 Depression and ageing. Neuropsychiatry, Neuropsychology and Behavioural Neurology 4(1): 24–35

Golding E 1989 The Middlesex Elderly Assessment of Mental State. Thames Valley Test Company, 7–9 The Green, Flempton, Bury St Edmunds, Suffolk IP28 6EL

Government Statistical Service 1992 1991 Census of Great Britain. CEN91 CM56. HMSO, London

Havighurst R J, Neugarten B L, Tobin S S 1968 Disengagement and patterns of ageing. Middle age and ageing. University of Chicago Press, Chicago

Hayslip B, Panek P E 1989 Adult development and ageing. Harper and Row, New York

Henderson A S 1988 The risk factors for Alzheimer's disease: a review and a hypothesis. Acta Psychiatrica Scandinavica 78: 257–275

Kitwood T, Bredin K 1992 Towards a theory of dementia care: personhood and well-being. Ageing and Society 12: 269–287

Lemon B et al 1972 An exploration of the activity theory of ageing: activity types and life satisfaction among in-movers to a retirement community. Journal of Gerontology 27

Lewis S C 1979 The mature years: a geriatric occupational therapy text. Slack, New Jersey

Livingston G 1994 Understanding dementia: the rarer dementias. Journal of Dementia Care 2(3): 27–29

Macdonald A 1980 Depression and elderly people. Mind, London

Maddox G L 1963 Activity and morale: a longitudinal study of selected elderly subjects. Social Forces 43

Mattis S 1988 Dementia Rating Scale. NFER-NELSON, Windsor

Midwinter E 1993 A voyage of rediscovery. Third Age, London

Perry R H, Irving D, Blessed G et al 1989 Clinically and neuropathologically distinct form of dementia in the elderly. Lancet 335: 166

Pinkney L, Barker P 1994 Snoezelen – an evaluation of a sensory environment used by people who are elderly and confused. In: Hutchinson R, Kewin J (eds) Sensations and disability. Rompa

Pitt B 1982 An introduction to the psychiatry of old age. Churchill Livingstone, Edinburgh

Rimmer L 1988 Reality orientation: principles and practice, 2nd edn. Winslow Press, Bicester, Oxfordshire

Roberts A 1989 Systems of life. Nursing Times 85(49): 57–60

Terry R D, Katzman R 1983 Senile dementia of the Alzheimer type. Annals of Neurology 14: 497–505

Turner J S, Helms D B 1989 Contemporary adulthood, 4th edn. Holt, Rinehart and Winston, Fort Worth, Florida

Twining T C 1988 Helping older people: a psychological approach. Wiley, Chichester

Zemke R, Gratz R 1982 The role of theory: Erikson and occupational therapy. Journal of Occupational Therapy in Mental Health 2(3)

FURTHER READING

Bender M, Norris A, Bauckham P (1987) Groupwork with the elderly: principles and practice. Winslow Press, Bicester, Oxfordshire

Bornat J (ed) 1993 Reminiscence reviewed: perspectives, evaluations and achievements. Open University Press, Buckinghamshire

Feil N 1992 Validation therapy: the Feil method. Edward Feil Productions, Cleveland

Midwinter E 1993 A voyage of rediscovery. Third Age, London

Rimmer L 1988 Reality orientation: principles and practice, 2nd edn. Winslow Press, Bicester, Oxfordshire

RECOMMENDED WEBSITES

www.alzheimers.org.uk
Information about Alzheimer's disease, the Alzheimer's Society and related websites

www.ccc.nottingham.ac.uk and link to lewyhom. html
Information about dementia with Lewy bodies

www.cjd.ac.uk
Information about new variant CJD

22

Child and adolescent mental health services

Lesley Lougher

INTRODUCTION

Child psychiatry and occupational therapy both have their roots in the mental hygiene movement of the early 20th century. This was a psychobiological approach to mental illness, which acknowledged that life events affect mental health and so extended the scope of psychiatry into community settings. Child psychiatry and child guidance clinics were established in order to prevent the development of some mental health problems in adulthood. Both child psychiatry and occupational therapy started from a belief in the importance of the context of an individual's life to his mental health. This is an area of practice where there is scope for development of a higher profile for occupational therapy. The Audit Commission (1999) found occupational therapists were 4% of all staff in child and adolescent mental health services.

There were major changes in child and adolescent mental health services in the UK in the late 1990s. The National Health Service (NHS) Health Advisory Service published a review of child and adolescent mental health services entitled *Together We Stand* (NHS Health Advisory Service 1995), in which greater recognition was given to the role of the primary health services. Health visitors, the school health service, educational services and voluntary organisations were seen to be the first line services in the prevention of, and early intervention in, children's emotional and behavioural difficulties. Child and adolescent mental health (CAMH) services now include community approaches to the mental health of children and multidisciplinary outpatient clinics as well as day and residential facilities. There are occupational therapists working in all these areas.

Child and adolescent mental health services work closely with other agencies, particularly social service and education departments , voluntary organisations, such as the National Society for the Protection of Children (NSPCC), National Children's Homes (NCH) and local projects. The Children Act (HMSO 1989), the Education Act (HMSO 1993), and the Police and Criminal Evidence Act (HMSO 1984) have all introduced changes in the law which have influenced the delivery of treatment for children with mental health problems. Government funding is only allocated to areas where there is evidence of joint working between agencies. For example, the Sure Start initiative provides community interventions to families with pre-school children (Department of Education and Employment 1999), Youth Offender Teams are multi-agency teams to reduce youth offending (HMSO 1998) and Looked After Children initiatives seek to provide better services to children in the care of local authorities. This chapter seeks to be an introduction to this changing area of work. The first two sections, concerning the life cycle of a family and child development, outline the context in which the child develops. The following section introduces the range of problems children experience and the final section considers occupational therapy assessment and treatment within the context of the multidisciplinary team and includes some discussion of clinical supervision.

THE LIFE CYCLE OF A FAMILY: CHANGES AND PRESSURES

A theoretical approach using the life cycle of an individual has been suggested by Llorens (1970) as one useful to occupational therapists. She described seven areas of development: neurophysiological, physical, psychosocial, psychody-namic, social language, daily living skills and sociocultural skills. These develop longitudinally, over time, and horizontally, in parallel. The family also has a developmental cycle in which each individual member requires different skills to negotiate each stage of the cycle. Dysfunction in one family member may signal family difficulty in moving to the next stage.

The stages in the family life cycle, as shown in Figure 22.1, overlap, in that the generations are negotiating different stages simultaneously, that is, the birth of a new baby creates new parents and grandparents.

The stages are defined as: adult couple, parent(s) and infants, parent(s) and schoolchildren, parent(s) with adolescents, parent(s) alone and young adults. Each stage requires the family to make certain changes in roles and occupations. If these are not accomplished, the family, or an individual within it, shows symptoms of distress. The symptom-carrier may be the person who is most aware of the pressure to change and resists it on behalf of the family, even to protect the family. That the family continues as a system is proof of its flexibility, since it must respond to internal and external changes and must be able to transform itself in ways that meet new circumstances without losing the continuity that

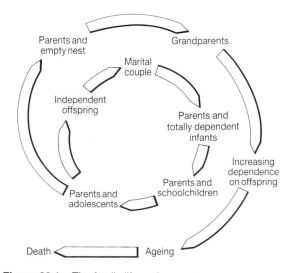

Figure 22.1 The family life cycle.

provides a frame of reference for its members (Minuchin 1974).

This section examines the natural development of a family but also shows the difficulties, which may lead to referral to a child and adolescent mental health service.

Adult couple

A marriage or committed partnership signifies the birth of a new family but one that is heavily influenced by the original families of the new couple. Cohabitation may be a smooth transition from one stage of the life cycle to the next, or it may signify a desperate move on the part of one or both partners to bring wholeness to their lives. Skynner (1976) suggested that 'Marriage is always an attempt at growth, at healing oneself and finding oneself again, however disastrously any particular attempt may fail for lack of sufficient understanding or external help'.

Changes

On marriage or cohabitation, the partners separate from their families of origin and establish a new adult relationship. The marital relationship requires a negotiation of gender roles and the development of a sexual relationship.

Difficulties may arise when these changes are not achieved. One or both partners may not be able to separate sufficiently from their own parents. The degree of separation required may vary, as in one marriage it may be acceptable that the woman maintains close emotional and supportive links with her mother, whereas in another this would be seen as dysfunctional.

Responsibilities for earning an income, household organisation, gardening and management of finances are allocated by decision or default. Gender roles within the marriage may differ from one or both families of origin. Either partner may feel anxious about being expected to perform a task she or he feels is in the province of the other sex. Sexual problems may have their origins in gender insecurity, inability to express emotions physically, fear of losing control or technical ignorance.

Building a marriage or partnership requires skill and persistence. Two people, possibly from very different types of family, have the task of creating a third family, which will be mutually satisfying and will, if required, provide a secure foundation for children.

Parent(s) and infants

Having begun to establish a marriage/partnership to their mutual satisfaction, the pair then changes to incorporate a third person. Pregnancy or adoption procedures may provide some preparation as the prospective parents fantasise about the presence of the child in their family, but few are fully prepared for the disruption in their lives. Some couples separate before the birth of the child.

Changes

- One parent, usually the mother, may reduce or cease outside employment, which reduces the family income, or return to work, having arranged for the child to be cared for by family, child minder or nursery.
- While at home, the baby's presence dominates all activities: the daily timetable revolves around the child's pattern of needs. A baby demands 24-hour care and a mother may find herself having very little sleep and no privacy.
- A working mother has to balance responsibilities between her family and employment. Household tasks may be reallocated between the couple.
- Both partners have the task of negotiating with their own parents the role of the new grandparents.
- In among the turmoil of so many changes, the mother begins to build a relationship with her child that will lay the foundation for his later development.

Difficulties may arise in the family. There is a third person to be loved and cared for, leaving less time and emotion for the adult relationship. The woman may miss her former independence and may have difficulty adjusting to the constant demands of motherhood. Oakley (1980) found that most women were less than satisfied with their new role and had mixed feelings about their babies. Some mothers may not love the baby as expected. This may be a transitory phase due to the trauma of the labour and the physical demands of early motherhood, or may be an early indication of a long-term problem. The act of parenting may remind the adults of their own childhood difficulties, particularly if they themselves were not adequately parented or even abused. There is an increased interest in offering support to parents and children at an early stage to prevent later problems developing.

Parent(s) and schoolchildren

This stage of development in the family life cycle requires yet more skills in parenting and a further change in the marital relationship.

Changes

- The child's increasing independence requires the parents to develop methods of controlling the child's behaviour for his safety and to ensure the behaviour is socially acceptable.
- The children start school and begin to move into a world outside home, learning new skills, meeting people other than family and beginning to bring in ideas and opinions from elsewhere.
- Grandparents may take a more active interest in their grandchildren, sometimes gaining more enjoyment from them than they had from their own children.

It is at this stage of development that children may begin to show evidence of emotional and behavioural problems. Typical problems of pre-school children are bed wetting, soiling and temper tantrums. School-age children may refuse to go to school or begin stealing. In some families, the children may be mentally, physically or sexually abused, or all three. Many problems may be a combination of the child's own personality and the parents' inability or difficulty in fulfilling their parental tasks. Some parents, having

survived a difficult childhood themselves, find themselves re-experiencing past emotional pain when passing through the same stage of family life cycle, as parents. In some families, the child's problem behaviour has the function of bringing into therapy parents who would otherwise be unable to ask for help.

Parent(s) and adolescents

Adolescence marks the transition from childhood to adulthood in both physical and emotional development. In the family, the parents need to mirror the child's development with their own ability to 'let go' and allow the new adult to emerge. Adolescence is a time of experimentation and learning by mistakes, which may be frustrating if not incomprehensible to some parents. The adolescent's search for identity may coincide with the parents' mid-life crises as they seek to come to terms with their own successes and failures. The grandparents' health may be failing and they may be becoming increasingly dependent on their children as the grandchildren move away.

Changes

- The adolescent becomes more involved in his peer group as a source of validation for his beliefs and opinions. Parental values may be scorned, at least temporarily.
- Having worked to keep the children within their control in previous stages, parents now have to relinquish some of this to allow their offspring to take more responsibility. Some limits are still needed so that the adolescent has freedom to rebel safely. An example of this could be the nightly curfew: if a time is set which is appropriate to the age of the child, the child may then argue about it, rebel occasionally by being late or put forward reasoned arguments for special considerations for particular occasions.
- Parents and grandparents may have to face making decisions as to whether the two households should combine if the grandparents are unable to cope alone.

Parents may feel undermined by the criticisms of their children, particularly if they lack confidence and support systems of their own. This may result in an inability to set some limits on the child's behaviour so that the child becomes increasingly challenging, in testing out non-existent limits. If the parental couple have had sexual problems, these may be highlighted in the emergent sexuality of the adolescent. There may even be envy of the young person.

The family may resist the move on to the next stage, and the child shows this by developing a symptom, such as anorexia nervosa or attempts at deliberate self-harm, which involves the parents in 'looking after' the child and the child being unable to move away.

One or both parents may be anxious that the child will repeat their own mistakes, such as failure in education or unplanned pregnancy. In an attempt to prevent this happening, parents may unwittingly increase the likelihood by putting on pressure for academic achievement or having unrealistically strict rules about boy- or girlfriends.

Parent(s) alone and young adults

In most families, children do decide to leave home and embark on an independent life. This may occur through education as the child leaves for college at around 18 years of age, or through work away from home. Others prefer to stay at home until they form a new partnership. The degree of separation between parents and children may depend on cultural beliefs and social values. The two generations may choose to remain in the same household or may live in separate households but geographically close, so that there is frequent contact. In others, either by choice or circumstance, the children may move far away and there is little contact between family members. Maturity involves a degree of separation between parent and offspring that cannot be judged by physical distances.

Changes

- The parents become a couple again and may well have the freedom of the house.

- Both parents and children begin to develop mutual respect for each other as adults, as they develop along their separate ways.
- The child takes on adult roles through work, sexuality and social life.
- The parents face retirement of the wage earner, with changes in the pattern of their lives and possible financial restrictions.
- The grandparents may become increasingly dependent or die.

This is a time of major change for all participants, the new beginnings are not just for the child. The parents may find they no longer wish to be a couple and may have to decide whether they want to stay together. A person who has valued the role of carer may feel bereft and useless. Retirement from paid employment may be an opportunity to engage in new occupations or may create a vacuum.

The young person may find it difficult to make the necessary sexual and social adjustments, and may become increasingly isolated, leading to attempts to resolve this through drug abuse, early pregnancy or even suicide attempts.

One-parent families

With a divorce rate of one in three marriages, there are many types of households raising children. Many children now grow up having intermittent contact with one parent. Some contact with a non-residential parent is usually preferable to none, however difficult the access arrangements may seem.

One-parent families are more likely to be families headed by the mother, but some fathers are also in this position. The reasons for this type of family system will affect the changes to be negotiated and, to some extent, the problems that arise.

Changes

- Death of one parent may leave the other parent to cope with bereavement, the children's loss and financial problems, while having to cope with the day-to-day tasks of running a family. The amount of support networks such as family, friends and child-care facilities will have an impact on the enormity of the task.

- Some families have always had only one parent, either by choice or by circumstances, and again the amount of outside help will influence the situation.

As women head most one-parent families, the family's income is generally reduced and some may require state benefits. However, in some families, this may mark an increase in their finances as the mother now has complete control of the income. Efforts by the state to make the absent parent provide financial support may create additional conflict between divorced parents. An only parent has, at least initially, to meet all the children's needs with no one else to fall back on. The separated parent may be supportive in the challenges of rearing children or may be critical. Where there is a difference in perception, the children may still be caught in parental arguments.

A single parent has very little time for herself. Babysitting, if affordable, may be difficult as many babysitters require transport home at night and this would involve either leaving the children alone or getting them up. It may be much more difficult for the single parent to make and maintain friendships. This is much improved where there are regular and reliable access arrangements.

Stepfamilies

This is a term applied to families where there has been a remarriage with children involved. A possible example would be where a divorced woman with children remarries a divorced man with children. The new household will then consist of mother, stepfather, mother's children and father's children who visit at weekends.

Changes

- The role of the new partner as to parenting responsibilities must be agreed.

- The children now have to share their mother with her new partner and have new step-siblings.
- The children may be in contact with father and stepfather and three sets of grandparents.
- The customs and habits of two households have to be coordinated in one family.

The natural parent is often unsure as to how much parental authority to accord to the new partner and over what time. If children are unsure about this, many will misbehave until the step-parent's position is clarified. Both partners and families, having experienced the breakdown of one relationship, may be unsure how far to trust this new one. Initially, at least, there will be rivalry between children and step-parent for the natural parent's affection. Step-siblings may also be jealous of each other.

The children may be members, if only part-time, of two households, which will have some different rules. It may take time to adjust to this or it may be exploited by insecure children. In families where there is no contact with the departing partner, children may need to grieve for that parent and may take out their anger on the remaining parent.

Many of these problems, relating to reconstituting families, exist because this is a fairly new form of family structure for which no rules have evolved. Each family has to negotiate its own terms. Most presumably manage to do this to their reasonable satisfaction, but it is perhaps not surprising that the divorce rate of second marriages is greater than that for first marriages.

CHILD DEVELOPMENT

Within the family life cycle is the life cycle of each individual. To describe and explain the changes inherent in the transformation of a new-born baby into a fully functioning, thinking, feeling adult has taxed the minds of many. These changes have been described in terms of physiological, cognitive and emotional development. The physiological stages of development are described elsewhere (Ch. 3). Occupational therapists working in child psychiatry require an understanding of some of the cognitive and affective theories of the human life cycle.

Theories of particular interest to occupational therapists are those which show how intrapsychic changes are perceived in terms of behavioural and thinking processes and in relationships with others. The stages of human development describe a process of attachment/ separation or inclusion/differentiation, as mentioned in the previous section. Figure 22.2 compares the theories of Erikson (1963) and Marcia (1979) concerning identity formation and those of Piaget (1932), Kohlberg (1981, 1984) and Gilligan (1982) who have conducted research into cognitive development and moral reasoning.

Identity formation: Erikson

The psychoanalyst, Erik Erikson, delineated eight stages of the life cycle. His is a psychosocial theory of development as it traces the individual's creation of self through relationships with others. Initially, this is through the mechanism of introjection, in which there is an incorporation of another's image, as in infancy, followed by identification, where the child enjoys 'being like' others, to the more sophisticated mechanism of identity formation in adolescence. Here, earlier identifications may be selected or discarded in accordance with present interests, abilities and values. Identity evolves and is reshaped throughout the life cycle.

By the end of adolescence and the beginnings of early adulthood, there should be a sense of well-being. 'Its most obvious concomitants are a feeling of being at home in one's body, a sense of "knowing where one is going" and an inner assuredness of anticipated recognition from those who count' (Kroger 1989).

According to Erikson, each stage in the life cycle represents a conflict to be resolved between a negative and positive pole (Fig. 22.2). A balance is achieved, preferably towards the positive end, which then becomes the turning point towards the next stage. The stages are sequential, in that one stage is resolved before movement on to the

next, and there are approximate ages within which each stage is achieved.

Erikson described the eight stages as follows:

1. Trust versus mistrust: hope

Stage 1 is set in the relationship between the infant and the care-giver. Here the quality of interaction between adult and child enables the child to achieve a sense of continuity, security and trust in itself and another. An ideal balance is towards the trusting pole, leading to hope which forms the basis for later secure development. However, a degree of mistrust of the world contributes to self-protection.

2. Autonomy versus shame and doubt: will

During the second and third years of life, the child gains an increasing sense of self in the control of bodily functions and development of motor and verbal skills. The search for autonomy can be seen in the toddler's use of 'I' and 'No'. Others' respect for the child's growing abilities contribute to the development of self-esteem. A sense of autonomy balanced by an awareness of fallibility is a healthy resolution of this stage.

3. Initiative versus guilt: purpose

During the pre-school years, more complex motor and language skills are learned. There is a greater awareness of sex roles and the development of imagination leads to a richer world of play. Initiative is the ability to translate thoughts into action and therefore to develop a sense of purpose. Social and sex roles can now be tried out. Guilt or fear may tip the balance negatively and act as a brake on the child's explorations. An optimal balance would be one of curiosity limited by social and cultural convention.

4. Industry versus inferiority: competence

The primary school years are important for the practice of skills which will be essential for achievements in adulthood. 'Industry has been described as an apprenticeship to life; feelings of

	1. Trust vs Mistrust	2. Autonomy vs Shame/doubt	3. Initiative vs Guilt	4. Industry vs Inferiority	5. Identity vs Role confusion	6. Intimacy vs Isolation	7. Generativity vs Stagnation	8. Integrity vs Despair
Erikson Identity formation	Infancy *Hope*	2–3 years *Will*	Pre-school *Purpose*	Primary school *Competence*	Adolescence *Fidelity*	Young adulthood *Love*	Adulthood *Care*	*Wisdom*
Marcia				Foreclosure Diffusion	Moratorium Achievement			
Piaget Cognitive development	Sensorimotor 0–2 years	Preoperational 2–7 years *Moral realism*		Concrete operational 7–11 years *Moral relativism*	Abstract operational 11 years →			
Kohlberg Moral reasoning		Level 1: Preconventional *Fairness based on individual need*			Level 2: Conventional *Fairness based on social agreement* Level 3: Postconventional or principled *Fairness based on principled understanding*			
Gilligan Ethics of care		1. Care for self to survive			2. Care for others: responsibility 3. Self and others as interdependent			

Figure 22.2   Comparison of human development theories.

competence and achievement are optimal results here' (Kroger 1989). Identification with adults, such as inspirational teachers, may influence areas of adult interest. A successful outcome of this stage would result in the child feeling rewarded and recognised for achievement, but with an understanding of the limits of competence.

5. Identity versus role confusion: fidelity

The task here is identity formation whereby the adolescent begins to have a stronger sense of self with beliefs, values, skills and sexual identity. James Marcia (cited in Kroger 1989) has expanded this stage to include four alternative outcomes: two types of committed identity and two of role confusion.

Identity achievement. This is a successful resolution to the crisis of Stage 5. It is demonstrated by a flexible yet strong manner of relating to the outside world. Those successful here may be thoughtful and introspective but are willing to listen and learn and are able to form close interpersonal relationships.

Foreclosure. This is an identity which is strongly influenced by others. Beliefs and values may have been taken on uncritically so that there is a rigidity of ideas, leading to an authoritarian standpoint. There is little differentiation from parents and intimate relationships echo the style of the parents.

Moratorium. A difficulty in detachment from parents may be present, along with avoidance of intimate relationships. Marcia described this identity status as an 'ambivalent struggle'. Individuals within this struggle demonstrate similar abilities to those who have achieved an identity and may well join them when the ambivalence is resolved.

Diffusion. There is difficulty in making identity commitment which may result in a drifting through life in an uninvolved yet carefree way. Others may experience great loneliness or severe psychopathology.

6. Intimacy versus isolation: love

Intimacy is only possible following the successful resolution of early stages. The ability to form a close relationship with another depends on a strong sense of self which can be committed but not lost in a relationship. A successful balance within this stage includes the possibility of being alone with an ability for genuine intimacy.

7. Generativity versus stagnation: care

This involves an ability to care and nurture both people and projects but to maintain a healthy self-interest.

8. Integrity versus despair: wisdom

Integrity 'is the acceptance of one's one and only life cycle as something that had to be and that, by necessity, permitted of no substitutions...In such final consolidation, death loses its sting' (Erikson, cited in Kroger 1989).

Moral reasoning: Kohlberg

As a graduate student in clinical psychology, Kohlberg had been an avid reader of Piaget. His research interests emerged from Piaget's concept of the development of autonomous morality. Kohlberg outlined three levels of moral reasoning with two stages at each level. Although there may be an optimal age to reach each level, some people may remain at the first level.

Level one: preconventional. The concept of fairness is based on individual need. This may entail satisfaction of the person's self-interest or physical needs. Some recognition may be given to another person in order to satisfy mutual needs: 'You scratch my back if I scratch yours.'

Level two: conventional. At this level, there is an awareness of group or social norms of fairness. This could be loyalty to a peer group or recognition of social institutions, sometimes termed as 'law and order orientation'. Actions and ideas are judged as to whether they meet the group rules or adhere to religious, political or cultural beliefs.

Level three: postconventional or principled. Reason is now based on ethical principles. There is an understanding of variable group norms and the possibility of a changing society requiring different laws.

The highest stage of moral reasoning is the belief that the equality and dignity of each human being is the essence of justice. The stages of moral reasoning can be summarised as follows (Kroger 1989):

Level 1 (i)   Obey rules to avoid punishment.
         (ii) Conform to obtain rewards, have favours returned.
Level 2 (iii) Conform to avoid disapproval, dislike by others.
         (iv) Conform to avoid censure by legitimate authorities.
Level 3 (v)   Conform to maintain the respect of the impartial spectator judging in terms of community welfare.
         (vi) Conform to avoid self-condemnation.

Kohlberg's research extended over 20 years and he found only about 30% of subjects reached level 3 type thinking. Kohlberg believed people could be educated to a higher stage of moral reasoning. Initially, he hoped a population could be taught to reason at the sixth stage (level 3). Eventually this was replaced by a hope that adolescents could achieve stage 4 (level 2).

Ethics of care: Gilligan

Carol Gilligan initially worked with Kohlberg, but became critical of the male bias of his samples. She also criticised Erikson, Marcia and Piaget for the same reason. Gilligan (1982) argued that female development is ignored, so that the above theorists had not taken into consideration girls' and women's experiences.

The issues of separation and attachment are different for men and women. Boys learn early to create a separate identity from their mothers, whereas girls confront this at adolescence. Instrumental abilities and individuation are valued highly in men. Girls' gender identity is defined by their attachments, so that expressive abilities and connectedness are highly rated. In adulthood, men are more likely to have problems with intimacy and women with separation.

Gilligan did not feel this was reflected in Erikson's theory.

She also argued that Kohlberg based his theory of moral development on the ethics of rights, whereas women operate within an ethics of responsibility; the difference being equality and equity. Men deal in hierarchies, women in webs.

From her research into women's decision-making processes when seeking an abortion, she outlined three levels of care:

1. care for self to survive
2. care for others, where responsibility for others outweighs care for self
3. self and others are interdependent so both need consideration.

Developmental theories and intervention

An understanding of some theories of child and adult development enables the therapist to understand the level of functioning of a child in order to match the intervention to that level. When working with adolescents, for example, it is important to understand that they are separating for the second time. The first separation was the physical separation of infant from carer, whereas the adolescent is struggling to form a separate identity. It may be worth looking at Erikson's stage four, the achievement of competence, to take the young person back a stage to increase their feeling of competence. Alternatively, the therapist may use Kohlberg's moral reasoning in order to stimulate movement from a more individualistic form of reasoning to one acknowledging the influence of peer group. Social skills training may be working towards both these aims. On the other hand, it may be inappropriate to teach assertiveness skills to an adolescent who is still struggling for peer group approval. Girls are more likely to work cooperatively in groups and find it easier to care than confront, whereas boys' groups are much more competitive.

Occupational therapists working with mothers and pre-school children may find Greenspan's theory of development useful, as he suggests activities for mothers to try with their babies to encourage both neurological development and the building of the relationship between mother and child (Greenspan 1999). These can be used with mothers who are struggling to establish good relationships with their children.

PRESENTING PROBLEMS

Children rarely initiate a request for treatment. Usually an adult, either a parent/carer or professional, decides that the child is suffering or is causing others to suffer. Some adolescents who have experienced trauma, such as sexual abuse, do ask for help in overcoming the effects.

While most children's problems can be understood in terms of developmental and family dynamics, some are precursors of schizophrenia and bipolar disorder (manic depression). For the purposes of treatment, clinicians tend to use a descriptive formulation of a child's difficulties, but for research purposes an awareness of a recognised classification of disorders is necessary. Both the DSM-IV, published by the American Psychiatric Association (1994), and the ICD 10, published by the World Health Organization (WHO 1992), describe mental disorders in children, and this section uses those listed in DSM-IV, although there are parallels between the two systems. DSM-IV uses a multiaxial assessment; the fourth axis describes psychosocial and environmental problems, both as contributory factors to disorder and as effects of it, and are of particular interest to occupational therapists.

Anxiety disorders

Children of all ages suffer from a wide range of anxiety disorders. They may have panic attacks, with or without agrophobia, specific phobias, such as fear of animals or the natural environment, for example, heights, or social phobia, where social or performance situations are avoided. Obsessive-compulsive disorder frequently starts in childhood, where the child may perform hour-long rituals before going to bed or leaving the house. Children can experience post-traumatic stress disorder and acute stress disorder. General anxiety disorder presents in children and adolescents as concern for performance. They may be perfectionists, worry about punctuality, or fear imminent disasters. It is thought that 50% of patients with this disorder first experience it in childhood.

Mood disorders

Major depressive episodes or disorders are found in children and are most frequently referred following social withdrawal, particularly from school, as these children do not elicit adult concern by being disruptive (Goodyear & Cooper 1993).

Adolescents also present with bipolar disorder or cyclothymic disorder where there are depressive and hypomanic symptoms. Cawthorn et al (1994) found a more positive outcome than for those children with schizophrenia.

Behavioural disorders

Attention deficit and disruptive behaviour disorders account for a large proportion of referrals to child mental health services:

1. Attention deficit/hyperactivity disorder describes the impulsive children who have difficulty being still at home or school unless given constant individual attention.
2. Conduct disorder accounts for a significant proportion of referrals, perhaps because of its social consequences. According to the DSM-IV it is 'Repetitive or persistent pattern of behaviour in which the basic rights of others or major age-appropriate societal norms or rules are violated.' This includes aggression to people, animals or property, deceitfulness or theft.
3. Oppositional defiant disorder is a 'recurrent pattern of negativistic, defiant, disobedient and hostile behaviour towards authority figures'. These symptoms are usually present at home, but not necessarily at school or in the community. These are the children parents often describe as 'having an attitude problem'. It may lead to conduct disorders.

Elimination disorders

- Encopresis is the repeated passage of faeces in inappropriate places, either voluntarily or involuntarily.
- Enuresis is the repeated voiding of urine during the day or night into the bed or clothes.

Eating disorders

Anorexia nervosa. In this condition, according to the DSM-IV, 'the individual refuses to maintain a minimally normal body weight, is intensely afraid of gaining weight and exhibits a significant disturbance in the perception of the shape or size of his or her body'. There is an absence of at least three consecutive menstrual cycles. Two subtypes are described:

- the 'restricting type' where weight loss is accomplished primarily through dieting, fasting or excessive exercise
- the 'binge-eating/purging type' where binge-eating is counteracted by self-induced vomiting, misuse of laxatives, diuretics or enemas.

Bulimia nervosa. According to the DSM-IV, this is associated with 'Binge-eating and inappropriate compensatory methods to prevent weight gain'. Bulimia is differentiated from anorexia in that weight may be within the normal range and/or menses are regular.

Sleep disorders

Children may present with nightmares or sleep terrors (no recollection of content on awakening) or sleepwalking.

Sexual and gender identity disorders

Although it may constitute a common concern to carers and professionals, under-age sexual activity does not constitute a mental disorder. The two disorders treated in child mental health services are paraphilia, more usually described as 'children who molest', and those with gender identity disorder.

Schizophrenia

This tends not to be diagnosed until late adolescence and has a poor outcome in work, relationships and activities of daily living (Cawthron et al 1994).

Dissociative disorders

Dissociative amnesia may be experienced by children who have had a trauma but have few memories of it. Survivors of sexual abuse may have only a vague recollection of events. The issue of false memory syndrome arises from allegations that psychotherapists have suggested the amnesia hides abusive experiences.

Survivors may also describe a depersonalisation disorder in that they coped with abuse by 'detaching from the body' and becoming an observer. This feeling of detachment may recur at other points of stress.

Somatoform disorders

Somatisation disorder. Many symptoms begin in childhood where the child complains of pain or gastrointestinal symptoms.

Conversion disorder. Children show disturbance of gait or are said to have seizures and yet do not seem unduly concerned by their symptoms.

Body dismorphic disorder. This is said to start in adolescence, although it may not be diagnosed until adulthood. This is an excessive preoccupation with a supposed body defect.

OTHER DISORDERS
Learning difficulties

Learning disorders occur when there is below expected achievement in standardised tests in reading, writing or mathematical ability. The child may present with low self-esteem and poor social skills.

Motor skills

Motor skills disorder includes the 'clumsy' children with poor motor coordination who are more regularly seen by paediatric occupational therapists.

Communication disorders

Communication disorders are mainly treated by speech and language therapists, but children who stutter may also be referred for psychological treatment.

Pervasive development disorders

Pervasive developmental disorders include children with autism or Asperger's syndrome.

Tic disorders

Tic disorders include children who present with repetitive, involuntary movements or sounds, for example Tourette's syndrome.

Other disorders of infancy, childhood and adolescence include the following:

Separation anxiety

Separation anxiety disorder describes children who have difficulty leaving the parent to go to school or develop independence and worry about possible harm to the family.

Selective mutism

Selective mutism is a disorder where a child refuses to speak in specific situations, such as school.

Reactive detachment disorders

Reactive detachment disorder of infancy or early childhood is described in the DSM-IV as 'markedly disturbed and developmentally inappropriate social relatedness in most contexts'. It begins before 5 years of age and is associated with grossly pathological care.

I. 'Inhibited type' includes the 'frozen watchfulness' of young children who anticipate being hurt by their carer.
II. 'Disinhibited type' describes abused children who are indiscriminate in their approach to adults. They will climb onto a strangers knee on first meeting, at an age when most children cling to their mothers.

Other problems requiring clinical attention

This heading applies to problems in relationships not covered elsewhere, including difficulties following abuse or neglect. Additional conditions may also include bereavement, problems of identity, acculturation or antisocial behaviour, which is insufficient to be termed a disorder.

This is a brief overview of the relevant mental disorders suffered by children, as described in DSM-IV. It is not possible in this section to mention all the criteria for diagnosis, but occupational therapists need to understand the use of the terms, not to provide diagnoses.

Knowledge of disorders does influence treatment, as in the following example:

A child may be referred for school refusal. This could be an indicator of one of the following:

- a learning disorder: the child is avoiding school as he is failing academically
- a conduct disorder: the child does not go to school as he prefers to burgle houses or to shoplift
- a separation anxiety disorder: the child is terrified to leave parents or home
- a major depressive disorder: social withdrawal as a symptom of depression leads to non-attendance
- a social phobia disorder: the child is afraid of mixing with others or of having his performance assessed
- a somatoform disorder: the child cannot go to school due to pains or sickness or is unable to walk.

OCCUPATIONAL THERAPY IN CHILD AND ADOLESCENT MENTAL HEALTH

Occupational therapy occurs within the context of a multidisciplinary team. A range of professionals may treat the child and family, either simultaneously or sequentially. The team may be working on a residential unit for children or adolescents, in an outpatient service or in a community team providing early intervention. The occupational therapy assessment forms a part of the general assessment for treatment and, to a lesser extent, for diagnosis.

The multidisciplinary team

The multidisciplinary team consists of health professionals as well as staff employed by social services departments (social workers) and education departments (teachers). The health professionals are typically:

- medical, that is, consultant child psychiatrist, specialist registrar and junior doctors
- nursing, either ward-based or community psychiatric nurses, and nursery nurses
- psychologists
- occupational therapists.

The multidisciplinary team is the single-handed occupational therapist's day-to-day support group. Teaching, clinical supervision and case discussion all occur within this context. The emotional challenge of working with deprived and abused children, or those who have suffered losses and bereavements, can only be met where each professional is able to count on the support and backing of colleagues.

Paediatricians, dieticians and speech and language therapists occasionally work with the team on specific problems such as anorexia nervosa or stammering, where there is both a physical and psychological component to the problem.

As children's difficulties are addressed by many agencies, an occupational therapist will find herself working alongside staff from other agencies, for example police and social workers investigating child abuse, or teachers and education welfare officers where the child does not attend school. The NHS Health Advisory Service (1995) and the Department of Health (1995) have endorsed the multidisciplinary team, and clarified levels of service delivery (Fig. 22.3). A summary of the tiered approach describes the levels of interventions (Table 22.1). A new role, that of primary mental health worker, has been adopted in many localities. Several occupational therapists, as well as social workers, nurses and teachers, have been appointed to these posts.

Occupational therapy assessment

Ambelas (1991), in analysing the flow of tasks within treatment, drew the distinction between assessment leading to diagnosis and assessment leading to the therapeutic hypothesis and, therefore, to therapy. Occupational therapy assessment generally falls into the latter category, as the task is to assess level of competence in skills or areas of occupation in which the patient is experiencing difficulty. In child psychiatry, diagnostic definitions are frequently behavioural descriptions and, in some teams, where the referring agent defines the problem clearly, an occupational therapist may be the only professional to assess or treat the child. It is of importance that the therapist is aware which elements she is intending to assess.

An advantage of formal assessments is that they can be used for measuring outcomes. Jeffrey (1993) discussed the use of standardised tests which are suitable for use with children. Most therapists working in a child and adolescent mental health service do not use these tests routinely and appear to use a more descriptive approach. Hoghugi (1992) developed the 'problem profile' to assess children's abilities in all aspects of their lives and remind therapists that 'the term problem can refer to unacceptable conditions which are *presented* or *suffered* by the child' (antisocial behaviour is an example of the former and being abused of the latter). Assessment of a child's problem includes discussion with carers and other professionals and collection of information from reviews and conferences, as it would be unnecessarily time-consuming to observe the child in all situations. Mocellin (1988) suggested that 'The guiding principle is that there should not be any assessment unless it leads to the development of competent behaviour in patients.' The purpose of assessment is to set therapeutic objectives which enable the occupational therapist to plan treatment and evaluate outcomes. Cook (1994) defined objective as 'a behavioural indicator of subjective change'. This enables an agreement to be drawn up between the child, family and the therapist, as well as taking into account the

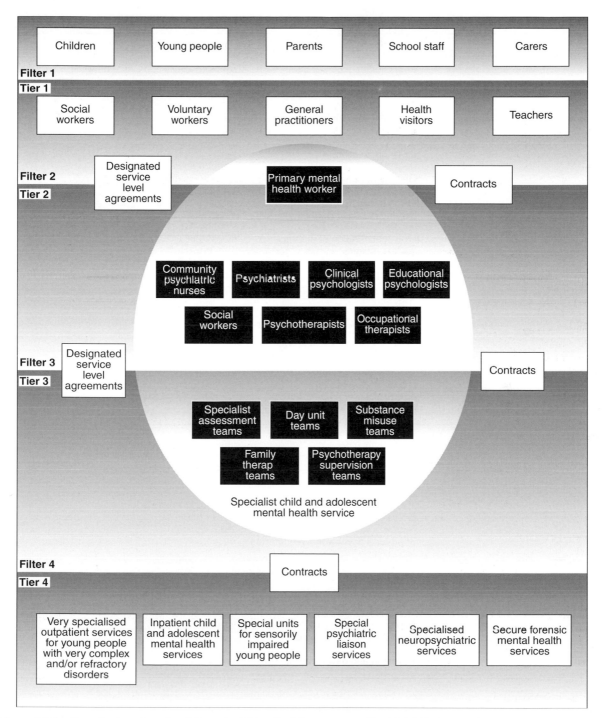

Figure 22.3 Organisation of service delivery in child and adolescent mental health (NHS Health Advisory Service 1995).

request of the referring agent. Some families bringing children for therapy request a general outcome, such as, the child should be happy. All parties must agree objectives, so the therapist

Table 22.1 Services offered in the tiered approach to child and adolescent mental health services

	Tier	Function	Professionals/agencies
	Health promotion	Promotion of good parenting: Parenting education in schools Contraceptive advice Antenatal education Postnatal support	Extended family and social network Personal and social education teachers School nurses Family planning advisors Midwives Health visitors
Tier 1	Primary care	Early intervention: General advice on child care/parenting Problem-solving approach Support in negotiating life events, e.g. bereavement, divorce Early identification of mental health problems	Health visitors School nurses Social services Voluntary agencies Teachers Educational welfare officers
	Filter between 1 and 2	Mapping Consultation Assessment	Primary mental health worker
Tier 2a	Network of professionals working independently	Community base Identification and treatment of mental disorder Training and consultation to professionals in tier 1 Assessment for another tier Outreach work to families who are unwilling to use other services	Paediatricians Educational psychologists Clinical psychologists Child psychiatrists Paediatric occupational therapists
Tier 2b	Multi-agency teams	Community base Mapping local services Training and consultation to professionals in tier 1 Joint work with primary care professionals Outreach work to families Short-term direct work with families and children	Health service staff School nurses Psychiatric nurses Occupational therapists Clinical psychologists Social workers Teachers
Tier 3	Specialist service-multidisciplinary team	Child mental health clinic Assessment and treatment of child mental health disorders Assessment for referral to tier 4 Contribution to training/consultation tiers 1/2 Research and development	Child and adolescent psychiatrists Clinical psychologists Occupational therapists Psychiatric nurse Possibly: Social workers Teachers Child psychotherapists Art, music, drama therapists
Tier 4	Tertiary services	Supra-district provision Adolescent/children's in-patient units Secure forensic adolescent units Eating disorder units Specialist teams for sexual abuse or neuropsychiatric problems	As above

may not always be able to include all the issues she believes pertinent (Box 22.1).

Occupational therapy for children and families

Occupational therapists in child and adolescent mental health services use a variety of frames of reference or theoretical approaches. In Britain, play therapy features in most published work whereas in the USA therapists describe the use of model of human occupation or the influence of occupational science (Lougher 2000). Although some occupational therapists may be using similar therapeutic interventions to other professions, there are opportunities to introduce an occupational perspective which is concerned with the changing roles of child and family, the child's balance of occupations and the family's use of the environment. This may be achieved in family work or individual sessions with the child or groupwork involving child, adult or both. Wilcock (1998) proposed a role for occupational therapy in health promotion which can be taken forward by occupational therapists working in the community (tier 2; NHS Health Advisory Service 1995). She cited the example of Olson's parent–child activity group in a programme focused on the prevention of mental health problems in pre-school children. In Britain, the Sure Start initiatives aim to support

---

Box 22.1 Case example 1

Mrs B brings her 13-year-old daughter, Sally, to the clinic. Mrs B wants her daughter to be as happy as she was before her parents' divorce 2 years ago. When asked how she would know Sally was happier, Mrs B replies that she would like to see her going out with her friends at weekends. Sally wants to stop crying when other girls mention their fathers. Sally's class teacher told the therapist that Sally was oversensitive to teasing by fellow pupils, so a third objective is agreed with Mrs B and Sally, that she should more assertive in classroom disagreements.

  The therapist then selects the type of treatment most likely to lead to positive outcomes on these objectives, although she may have observed other areas of difficulty the family prefer not to address at the moment. Mrs B refuses counselling for her own sadness following the divorce, so any change in her mood is not included in the objectives.

---

families with pre-school children and so may provide occupational therapists with opportunities in health promotion as well as treatment.

Child-focused therapy

Although children are invited to attend the clinic with their carers initially, it may be decided that they would benefit from individual treatment sessions. The following factors are important when setting objectives and selecting activities:

1. An assessment of the child's psychological and physiological development, as outlined in the section on child development.
2. A consideration of whether the child has difficulty expressing emotions, or a tendency to erupt uncontrollably and require containment.
3. An awareness of the stability of the child's living arrangements. Children in temporary accommodation feel very vulnerable and treatment should not be too challenging.
4. An understanding of local child protection regulations and knowledge of the progress of any ongoing child protection investigations.
5. The level of cooperation and support of the carers.

Individual therapy

The depth of individual work takes into account the child's level of support from family or carers and the child's own capacity to work towards change. There are three possible levels of intervention:

1. Skills acquisition, for example, personal care, social skills, assertiveness techniques and anxiety management. Specific deficits in the child's areas of competence in performance are identified and the child is taught the necessary skills. This is likely to take place within a time-limited programme. Sensory integration could also be included in this group.
2. Problem resolution using directive play therapy or the use of media to aid self-expression. The child's disturbance of behaviour and/or mood is thought to follow specific unhappy or traumatic experiences so that the aim of therapy is to facilitate understanding or expression of

emotions. This may be a time-limited or a longer-term treatment programme (see Ch. 7).

3. Explorative psychotherapy, for example, non-directive play therapy or psychodynamic psychotherapy. These therapies focus on problems which are not available to the conscious mind, and entail further training for occupational therapists.

Groupwork

From the age of 5 years, children are accustomed to working with their peers. During adolescence, the peer group increases in importance and is valuable to therapeutic interventions. Groupwork may also be concerned with skills acquisition, problem solving and exploration, as with groups for adults (see Ch. 14). Children with similar problems are able to support each other, such as survivors of sexual abuse, victims of bullying and children suffering bereavement.

Figure 22.4 shows the range of interventions used by occupational therapists working with children.

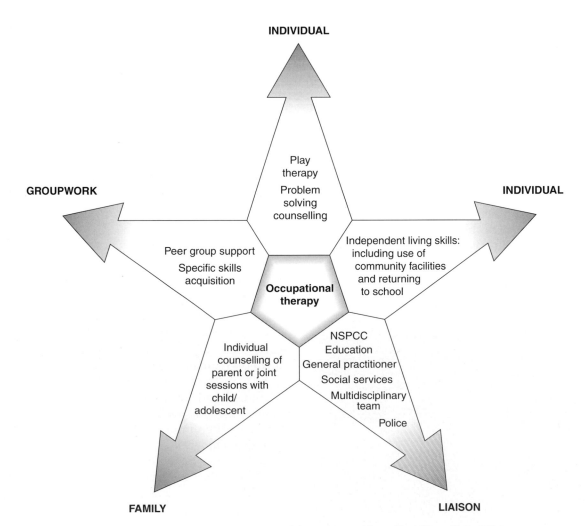

Figure 22.4 The range of interventions used by occupational therapists working with children (Cole 1994).

Therapy for adult family members

Therapeutic support for parents is given to enable them to improve their ability to care for the child or to empower them in negotiations with the necessary agencies or, indeed, with their children. Referral to adult services is indicated where a parent requests therapy for their personal issues or is thought to show signs of mental ill-health. Groupwork is valuable for mothers, parents and families. Marital therapy enables parents to address the difficulties in their own relationship, as some children express the stresses they perceive between parents.

Family work

The behaviour and emotions of a child are affected, if not caused by, difficulties in interactions between family members. Certain patterns of family organisation appear to be transmitted across generations. It is valuable to meet the child and the people with whom he is living, as any change in one person will affect others in the family. All therapy for children takes place in the context of the family, as individual work with the child is only effective when the family is able to adjust to change in the child. It is essential that therapists are able to talk to parents/carers, including them as partners in therapy (Box 22.2). Families attend clinics already believing they have failed, so it is important they leave feeling they have been listened to and their opinions valued.

Occupational therapists may work with parents to develop strategies in managing their children's difficult behaviour or, by the use of activities, enable a parent to build a closer relationship with their child. Family therapy is a specific form of therapy which some occupational therapists use after further training.

Not all children live with their own families; some children will be living in children's homes, others with foster carers. Members of their support network, key workers or foster parents are included in therapy, as a shared responsibility for treatment is essential.

Clinical supervision

A therapist working in child and adolescent mental health services is constantly drawing on her own emotional resources. This is true in all areas of occupational therapy, but working with children who have been abused or deprived of

---

Box 22.2 Case example 2

Anne C, aged 15, is referred to the clinic by the physician. Anne has poorly controlled diabetes. This has led to her staying away from school and losing friendships. Mrs C works long hours as a cleaner and her husband has been unemployed for a year.

The family is seen initially by a consultant psychiatrist and occupational therapist. They draw up a genogram with the family (Fig. 22.5). This shows that Anne was the result of the third pregnancy. Mrs C's previous pregnancies had resulted in miscarriages, so that Anne had always been a particularly precious child to her parents. When she was found to have diabetes, aged 1, both parents played an active role in managing the condition.

Mr C's sister had died, aged 15, of an asthma attack, so that Mr C is particularly anxious about his daughter's health. He has also been distressed and frustrated by his year of unemployment. Mrs C tends to leave the supervision of Anne to her husband and has only recently worked through the loss of her father. Anne resents her father's constant worrying about her health and will deliberately mislead him about her insulin intake.

It is felt that Mr C does not allow Anne sufficient responsibility for managing her own diabetes. It is suggested Mrs C could support him in coping with his anxieties about Anne's health. Anne is also concerned about dad's misery and, in part, stays at home to cheer him up. The parents agree to try to give Anne more responsibility and the occupational therapist agrees to see Anne.

Initially, Anne has individual counselling where she can express her frustrations at having diabetes. She is then offered a place in a girls' group run by the occupational therapist and a teacher. Anne is able to discover that other girls can also feel different and isolated and is able to establish new friendships. The teacher arranges a programme at the local college and an occupational therapy assistant takes her to visit the building and to practise bus routes. As Anne is returning to education, Mr C finds a job as a skilled craftsman.

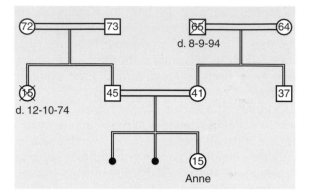

Figure 22.5 A family genogram for Anne C.

affection is especially demanding. Clinical supervision is the process by which the therapist is able to review her work with other professionals.

Hawkins & Shohet (1989) suggested that supervision may include elements of education, support and management. An essential component is an exploration of the dynamics of the patient's difficulties and how these affect the relationship between therapist and patient. Failure of the therapist to monitor her level of involvement with her patients may lead to stress and burnout as the needs of deprived children can seem infinite.

Supervision needs to be regular, reliable and supportive and is beginning to be seen by some organisations as necessary to ensure a high quality of therapy.

Child protection procedures

All staff working with children should be aware of their local child protection procedures. These should be available in all departments so that each occupational therapist is confident about how to respond to an allegation of child abuse. Professional confidentiality is not absolute where the safety of a child is at issue.

Occupational therapists are not responsible for the investigation of possible child abuse. This is the role of the social services department and the police.

SUMMARY

Occupational therapists in the field of child and adolescent mental health need to be keenly aware of the contexts within which they work. They form part of a multidisciplinary team which must itself be able to coordinate its function with social services departments, the local education authority, and other agencies. The family influences children, even where the family is largely absent. Whoever cares for the child, relatives, foster parents or the local authority, must be involved with the therapeutic programme.

In this chapter, I hope to have shown the occupational therapist at work within the wider network, as well as having the knowledge to treat individual patients. An understanding of the purpose of the other agencies, followed by an awareness of specific roles within the multidisciplinary team as well as the overlap, is a prerequisite to the delivery of treatment.

Assessment of the patient requires familiarity with the life cycle of the family and theories of child development. The most important skill needed is the ability to engage with children as well as their families.

This can be a very emotionally charged field of work and many occupational therapists are single-handed. It is, therefore, essential to have a good system of supervision and informal support. Organisations such as the National Association of Paediatric Occupational Therapists (NAPOT) have local groups and organise national conferences. The Association for Child Psychology and Psychiatry (ACPP) publishes regular newsletters and a journal, which includes recent research.

In spite of the difficulties, this is an exciting and quickly moving area of work. Where else could you be crawling around the floor helping a teddy talk to a rabbit in the morning, discussing the programme for an anorexic patient on a general ward before lunch and then liasing with NSPCC and police in the afternoon? It is perhaps not a job for a newly qualified occupational therapist but allows plenty of scope for a more experienced therapist.

REFERENCES

Ambelas 1991 The task of treatment and the multidisciplinary team. Psychiatric Bulletin 15(2): 77–79

American Psychiatric Association 1994 Diagnostic and Statistical Manual IV. American Psychiatric Association, Washington

Audit Commission 1999 National report: children in mind: child and adolescent mental health services. HMSO, London

Cawthron P, James A, Seagroatt V 1994 Adolescent onset psychosis: a clinical and outcome study. Journal of Child Psychology and Psychiatry 35(7): 1321–1332

Cole 1994 Personal communication

Cook 1994 Workshop. National Association of Paediatric Occupational Therapists' Conference, guildford, 8–9 September

Crime and Disorder Act 1998 Youth Justice Board interdepartmental circular: establishing youth offender teams. 22 December 1998

Department of Education and Employment 1999 Sure Start: making a difference for children and families. Department of Education and Employment Publications, London

Department of Health 1995 A handbook on child and adolescent mental health. HMSO, London

Erikson E H 1963 Childhood and society, 2nd edn. W W Norton, New York

Gilligan C 1982 In a different voice: psychological theory and women's development. Harvard University Press, Cambridge, Mass

Goodyer I, Cooper D J 1993 A community study of depression in adolescent girls. II. The clinical features of identified disorder. British Journal of Psychiatry 163: 369–380

Greenspan S 1999 Building healthy minds. Perseus Books, Cambridge, Mass

Hawkins P, Shohet R 1989 Supervision in the helping professions. Open University Press, Milton Keynes

Hoghugi M 1992 Assessing child and adolescent disorders. Sage, London

Jeffrey L 1993 Aspects of selecting outcome measures to demonstrate effectiveness of comprehensive rehabilitation. British Journal of Occupational Therapy 56(11): 394–400

Kohlberg L 1981 Essays in moral development, vol. 1. The philosophy of moral development. Harper and Row, San Francisco

Kohlberg L 1984 Essays in moral development, vol. 2. The psychology of moral development. Harper and Row, San Francisco

Kroger J 1989 Identity in adolescence: the balance between self and other. Routledge, London

Llorens L A 1970 Facilitating growth and development: the promise of occupational therapy. American Journal of Occupational Therapy 14(2): 93–101

Lougher L 2001 Occupational therapy in child and adolescent mental health services. Churchill Livingstone, London

Marcia J E 1979 Identity status in late adolescence; description of some clinical implications. Identity Development Symposium, Groningen, Netherlands, June

Minuchin S 1974 Families and family therapy. Tavistock, London

Mocellin G 1988 A perspective on the principles and practice of occupational therapy. British Journal of Occupational Therapy 51(1): 4–7

NHS Health Advisory Service 1995 A thematic review of child and adolescent mental health services: together we stand. HMSO, London

Oakley A 1980 Women confined. Martin Robertson, Oxford

Piaget J 1932 The moral judgement of the child. Kegan Paul, London

Skynner R 1976 One flesh: separate persons: principles of family and marital psychotherapy. Constable, London

Wilcock A A 1998 An occupational perspective of health. Slack, New Jersey

World Health Organization 1992 The ICD-10 classification of mental and behavioural disorders: clinical descriptions and diagnostic guidelines. WHO, Geneva

FURTHER READING

Black D, Cottrell D (eds) 1993 Seminars in child and adolescent psychiatry. Royal College of Psychiatrists, London

Dwivedi K N (ed) 1993 Groupwork with children and adolescents. Jessica Kingsley, London

Greenspan S 1999 Building healthy minds. Perseus Books, Cambridge, Mass.

Wilcock A A 1998 An occupational perspective of health. Slack, New Jersey

USEFUL ADDRESSES

National Association of Paediatric Occupational Therapists (NAPOT), Barton's Cottage, Prestbury Road, Wilmslow, Cheshire SK9 2LL
(*publish 3 journals per year*)

Association for Child Psychology and Psychiatry (ACPP), St Saviour's House, 39–41 Union Street, London SE1 1SD

(*publish Journal of Child Psychology and Psychiatry; Child Psychology and Psychiatry Review*)

Young Minds, 102–108 Clerkenwell Road, London EC1M 5SA
(*publish a magazine every 2 months which covers news on issues affecting children's emotional and mental health*)

23

Learning disabilities

Anne Fleming   Mhairi McAughtrie
Ruth Mitchell   Lesley McNaughton

INTRODUCTION

This chapter is intended as a practical guide to those entering this specialty. It is not intended to be either definitive or prescriptive in content. The text aims to serve as a reference and to direct the reader to other information which has been adequately provided and discussed elsewhere.

The focus of the chapter is on the application of occupational therapy skills with this client group. Ward (1990) defined this population, for legal purposes, as characterised by intellectual functioning which is significantly below average and having marked impairment in the ability to adapt to the cultural demands of society. Both characteristics must be present.

The authors have chosen to adopt a case study approach in order to illustrate the clinical reasoning involved in any period of intervention regardless of the setting. The intention is to bring the reader up to date with the current philosophy of care and service provision, as determined by legislation and social policy, and to demonstrate some of the factors which make working in this specialty so challenging and interesting.

A HISTORICAL PERSPECTIVE

Historically, people with a learning disability were held to be of little value to society and custodial models of care were the norm. The inception of the National Health Service in 1948 continued this custodial model and encouraged the belief that people with learning disabilities required treatment, as opposed to education and social care. Over the past century there has been a dramatic change in both care and attitudes towards people with learning disabilities (Wright & Digby). Some of the legislation which has driven these changes is detailed in Box 23.1 Since the 1970s, a steady development of a social model of care has occurred which reflects the belief that people with learning disabilities are individuals who have needs, wishes and responsibilities in common with the rest of society. Current policy is that people with learning disabilities should live in the community, accessing mainstream services, with additional support as required. At the time of writing, the Mental Health Act (Scotland) 1984 and the Mental Health Act are under review, and the Learning Disabilities Strategy Review is nearing completion. The impact of these will continue to influence the way in which services are provided.

Box 23.1	Legislation concerning people with learning disabilities	
Year	**Legislation**	**Statutory requirements**
1913 1914	Mental Deficiency Act Mental Deficiency Act	Local education authorities to determine the mental ability of all school-age children and provide appropriate social education for those seen as 'defective' but 'educable'.
1957	Report of Royal Commission on the law relating to mental illness and mental handicap	Recognised the need for a reversal of policy which relied on institutional care, towards a policy of 'community care'.
1959	Mental Health Act	Followed recommendations from 1957 report. Many people were given the status of 'informal' admissions.
1970	Education Act	Local authorities were now responsible for the education of all children with a mental handicap, bringing them closer to using mainstream services.
1971	White Paper: Better Services for the Mentally Handicapped	This proposed that hospital populations should be reduced and attempts made to avoid segregation from local community and services.
1978	Warnock Report: Special Educational Needs	Special educational needs laid down the rights of previously uneducable children to education within ordinary schools.
1979	Jay Report	This report indicated the need for a different approach to training staff. Emphasis was placed on social rather than on clinical aspects.
1981	Education Act	Implemented recommendations of Warnock Report.
1988	Griffiths Report: Community Care Agenda For Action	Recommended assessing community care needs and care management and the purchasing and provision of services to maintain or establish people in their own homes.
1989	White Paper: Caring for People: Community Care in the Next Decade and Beyond	Claimed to offer a coherent programme to meet present and future challenges, to give people the services they need, utilising public agencies, thus providing more efficient care.
1990	NHS and Community Care Act	Implemented the recommendations of the 1989 White Paper.
1998	Modernising Community Care: An Action Plan	A plan to provide better and more timely results for people needing community care. Key themes were working together, best value, user involvement and faster decision-making.
1999	Aiming for Excellence	Proposals to strengthen the protection of children and vulnerable adults through service standards and regulation.

Terminology

The change in attitude towards people with learning disabilities within general society is reflected in the revised definitions of this group of people.

It was not until 1913 that mental handicap was recognised as being different from mental illness, when the Mental Deficiency Act (1913) categorised mentally defective people as:

- idiots
- imbeciles
- feeble-minded
- moral defective.

In the 1970s the term 'people with a mental handicap' was used, emphasising that clients are people first who happen to be handicapped. This drew heavily upon the ideas of normalisation and social role valorisation (Wolfensberger 1972).

Earlier classifications have now been superseded: for example, the DSM-IV (American Psychiatric Association 1995) classification system uses the following terms:

- *Mild (IQ 52–67).* This may be only a matter of delayed development and adults may lead independent lives and never be classified as mentally handicapped.
- *Moderate (IQ 36–51).* Affected persons are obviously handicapped, but may learn self-help skills and work in sheltered employment, adapting well to life in the community, usually in supervised settings.
- *Severe (IQ 20–35).* There may be delayed development, or failure to develop physical and communication skills. Often affected people are also physically handicapped, but they can still show limited independence.
- *Profound (IQ 0–19).* Most individuals with this diagnosis have an identified neurological condition. Optimal development may occur in a highly structured environment with constant aid and supervision and an individual relationship with a care-giver.

This classification is based not only on IQ, but also recognises the importance of adaptive behaviour in relation to environmental demands as a predictor of level of ability.

The reader is referred to the World Health Organization (1980) classification of impairment, disability and handicap:

- *Impairment*: any loss or abnormality of psychological or anatomical structure or function.
- *Disability*: any restriction or lack (resulting from an impairment) of ability to perform an activity in the manner or within the range considered normal for a human being.
- *Handicap*: a disadvantage for an individual resulting from an impairment or disability that limits or prevents the fulfilment of a role that is normal (depending on age, sex, social and cultural factors) for that individual.

Figure 23.1 shows how handicap is imposed on people socially; whatever the nature of their disability, the extent to which it handicaps them depends on the social conditions in which they live. Although it is usually impossible to restore an impairment, it is recognised that, with advances in treatment and technology, it is possible to reduce a disability, and a combination of technology and social attitudes can reduce and avoid handicap. It is therefore necessary to alter society's perceptions of people with learning disabilities in order to block the route to handicap.

Looking at these definitions it becomes clearer why we have moved away from the term 'mental handicap'. 'Mental' is a term which fits more accurately within psychiatry, and the problems experienced within this group of people are more commonly associated with the process of learning. The use of the term 'disability' as opposed to 'handicap' focuses attention on the need to enable the person to reach his fullest potential by utilising whatever means are possible.

Currently, the most frequently used term is 'people with learning disabilities'. This description has been adopted by the Department of Health and most agencies within this area of work, for example, the British Institute of Learning Disabilities.

There is a recognition that a consensus in terminology is required for representing people with a learning disability. As professionals we

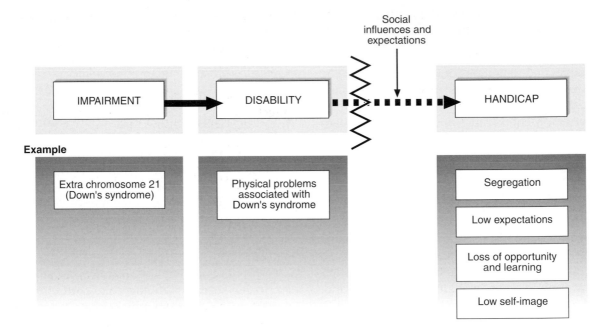

Figure 23.1 The route to handicap.

have a responsibility to promote the most favourable impression of this client group, and we must recognise the power of the words that we use to describe them.

Labelling

Labelling is the process of categorising, by their most predominant characteristic or characteristics, a group of people who behave outside the norms of society and can therefore be identified as different. Labelling, or diagnosing, is not only a process of description and classification but also comes with assumptions about appropriate treatment methods to be employed and the types of outcome that may be expected. Franco (1982) and Rowitz (1981) have identified that a primary motivation behind identifying a group of people as having 'mental handicap' is to draw attention to their special needs and thus to facilitate the provision of support, services or special treatments for them. Box 23.2 shows positive and negative aspects of labelling.

It is recognised that all labels will eventually become dated and deemed inappropriate, as has

been seen throughout history. Although it is important to continue to recognise the positive aspects of labelling, we must also be aware that we are dealing with individuals whom it is difficult to categorise using a non-specific label. People referred to occupational therapy have individual needs and should not be seen in terms of a rigid diagnostic label. This type of classification does not reflect the potential variations of individual complexities and needs which develop in respect of life experiences.

The adoption of labels with the most positive or least negative connotations may be the first

---

Box 23.2 Aspects of labelling

Negative
- Promoting a negative view of this group of people within society
- Low expectations
- Opportunity deprivation
- Negative or diminished experiences
- Prejudiced beliefs

Positive
- Highlights the need for specific treatment or care
- Protects legal rights

step in encouraging more positive attitudes towards people with learning disabilities (Hastings & Remmington 1993).

PREVENTION OF LEARNING DISABILITIES

Generally speaking, there are two main types of factor responsible for learning disabilities: genetic and environmental. The latter are factors that affect mother and/or child during pregnancy, delivery or after birth. The causes of learning disability are shown, proportionately, in Figure 23.2.

Despite significant advances in molecular biology and genetics, medical scientific knowledge about the cause of learning disabilities is still incomplete, and in as many as one-third of all cases no specific cause can be identified.

Due to the progress made in medical science and to increased awareness of the influence of environmental factors, there has been a reduction in the number of children being born with impairments, but the factors giving rise to learning disability are often difficult to prevent.

Genetic disorders

Some genetic disorders can be detected through screening tests during early pregnancy. Amniocentesis is one such test, carried out during the 18–20th weeks of pregnancy to detect chromosomal abnormalities such as Down's syndrome. Chorionic villus sampling (CVS) has recently enabled a diagnosis to be made as early

as 8 weeks, allowing the option of termination to be open to the mother. The 'fragile X' syndrome is now second only to Down's syndrome as a cause of learning disability. Despite this, between 2 and 20% of males with learning disabilities have this disorder undiagnosed. Identification of affected males is vital to enable the determination of risk in other family members. Through genetic counselling, it should be possible to prevent this form of learning disability.

Genetic counselling plays a large part in reducing and preventing the incidence of learning disability in all identified genetic conditions. With advances in medical science, more genetic conditions will be identified and therefore more will ultimately be prevented.

As yet, there is no method for correcting primary gene defects, despite rapid advances in genetic engineering. Substantial technical and ethical issues remain to be overcome. However, some methods of treatment are now available which can reduce or alleviate the consequences of genetic defects (Box 23.3). For instance in phenylketonuria (PKU) which, if undetected, leads to severe learning disabilities, neonatal screening (Guthrie test) allows a restriction of the phenylalanine intake in affected children, preventing both the intellectual and neurological deterioration.

Environmental factors

Much can now be done to limit environmentally caused abnormalities, that is, those occurring because of events during pregnancy, delivery and shortly after birth.

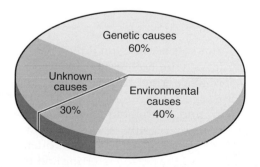

Figure 23.2 Causes of learning disability.

Box 23.3 Reducing the occurrence of genetic defects	
Risk factors	**Limitation/prevention**
Blood relatives, e.g. aunt, grandparent, parent with inherited genetic condition	Genetic counselling Screening tests Amniocentesis Chorionic villus sampling Termination
Woman already with a disabled child	
Woman over 35 having first child	

Low birth weight is often associated with an increased risk of abnormality. Improved antenatal care, targeted at factors which contribute to lower birth weight, is now common practice. This includes education about maternal diet, alcohol, smoking and poor social conditions. In addition, there is now better monitoring of diabetes and other medical conditions in women contemplating pregnancy.

Maternal infection during pregnancy, and early childhood infection, increase the risk of a child becoming impaired. Immunisation plays a large part in reducing the occurrence of infections such as rubella, meningitis, whooping cough and measles. The interventions described in Box 23.4 help to reduce the risk of environmentally caused defects.

Other environmental factors which influence the incidence of abnormalities are obstetric and neonatal care. Obstetric complications and birth injuries at time of delivery are thought to account for 10% of all cases of severe learning disabilities.

Other factors are the prevention of accidents, in the home or on the road, and child abuse.

Relevance to occupational therapy practice

In order to inform occupational therapy practice, it is essential to have an understanding of the factors causing the learning disability. Symptoms produced by genetic conditions will remain fixed, and it is part of the challenge for the occupational therapist to find ways to modify or compensate for these symptoms (Gilbert 1996). This is perhaps now even more important as people with learning disability increasingly lead more independent lives, contemplating their own relationships and having children of their own.

As occupational therapists, we may become involved in health promotion and counselling on issues described in Boxes 23.3 and 23.4.

THE OCCUPATIONAL THERAPY PROCESS IN LEARNING DISABILITIES

There is no theoretical framework that cannot be applied to this population. Models of intervention are adequately addressed elsewhere (for example, Chapter 13 and Hagedorn 1997) and each therapist will choose an approach from which to work. This will probably be arrived at and applied by following the occupational therapy process as shown in Figure 23.3.

A case study format has been used to clarify the different stages of the occupational therapy process in a practical way.

Referral

Mary was referred to occupational therapy by a community learning disability nurse, through the Community Learning Disability Service. The referral requested 'an assessment of her domestic ability, with a view to increasing her participation in meal preparation for her family'. Mary is a 32-year-old woman, with moderate learning disability, experiencing difficulties in daily living activities due to rheumatoid arthritis and obesity. She has been married to Tom for 6 years and they have a 7-year-old daughter, Jane. . . .

This referral was accepted in duty of care terms, in accordance with both national and local standards of practice. Referrals can be very specific as in this instance, however, as can be deduced from the background information, there is often scope for the therapist to apply more skills than initially indicated by the referral. Referrals often reflect the priorities of the person referring and the therapist will need to apply her interview skills

Box 23.4 Environmental factors	
Environmental causes	**Limitation/prevention**
Poor maternal diet	Health education
Smoking, excess alcohol in pregnancy	Improved living and social conditions
Poor social conditions and low income	Primary health care
Inadequate education	Immunisation
Damage during birth	Improved obstetric and neonatal care
Maternal or post-natal infection	
Accidents or abuse	

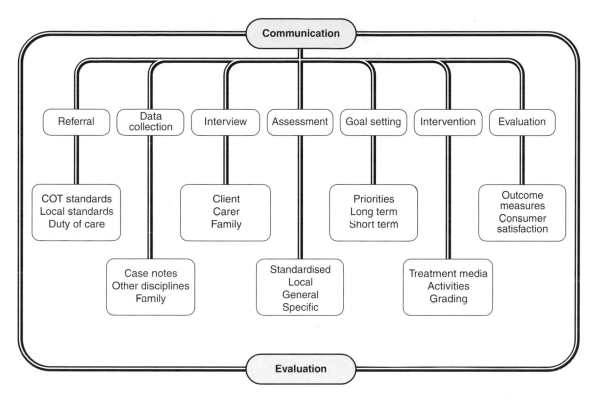

Figure 23.3 Stages in the occupational therapy process.

effectively when identifying and incorporating the wishes of her client. Clinicians should make themselves aware of the assessment tools available.

Data collection

> . . . Professionals already involved with Mary were contacted and asked for any relevant information relating to their past or present input. In general there appeared to have been a lot of intervention from various professionals and support workers, especially after the birth of her daughter, and it became apparent that there was very little coordination of input. The professionals who had been involved with the family over a long period of time had seen little progress and, as a result, were suffering from burnout (Edwards & Miltenberger 1991). . . .

Data collection is closely linked with, and may include, interview. As well as revising her know-

ledge of any conditions detailed, the therapist will want to evaluate the information gathered and take into account the perspective from which it has been gained.

Interview

> . . . An initial visit was arranged to meet Mary and begin developing rapport with her. A semi-structured interview elicited the following information.
> Mary was in severe pain from her rheumatoid arthritis and reported having problems with her neighbours. She felt she was isolated in her home, and said she did not go out much. She felt that her daughter was difficult to cope with and she complained that her husband went out and left her on her own. She stated that her mother regularly interfered in matters between herself and her husband and was a dominant force in the family home. She felt her family expected her to take on a more active role in the home but they gave her no support to do so. She was overwhelmed by negative feedback, especially from her mother. Mary said the relationship with her husband had deteriorated

to a point where they were having no sexual relationship and it appeared their communication was poor and ineffective. This was adding to the stress and there was pressure on her from her mother to leave Tom. However, she appeared not to grasp the reality of her marital problems and expressed the desire to have another baby. Overall, Mary felt helpless and dissatisfied with her lifestyle but could not identify any strategies to change her situation. Prior to the birth of her daughter, and while living with her parents, she had an active social life, attended a training centre and was a member of a sports club. . . .

Although the interview format was used successfully with this client, it may be necessary to interview carers as representatives of the client. However one should be cautious about relying solely on this information and alternative methods of gaining information directly from the client should always be attempted. Interview need not be restricted to questionnaires or pen and paper exercises. Careful clinical observation and reflection are as essential to successful interviewing as the ability to listen (Remington 1997). When interviewing clients with profound or multiple handicaps, the careful selection of activities taken for the interview can yield useful information. Some musical instruments, a small torch and a ball or beanbag can be used to indicate much about the client's interactional skills, leisure interests, previous experiences and opportunities. The therapist should try to ensure that the activities and equipment are appropriate to the age of the client. It is not necessarily wrong to use play, as adults also play, although often with more structure, more rules and more players than children.

It is worthwhile to prepare an interview schedule, that is, listing what information you want to exchange with the client. Box 23.5 shows an example of an initial interview format which readers may wish to adapt for themselves. Determining what it is she wants to know brings the therapist closer to deciding how to elicit the information.

Assessment

. . . From the initial interview, the priorities for assessment were Mary's physical condition and her mental health. The plan was to assess her physical functioning, within and outwith her home, and also to gain an overall picture of her life, past and present; how her rheumatoid arthritis had affected it, and how she herself felt about the present and the future. The general impression from the assessment period was that Mary was in a maladaptive cycle, as shown in Figure 23.4, in which she felt her limitations were completely insurmountable, which contributed greatly to her low mood (Box 23.6). . . .

Box 23.5 An example of an initial interview format

One of the main reasons for interview is to commence building rapport. Where possible, the therapist should explain the purpose of the interview, who requested occupational therapy intervention, and the client's rights to agree/disagree with that intervention. An initial interview may last approximately 5 minutes to half-an-hour, and should give direction to further intervention. The next step may be selected from diverse objectives such as (a) further development of the therapeutic relationship; (b) functional assessment; and (c) the closure of an inappropriate referral.

Physical condition. The therapist may wish to assess posture, gait, movement through position, tremor, deformity, muscle tone, vision, hearing, gross coordination and build. Asking the client if he would like to move to a quiet/seated/tabletop area provides an opportunity for observing many of these points as well as adding insight concerning the client's orientation/familiarity with his environment.

Mental state. This may include emotional stability, mood, attention span, interests, motivation to participate in activity and the client's own perception of his difficulties. If the client is non-verbal or non-vocal, then photographs, foodstuffs, and simple remedial games can indicate much about his previous experiences and reaction to them. The client's own possessions can aid the information seeking process.

Communication/interaction. Attention should be given to both non-verbal and verbal skills. Hearing, comprehension, response to touch and to sound should be considered as factors influencing interactional ability. Insight into behaviours, relationships and interests may be gained both through discussion and observation of responses to environmental distractions. A variety of media such as photographs, pen and paper, music and the therapist can be used to elicit responses.

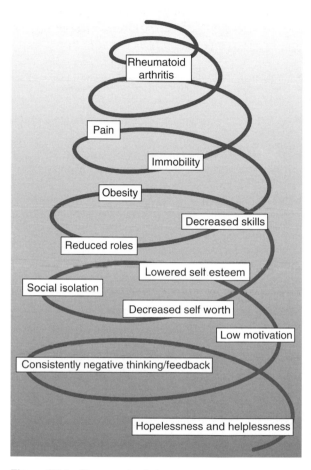

Figure 23.4   Downward spiral.

The clinician should also consider who else is assessing the client. It is frustrating for the client to be repeatedly assessed by people from different disciplines and it may be possible to decrease the overlap in an effective team by sharing results. An assessment is useless (especially from the client's perspective) unless it leads to interventions which address needs. The history and development of assessment can be found in Hogg & Raynes (1987) and Dickens & Stallard (1987).

Goal setting

.... It was recognised that gaining Mary's cooperation and sustaining her motivation to participate in treatment could be difficult. This was due not only to her mental state and her level of understanding but also to her past experience with professionals whom she felt had interfered with her life, but not really helped. Mary was encouraged to take an active part in goal setting; however, this was something she found very difficult. This was reflected in her vague long-term goals, identified within the Occupational Case Analysis and Interview Rating Scale. She understood that to make improvements in her life she had to effect the change, but she required a lot of help identifying realistic and achievable goals. The occupational therapist decided to focus initially on developing her practical skills. This would have the effect of increasing her level of independence and her participation in activities within the home. The other purpose of focusing on such skills was that they were highly visible and would affect not only her own self-perception but also her relationship with her mother and husband (Box 23.7). ....

Box 23.6   Assessment procedure

Assessed area	Potential tools	Actual tools	Result
Rheumatoid arthritis/obesity	Assessment of motor and process skills. Jebson hand function test	Local, non-standardised tests	Constant pain, limited range of movement
Social functioning	Assessment of communication and interactional skills. Role checklist. Volitional questionnaire	Assessment of communication and interactional skills. Volitional questionnaire	Poor social skills. Social isolation and low motivation
Occupational performance	Occupational case analysis and interview rating scale. Canadian occupational performance measure	Occupational case analysis and interview rating scale.	In a maladaptive cycle and a downward spiral of apathy (Fig. 23.4). Lost role identification as mother, wife. Many other negative roles. Poorly defined routine with no meaning.

Box 23.7 Treatment aims and methods

Treatment aims	Method/activity
Provide necessary aids and equipment within the home environment	• Provision of aids as identified by assessment • Liaison with the social work occupational therapist re larger equipment and adaptations
Increase housework skills	• Specific teaching programmes aimed at developing skills in dusting, hoovering, laundry, kitchen cleaning • Occupational therapist to work with home help discussing what Mary can do in the house and how this can be facilitated
Increase cookery skills	• One-to-one sessions for 6 weeks with the occupational therapist at home, preparing an evening meal for the family • Attendance at a weekly healthy eating group run jointly by an occupational therapy assistant and dietician, on days when she attended work project
Increase ability to attend sessions outwith the home	• Health eating group • Women's group • Work project
Improve decision making skills	• Participation in women's group
Increase self-confidence	• Achievement in acquiring new skills • Positive feedback from occupational therapist, family and other members of the treatment team
Improve parenting skills	• Role modelling through sessions with the occupational therapist • Voluntary work in local nursery • Sexuality counselling
Provide employment opportunities within a supported environment	• Occupational therapist-run sheltered work project • Voluntary work in local nursery • Sheltered work placement in college nursery

---

Goals do not remain static, instead they reflect the evaluation of the assessments and intervention, and must be redefined constantly. Goals may be long-term, with various short-term objectives being set for their eventual achievement. Even long-term goals should be reviewed regularly to ensure their continuing relevance to the client. Goals should reflect the values of the client and be achievable.

Intervention

The period of intervention lasted for 6 months with continuing support meetings to the time of writing.

. . . Initially, occupational therapy intervention took place within Mary's home, enabling the therapist to establish relationships with Mary, her husband and daughter. It also allowed informal observation of the family dynamics, with special interest in the relationship between Mary and Jane. This facilitated an assessment of Mary's parenting skills. During the initial sessions, the intervention was of a counselling nature, where Mary discussed her past and present problems, most of which centred around family issues. In this situation, the therapist was careful not to be simply a problem solver but rather used techniques to encourage Mary to identify her own future goals.

To achieve these identified goals, intervention focused on four specific areas: supply aids to daily living, domestic work, women's group and work placement. These four areas were worked on concurrently, although some were time limited, such as domestic work, while others had longer-term implications.

1. Aids and adaptations. It was essential that Mary saw immediate effects of the occupational therapist's involvement, so that she felt the intervention was going to produce results. This was therefore the first area of intervention.

Due to her obesity, Mary was experiencing significant problems in personal care. This had led to her becoming unkempt with problems of body odour. Liaison with the local community occupational therapist enabled the supply of various bathing and toilet aids to overcome immediate difficulties. It was also suggested that a shower cubicle would be more suitable for Mary's needs. A perching stool and other kitchen aids were supplied and utilised during domestic sessions. These assisted in overcoming the constant pain which Mary experienced when standing, which had contributed to her previous reluctance to participate in household chores.

2. Domestic sessions. Initially all domestic sessions took place at home over a period of 6 weeks, and were carried out by an occupational therapist. Initial focus was on basic food preparation, such as making a sandwich for her daughter when she returned from school. In this way, not only did Mary develop cookery skills, but also received positive feedback from her family. This activity was also used to teach positive parenting skills. It encouraged interaction between Mary and Jane, and focused on something positive rather than on Jane's behaviour. During these sessions there was a notable increase in positive interactions and a decrease in Jane's attention seeking behaviour. Also, these sessions facilitated work on topics such as healthy eating (utilising information and resources from the dietician), health and safety and menu planning/budgeting. The menu planning and budgeting sessions also involved her husband since they did the shopping together. The development of cooking skills became more complex as Mary's motivation and skills increased. Eventually she was able to prepare an evening meal for her family during the sessions. The issues of cooking in bulk and freezing were also introduced as this appeared to suit the needs of the family.

The occupational therapist worked alongside the home help, who came to the house two mornings per week, educating her as to how to engage Mary in housework tasks, and together they identified key tasks that Mary could carry out independently. Mary also worked alongside the home help and learned how to do other chores. Although Mary's physical problems limited the number of household chores she could realistically do, it was important that she assumed some responsibility in this area.

The final element in the development of her domestic skills was her attendance at a weekly food preparation group run by an occupational therapy assistant. This reinforced the skills she had developed in one-to-one sessions and also provided a social setting where she worked cooperatively with others. Mary enjoyed these sessions and appeared highly motivated to participate. The group also included a module on healthy eating, which was a joint intervention with the dietician. This introduced Mary to low fat/diet products which she had previously never used, and she learned how to incorporate these into her family's diet.

3. Women's group. This group was facilitated by an occupational therapist and held in a local health centre. In total, eight women with learning disabilities attended and the group ran over a 3-month period. The topics within the group were varied, and latterly were directed by the group members as their confidence increased. Topics included: relationships, safe sex, decision making, self-image and leaving home.

Mary was reluctant to attend this group at first, but was collected by the occupational therapist for the first session. Other professionals raised concern that by collecting Mary this could lead to a dependence on the occupational therapist. However, the rationale behind the action was that by enabling Mary to attend, she could then make an informed choice regarding her participation. In fact, she became highly motivated to attend and was able to travel independently.

For Mary, this group met her social and emotional needs. She was enabled to explore her feelings, as well as receiving feedback from not only the occupational therapist but, more importantly, her peers. Her experiences as a wife and mother were different from those of the other group members and she was able to discuss how these factors affected her life. Interest and praise she received from the other group members improved her self-esteem, and some of the difficulties she talked about relating to being a parent were used by the occupational therapist to illustrate to the others the responsibility and work involved in taking the decision to have a child. Mary herself had intimated that she wished for another child, but through such discussions she began to realise how this would impact on her life and existing problems.

Over the 3-month period, there was a considerable change in Mary, both physically and psychologically. She became more concerned about her appearance and there was a noticeable improvement in her personal hygiene and her clothes. She also became more confident in this social setting, often going for a coffee after the group with other members. Her mood showed a major improvement within these sessions where she appeared animated and keen to participate in group discussion. This was partly due to the change in environment but, more importantly, she had been given the chance to meet with a peer group who accepted her as herself and gave her a sense of self-worth.

4. Work. After 3 months, Mary began attending a sheltered work placement run by the occupational therapy service. She attended 2 days per week, thus she had opportunity to be out of the house and was engaged in activity. During these days, she also attended a food preparation group with an occupational therapy assistant and was able to use the swimming pool, which provided exercise.

As her physical stamina for work increased, the occupational therapist arranged a voluntary work placement within a local nursery for 2 days a week. Mary received regular support and on-site skills training from the occupational therapist, who also liaised with and supported staff involved in the project. After 3 months, a sheltered work placement was arranged with the local college crèche. Again, the occupational therapist provided regular support and skills training until Mary was competent in the tasks she was required to do. Latterly, a weekly support visit was all that was required. . . .

Competence versus independence

'To be competent means to be sufficient or adequate to meet the demands of a situation or task' (White 1971). This definition reflects the person-centred approach advocated by occupational therapists, in that excellence is not a prerequisite for an optimal level of independence.

There is a potential misunderstanding that occupational therapists are seeking total independence in all interventions. The aim of occupational therapy intervention does focus on enabling the individual to reach his own optimal level of independence, but the reader must be aware of great differences in the potential levels of independence among people with learning disabilities.

Medley (1984) offered the following definitions:

- A competency is 'a single knowledge, skill or professional value'.
- Competence is 'the repertoire of competencies'.

The occupational therapist assists the individual by teaching specific competencies, leading to an overall level of competence which is effective and has relevance to the client's specific environment. The reader will be aware, however, that this may not reflect an ability to function with complete independence.

Mocellin (1988) advocated that the focus of intervention should be on 'small wins', illustrated in Figure 23.5. A small win is a 'concrete, complete, implemented action of moderate importance'. These small wins, or competencies, are built on by the occupational therapist to enable the person to reach a realistic level of competence in a specific area.

Some people may never realise the optimal level of independence as dictated by professional judgements. However, competence is specified for each person at a level which is realistic and relevant to individual needs and the environments in which they function.

Treatment media

It would be impossible within this section to outline all the possible activities that could be utilised within this field. What is intended is for the reader to realise that any activity can be selected. Grading the activity enables the therapist to meet individual needs or treatment goals. Analysis, application and grading activities constitute the art of our profession and make us unique among other professions within the health care environment.

While Neistadt (1986) and Llewellyn (1991) referred to 'remedial' and 'adaptive' treatment methods, within this text we will refer to 'experiential learning' and 'skills-based learning'. The use of the terms 'remedial' and 'adaptive' could be construed as negative when considering this

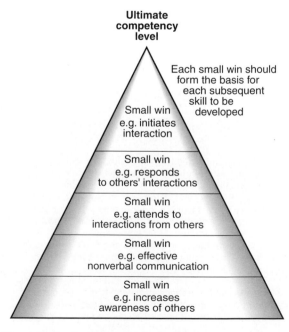

Figure 23.5 Illustration of 'small wins' theory.

client group. They also imply the use of a formal teaching strategy, which may not be the primary method of intervention chosen by the occupational therapist. 'Experiential learning' and 'skills-based learning' are terms more descriptive of the developmental process through which an occupational therapist can provide stimulation, opportunities and positive experiences for the client group.

These two approaches can be used exclusively or in conjunction with each other, as neither precludes the other from occurring spontaneously. As mentioned earlier, people with learning disabilities may have pockets of particular skills which are not reflective of their overall performance. For this reason the mix of experiential and skills-based learning is particularly effective within the field of learning disabilities. It should be noted that experiential learning can produce skills development although this may not have been the primary goal of intervention. Experiential learning gives people opportunities to develop positive concepts relating to interaction with others and the environment, and this engenders confidence and the motivation to develop further.

Evaluation

... After a 6-month period, the OCAIRS Rating Scale was used to evaluate the outcomes of the intervention. Significant progress had been made in that Mary's range of roles had increased, domestic skills had improved and her participation within the household had expanded. It was agreed that although ongoing support would be offered, this would be reduced over future months and, unless there was a significant life change when intervention may need to be more intense, liaison with the home help and other agencies would provide sufficient information about whether Mary and her family were continuing to develop and mature.

No intervention can be shown to be beneficial for the client if evaluation does not occur. Evaluation must happen throughout the occupational therapy process in order for it to be effective; for example, evaluation of the referral should enquire whether it is appropriate. Many assess-

ments now supply individual learning packages which include criteria for evaluating progress.

Little is available, however, for evaluating the client's satisfaction with treatment, particularly the client with severe or profound learning disability. A possible solution is to interview the carer, although the therapist should be aware of any bias that may be present. Another possible solution is to agree with other agencies a checklist of behaviours thought to represent interest and pleasure, and to sample for these behaviours at varying intervals. This can then be used to infer satisfaction or otherwise on the client's behalf. More able clients can choose not to attend or vocalise their dissatisfaction.

When designing evaluation tools the therapist must be careful not to lead the client by verbal or non-verbal cues. Also, the language must be appropriate to the client's communication abilities and relevant to their sphere of experiences.

EVOLVING SERVICE AREAS

The specialist label which this area of work often attracts could be considered a misnomer, as an occupational therapist will utilise all the core skills of the profession and many of the peripheral competencies which are developed during and after training. As discussed earlier in the chapter, the approach used by occupational therapists is primarily person centred. Quality of life is considered at all times and the individual is assisted to function at his optimal level, dependent on a range of factors identified in the assessment process.

The knowledge base in medical and psychiatric conditions facilitates understanding of the behaviours presented, contraindications for treatment planning and implications of drug side-effects. Skills in assessment provide sound baseline information from which to develop realistic aims and objectives to assist learning and development.

The creative approach of occupational therapists assists individuals to overcome physical disabilities through the teaching of compensatory methods of functioning. Aids and equipment can be provided to assist functional independence.

Occupational therapists are skilled in communication which will assist the development in clients of awareness, interaction and social skills, leading to increased levels of motivation and participation. The ability to grade activity is the factor which most contributes to the success of the occupational therapist as a clinician. This is particularly true in the field of learning disability where developmental delay, combined with erratic expectations from carers, can cause pockets of skills among major learning deficits. It must be emphasised, however, that the activity chosen, and the setting, are only justifiable if they reflect the needs and wishes of the client. If the occupational therapist is doing more in the session than the client, then either the grading or the activity itself is wrong and a reevaluation of the client and the programme should be undertaken. The occupational therapist must be clear about specific goals and about the teaching necessary for optimal independence and readjustment into mainstream society, if this is the target.

Clients with multiple disabilities

The developmental problems experienced by people with learning disability often combine with auditory and visual impairments to create serious difficulties for those affected. When someone has limited awareness and response to contact, the process of development is slow and laborious. The lack of feedback can demoralise carers, who are unsure how to stimulate these people effectively. The occupational therapist can assist in revising the expectations of carers and others to realise the individual's potential for interaction and participation. When learning is organised into sequentially graded steps that can be accepted and understood by the individual, it becomes clear that the techniques for this group of clients are similar to those used for other groups, that is, physical intervention and support, practical demonstration, verbal instruction and physical and verbal cueing, reducing as independent sequencing of activity is achieved. In practice, it is the timescale for achievement

which varies from one individual to another. The reader is referred back to Figure 23.5 (p. 426) where the small wins theory is illustrated. Small wins may indeed be very small but, if tasks are graded carefully, progress can be clearly identified, sustaining the therapist and carer and ensuring that the individual's development is consolidated.

This client group has specific needs for:

- a structured environment to facilitate understanding, using environmental cues and referencing whenever possible
- consistency of approach to allow trust and self-confidence to develop – random input will only serve to fuel apprehension and encourage withdrawal from situations
- explanation and assistance in exploration of own potential and of the environment
- time, without which little can be achieved
- identification of alternative communication systems that may be necessary to ensure that information is exchanged between the therapist and the client.

Often, the most important piece of equipment is the therapist herself. In establishing rapport and facilitating awareness and understanding of the environment and its opportunities for learning, the therapist may initially need no more than herself, a creative mind and sound observational skills to identify areas where reaction and interaction is positive. Thereafter, equipment can be introduced to allow exploration to develop along more structured lines. In creating dynamic, structured programmes for individuals with multiple disability it is important to remember that a 24-hour approach is the only way to offer true consistency and it will therefore be necessary to liaise closely with parents, carers and other professionals when coordinating input for these individuals.

The ageing process in people with a learning disability

It is important to consider the long-term future of the people who are at present successfully and happily placed in the community. We must be aware that the needs of the person with a learning disability can change considerably as they grow older and that community resources may no longer be appropriate for them. This is already apparent in the case of people with Down's syndrome who have a much higher than normal risk of pre-senile dementia from the age of 40. Other significant changes can be physical, the onset of mental health problems or even the loss of support from family/friends (such as the death of parents) which can reduce the person's ability to remain where they previously lived. At present many are returning to hospital or residential/nursing homes but this may not be a move which best meets their needs, nor is it the long-term solution to what will be a growing problem. Occupational therapy has a significant role in anticipating future needs and can play a large part in designing and implementing care facilities which at present do not exist.

Dual diagnosis

Historically, services have been delivered from either a mental health perspective or a learning disabilities perspective. Over the last ten years, and particularly since the National Health Service and Community Care Act (1990), there has been increasing recognition that many people with a learning disability also have one or more mental health disorders (Gravestock 1999). Occupational therapists can make a significant contribution to diagnosis and to intervention, both through direct client contact and advice and training for carers and other agencies. Therapists may find themselves working within different service models – community-based dual diagnosis teams, in-patient assessment units with outreach function, or in-patient mental health acute admission units with designated dual diagnosis beds. At the time of writing there is little research or evaluation as to which model is most effective. Currently there is much discussion as to whether staff should be experienced and trained in both mental health and learning disability or whether staff teams should consist of a mix of members experienced in each specialty.

Work programmes

In both the UK and the USA an increasing demand for employment from people with a learning disability and their carers has accompanied dissatisfaction with traditional adult training centres. The reasons for this and some models of employment are discussed by Bayer & Kilsby (1997) and Pratt & Jacobs (1997). Occupational therapists recognise the value of people being engaged to their optimum capacity in purposeful activity which for most people includes productive work. Wilcock (1993) stated: 'Occupation is a central aspect of human experience. Health and survival are strongly related to the innate need to engage in purposeful occupation.' From this fundamental, professional belief, with the professional skills of activity analysis and prescription of activities, occupational therapists are ideally placed to provide opportunities that will enable skills development while encouraging both physical and psychological well-being.

Day services

Occupational therapists have a role to play in the provision of day services, whether in a more traditional day centre or working to enable people to access community facilities and integrate more effectively. Many clients live alone or with a few hours support each day. Working with the staff either from social services, voluntary organisations or housing associations, occupational therapists can help to increase clients' self-confidence through broadening their leisure opportunities, offering opportunities for personal development and helping to create work roles, reducing their reliance on traditional support centres. Training or advice to carers may help alter the perception of their role to one that facilitates individual development and encourages more independence. For individuals requiring increased levels of care and support, the occupational therapist can grade activity, use compensatory techniques to minimise physical limitations and promote interaction and communication to further development. The occupational therapist may also take an advisory role, advising and training staff to develop their own programmes for clients which can be adapted as individual needs dictate.

SUMMARY

Occupational therapists will always have a role within the area of learning disabilities. However, in the future they may see their role widen and change due to the changing pattern of incidence of learning disabilities previously described.

As more genetic conditions are identified, for example 'fragile X' and Rett's syndrome, the occupational therapist will meet more definite patterns of presentation. Although each person must be dealt with as an individual with specific needs, this gives a firmer baseline for treatment and more realistic insight into both the scope and limitations expected of the person.

At present, the main role of the occupational therapist is to treat people as they are, providing opportunities and limiting the effects of their learning disability. In the future, the occupational therapist will find herself involved at different levels of the process of limiting and preventing learning disabilities. As the occupational thera-

pist's role grows within community care teams, there will be opportunities to be involved in health education and primary health care. She may also find herself involved, at some level, with genetic counselling.

There is now wide scope in this area for occupational therapists to be involved in research and pioneering work in identifying and diagnosing symptoms. Autism and fragile X syndrome are just two conditions which have, until recently, been undiagnosed in many people. Due to advanced technology and easy access to and availability of statistics, it is easier to recognise common symptoms and behaviours in a wide range of people, both nationally and internationally. Much of this identification had its origins in clinical observation and this remains important today.

However, research is required not just for diagnosis. Much work needs to be done in evaluating the use of techniques such as sensory integration with this population, and developing new treatment models and methods of intervention to assist their development. Similarly, more research and education should be carried out within the population at large, in order to dispel continuing prejudices and to foster successful integration.

REFERENCES

American Psychiatric Association 1995 DSM-IV. Diagnostic and statistical manual of mental disorders, 4th edn. American Psychiatric Association, Washington

Bruce M A, Borg B 1987 Frames of reference in psychosocial occupational therapy. Slack, New Jersey

Dickens P, Stallard A 1987 Assessing mentally handicapped people. NFER-Nelson, Berks

Edwards P, Miltenberger R 1991 Burnout among staff members at community residential facilities for persons with mental retardation. Mental Retardation 29(3): 125–128

Franco V W 1982 Labelling the mentally retarded: ethical analysis. New York State Journal of Medicine 82: 1377–1382

Gilbert P 1996 The A–Z reference book of syndromes and inherited disorders, 2nd edn. Chapman and Hall, London

Gravestock S 1999 Tizard Learning Disability Review, Pavilion, Brighton 4(2): 6–11

Hagedorn R 1995 Occupational therapy: perspectives and processes. Churchill Livingstone, Edinburgh

Hastings P, Remington B 1993 Connotations of labels for mental handicap and challenging behaviour: a review and

research evaluation. Mental Handicap Research 6(3): 237–247

Hogg J, Raynes N V (eds) 1987 Assessment in mental handicap. Croom Helm, Kent

Llewellyn G 1991 Occupational therapy treatment goals for adults with developmental disabilities. Australian Journal of Occupational Therapy 38(1): 233–236

Medley D 1984 Cited in: Ellis R (ed) 1988 Professional competence and quality assurance in the caring professions. Croom Helm, London, pp. 43–58

Mocellin G 1988 A perspective on the principles and practice of occupational therapy. British Journal of Occupational Therapy 51(1): 4–7

Neistadt M E 1986 Occupational therapy treatment goals for adults with developmental disabilities. American Journal of Occupational Therapy 40(10): 672–677

Pratt S, Jacobs K (eds) 1997 Work practice: international perspectives. Butterworth-Heineman

Remington R 1997 Verbal communication in people with learning difficulties, an overview. Tizard Learning Disability Review, Pavilion, Brighton

Rowitz L 1981 A sociological perspective on labelling in mental retardation. Mental Retardation 19: 47–51

Ward A 1990 The power to act. Churchill Livingstone, Edinburgh

White R 1971 The urge towards competence. American Journal of Occupational Therapy 25(6): 271–274

Wilcock A A 1998 An occupational perspective of health. SLACK, New Jersey

Wolfensberger W 1972 Normalisation. National Institute of Mental Retardation, Bethesda, Maryland

World Health Organization 1980 International classification of impairments, disabilities and handicaps. WHO, Geneva

Wright D, Digby A 1996 From idiocy to mental deficiency. Routledge, London

FURTHER READING

Booth T 1994 Parenting under pressure, mothers and fathers with learning disabilities. Open University Press, Buckinghamshire

Christiansen C, Baum C 1991 Occupational therapy: overcoming human performance deficits. Slack, New Jersey

Forsyth K, Lai J S, Keilhofner G 1999 The assessment of communication and interaction skills (ACIS). measurement properties. British Journal of Occupational Therapy 62(2): 69–74

Kaplan K L, Keilhofner G 1989 Occupational case analysis interview and rating scale. Slack, New Jersey

Magalini S I I, Magalini S C 1997 Dictionary to Medical Syndromes, 4th edn. Lippincott-Raven, Philadelphia

Scottish Office 1998 Modernising community care: an action plan. Stationery Office, Edinburgh

Scottish Office 1999 Aiming for excellence. Stationery Office, Edinburgh

Smith S, Cooke D 1990 A study in the use of rebound therapy for adults with special needs. Physiotherapy 76(11): 734–735

Whitman B, Accardo P 1990 When a parent is mentally retarded. Brookes, Baltimore

24

Community

Penny Lewis   Tom Miller

INTRODUCTION

Community care is now a well-established field of work for occupational therapists in the UK. Occupational therapists have moved from working solely in traditional settings to take part in providing community services and alternatives to hospital. Therapists continue to question and define practice, both within the profession and in response to external social and political expectations. The experience serves to illuminate an understanding of the principles behind the profession. Occupational therapy has had to address and resolve issues of role identification and of the value and effectiveness of the occupational therapy process. Developments have also challenged the management and governance of therapists often working alone in a broad range of clinical environments.

This chapter identifies the aspects of occupational therapy pertinent to community work:

- What is community care?
- Beliefs of the profession
- Settings and methods of delivering occupational therapy
- Practising community occupational therapy
- Resources available to the occupational therapist
- Common problems related to community work
- Management of the service
- Summary.

Many of the methods used are the same as those used in institutional settings but the method of delivery and level of responsibility are different.

WHAT IS COMMUNITY CARE?

Barris et al (1988) suggested that 'Community mental health is less a distinct body of knowledge than it is a political movement and commitment to certain beliefs.' The beliefs underlying community mental health centre around the impact the environment (including social factors) has on the individual. The move is away from traditional, institution based treatment towards providing services within the community setting. It seeks to find alternatives to admission to hospital and to provide effective support for people with mental health problems living within the community. Barris and colleagues emphasised the view of health propounded as one of successful adaptation to the environment. In their summary of the field they commented that: 'Although occupational therapists clearly have a place in community treatment, they have frequently assumed the roles created by other mental health workers instead of capitalising on their own strengths . . . . Bockoven suggests that the future of community mental health lies with occupational therapists.'

Politically and practically, community care involves the replacement of care previously delivered in large institutions by a wide range of services and facilities provided locally in collaboration between health, local authority and voluntary bodies. The time-scale of this development has meant that current clients will rarely have experienced the more traditional style of care.

The division between health and social care has created much debate about various interventions provided for people with mental illness but particularly about occupational therapy. There are no hard and fast definitions, local health and social services authorities making their own arrangements, however, the following is a typical example: 'Health care is mainly a treatment-orientated short-term activity, under the direction of a medical practitioner. Social care is broadly those personal tasks which would be reasonable for an informed relative to undertake' (Devon County Council 1993). More recent thinking has seen the necessity to integrate and coordinate services and agencies:

evidence and experience has demonstrated the benefits of well co-ordinated care to those with mental health problems. Mental health service users, particularly those with the most complex and enduring needs, can require help with other aspects of their lives, e.g. housing, finance, employment, education and physical health needs. Mental illness places demands on services that no one discipline or agency can meet alone. It is logical that a system of effective care co-ordination is required if all services are to work in harmony to the benefit of the service user. (DoH 1999c)

Occupational therapists are trained to adapt to the resources available. Community care calls on the therapist to make full use of the resources existing in local areas and, if necessary, to create appropriate situations. The changes in services have forced occupational therapists to address many professional issues and extend their practice rather than change it dramatically. This style of working across organisational boundaries is now normal practice for occupational therapists in mental health.

'Most people who need long-term care can and should be looked after in the community. This is what most of them want for themselves and what those responsible for their care believe to be best' (DHSS 1983). Psychiatric services have undergone considerable changes in style, gradually moving away from institutional care from the 1960s onwards. This move was accelerated with the White Paper *Better Services for the Mentally Ill* (DHSS 1975). As a result of the paper there has been particular emphasis on developing community resources for the mentally ill. In many parts of the Western world, community services offer a viable alternative to hospital and provide services which support a normal, appropriate living pattern for the individual suffering from severe mental illness. Further legislation followed in the *National Health Service and Community Care Act 1991*. One aspect of this was to change the terminology from the impersonal 'case management' to 'care management'. Further Department of Health guidance has been issued on the Care Programme Approach, and more recently *Effective Care Coordination* (DoH 1999c) and the *National Service Framework for Mental Health* (DoH 1999b). The finite resources of both health and social services have led to targeting the needs of people with serious mental illness.

Modernising Mental Health Services (DoH 1998b) summarised the key themes:

- Improving services
  — 24-hour access, needs assessment; good primary care; effective treatment; and effective care processes
- Improving safety
  — good risk management; early intervention; enough beds; better outreach, integrated forensic and secure provision; and a modern legislative framework
- Involving patients, users and carers
  access to employment, education and housing; working in partnership; better information; promoting good mental health and reducing stigma.

This key document identified the direction of development for both health and social services.

There is evidence that if the movement away from in-patient care towards community care is to be successful, a range of rehabilitation and support services must be developed (McCreadie et al 1985). The 'Italian experience' of the fast closures of mental hospitals was highly praised by some British observers but it highlighted the fact that clients do not automatically become well when they are discharged from the institution. Clients and families need help from planned community services (Jones & Poleti 1985). There has been strong user and carer pressure on government, purchasers and providers about the provision of adequate community care facilities and resources. A shift in planning and practice takes place when community services are seen as the core method of service delivery with appropriate and adequate support through the use of in-patient and alternative residential accommodation. A review of case manage-

ment arrangements undertaken for the Cochrane Library (Marshall et al 2000) identified that, while maintaining contact with clients, case management did not reduce the likelihood of admission, nor is it more effective than standard care in terms of outcome. A more efficient and effective approach may well be assertive community treatment. Measuring effectiveness is limited by the scope and minimal validity of current measures or instruments.

The supportive and robust network of care needed for service users with a serious mental illness means it is necessary for thorough plans to be made and implemented for successful discharge from hospital. *Effective Care Coordination* (DoH 1999c), the *National Service Framework* (DoH 1999b) and *Revised Code of Practice Mental Health Act* (DoH and Welsh Office 1999) require that anyone with a severe and enduring mental illness who is discharged from hospital should be subject to the Care Programme Approach (CPA). Both CPA and Section 117 of the Mental Health Act ensure that preparation and arrangements for discharge are in place prior to discharge from the hospital and a care coordinator (key worker) must be named and responsible for the implementation and follow-up after discharge. The aim is to ensure support for people once in the community. Appleby (1999) has identified that people are at their most vulnerable in the first 3 months after discharge. The National Centre for Health Outcomes Development has published suggested health outcome indicators for severe mental illness (SMI) (Charlwood et al 1999). These service measures recognise the complex composite picture of effectiveness SMI outcomes.

The problem areas covered by the initial care management assessment include many familiar to occupational therapists (Thornicroft et al 1993). *Modernising Mental Health Services* (DoH 1998b) places a strong requirement on services and practitioners to assess risks to the individual client, to the informal carers and to society. This has now become a more explicit role of all staff, occupational therapists included. Occupational therapists may be involved in a generic mental health assessment or specialist assessments of function and occupation (in the fullest sense of the word), for example self-maintenance, work activity, coping strategies and problem solving. Health and local authorities nominate staff to be care coordinators; occupational therapists may be included in this arrangement. A range of individuals and professionals from within health, social services or voluntary and independent providers may actually supply the agreed services for the client. Primary care groups (on behalf of the health authority) and local authority social services departments commission a range of services. In addition, the care coordinator may be able to access social services funding for specific care packages for an individual client.

General practitioners retain the medical responsibility for people with less severe mental illness or mental health problems. Consultant psychiatrists may share responsibility with general practitioners for people with severe or enduring mental illness. This shift in practice has consequences for occupational therapists. The emphasis in mental health secondary care is clearly being placed on those with serious mental illness. Occupational therapy for people with less severe problems becomes a complex arrangement with primary health care or a care coordinator. Therapists now need to relate to more medical practitioners and within both primary and secondary care. Limited financial budgets mean that care coordinators, regardless of their professional background, have to be able to argue the priority given to their client.

Authorities throughout the country have been developing a range of services. The demands on occupational therapy services have changed accordingly. This has proved an opportunity for therapists in mental health to review their practice, improve on the delivery of the service and demonstrate the effectiveness of interventions used.

BELIEFS OF THE PROFESSION

Occupational therapists believe that a person can be seen as an open system (Kielhofner 1985), constantly relating with the external world. This is a two-way process, in which the person influences others and is also influenced. This is thought to be sequential although it may, at times, appear simultaneous.

Independence and autonomy

Powell-Lawton (1972) suggested that competence and functional ability have two components:

1. *Autonomy*: the ability to function as an individual
2. *Environmental control*: the ability to function within a particular situation.

This can be summarised as people as initiators of action and people as social animals.

Occupational therapists value the right of each person to act as an individual if they choose to do so. The therapist is concerned with the individual's belief in himself, his motivation, and his belief in control over himself and over external forces, in addition to developing, where necessary, the skills to carry out the planned action. In a community setting there is even greater emphasis on the individual client sharing the responsibility for devising and implementing his own treatment programme.

The external world

The external world consists of objects and people as well as space (Dunning 1972). The individual can use objects to impinge on the environment, for example by painting with a brush, or the environment can impinge on the individual, for example the steps up to a house force certain physical movements to be taken. In the same way, other people influence this process of interaction, as when they show appreciation for a meal cooked or listen to a conversation.

A system can be defined as a set of parts interconnected and organised into a complex total, which works as a whole. The external world can be seen as a system. Society and the pattern of relationships experienced by the individual form a complex, ever-changing picture. People with mental health problems are interacting with three systems:

1. The health system, which may have one set of values
2. The family and informal support network, which could have another set of values and expectations
3. The wider system of society with its cultural norms and expectations of the individual.

Adaptation, in order to function within these possibly contradictory groups, calls for a high degree of skilled behaviour.

In institutional settings, the occupational therapist enables the person to function within the sheltered environment of the hospital. In the community it is the normal everyday situation shared by the majority that is the milieu. This forces the therapist to consider more deeply the particular facets of the environment with which the individual has to cope. Interventions often have to take into account prejudice and poverty as well as the factors that enable integration with many different ideological groups (Etcheverry 1979).

A tension held within the practice of occupational therapy is the need and obligation to analyse the consequence of the individual's actions on his physical and social environment. While using a client centred approach to solve problems or to create better insight, the occupational therapist still has an obligation to act for the greater good of others. This may not be seen by the client as in his immediate best interests. Examples might be:

- A lady showing confusion, who is unable to use a gas cooker safely and is waiting to return to live in a block of flats
- A man with long-standing paedophile history wanting to create a scrapbook of pictures of children from the local papers
- A young man with treatment resistant schizophrenia living at home, with a history of aggression directed towards his parents, suddenly showing an interest in martial arts.

The individual

An individual can be seen as a combination of values and beliefs, abilities (both motor and perceptual), emotions and experience. Time also affects the individual; life is a continuing and developing process. Occupational therapists regard the person in the light of life stages as well as abilities and beliefs. Working with someone in the community results in assisting them to function in a wide range of life's roles as they occur.

In order to interact and function, the person must have the ability and desire to do so. Ability consists of movement, perception and thinking. The desire to achieve function consists of motivation, beliefs and past experience of success.

Skills can be seen in patterns of behaviour that can be used to achieve a desired outcome. For example, riding a bike consists of motor and spatial performances. Once learned, they become routines that can be produced with little effort and are then known as 'habits'. Dysfunction in interpersonal activities can be caused by a disruption in skills (Fig. 24.1).

Occupation

Occupational therapists are primarily concerned with the interaction between individuals and the environments or systems within which they live. This area of interaction is the area of occupation and function. There can be no interaction without some form of activity. It follows that activity and occupation are very broad concepts. Occupational therapists work with an enormous range of problems in functional ability.

Maslow's hierarchy of needs (Maslow 1970) is often used to illustrate how areas of dysfunction are prioritised (see Ch. 7 p. 131). Using this framework, aspects such as personal activities of daily living are more essential than creativity and are addressed first. Once a need has been met, or largely met, it is possible to move on to the next driving force or need. Occupational therapists aim to enable people to meet their own needs and therefore to be independent. This is easier in the community than in a hospital setting since the opportunities for choice and normal lifestyles are increased.

The fundamental idea is that humans engage in activity and benefit both themselves and others by this active participation. The mores of society dictate which activities are acceptable.

Cause of dysfunction	Example
Lack of opportunity	Never leaving the house and therefore never meeting people
Adverse reaction when carrying out the behaviour	Attempts at establishing relationships fail
Social pressure	Pressure from family to remain dependent
Physical dysfunction	A speech impediment
Perceptual difficulties	Incorrect perception of non-verbal communication shown by others
Low self esteem	A fear of failure
Emotion and mood	Depression

Figure 24.1 Dysfunction in interpersonal activities.

Occupational therapists remain within the standards of the relevant society and its cultural norms; the aim is to aid the person to relate to and function within the immediate environment.

The pattern of occupation

Throughout the day, and throughout our lives, we engage in many different activities and occupations. These fall roughly into the following categories:

- personal and self-maintenance activities
- social activities
- intellectual and creative activities
- work activities.

The occupational therapist looks at the whole pattern of the individual's day – the balance between work, leisure and play – taking into account subjective perception. One person may feel shopping is leisure, another that it is work. The pattern of occupation reflects the expectations of the individual (Parker 1976) and of the community. Working in the community gives the therapist the opportunity to use normal activity to reinforce the skills shown by the individual. It challenges and utilises the person's beliefs and expectations in a way that is difficult to simulate in the unnatural environment of a hospital.

Activity analysis

An occupational therapist studies not only the combination of the individual and the system (both physical and human) in which he interacts, but also the interaction and activity itself. An occupational therapist undertakes an analysis of the activity. This includes the skills required of the individual as well as the physical, social and emotional environment (see Ch. 7, p. 126). Through this analysis, the therapist is able to identify suitable adaptations to the way the task is achieved so that the person is able to perform effectively.

In community settings, adaptation and grading of activity can be difficult to achieve because the therapist cannot control and alter all the experiences of normal life. An alternative approach is to identify whole activities that call for the desired outcome. The whole activity is graded, not the components of the activity. Activities can be established to facilitate and utilise different abilities, for example different levels of confidence and social behaviour are needed to attend a structured day centre and a local evening class.

Setting achievable goals

The occupational therapist analyses the tasks and the skills necessary to accomplish an activity. The activity is then divided into achievable parts, taking into account the abilities and motivation of the individual. Consideration is given to establishing realistic goals for the individual. The person must feel able to reach the goal and yet it must not be so easy that it diminishes the importance of the task (Yerxa 1988). This area highlights occupational therapists' particular professional skills. It is a matter of using the right activities at the right time and in the right way for the right person – the 'just right' challenge (Box 24.1).

As used by occupational therapists, activities are offered with a remedial aim in mind.

Hagedorn (1992) suggested the following definition of occupational therapy: 'the prescription of occupations, interactions and environmental adaptations to enable the individual to regain, develop or retain the occupational skills and roles required to maintain personal well being and to achieve meaningful personal goals and relationships appropriate to the relevant social and cultural setting.' Within the context of the community, activities are the actions of everyday life. The therapist will highlight the importance of specific activities and will reinforce achievement and functional ability, all in relation to the individual client's view of the world.

The occupational therapist may not always use activity as a medium but it remains the aim of intervention. Community work uses goal directed activities which form part of daily living. The client centred approach of occupational therapy means that the individual plays a very large part in selecting the goal and the medium for achieving it.

The occupational therapist, therefore, works with an interconnected and dynamic combination of the person, the activity and the

---

Box 24.1 Case example 1

Mrs Andrews, aged 52, was married with two sons both in their twenties, one still living at home.

She came from a large family. She was the only one to go to the grammar school and had always felt isolated. Her parents were very strict and did not show affection or give praise. At the age of 13 she was sexually abused by a man who worked for her father. She never told anyone about this but tried to commit suicide by drinking weedkiller.

Fifteen years ago, Mrs Andrews was admitted to the in-patient unit for 3 months when she was found to be depressed and suicidal. During this admission she told a doctor about the rape but couldn't bring herself to talk about it in depth. She continued to attend as a day patient for several years. Mrs Andrews was employed as a cleaner in a shop during week-day evenings; her responsibilities included securing the premises. She had been much better for the last 3 years until recently when her feelings of agitation and depression returned.

Her general practitioner referred her to the community mental health team and she was allocated to the occupational therapist.

The long-term aims of treatment for Mrs Andrews were:

- To help keep her out of hospital
- To give her the opportunity to express her feelings
- To assist her to feel more positive and to gain feelings of self-worth
- To support her in her return to work.

The short-term objectives were:

1. To meet on a regular (weekly then fortnightly) one-to-one basis while she was feeling depressed
2. To encourage her to talk about her feelings of bereavement and loss
3. To help her to find a way to ask for what she wants, particularly from the family
4. To encourage her to take up writing again (which gives her great pleasure)
5. To increase her self-esteem by helping her to establish the positives of her personality and aspects that give her satisfaction. To discuss the possibility of voluntary work in the future
6. To identify strategies to help her to sleep and relaxation techniques to still the mind
7. To help her to explore feelings about the abuse (when she was ready). To discuss the possibility of attending a community art or writing group.

environment. In institutional settings, emphasis is placed on adapting the interaction or activity to meet the needs of the individual. In community settings, the emphasis of change is either with the individual or with the environment and system. The balance between activity centred and client centred analysis is altered (Meeson 1998). However, the aim is always towards improvement in function.

SETTINGS AND METHODS OF DELIVERING OCCUPATIONAL THERAPY

Community occupational therapists work in a variety of settings such as:

- community teams
- day hospitals or day treatment centres.

Approaches include:

- planned sessional work, for example, a weekly stress management group
- planned individual treatment programme as member of a team such as care coordinator and provider of care for client
- assess and respond crisis intervention duties.

Community teams

It has become commonplace for therapists to be part of a multidisciplinary team. A typical team consists of:

- medical staff
- community psychiatric nurses
- psychologist
- social worker
- occupational therapist
- community support workers.

The development of teams has posed challenging questions about the role of the individual professions in community psychiatric services. There is a danger that occupational therapists in multidisciplinary teams develop their identity as team members at the expense of their professional expertise. The roles of team members merge to produce mental health workers who are multipurpose practitioners, each carrying similar caseloads that do not necessarily reflect specific professional skills. Patmore & Weaver (1991) recognised that a single worker could not always meet client needs and that quality services occur when the core skills are emphasised and used fully within a multi-professional team. Care coordination calls for various professionals to augment their core skills with more generic skills to ensure a comprehensive approach for the client. The challenge for all is to retain the core skills as well as developing a broader perspective.

An occupational therapist working in a team must have a thorough and firm understanding of occupational therapy to ensure that the team has a valuable and viable resource that can be appropriately used. This calls for professional maturity – a belief in the strengths and core skills of the profession but also an understanding of the limitations. Professional maturity is supported and maintained by clear, positive, professional leadership and supervision.

Expectations of other members of the team will also influence the application of occupational therapy. At times, a dilution of skills has been avoided by occupational therapists working as specialists rather than as care coordinators. This enables them to address specific referrals for occupational therapy and provide a service that can be used by care coordinators, such as group-work on various topics, contact clubs, functional assessment and treatment.

The therapist will assess and carry out treatment in a variety of places, but usually either in the mental health centre or in the client's home. Other venues include leisure facilities, normal community facilities and health centres.

The clients seen reflect the expertise of the therapist and the needs of the team. In general, occupational therapists are particularly skilled in assisting someone who is having difficulty in functioning, whether it is in the area of self-maintenance, work or leisure. The broad training of occupational therapy allows staff to work with clients showing a range of problems of varying degrees of severity.

In the past, a community was seen as a resource for the hospital which usually became active after the patient was discharged. Current emphasis and the development of community services has turned this around to view hospital beds as a resource for the community team who use admission as a contingency plan within the overall community care plan.

In addition to the traditional community mental health team described above, there are also specialist teams either working with a defined population, for example in a drug and alcohol team, or for a prescribed period of time, for example with a post-discharge team, or a particular approach, as in an assertive outreach team. It is also possible to have a profession-specific team based in the community; occupational therapists may form teams to deliver a viable service to numerous small units. Local practice will determine whether any of these specialist teams have responsibility for care coordination.

Day hospitals/day treatment services

The use of day hospitals varies throughout the country; some areas are opening them for the first time, others closing them in favour of other methods of delivering the service. There is often a debate (for funding purposes) as to whether the need is for medically orientated day hospitals or for socially orientated day centres. Social day care is now provided by the voluntary and independent sector through contracts with social services. Another option is emerging, the development of day treatment services which offer specific interventions on a sessional basis. These are sometimes known as day treatment services.

To have occupational therapists attached to individual units is a logical and well-accepted approach to service delivery. This method, however, does have the disadvantage that the therapist is often forced to work in isolation from occupational therapy colleagues. Support and good supervision are essential to avoid the reduction of specialist skills and to ease role conflicts for the individual therapist. In such settings occupational therapists have often been trapped by the requirement to devise and implement programmes for groups of attendees rather than for individuals. While therapists have the necessary skills, it restricts their practice and may result in professional stagnation.

Community based sessional groupwork

This is becoming a more popular method of service delivery. Occupational therapists provide therapy in a number of different settings, giving a viable service to numerous small units while allowing professional support and supervision to be maintained. Therapists work together in carrying out appropriate treatment sessions in individual units and also in providing independent venues to which clients from many units may be referred. This method increases the autonomy of the occupational therapy service and enables greater flexibility in treatment programmes. One drawback is that it is harder for the therapist to bring about changes to the environment and approaches of the unit as treatment and interventions are directed at the individual. It is easier to alter the approaches of other staff or the unit environment if the therapist is seen to belong to the staff group.

The venues used may be health premises or may be hired from other agencies, for example the arts centre. While the use of public facilities is very important, it should be noted that this complicates the treatment planning and implementation process. Time is taken to arrange facilities and transport resources, and arrangements are often cancelled without prior notice.

Delivering a service in this manner means that the occupational therapist has to relate to a large number of staff and clients. Clear communication channels are essential. It is vital to develop an effective method of participating in case discussions and decision making.

If these difficulties can be overcome, an efficient and effective occupational therapy service can be provided. The individual therapist has professional support and supervision, professional role models and a greater opportunity to mature professionally.

Structured leisure facilities

One of the roles of traditional occupational therapy departments was to promote the constructive use of leisure time and to provide leisure or hobby activities for therapeutic purposes and for pleasure. Community care has provided the opportunity to develop a wide range of leisure facilities, day centres, drop-in centres and clubs. Occupational therapy helpers, voluntary organisations or the clients themselves may run these. They may be part time or full time, in a variety of locations. If they are planned with care, clients can be given much greater choice in the type of day care they use.

PRACTISING COMMUNITY OCCUPATIONAL THERAPY

The trend towards community care involved a move away from the pathological model of practice previously held by most health care professions. This resulted in the rejection for many of the label 'illness' in favour of the term 'mental health'. However, the individual or others still complain of feelings or behaviours which are perceived as not normal. Society is constantly moving the line between normality and abnormality. Current government guidance and terminology has returned to emphasising the term 'mental illness' and the needs of those with serious difficulties. This is the main client group for whom services are purchased by health or by social services. There remains in practice the need for all staff to balance an awareness of the abnormal needs experienced by people with mental illness with a service delivered in the most normal way possible.

Tasks and activities

The occupational therapist in the community strives to use tasks and activities that are available to the public (for example clubs, classes and sports centres) or to adapt and create activities that are as normal as possible. This has to take into account the priorities of individuals and the environment in which they wish to act.

The objective is to facilitate tasks that demand the right level of challenge for the person, are achievable and contain no more than an acceptable level of risk. Freedom of choice carries with it the freedom to take risks. This requires informed choice. People need to demonstrate the ability to appreciate and evaluate options and to realise the consequences of taking a certain action. The therapist may have to take some decisions on behalf of people whose cognitive abilities or insight make it difficult to understand possible danger or consequences. In community settings the occupational therapist has very little control over activities and tasks. This entails the individual client taking greater responsibility for the occupations performed.

The environment

The aim of treatment is to provide opportunities for the individual to interact with the environment. The approach of the occupational therapist does not just rely on the person to adapt to a fixed situation but also views the outside world and social system as adaptable. The focus of adaptation depends on the abilities and motivation to change of all concerned. The service may need to create situations that enable this interaction, as well as utilising public facilities, for example, a coffee club where social skills can be learned and practised. The social support system may need to be adapted to understand and accommodate the needs of the person.

Assessment

The occupational therapy process begins with a thorough assessment of the person and situation. Assessment procedures in the mental health field are often difficult to identify and in community work become even more complicated. The content of the assessment varies from person to person and, to a certain degree, from therapist to therapist. On top of this there is the concept of the mental health worker which ostensibly negates the professional assessment.

Assessment is 'the process of collecting information systematically and organising it in a relevant and useful way' (Willson 1983). Care coordination requires a common assessment procedure to be carried out by all members of a team, particularly when members act as representatives of the whole team, for example at an initial assessment or when acting as a care coordinator. The concept of a common assessment enables the group to identify the crucial elements of information and the results are structured in a way that can be used by any of the members. *Effective Care Coordination* (DoH 1999c) and the *Mental Health Minimum Data Set* call for the use of Health of the Nation Outcome Scales (HoNOS). This forms a simple rating of the severity of difficulties experienced.

Since all health care professions use interpersonal communication as a prime skill in working with clients, it follows that an assessment is conducted along fairly similar lines for the majority of workers. Often a team will agree the manner of communicating any results, usually in predetermined report form. The decision-making process involved in establishing a common approach enables members to explore issues of philosophy and policies, and of the values held by the individual professions. It may be important to the working of the team that this process is continually repeated, resulting in a reaffirmation of the common philosophy and an inauguration of new members. Again, *Effective Care Coordination* provides the basic framework for recording the assessment.

The dilemma of a common assessment procedure is whether or not to retain the specific professional approaches and techniques. Occupational therapy may have an advantage over many of the other disciplines as the ability to view the person, task, and the surrounding situation enables the therapist to undertake a comprehensive assessment without stepping outside the approaches commonly used by other occupational therapists (Box 24.2).

The initial assessment

From the occupational therapy perspective, the initial assessment is very similar in method to those conducted in other settings. It usually

---

Box 24.2   Case example 2

Mr Brown was 33. He had recently been diagnosed as suffering from schizophrenia. He had been living with his parents for the last 8 years but prior to that he had lived in his own flat. Mr Brown had always been 'a bit of a loner' since his teens, but had done well at school and, although he had left university without finishing his degree, he had run a successful small business. However, his business began to fail and family and friends had become concerned about his increasing isolation and odd behaviour.

At the time of the referral, Mr Brown had been admitted to hospital under Section 3 of the Mental Health Act (1983). He showed signs of paranoia, aggression and delusions, although medication was keeping these under control. He was soon to be moved to a staffed hostel. The long-term aim for Mr Brown was to enable him to move from the hostel to more independent living in a supported satellite house supervised by a voluntary organisation.

Mr Brown had been allocated a care coordinator who was a social worker. He was thought to need remotivation and the opportunity to engage in constructive and useful activities. The care coordinator referred him to the community occupational therapist for assessment and a programme of suitable activities.

Mr Brown was assessed by the occupational therapist on the community rehabilitation team. A number of informal meetings took place to exchange information and to build up trust. A number of self-assessment checklists were used to gain further information and to ascertain Mr Brown's perception of his difficulties. These included leisure and work interests and present, past and possible future social roles.

The occupational therapist also undertook formal assessments of Mr Brown's abilities in the fields of personal and domestic activities of daily living. As Mr Brown often appeared to be anxious and under stress he was encouraged to keep a diary of his daily activity and record his levels of anxiety on a self-rating scale.

After assessment, the following aims of treatment were formulated:

1. To improve understanding of anxiety and develop appropriate coping strategies
2. To increase motivation by facilitating the accomplishment of activities that he had defined as important, for example gardening, darts and swimming
3. To increase independence by providing the opportunity to develop skills, for example, social skills, work skills and domestic activities.

consists of ascertaining the client's or carer's view of the problem, introducing the service and establishing rapport. The key elements are:

- frequency of problems
- intensity or severity of problems
- duration
- onset and history.

It is necessary to gauge the severity of the problem, with particular reference to the safety of the individual and of others. This is known as a risk assessment. This is an added responsibility for the therapist that does not always arise in an institutional setting. The occupational therapist is representing the team and not only the profession, acting as the first point of contact with the service and deciding whether or not the referral to the service is appropriate. The case may have to be passed on to another member of staff.

The occupational therapist is well equipped to assess the global situation of the individual in the community: the abilities of the individual in the community, the difficulties, the task or activity causing concern and the situation (both physical and social) within which the person functions. In addition to the more detailed assessments (the individual, tasks, the environment and support system) described elsewhere, it is necessary to gather information about medication, financial circumstances and existing support systems.

The occupational therapist also carries out assessments of specific areas of dysfunction, for example assertiveness, work skills, social interaction and the daily pattern of activity (see Box 24.2).

Location

The location of the initial meeting will differ from professional to professional and from team to team. Economics may advocate that the person is seen at the mental health centre but a much better picture of the situation is gained from an assessment conducted in the home.

The ability to observe functional behaviour when carrying out an assessment in someone's own home requires a mixture of diplomacy, great sensitivity and opportunism, as well as sophisti-cated observation and communication skills. The community setting reduces the opportunity to use activities to assess function. Great reliance may be placed on self-reporting by the individual or carer. This can, however, provide the chance to identify the perceptions of the individual and to examine aspects such as motivation, beliefs and autonomy.

The individual

The performance skills and abilities of the individual are assessed where necessary. Interactional dysfunction is a problem area for many people who are functioning satisfactorily in the areas of self-care and domestic activities. For others, such as the confused or those showing behavioural disturbances, the ability to perform basic self-maintenance tasks may be in question. Other agencies or facilities may be used to assess precise performance skills, for example assessment of work skills undertaken by government employment schemes.

The role and expectations of the person are an important part of the assessment and help to ascertain how they hope to interact with the outside world. The traumatic phase of transition from one role to another, with the incumbent changes in personal adjustment, often causes the referral to the service. The professional's view of life events assists in identifying problem areas and possible remedial action. Occupational therapy works within the individual's belief system and satisfaction with performance. A picture of the daily pattern of activity will be formed with reference to the degree of fulfilment it gives. The concepts of autonomy and choice are very important. Assessments include the locus of control and perceived personal effectiveness, as reported by the person.

The occupational therapist also identifies the degree of motivation shown. This may relate to the way the person needs to adapt or change or to the desired outcome that will result in the environment changing. The difficulty stated by the individual is the primary problem assessed. This allows the treatment process to progress at the appropriate rate and within the client's motivational drive.

Assessing tasks and activities

The exact situation in which the individual feels dissatisfaction and dysfunction is identified and examined. In addition, the occupational therapist will establish circumstances in which the person feels competent. This enables effective skills to be both recognised and utilised. Analysis of the activity requires the therapist to have a thorough knowledge of all occupational roles and many fields of employment. For example, many women referred as showing depressive behaviour are going through the ordeal of adjusting from being an autonomous adult to being a partner and a parent, or adjusting to the reverse situation.

Tasks that may be identified as problems are varied, life for the majority of society is made up of many different tasks and some of these may cause degrees of difficulty for anyone. Common problems are adjustments to changes in roles and the skills needed to carry them out, for example child rearing or retirement. Other common problems are lack of assertiveness or the task of handling conflict, such as marital disharmony. Another difficulty could be in coping with the bureaucracy of the benefits and welfare system. The assessment ascertains what it is that is required, whether information, skills training or emotional support.

Assessing the environment and support system

If relevant, the physical environment is assessed, particularly when it is preventing autonomy. The assessment may examine the physical attributes of the situation or it may consider the whole environment, for example assessing accommodation need and deciding between a hostel, bed and breakfast and the family home.

The support system is an important component of community work. Family, friends and colleagues give informal support. Members of a service, including other staff in the health service, social services, the primary health care team, voluntary workers and private care schemes, give formal support.

Expectations of the support system greatly influence function. Just as the values and beliefs of the individual are assessed, so it is part of the therapist's task to assess the beliefs and motivation of the support network. Gaps in the network are identified, for example periods of time without help, a lack of emotional support or little motivation for change (Box 24.3).

RECORDING INFORMATION

The object of recording assessment and treatment is to convey information about aims, process and progress. This is communicated internally, as a memory jogger to the professional dealing with the case, and to other members of the team when the need arises. Information is also conveyed externally to the primary health care team, to other sections of the secondary health care service and to other agencies.

One of the basic differences between traditional practice and working in the community is in the role of care coordinator. In this role staff are taking responsibility for the overall case notes, whereas in other settings each profession may formulate their own records, which can result in duplication of information. In the community the onus is on the care coordinator to keep notes that are up to date, comprehensive and accurate. The standards of practice are those of occupational therapy but, in addition, standards held by other mental health workers must be borne in mind since they influence team policy. Areas of conflict should be discussed openly and fully. It is important to understand the values of different disciplines but the occupational therapist must also adhere to the standards set by the profession.

Records should be of a standard that can stand up to scrutiny. They should be dated and signed. They should document the process of intervention as well as the progress. Occupational therapists are familiar with using observable behaviour as the basis of their records. In addition, as well as behaviour seen, care should be taken to detail behaviour *not* seen. Motivational drives should be noted since these are frequently the reason for choosing one treatment medium over another.

Box 24.3 Case example 3

Mrs Campbell was 76 years old and suffering from Alzheimer's disease. She lived with her 78-year-old husband in their own bungalow. At the time of the referral they were experiencing a wide variety of functional, social and financial problems.

Mr Campbell was very concerned about his wife's deterioration. He had to deal with all the daily problems alone, including personal and domestic activities, and dealing with his own feelings of bereavement, guilt and frustration. He was socially isolated as he was unable to leave his wife for more than 30 minutes and could manage only short trips to the local shops. He had no one with whom to discuss his situation and did not know what help, if any, was available. Mrs Campbell had recently developed nocturnal incontinence and, in addition, the skin on her thighs had become inflamed.

The general practitioner referred Mrs Campbell to the local community mental health team for the elderly. She was allocated a care manager who collated all the assessments and recommendations. The majority of the work fell to the occupational therapist. An initial assessment was carried out in the couple's own home. Mr Campbell identified the problems and the

occupational therapist helped him to place them in priority order.

A day assessment was arranged at the local specialised unit for older confused people. During the day Mrs Campbell was examined by a doctor and she spent time in a variety of sessions in the unit's day care facility to observe her interactional and conversational skills (this was undertaken by the occupational therapist). With the assistance of Mr Campbell, the therapist administered the Clifton Assessment Procedure for the Elderly in order to establish both a behavioural and cognitive baseline.

The agreed aims of treatment for Mrs Campbell were:

1. To maintain her level of physical, mental and social function, and to slow down her rate of deterioration
2. To involve her more actively in her own self-care
3. To encourage her to be as mobile as possible
4. To support Mr Campbell by offering advice and help over practical tasks and the wide variety of resources available
5. To offer Mrs Campbell the use of periodic planned admissions in order to assess her function and to provide respite care.

Any advice or information given, or action taken by the therapist, should also be noted.

Internal recording

There are no hard and fast rules on how the professional should record the information as it occurs. Some people make notes at the interview, others prefer to wait until the session is completed and others record only changes observed. Actions that arise from the assessment should be documented.

The service may devise a common structure to accommodate the information gathered. This usually details contacts made, actions to be undertaken and a review date. There may also be a common review format in line with care coordination.

In general, the standards of practice adhered to by occupational therapists are appropriate to community work, although the onus on the therapist to keep accurate records is even greater in the community than in a traditional hospital setting. Most occupational therapists (in any field or setting) write notes on the basis that they may be

read by the client one day. Descriptions tend to be of the situation from the individual's perspective and contain clear behavioural statements rather than speculation. The rights of clients to see what has been recorded about them are now defined by legislation.

Recording information for use outside the team

General practitioners should be regularly kept informed about clients. This is usually done by means of a summary letter describing assessment findings, progress to date and the future plan of intervention. Other members of the primary health care team involved with the care, for example district nurses, must also be advised of any changes to the intervention plans.

Information is usually conveyed to other involved sections of the secondary health care service by attendance at decision-making meetings, for example ward rounds after the admission of a client or a care coordination review. The decision about future care becomes a joint responsibility between the hospital and the community; however, it is the community therapist who has to implement the decisions after the client is discharged from the institution. When the responsibiity for care moves from one part of the service to another, a summary of the situation and approaches used should accompany the individual.

Where other employing agencies and organisations are involved, thought should be given to the amount of information needed. There should be no breach of confidentiality, as there is no control over the way in which non-NHS agencies handle data. Files may be accessible to the client or carer in the future, if not now. Occupational therapists must conform to the guidelines set down by the service. Most occupational therapists would approach the problem of communicating information outside the NHS by encouraging the individual client or carer to give the relevant information personally. *Effective Care Coordination* (DoH 1999c) identifies the need for all those delivering the care to have the appropriate information.

Confidentiality

It is essential that the service and professions adhere to the standards of confidentiality detailed in service guidelines and those laid down in the professional code of ethics. Conflicts can arise from work in the community, for much of the time the therapist is assisting the client to interact within a social environment. Care has to be taken that in attempting to change the social network no confidentiality is breached; for example, when working with a wife and husband it would be important not to refer to information given in confidence by one or the other.

Some disciplines advocate different levels of confidentiality and privacy, suggesting that people in socially sensitive jobs (such as police, teaching and the health service) require greater confidentiality than others. In general, occupational therapists would hope to apply the highest standards to all, regardless of their employment status. When information that does demand additional privacy is given, it should be kept in a manner that reduces the likelihood of its being

unnecessarily or accidentally obtained, for example in a sealed envelope in the notes. Some professional workers do not record the information, but this can lead to future difficulties, both for the individual and for any other professionals involved. Where there is doubt, the standards of the profession should be identified and followed.

Decisions have to be taken to identify the role and responsibilities of support staff, particularly in relation to access to information. This should include how the appointment system can be kept private.

Diaries are often used to record names and addresses, as well as events. It should be considered whether or not this could lead to potential breach of confidentiality. Diaries can be misplaced or read accidentally by others. The therapist should use a form of code to record appointments and should ensure the security of any information.

Ideally, occupational therapists would discuss the issue of confidentiality at the early stages of engagement with the client so that the limits are clear. There will be times when the right of confidentiality is overridden in order to protect the safety of the individual or others.

RESOURCES AVAILABLE TO THE OCCUPATIONAL THERAPIST

A resource can be defined as a source or possibility of help. The occupational therapist is concerned with shaping the actions performed by the client. Dysfunction may require help with learning new skills, in changing the task or in creating a suitable environment and system (physical and social) within which to interact. The resources available to an occupational therapist working in the community reflect these different approaches to intervention.

The support system around the client is often the most effective resource. This includes both informal and formal networks (Box 24.4). The individual's perception of the adequacy and efficacy of the system is vital.

The process of occupational therapy actively uses people and normally available services to

---

Box 24.4 Resources available to the occupational therapist working with Mrs Andrews

- Individual sessions with key worker occupational therapist
- Support from family and two friends
- Supportive general practitioner
- Women's group
- Stress management group and individual relaxation instructions
- Creative writing through local arts centre
- Volunteer bureau, occupational therapy support worker for those with special needs
- Creative therapies, individual sessions offered in music, drama, dance and art

---

meet the needs of clients, therefore occupational therapists work with an enormous range of resources and media so that the most effective approach for any individual is available (Box 24.5). The activities used are not focused on single muscle movements or behavioural responses but rather on the set of routine skills used by the majority of the population. The individual client may require skills practice and support, skills training or the adaptation of the task to make the best use of remaining skills.

The emphasis on partnerships and joint working across organisations and agencies allows packages of care that meet the complex needs of people with serious mental illness. Occupational therapists find themselves part of the provision, accessing resources and also often coordinating the care.

The expertise of occupational therapists is a vital resource for the planning and development of environments and projects, which can be used for a number of clients. The occupational therapist is able to recognise the treatment potential of alternative settings.

Activities of daily living

- Community living groups, usually available to people with long-term mental health problems, are run to identify the necessary skills and approaches that people have to take into account when planning to coexist with others. They include topics such as personal hygiene and looking one's best. Peer-group pressure, from inside and outside the group, is a powerful shaper of behaviour.

- Various services can be brought into the home to assist with personal activities. These include community nursing, voluntary and private nursing care schemes, mobile hairdressers and chiropodists. Assistance may be obtained when attending a day hospital, for example help with bathing.

Box 24.5 Resources available to the occupational therapist working with Mr and Mrs Campbell

NHS provision consists of:

- The community mental health team for the elderly offering domiciliary assessment and support from a group of professionals: community psychiatric nurses, occupational therapist and social worker
- The local specialised unit for the elderly confused providing facilities such as day care, night care, holiday relief and assessment
- The primary health care team, including the general practitioner and district nurses
- Disability service centre for the provision of a wheelchair
- Physiotherapy to help Mr Campbell to improve his wife's mobility
- Memory clinic run by a psychologist

Social service provision consists of:

- Specific rehabilitation equipment supplied by the occupational therapist

- Home helps and laundry facilities
- Day centre
- Respite care
- Financial advice on benefits

The voluntary sector offers:

- Local carers' group and Alzheimer's Society to support Mr Campbell
- Sitter register
- Publications and information

The private/independent sector offers:

- Sitting service
- Night care
- Home helps and nursing assistants
- Respite care
- Day care

- Simple equipment such as toilet and bathing aids can be of great help to both clients and carers. The use of non-slip mats can simplify a task to make it achievable. Labour-saving methods such as easy-care clothes or dry shampoo can drastically reduce the burden of care. Occupational therapists are skilled in the precise use of equipment to facilitate, but not eliminate, a task to provide the just right challenge for the individual. As with all disciplines, it is the ability to reject inappropriate treatments that marks a true professional. The provision of equipment depends entirely on the functional needs of the individual and not on the diagnostic label.

Stress management and relaxation

Many occupational therapists in the community are teaching stress management skills, either to groups or to individuals. Relaxation tapes are used to augment the treatment. The ability to cope with stress is crucial to coping with daily life; many people are prevented by their fears from gaining more out of life. The service sets up many different ways of meeting this need, including the use of adult education classes.

Mobility

- Sports activities, fitness and swimming groups can be run in the community. Public facilities may be used or, if a more sheltered environment is needed, halls or pools can be hired. With enthusiasm from staff it is possible for people to join in organised events such as sponsored walks or marathons.
- Small pieces of equipment, such as chair raisers and rails, can improve the quality of life for all concerned. Advice can be given to other disciplines on the appropriateness of certain items, for example the effect of a self-lifting ejector seat on someone who is confused.
- Where necessary, wheelchairs may be provided, either on short-term loan from voluntary organisations or by prescribing the long-term use of a wheelchair for the individual. Care should

be taken by staff to instruct on the safe use of the equipment and factors to monitor, such as tyre pressure.

Transport to facilities is a crucial consideration when planning a treatment programme. Availability, accessibility and financial cost to the individual and the service all need to be identified. People with mental health difficulties may find dealing with transport problems beyond their abilities. Facilities that specifically aim to help those with poor motivation need particular support with transport.

Domestic activities

- Many people have domestic skills but are not able to put them into practice – the tasks seem overwhelming. In this case the occupational therapist assists with setting priorities. Aims are then broken down into small steps which *can* be achieved. Depending on the need of the individual, there is either help with the task or, preferably, success is reinforced when it occurs.
- Community living groups are instrumental in teaching skills. The groups may be run in health service property, hostels, colleges of further education or community centres. The group provides knowledge and the opportunity to practise budgeting and cooking activities. Encouragement is towards healthy living.
- Assistance can be offered to those who find domestic tasks impossible or have placed them as a lower priority than other activities. Meals on Wheels may be provided, but provision at weekends needs to be considered. Home helps are a great boon, particularly when they are encouraged to take a wider view of their job to include, for example, shopping and the preparation of food. Laundry services and the use of easy-care fabrics reduce the burden of heavy washing.

Social activities

- Many people need help with joining a social group. Befriending schemes can assist people over this initial hurdle. The occupational therapist needs to be familiar with the various facilities and organisations. This ensures the correct medium is chosen to provide the correct amount of challenge and satisfaction. An activation team, consisting of unqualified occupational therapy staff or other support workers, can support people in using facilities, offering help either in the home or in the local community.

• Skills training, both in interactional skills and in community living, can enable people to practise successful behaviour. Individual, as well as group, facilities need to be available. Feedback, often in the form of peer group response, is given on the behaviour seen. Consideration needs to be given to the venue used, as appropriate behaviour is most likely to be seen in appropriate settings.

• Environments that make best use of existing skills need to be harnessed by the therapist. The interest and abilities of the clients dictate the exact nature of what is developed. The service needs to access a range of different options which cater for different groups of people with different abilities. The range should go from structured leisure facilities offering social contact without the label of illness to intensive input, as in a day hospital, and to the use of ordinary social events open to all. Drop-in coffee clubs or contact clubs can offer a less structured but supportive atmosphere that suits the needs of many (Box 24.6).

Work activities

All occupational therapists will be aware of the many different motivational forces behind the drive for purposeful occupation, commonly called work. These include social acceptance and contact, a feeling of achievement, financial need, and intellectual and creative stimulation. Currently, employment is not available for all, particularly those with functional difficulties. The therapist needs to create and use opportunities to meet the need for work activities.

An assessment of work-related skills must be undertaken. The method is dependent on the individual and the nature of the work preferred. Government schemes at present in operation

---

Box 24.6 Resources available to the occupational therapist working with Mr Brown

• Multidisciplinary community mental health team: medical staff, nurses, social worker, occupational therapist
• Residential care and supported housing – independent and voluntary
• In-patient facilities
• Leisure opportunities: day centre, drop-in coffee club, weekend social clubs, swimming group, sports group, activities club
• Skills training groups: life skills, social skills, confidence and assertion groups
• Community support team (community based occupational therapy/nursing support staff who enable people to function in their home setting and to use facilities available in the community)

---

offer this facility. The employment re-ablement officer is a useful ally for an occupational therapist. Occupational therapists need to ensure that a variety of work activities is established to meet the different needs of individuals. These should reflect the varied work pattern shown by the local community.

Schemes and projects offering suitable activities may involve gardening, decorating, printing, furniture restoration, cashier work, routine office work and information technology skills. The extent to which the occupational therapist is responsible for the establishment and running of these various facilities depends on local structures. Sheltered employment projects and training schemes may be run by either the statutory or the voluntary sector. Wherever possible, the activities should be presented in as ordinary a manner as possible.

Leisure activities

• As with social activities, some people require direction and support to undertake leisure activities. The therapist will attempt to find or organise activities that suit the individual needs of the client. Locally run classes usually allow a reduction in fees for the unwaged.

• Projects and clubs can be set up for those who need more active assistance. Hobbies clubs can enable crafts and creative activities to be undertaken in a sheltered environment, ensuring an appropriate task and social support. The venue should not be in hospital accommodation.

• While the specialist therapies (drama, music, art and dance) are not leisure activities, they do call on the creative ability common to many. Such therapies require equipment and space. They can be provided in specialist units accessible to people living in the community.

COMMON CONCERNS IN COMMUNITY WORK

While this is a challenging and exciting field of work, its comparative newness means that occupational therapists need to review their philosophy and practice. The service and the profession have to work together to ensure that an efficient and effective pattern of care is offered to the client within governmental guidance.

Setting priorities

The service and professional managers must define the target client group, to ensure correct referrals and the identification of priorities. One role of the professional manager is to foster a special interest in the needs of the defined group. Ideally, personal interests and ambitions should enhance care in the service and not conflict with it.

Occupational therapists need to identify professional priorities. This requires an appreciation of the therapeutic process used and support in the decision reached.

Community work does not impose a structured framework onto the working week, so all team members must devise methods of managing time effectively. Cases and other duties have to be placed in order of priority. The needs of the client extend beyond the usual 9 to 5 working day. Occupational therapists may have to enable their time to be accessed in a more flexible manner than previously recognised within the profession, for example support and interventions for clients who are able to maintain their working life may need to be in the evenings.

Identifying the appropriate use of skills

In establishing priorities, the therapist has to define and describe the contributions of the profession. This may be to other team members, referrers or clients and, most importantly, to oneself. The therapist will need to gain confidence in the work and what can be offered under the name of occupational therapy. Occupational therapy does not have the advantages of some other disciplines, such as medicine and social work, whose skills and involvement have been defined by legislation. It is important for occupational therapy staff to link together and identify a common approach.

The novelty of the community setting at first suggested that it called for a complete break with traditional practice. Experience has shown that this is quite incorrect. Community work in mental health has enabled a return to the basic beliefs and skills of the profession.

Support and supervision

Occupational therapy is in its early stages as far as identifying the various methods of supervision. Traditionally, the doctor in charge held the final responsibility for a case but, as the pattern of health care changes, this changes, too.

There is a need for clinical case supervision of an occupational therapist by an occupational therapist in order to ensure effective professional approaches are used. Many occupational therapy managers have felt they do not have the knowledge of such a new field; however, they do have the knowledge and experience of occupational therapy. Case supervision requires an understanding of the system in which the therapist is working and of the principles underpinning the profession, no matter what the field of work. Reference should be made to the current standards, policies and procedures laid down by the College of Occupational Therapists as well as local service directives. It is the responsibility of the professional clinician to seek appropriate supervision and ensure her practice is within the expectations of the profession.

More general managerial supervision and support need not be delivered by a fellow occupational therapist. Often the key issue is how the professional fits with the team and the demands placed on it.

All singleton professionals, such as psychologists and occupational therapists, require support in maintaining their approach and in dealing with being alone in a group setting. Occupational therapists have a particular need since the harmonising skills often shown may result in the lessening of the obvious differences between disciplines. New and established staff need support in their work. Any changes within the setting can result in transitional strain.

Occupational therapy requires a problem-solving ability in order to be effective. Contact with other occupational therapists can enhance creativity. Unfortunately, some therapists find it difficult to resolve the conflict of long-term gain over short-term loss, and for them, time spent with colleagues is in conflict with time spent with clients. The role of the manager is to point out the consequences of this belief.

Professional role models

Traditional settings consisted of a department with a mixture of grades of staff. There were senior staff who could act as role models for juniors. The move into the community and the dispersal of personnel has altered this practice. New staff may use other disciplines as models, which results in a further blurring of roles. Professional networks need to be established to provide all staff with the ability to learn from others. Experienced staff need to be encouraged to take on a mentor role with colleagues and guide them through difficult situations.

Evaluation

Occupational therapists are identifying the need to question practice, to evaluate the work undertaken and to communicate this to others. Owing to the increasing emphasis on the evidence base of interventions, therapists should be encouraged to pursue specific topics, judiciously use the literature and learn the skills of evaluation and research.

Clinical audit is a method of examining practice which can be undertaken within a single professional field or together with other professions. The results should identify action arising from the audit, which leads towards improving the service.

Contractual audits centre on whether the contractual obligations have been met. Current measures are the *National Service Framework* (DoH 1999b), *Serious Mental Illness* list and the *Patients Charter*.

Some research methods, such as clinical trials, are initially difficult to apply to community settings. There is an increasing use of qualitative methods such as sociological models and single case studies. These can be used to good effect.

MANAGEMENT OF THE SERVICE

The introduction of clinical governance to the health service has highlighted the need to assure and monitor the quality of professional actions (DoH 1998a, 1999a). The professional manager must be responsible for maintaining professional standards and ensuring effective methods of service delivery. The staff of a community occupational therapy service are its most important resource. The manager must be able to motivate them and allow them to develop and mature as professionals. Effective management harnesses the creative and enthusiastic energy of staff.

Helpers and technical instructors can provide a flexible workforce to set up and run a variety of leisure-related facilities and groups. Good management and support of staff is vital. Staff should be appointed to one of the support services and not to a particular club or centre, to allow for greater flexibility.

Professional management can create a team spirit which enables occupational therapists to share their expertise and skills and to work more confidently in the knowledge that they have their colleagues' support. This is increasingly import-ant in community work, where therapists are working in isolation and have to respond to the changing needs of a new service.

SUMMARY

In conclusion, it will be seen from this chapter that occupational therapists working in the com-munity reflect the practice of their colleagues in hospitals but show a greater emphasis on the environment and system the client uses. Activities used to promote function are based on the normal activities performed by the majority of the population. Where it is not possible to use public facilities, effort is taken to present options as close to normal as possible. Community occu-pational therapists teach skills and routine sets of behaviour to allow people to make use of com-munity resources.

The holistic, flexible approach used by occupa-tional therapists is ideally suited to community work in the field of mental health. Therapists already work in social services and other fields that are primarily set in the community. The phil-osophy of the profession fits well with the concepts and goals of community care. Occupational thera-pists need to build on the strong, wide foundation of the profession. This may be a new direction for mental health but it is familiar ground which allows full use to be made of the comprehensive skills shown in occupational therapy. Individual practitioners need to be well supported, encou-raged and supervised in order to contribute to the community mental health teams as occupational therapists. Community work calls for the creativity of occupational therapy.

No doubt the pattern of health care will con-tinue to change. Occupational therapists are more than able to develop their practice to meet the needs of the current and future situations.

REFERENCES

Appleby L 1999 Safer services: national confidential inquiry into suicide and homicide by people with mental illness. Department of Health, London

Barris R, Keilhofner G, Watts J H 1988 Bodies of knowledge in psycho-social practice. Slack, New Jersey

Charlwood P, Mason A, Goldacre M, Cleary R, Wilkinson E (eds) 1999 Health outcome indicators: severe mental illness. Report of a working party to the Department of Health. National Centre for Health Outcomes Development, Oxford

Department of Health and Social Security 1975 Better services for the mentally ill. DHSS, London

Department of Health and Social Security 1983 Care in the community: a consultative document on moving resources for care in England. DHSS, London

Department of Health 1998a A first class service. Department of Health, London

Department of Health 1998b Modernising mental health services: safe sound and supportive. Department of Health, London

Department of Health 1999a Clinical governance: quality in the NHS. Department of Health, London

Department of Health 1999b National service framework for mental health; modern standards and service models. Department of Health, London

Department of Health 1999c Effective care coordination in mental health services: modernising the care programme approach. Department of Health, London

Department of Health and Welsh Office 1999 Mental Health Act 1983 Code of Practice. Stationery Office, London

Devon County Council 1993 Community care in Devon 1993–1994. Devon Social Services, Exeter

Dunning H 1972 Environmental occupational therapy. American Journal of Occupational Therapy, 26 (6): 292–298

Etcheverry E 1979 Curriculum planning for community occupational therapy. Canadian Journal of Occupational Therapy 46(5): 210–205

Hagedorn R 1992 Occupational therapy perspectives and processes. Churchill Livingstone, London

House of Commons 1990 The National Health Service and Community Care Act 1990. HMSO, London

Jones K, Poleti A 1985 Understanding the Italian experience. British Journal of Psychiatry 146: 341–347

Kielhofner G 1985 A model of human occupation. Williams and Wilkins, London

Marshall M, Gray A, Lockwood A, Green R 2000 Case management for people with severe mental disorders (Cochrane Review). Cochrane Library, Issue 1. Update Software, Oxford

Maslow A H 1970 Motivation and personality. Harper and Row, New York

McCreadie R G et al 1985 The Scottish survey of psychiatric rehabilitation and support services. British Journal of Psychiatry 147: 289–294

Meeson B 1998 Occupational therapy in community mental health. Part 2. Factors influencing intervention choice. British Journal of Occupational Therapy 61(2): 57–62

Parker S 1976 The sociology of leisure. Allen and Unwin, London

Patmore C, Weaver T 1991 Community mental health teams: lessons for planners and managers. Good Practices in Mental Health, London

Powell-Lawton M 1972 Assessing the competence of older people in Kent. Action for the elderly. Behavioural Publications, Kent

Thornicroft G, Ward P, James S 1993 Care management and mental health. British Medical Journal 306: 768–771

Willson M 1983 Occupational therapy in long-term psychiatry. Churchill Livingstone, Edinburgh

Yerxa E J 1988 Personal communication.

25

Occupational therapy in primary care

Jennifer Creek   Sue Beynon
Sarah Cook   Tania Tulloch

INTRODUCTION

The profession of occupational therapy came into being because of a perceived need for activity programmes in long-stay mental institutions (Hopkins 1988). It had been observed that people who are incarcerated, without access to the normal range of human choices and activities, become disturbed and distressed, whether or not they have a mental illness. Many of these long-stay institutions have now closed down as patterns of care have changed. However, the profession continues to grow and develop in the context of a continuing human need for support and help in carrying out a balanced and satisfying range of activities when disease, disability or circumstances interfere with normal function.

In order to fulfil their professional purpose, occupational therapists have developed theories to explain the relationship between health and activity (for example, Wilcock 1998) and skills in helping clients to overcome performance deficits. Earlier theories and skills were appropriate for application within institutions. More recent approaches have been developed for use in community settings. With our wide knowledge base and extensive range of techniques for intervention, occupational therapists are able to work confidently in a range of treatment settings, from long-stay institutions, such as special hospitals (see Ch. 27), to community mental health teams (see Ch. 24).

As patterns of care change in response to social changes and the policies of successive governments, occupational therapists adapt their approach and move into new areas of practice.

Over the past few years, the status of primary care services within the National Health Service (NHS) in the UK has been changing rapidly. The first major changes, in the 1980s, saw general practices becoming fund holders. General practitioners (GPs) could decide what services they wanted to purchase for their patients and include more services within their practices if they chose to.

In 1996, the government published a White Paper, *Choice and Opportunity*, which set out proposals for new primary care legislation. This allowed for the development of new models and arrangements for providing care to address local problems and bring about improvements. In 1997, more than 80 practices took part in the first wave of personal medical services pilots, ranging from practice based pilots, some with GPs and nurses working in partnership together, to nurse led pilots and pilots with salaried doctors employed by an NHS Community Trust.

This chapter discusses a few of the many services that occupational therapists have set up in response to these changes. The five projects described here illustrate different ways in which the profession has adapted its practice to fit in with service changes.

The first section, Penny Meadow, describes a pilot project which was started in 1990 and represents a scheme to establish occupational therapy in a fund-holding practice. The second section, Portsmouth, describes a project in which occupational therapists were able to accept direct referrals from general practitioners. The third section, Church Lane, describes another pilot scheme in which staff from a community mental health team held sessions in a GP surgery. The fourth section, Pitsmoor, describes a very different occupational therapy service which was set up to support people with severe, enduring mental illness at primary care level. The final section, Pennywell, describes a mental health promotion service developed by an occupational therapist working in a first wave pilot personal medical service.

PENNY MEADOW: SESSIONAL OCCUPATIONAL THERAPY WITHIN PRIMARY CARE

In 1989, a commission of enquiry, chaired by Blom-Cooper published its findings about the role, function and organisation of the profession of occupational therapy. One of the recommendations of the report was that the College of Occupational Therapists should 'accelerate the pace of change, already taking place, towards a redeployment of occupational therapists to work in the community, rather than in hospitals' (Blom-Cooper 1989, p. 85).

Inspired by this report, two occupational therapists based in a psychiatric unit within a district general hospital decided to attempt to set up a community based service for people with mental health problems. The decision was taken to pilot a small scheme, offering occupational therapy sessions within a local general practice. The aims of the scheme were:

- to see if there was a role for occupational therapists working with people with mental health problems in a primary care setting
- to demonstrate to the GPs that an occupational therapy service could free some of their time and provide an alternative to prescribing certain drugs
- to give patients access to occupational therapy services without having to attend the hospital
- to see if such a service could reduce the number of GP referrals to the outpatient psychiatric department at the hospital.

Due to limited resources within the department, only two half-day sessions were offered, for an initial period of 1 year. In order to market occupational therapy effectively to the GPs, each therapist selected a particular client group to work with and wrote clear referral criteria so that the doctors would find it easy to make referrals and there would be a natural limit to the number.

A letter was sent to a local practice of seven doctors, explaining the role of occupational therapy in mental health and offering the two sessions. The therapists were invited to a practice meeting to discuss the scheme with the GPs. At this meeting, it was agreed that the 1-year pilot scheme would be implemented. Each GP was given a written description of the service offered (Box 25.1) and a list of referral criteria (Box 25.2). One therapist offered a stress management group and the other a women's group. The practice provided sessional time in a small suite of rooms, which included a kitchen and storage space for records. The occupational therapists planned to see people individually for the first few weeks, until enough referrals were collected for the groups to start.

The stress management group folded after a short time and the therapist stopped going to the practice. The other therapist was able to adapt her practice and continued to offer a weekly session for the full year.

How the pilot project worked

A diary was left at the practice reception, giving appointment times for the occupational therapist, and referral cards were left for the GPs to fill in. The procedure for making a referral was that the doctor would discuss it with the patient who could then make an appointment through the receptionist. The GP would leave the referral card in the occupational therapy diary. The occupational therapist could have access to a patient's notes if the patient's verbal permission was obtained. An hour was allowed for each patient so that three people could be seen every week.

The intention had been to run a group for women having problems such as depression, tranquilliser dependency or social isolation. Within a few weeks of the scheme starting, it became apparent that only one of the women seen would benefit from group intervention at that time. It was therefore agreed that patients would be seen individually and anyone needing group intervention would be referred directly to the occupational therapy service at the hospital.

Referrals

Between November 1989, when the scheme started, and December 1990 when it was due to finish, 27 new referrals were made. The majority of these were for anxiety or related problems, although anxiety was not one of the stated

---

Box 25.1   The occupational therapy service offered at Penny Meadow

WHAT WE ARE OFFERING

- two experienced occupational therapists for a half day each
- groups or individual sessions for people with social and emotional problems
- a 1-year pilot scheme
- evaluation of the scheme

WHAT YOU PROVIDE

- appropriate referrals
- premises
- support
- access to information about patients

POTENTIAL ACTIVITIES OF THE WOMEN'S GROUP

- time structuring
- exploration of local resources
- exploration of personal skills and roles

- opportunities for shared feelings and experiences
- supportive psychotherapy
- development of new skills/roles/interests

BENEFITS TO YOU

- reduced time seeing patients with social and emotional problems
- reduced prescriptions for anxiolytics and antidepressants
- status in offering an extra service to patients

BENEFITS TO PATIENTS

- more staff time
- immediate access to specialised help without hospital attendance
- opportunities to learn skills to manage own problems
- improved quality of life

Box 25.2 Referral criteria for the women's group at Penny Meadow

- Female
- Aged 40–60
- Problems such as:
  — loneliness
  — boredom
  — depression
  — an 'empty nest'
  — lack of confidence
  — transquilliser dependence

referral criteria (see Box 25.2). The range of presenting problems is shown in Table 25.1. These have been categorised as: anxiety-related, depression, specific events requiring counselling, lifestyle problems and lack of self-confidence. A child abuse case has been included in the lifestyle category because the single incident of abuse was a response to long-term stress within the family.

Of the seven doctors in the practice, four made referrals for occupational therapy and three did not. This is partly explained by patients saying that they chose to see doctors who had a reputation for being sympathetic to mental health problems. Two GP trainees with recent psychiatric experience also made referrals. The most patients referred by one doctor was eight and the least was one.

Twenty-four of the referrals were for women and three for men, although the original referral criteria stated women only. The first man was referred and accepted when the scheme had been running for 8 months and was well established.

The ages of people seen ranged from 21 to 76 (Table 25.2). The ages of seven of those seen were unknown, but are estimated to have been between 50 and 60.

Ninety-five appointments were kept during the year. The least number of times any individual was seen was one and the most was 28 (Table 25.3). Three people did not keep their first appointment and were never seen. One person did not keep her first appointment but subsequently made another one and was seen. Four people terminated the intervention by missing an appointment and not making

Table 25.1 Presenting problems at Penny Meadow

Presenting problem	No. of referrals
Long-term anxiety	8
Recent onset anxiety	6
Stress	3
Obsessional ideas	2
Tranquilliser dependency	2
All anxiety related problems	21
Postnatal depression	2
Depression	1
All types of depression	3
Marital disharmony	1
Bereavement	1
Unresolved guilt over termination of pregnancy	1
All problems requiring counselling	3
Loneliness	1
Unsatisfactory lifestyle	1
Child abuse	1
All lifestyle problems	3
Lack of self-confidence	4

Table 25.2 Age range at Penny Meadow

Age	No. of referrals
20–24	2
25–29	1
30–34	2
35–39	3
40–44	3
45–49	5
50–54	0
55–59	3
60–64	0
65–69	0
70–74	0
75–79	1
Unknown	7

Table 25.3 Number of times people were seen at Penny Meadow

Number of sessions	0	1	2	3	4	5	6	12	28
Number of people	3	9	5	3	0	3	2	1	1

another one. Altogether, 10 appointments were not kept and 12 were cancelled during the year.

Results of the Penny Meadow pilot

When the pilot year ended, two people were being seen by occupational therapists at the hospital as outpatients rather than at the practice, four people were still being seen at the practice, four had terminated contact with occupational therapy, five had transferred to occupational therapy groups at the local hospital and the remainder are unaccounted for.

The GPs expressed appreciation of the occupational therapy service and wished to continue it when the pilot year ended. As they became a fund holding practice at that time, they were able to pay the hospital for future services.

Most people who were referred were very positive about being seen at the practice rather than having to attend the hospital. Several declined the offer of a group at the hospital because they did not want to be seen there by anyone who knew them. However, two people agreed to be seen individually at the hospital because the session time at the clinic was not convenient. Four people stopped attending without any explanation and one declined any further intervention because she did not find it helpful. The others said that they found the service accessible, convenient and useful.

An unexpected development was an increase in direct referrals to the occupational therapy department at the hospital from other general practices. Patients said that they had been told about the occupational therapy service at Penny Meadow by friends and relatives who had used it and had asked their own GP to make a referral.

The occupational therapist at first had some difficulty in adjusting to working in the practice. Most people referred did not have psychiatric diagnoses and their problems were stated very briefly on the referral form. There was no multidisciplinary team with whom to discuss problems, and there was a higher rate of missed appointments than at the hospital. An unexpected discovery was that the resources of the hospital were missed. The therapist had not previously been aware of how much she relied on the materials and space available in an occupational therapy department.

However, the advantages of working in the primary care setting far outweighed any disadvantages. Most people needed to be seen fewer times than they would have in hospital because they were seen at an earlier stage, when they were not so acutely distressed. People were able to retain their sense of autonomy and personal responsibility to a greater degree than either inpatients or outpatients at the hospital. They would listen to the therapist but make their own decisions about what action to take. Also, the range of problems seen was varied and interesting, including problems that would not usually be seen within secondary mental health services, for example, premenstrual syndrome.

Not all the work was specific to occupational therapy, as several people required more general counselling. However, all the referrals were appropriate and the occupational therapist was able to offer some form of intervention to everyone, even if the offer was not taken up.

At the beginning of the scheme, the therapist did not set a limit to the number of appointments offered. Later, she made a contract with each patient, offering a set number of appointments with clear agreement about what the time would be used for. This was partly due to pressure of new referrals and partly to a need to let the GPs know exactly what interventions their clients were receiving.

The original plan for the Penny Meadow pilot was substantially modified during the year, but most people involved felt that it was of benefit to them. The two main factors which contributed to its success are considered to be:

1. the well defined referral criteria which helped the GPs to decide who might benefit from the service
2. a willingness on the part of the occupational therapist to be flexible and respond to perceived needs rather than continuing with the original plan.

PORTSMOUTH: DIRECT REFERRAL TO OCCUPATIONAL THERAPY

A primary care occupational therapy service was provided in the Havant and Petersfield locality of

Portsmouth Healthcare NHS Trust from 1993 to 1997. Primary care mental health occupational therapy was provided from occupational therapists working within community mental health teams (CMHTs). These therapists accepted referrals from all CMHT members and other professions working within the community, including health visitors, probation officers and general practitioners. The service ceased when the Trust set up a primary care counselling service and the occupational therapy management structure changed.

How the service was set up

There had been no mental health occupational therapy service in this locality for approximately 18 months, following the closure of a day hospital and the allocation of the premises for a CMHT base. A Head III occupational therapist was then appointed to manage all occupational therapists in the locality, which included peripatetic occupational therapists and a service for people with learning disabilities. Part of the remit for this post was to determine what mental health occupational therapy services were needed.

Following a survey of service users, members of the CMHT and GPs, it was decided that the mental health occupational therapists would work to the same model as their community counterparts, accepting direct referrals from agencies external to the core CMHT, from GPs and from patients themselves if this was appropriate and the GP was in agreement. Referrals were also taken from within the CMHT.

Primary care mental health occupational therapy became an extension of the existing peripatetic community service. Staffing consisted of 0.5 whole time equivalent (WTE) Head III, two WTE Senior I and 0.5 WTE Senior II occupational therapists, all working as autonomous practitioners with their community colleagues. Referrals were taken from all general practices within the locality.

Types of intervention used

Occupational therapists worked with people suffering from a range of conditions, as shown in Box 25.3. Treatment was offered on either a group or an individual basis and was time limited. Groups were closed and time limited. Treatment could take place in the client's home, in the GP surgery, on CMHT premises, in the GP hospital or in other community settings.

Anxiety management groups were run on primary care or CMHT premises, either during the day or in the evening. A group would run for 2 hours on 6 consecutive weeks. Patients were allocated to these groups following assessment. A cognitive behavioural approach was used, and weekly goals and homework tasks were set.

Anger management groups were run at the CMHT site during office hours. They would run for 2 hours over 4 consecutive weeks. A cognitive behavioural approach was used, although therapists required a working knowledge of psychodynamic theory to explore some of the group and individual processes. Homework tasks were set, along with individual goals, and this group often used creative techniques such as writing and life maps.

Groups for survivors of sexual abuse were run at both CMHT and primary care sites. The head occupational therapist had experience in this area and led the groups, with senior therapists acting as co-facilitators. The group focused on the effects of the experience of abuse on self-esteem, confidence, assertiveness skills and communication skills, rather than on the experience itself. This

---

Box 25.3 Range of patients seen at Portsmouth

- Anxiety conditions
- People dependent on benzodiazepines or barbiturates
- Women going through the menopause
- Depression, both reactive and chronic
- Problems with anger management
- Communication/relationship difficulties, including people with poor assertion or social skills
- Survivors of sexual abuse
- Physical dysfunctions, e.g. rheumatoid conditions, ME, chronic fatigue syndrome
- Multiple sclerosis
- Myocardial infarction (for stress management and lifestyle changes)
- Low self-confidence/self-esteem
- Bereavement/loss or change of role
- Employment and unemployment issues
- Post-traumatic stress disorder

was generally worked through with an individual counsellor or community psychiatric nurse. Groups ran for 2 hours over 10 consecutive weeks.

Groups for teaching assertiveness skills, social skills or communication skills were run at either the CMHT base or primary care sites. A psycho-educational approach was used, looking at reasons for difficulties together with introducing coping strategies. Skills were taught and practised using role play techniques prior to trying them out in real situations. The treatment was goal-focused and homework tasks were set. The groups ran for 2 hours over 6 consecutive weeks.

The young person's group aimed to provide young people with a chance to develop social and interactional skills. It used debates, problem-solving exercises, decision-making games and techniques for reducing anxiety and increasing assertion. The group ran for 2 hours over 8 consecutive weeks.

A self-esteem and confidence building group ran for 2 hours over 4 consecutive weeks or in a single-day, workshop format. The all day session would run from 9.30 a.m. to 4.30 p.m.

Other groups were run in response to need, for example, a group for people who felt stuck, helping them to explore alternative ways of coping and to make changes.

People referred to any of these groups were offered an initial assessment before they joined the group. There would be a choice of individual work for those who did not feel able to work in groups. Help was given to people with poor verbal or writing skills. On occasion, a group would run for a longer period of time if participants felt it would be helpful.

The overall aim of all these interventions was to improve the individual's ability to cope, providing strategies for self-development and management. Cognitive behavioural, psycho-dynamic and rehabilitative models were used within groups, and problem-solving, goal-setting and behavioural approaches were all incorporated. Creative therapies were used extensively in all groups. Individual treatment aims were negotiated with group participants and the achievement of these individual aims was used as an outcome measure.

Individual work was also time limited, but could take place in the patient's home as well as in the other settings. Areas targeted for individual intervention included daily living skills, the home environment, coping with surgery, self-care, health promotion, anxiety and community involvement. Specific techniques were used, such as anxiety management, relaxation and cognitive behavioural techniques.

Evaluation of the service

Patients were asked to complete questionnaires following their attendance at a group. There was also a follow-up session, usually 6–8 weeks after the group, to review progress. The occupational therapy department produced goal-focused work sheets on anxiety management, anger management, developing assertion skills and developing self-esteem, for use with groups and individuals. Patients reported that they found these useful both during groups and afterwards when they served as a reminder of what had been learned and the progress made. The occupational therapists also produced a relaxation tape of four different relaxation methods, in response to demand from patients. The work-sheets and tapes are still in use by the mental health services both within and outside the Trust.

General practitioners were also asked for their views on the service. The feedback was very favourable and the consistently high referral rate to occupational therapy suggested that the service was considered to be useful.

GPs said that patients were asking to be referred because their friend, neighbour or family member had found occupational therapy useful.

Problems with the service

The consistently high demand for the service resulted in a waiting list in excess of 3 months. There was tension between the demands of the CMHT and of the local GPs, in terms of prioritising the service. Travelling between sites was time consuming and understanding the room booking systems and security procedures on different sites was demanding. The occupational therapists found that they were often the last staff to leave premises and had to take responsibility for locking up.

Storage of notes was a major issue. If the patient had no hospital file, the notes would be kept in the CMHT premises.

People were referred for anger management by social workers or probation officers, because the professional felt that they needed help, but several people failed to keep appointments or engage with therapy because they did not own the problem.

There was also a problem of inequity, as this service was provided only within one locality of Portsmouth. The other two localities had CMHTs but the difference created tensions within the occupational therapy service overall.

Strengths of the service

Most people referred to the occupational therapy service had no psychiatric history and so no psychiatric case notes. This helped to avoid the stigma of a mental illness diagnosis and may have been one of the reasons why people would ask their GP to refer them. People did not mind coming to the CMHT premises to see an occupational therapist. People with severe and enduring mental illnesses found themselves working in groups with patients from primary care and this served to normalise the experiences they had.

A biopsychosocial model was used, with GPs and psychiatrists readily accessed as necessary. This allowed for flexibility and joint working with other agencies and primary care workers. These included district nurses, health visitors and occupational therapists working in the physical field. Patients received a well rounded, multi disciplinary service that was locally based and responsive to their needs. People could be seen in the GP surgery and avoid having to attend mental health service premises. They could be seen at hours to suit them, which was not the usual practice of the CMHTs.

Another feature of this work was the health promotion aspect. People were helped to deal with stress and the demands they had

to deal with so that they made time for themselves and were more nurturing.

For the occupational therapy staff, this way of working allowed for professional autonomy, flexibility and creativity in improving the quality of people's lives.

CHURCH LANE: BRIEF INTERVENTIONS WITHIN PRIMARY CARE

Ripon Community Mental Health Team is a multidisciplinary team which serves eight general practices in its catchment area. It is made up of two distinct staff groups, one focusing on the 16–65 age range (18 if still in full time education) and the other on people aged 65 and above.

Staff working in the former group include: one whole time equivalent (WTE) occupational therapist, one WTE community psychiatric nurse and one social worker who also carries out duties on the ASW rota. Staff working in the latter group include: one WTE occupational therapist, one WTE community psychiatric nurse and 0.5 WTE social worker who also carries out duties on the ASW rota. The whole team is served by 1.12 WTE team managers, job sharing, who also share the responsibility of being head occupational therapist for mental health services within the Trust. There is secretarial and administrative support.

A physiotherapist specialising in mental health is based with the teams. She also offers input to the Community Unit for the Elderly in both the residential and day unit sectors. The teams have access to a consultant psychiatrist for people aged 16–64 and one for people aged 65 and over.

The Ripon CMHT receives a high percentage of referrals from Church Lane surgery, based in the market town of Boroughbridge. This fund holding general practice covers a mainly rural area, including the Dishforth army base. It has 9100 registered patients. There are seven partners, one of whom is a salaried GP. The practice also has practice nurses, health visitors and midwives. Services provided by secondary care staff include chiropody, speech therapy, physiotherapy and psychology. There is no practice counsellor.

Setting up the project

The Boroughbridge project was set up in response to a request from Church Lane surgery for a mental health service which could act as a bridge between primary and secondary care while giving patients access to the skills of both. This was partly as a result of referrals to the CMHT increasing when the practice ceased to be a fund holder. The GPs felt that the CMHT could easily access the psychiatrist on their behalf, should they need to. They were also in favour of a single point of entry into the service through the CMHT gateway, as recommended by the Audit Commission in 1995.

It was decided to offer sessions from a member of the CMHT staff, one of the occupational therapists, at the surgery for selected patients, initially for 6 months. The clinician was available for 17 weeks during this time, allowing for bank holidays, annual leave, sickness and other work commitments.

The design of the project was based on an established service in Dewsbury, where patients are seen for up to four sessions within an allocated time slot at the practice. Should they require further intervention, they move from that allocated slot into time available in the remainder of the clinician's working week.

The aims of the project were to:

- improve access for mental health assessment within the familiar surroundings of the practice
- provide timely and effective brief intervention for selected patients
- develop closer links with staff in primary care teams, in line with the health improvement plan.

Following discussions between all staff involved, it was agreed that referrals would be sent to the CMHT in the normal way and patients would be selected by them for inclusion in the pilot project. This system allowed the clinician to control appointments and keep her own diary and did not create extra work for support staff employed by the primary health care team.

Records were kept according to the standards already established within the CMHT. This means that:

- all patients are given a documented mental health assessment
- a letter is sent to the referrer which includes a summary of the assessment and a treatment plan
- all patients are put on the Care Programme Approach
- all interventions are recorded with an outcome code
- all referrers are sent a discharge letter, which includes a summary of the treatment received by the patient.

Assessment

Referrals to the service from GPs were, on the whole, appropriate. During the 6-month period, 16 people were offered an assessment. Five of these referrals had been marked as urgent. (The CMHT standard is to respond to urgent referrals within 5 working days.) One person had been assessed by another member of the CMHT and recommended for a brief intervention.

Three people declined the assessment and, following a letter from the team, stated that they did not wish to be seen. The GPs were keen that a questionnaire should be sent to this group in order to ascertain their reasons for refusing the assessment. None of the other 13 people failed to attend the assessment appointment that they were offered.

Treatment

Ten people were offered treatment following assessment. Two others required some advice and signposting to other non-statutory services after assessment.

Treatments carried out within the surgery included:

- solution-focused brief counselling
- assertiveness training

- depression management
- creative therapies, for example art and psychodynamic sculpting
- goal setting
- problem solving.

Carrying out treatments within the surgery provided an opportunity to offer explanation and education about the various treatment methods being used.

Five people completed their treatment having seen only the dedicated clinician. Three defaulted from treatment and failed to respond to the default letter sent from the team. Patients are informed that they will automatically be discharged should they fail to reply.

Seven people were referred by the dedicated clinician to the wider services of the CMHT. These included:

- two for a self-awareness and self-esteem group
- one for a stress management group
- two for physiotherapy with the mental health physiotherapist
- one to the consultant psychiatrist
- one for cognitive behavioural therapy by the CPN on the team who was more skilled than dedicated clinician in that particular therapeutic intervention
- one to a male worker in response to gender preference from the patient.

Outcomes

All of the patients seen during the pilot project fell into the 16–65 age range.

The number of referrals to the CMHT rose dramatically during the project, as shown in Figure 25.1. Higher caseload numbers for all clinicians in the team resulted in urgent referrals and potential child protection cases having to be prioritised.

Apart from patients seen as part of the project, the GPs and health visitors discussed approximately 16 further patients with a view to referral or to gain more information about other services that may be appropriate and available.

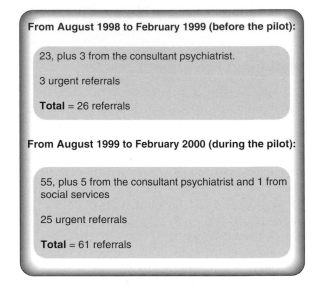

From August 1998 to February 1999 (before the pilot):

23, plus 3 from the consultant psychiatrist.

3 urgent referrals

Total = 26 referrals

From August 1999 to February 2000 (during the pilot):

55, plus 5 from the consultant psychiatrist and 1 from social services

25 urgent referrals

Total = 61 referrals

Figure 25.1 Referrals to the community mental health team: Church Lane project.

Other members of the CMHT began using the surgery more often to see patients and felt welcomed by the staff there.

During the pilot project, it became apparent to the occupational therapist that access for patients to the wider services of the CMHT and secondary care, with its multidisciplinary nature, was invaluable. Patient views were sought via a questionnaire which was sent out by the practice manager. Patients were asked to consider:

- the usefulness or appropriateness to their needs at the time
- whether they were helped to move on from the presenting difficulties
- convenience of location and access to the service.

The responses indicated that clients would like to have been referred sooner and seen sooner if they were on a waiting list. An out-of-hours service would have been helpful for those in education or full-time work. However, attending the surgery was convenient and less stressful than going to another location. One person would have preferred to have been seen at home. All respondents had managed to move on from their presenting difficulties.

Following completion of the project, the teams had to decide whether to roll this service model out to all the general practices that they served. This would require them to find a fair way of assigning staff to practices. Looking at numbers registered with a practice in order to be equitable with resources may be the best way to do this. One option is to rotate clinicians so that each practice can enjoy the range of skills that is available from the CMHT. However, the GPs are not in favour of this option, as they would prefer to have one person as their link person to relate to.

It was agreed that, in the meantime, other team members would continue to use the surgery to see clients as appropriate.

PITSMOOR: SUPPORTING PEOPLE WITH SEVERE, ENDURING MENTAL ILLNESS

A high prevalence of people with long term psychotic conditions (1.98% of adult patients) was found to be registered with one inner city GP surgery in Sheffield. This was due to the social drift of disabled people to areas of unemployment, poverty and cheap housing (Freeman 1994). The surgery had employed a research occupational therapist to survey this group's health and social care needs. The results revealed a wide range of unmet needs, especially for information, daytime activities, help with benefits and social company. The survey also produced evidence that, although 95% of psychotic patients were in contact with their GPs, only 60% received care from community mental health professionals and only 7% were receiving a care programme. Following the survey and consultation with local agencies, the health authority agreed to fund a primary care based mental health service that was managed by the GPs rather than introducing secondary care. The GPs employed the research occupational therapist to develop and deliver the new service.

The aim of the service was to improve the quality of life of a group of severely disabled people who, prior to the new GP based service, were not receiving support from any specialised

mental health services. Occupational therapy aimed to improve people's roles, function (in self-care, leisure and work) and social relationships within their local environment.

The occupational therapy service

The service was funded for one full-time occupational therapist and was delivered by a senior occupational therapist working 4 days a week and a support worker working the equivalent of 2 days a week. Clients of the service did not see any other mental health professional except the psychiatrist who visited the surgery for one session every 2 weeks.

Referrals were restricted to patients of the general practice who were not receiving support from community mental health professionals, were over 18 years old, had a diagnosis of a psychotic condition, such as schizophrenia or affective psychosis, and had social disabilities as defined by Kendrick et al (1994, p. 304): 'the patient is unable to fulfil any one of four roles: holding down a job, maintaining self-care and personal hygiene, performing necessary domestic chores, or participating in recreational activities.'

People had previously lost their support from secondary care because their suspiciousness or delusional paranoia made them difficult to engage (Sainsbury Centre 1998) or because they lacked the skills and motivation to request help. The clients were mostly men, aged between 30 and 80 years. All were unemployed. Many lived in private residential homes where they had been housed following hospitalisation, homelessness, debt problems or a period of poor self-care.

The service model used was one of coordinated and comprehensive care, combining case management, care programming (DoH 1996) and assertive outreach (Gauntlett et al 1996). The interventions were grounded in two systems-based models:

1. the vulnerability–stress model for people with psychotic conditions (Zubin & Spring 1977)
2. the person–environment–occupation model of occupational therapy (Law et al 1996).

The consequent psychosocial interventions are listed in Figure 25.2.

Evaluation of the service

The new service was formally evaluated with a pre-post test research design using standardised tests of symptoms (Lancashire 1994), function (Birchwood et al 1990) and problems (Wing et al 1994). Each client's treatment was evaluated using goal attainment: the Binary Outcome Measure was integrated with the client records (Spreadbury & Cook 1996). The perceptions of clients were surveyed with a patient satisfaction questionnaire, VSSS-32 (Ruggeri et al 1994), that has been developed as a valid and reliable measure of community mental health care.

The mean averages for social functioning after 12 months of intervention showed very high statistically significant improvement. There was improvement in all the sub-areas of social functioning, but the scores for employment were still low.

Before therapy, people's most severe symptoms were anxiety and depression as well as psychotic symptoms such as hallucinations and delusions. After a year of interventions there was statistically significant improvement for anxiety, depression, incongruity and overactivity, but not for suicidality and elevated mood. It is suggested that as some people recovered from incapacitating depression they either became suicidal or manic. With psychotic symptoms the only significant improvement was in communication related symptoms such as poverty of speech. It may be that people learned to manage their psychotic symptoms rather than reduce them.

Mean averages suggest that people's problems were statistically significantly reduced in most areas. There was a very highly significant

Psycho-social occupational therapy

Assessment of function, problems and symptoms

Selection, grading, and adaptation of therapeutic activities

Adapting the environment
• Developing partnerships in the local community
• Adapting the physical and social environment

Enhancing coping skills and strategies:
• Self care (budgeting, shopping, hygiene, etc.)
• Social skills
• Anxiety management
• Living with hallucinations and delusions

Other psycho-social interventions

• Engagement
• Supportive counselling
• Family interventions
• Cognitive-behavioural therapy
• Information and education about conditions and treatment

Case management/ care co-ordination

• Full needs assessment
• Help with benefits and finances
• Securing suitable accommodation
• Access to day care and support services

Figure 25.2 Interventions provided by the primary mental health care service.

reduction in problems with living conditions and problems with occupation and activities.

When asked how much their psychiatric treatment was right for them, 66.5% of people replied that it was between 8 and 10 out of a 10-point scale. The aspects most liked were:

- the helpfulness, the listening and understanding and the manner of doctors and occupational therapy staff
- help with dealing with problems, benefits, recreational activities, work, self-care and the home
- psychotherapy (counselling, group activities, cognitive behavioural therapy)
- support and education for carers and residential care staff
- the GP surgery in general and the comfort of the facilities.

Problems and barriers

Considerable time was needed to work effectively with this client group and to set up partnerships in the local community. The caseload was limited to between 20 and 25 people at any one time.

Working in a GP surgery could be isolating for an occupational therapist but this was overcome by securing excellent clinical supervision, continuing professional development and setting up collaborative networks with other mental health workers.

There was a danger of trying to be all things to all people, as shown in the list of interventions. The role of the occupational therapist would have been more focused if there had been a small team of an occupational therapist, social worker and nurse (trained in psychosocial interventions) working with GPs.

Strengths of the service

Being based in a local GP surgery:

- Made it possible to engage with people who were very reluctant to have contact with psychiatric services.
- Facilitated a close working relationship with the GPs and primary care staff who were the

people who had most contact with this client group.
- Helped the work with the neighbourhood, as the surgery was respected and liked in the local community.
- Provided effective project management. The small organisation and ring-fenced funding led to responsive and quick decision making and service improvements. There was a feeling of ownership and collaboration.

The ethos of a service set up to meet people's needs encouraged a client centred approach to therapy.

The occupational therapist based in primary care was able to develop initiatives within the local community that succeeded in socially integrating previously excluded people. A gardening group took over an allotment, a befriending scheme was started and a community café was helped to get funding. Training was provided for relatives and residential care workers to develop their skills and knowledge, and local shops, pubs, clubs and churches were encouraged to become accepting and welcoming.

Within the first 2 years, the new service successfully improved the quality of life of a group of vulnerable people, by responding to local needs with local resources. A further success has been the introduction of a social and occupational agenda within the medical arena of a GP surgery.

PENNYWELL: PROMOTING GOOD MENTAL HEALTH

Pennywell is a housing estate in one of the most deprived areas of the city of Sunderland, which itself has one of the poorest socioeconomic profiles in the UK.

The Pennywell pilot project is one of the first wave personal medical service pilots. It started in 1997 with a salaried GP and an integrated primary health care team consisting of nurses, administrative and clerical staff and sessional staff such as a community dietician. One session a week of occupational therapy time was also included.

The head occupational therapist of the NHS Trust seconded an experienced occupational therapist to Pennywell Medical Centre to undertake the weekly session. It became apparent that more information about patient needs would be necessary in order to make best use of this time. The occupational therapist therefore carried out a survey of needs which identified clearly the areas of unmet need in Pennywell and matched them to the skills of the occupational therapist.

In December 1999, an occupational therapist was employed half-time for 6 months to implement some of the mental health input suggested by this needs survey and to evaluate the effect an occupational therapy service could have. In January 2000, the medical centre moved into a new, purpose-built building shared with the Pennywell Neighbourhood Centre.

The occupational therapist held discussions with the community psychiatric nurse (CPN) on the primary health care team and with the senior GP to identify what her role might be within the practice. It was felt that the CPN could manage any patients needing individual sessions and that the occupational therapist should set up two groups, one for people with depression and one for people needing help with coping skills. The groups were planned and advertised to all staff in the medical centre. No referrals were received for either group.

A women's health promotion group

While waiting for referrals, the occupational therapist visited local community organisations such as the Neighbourhood Centre, the nursery school and the Youth Project. The manager of the Neighbourhood Centre asked if she would be willing to take over a women's creative activity group that had been run for some time by centre staff. They had identified that the women had needs which were not being met by this group. When the new building opened, the occupational therapist began a 6-week pilot of the women's group on Monday mornings. This proved so popular that it was continued for a further year.

The aims of the group were:

1. to offer opportunities to engage in a range of creative activities, with or without an end product
2. to provide a safe forum for women to explore their own creative potential
3. to broaden the experience of activity of women with social and/or mental health problems.

The group met for 2 hours a week with between six and ten participants. For the first few months, everyone did the same activity every week. The activity was carefully selected so that it could be completed within the 2 hours, with a coffee break in the middle. Having an end product was seen as key to the value of the group. The women fed back to the group the praise they received at home for items they had made. They were initially very keen to attend but were anxious about their performance. As they became more confident, people began to ask to continue projects, or to take their work forward in different ways, so that it was not necessary to introduce a new activity every week.

Activities for older people

Staff from the Neighbourhood Centre ran a creative activity session, called 'Young at Heart', once a fortnight in the local sheltered housing complex. The occupational therapist was invited to join the worker at these sessions and introduce some new activities. These were popular and the warden invited the therapist to run a full day of activities during the week when sheltered housing schemes were being promoted nationally.

A bid was submitted for funding to continue the project under the Healthy Ageing initiative, but this was unsuccessful and occupational therapy participation in the scheme ended when the first 6-month contract finished.

Young people's mental health

The manager of the Neighbourhood Centre and the CPN from the medical centre made a successful bid for funding to do research into the mental health needs of young people in Pennywell. They invited the occupational therapist to take part in the project, 'Young Minds Matter'.

Young Minds Matter is an innovative mental health project funded with health action zone money. The first phase of the project was to recruit 10 volunteers between the ages of 12 and 17 and train them to carry out research into the mental health needs and opinions about mental health care services of other young people in Pennywell. The project was advertised locally, interviews were held, and 10 young people were appointed. The occupational therapist planned a training programme which was carried out by herself and the CPN, with support from two youth workers, over seven Saturdays. The volunteers then carried out the survey, produced a report and presented their results to an invited audience of stakeholders in Sunderland.

Activities for children

In July, Pennywell held a carnival. The occupational therapist was asked to lead a group of eight children in designing and building a model of the Lambton Worm and Penshaw Monument for the float. This was a full-day activity which was held in an empty unit in the Pennywell Business Centre. It proved popular and the therapist was then asked to work with Neighbourhood Centre staff running activity groups in local schools as part of the summer activity scheme.

The activities were carried out with up to 30 children at a time, between the ages of 8 and 12, in several local schools. Activities were chosen after a survey of preferred activities among local schoolchildren. These were glass painting, T-shirt design and making dream catchers. Attendance at these sessions was higher than at previous summer play schemes and the therapist was asked to take part in future holiday activity programmes.

Discussion

The original remit for the occupational therapist at Pennywell medical centre was to work with people suffering from mental health problems. It was found that, in this small practice of only 2000 patients, the CPN could manage the mental health problems that were presented. With agreement and support from the GP and head occupational therapist, the occupational therapist in post was able to move out of the medical centre and work with community organisations to develop a range of activities for different age groups that would help them develop the coping skills to support positive mental health in people living in conditions of social deprivation.

One of the most positive aspects of the project was the response of local community organisations to having access to an occupational therapist. Without any advertising or education about the skills of the occupational therapist, they recognised the value of the way in which activity is applied by a skilled professional and were able to identify appropriate areas for intervention.

SUMMARY AND CONCLUSION

This chapter has described five projects in which an occupational therapy service has been introduced into a primary care setting. The first three schemes, Penny Meadow, Portsmouth and Church Lane, describe how the skills of the mental health occupational therapist were made available to people as part of a primary care service. The strengths and weaknesses of the three projects were evaluated, and the conclusion drawn is that providing occupational therapy input into primary care is of benefit to everyone concerned.

The last two schemes, Pitsmoor and Pennywell, are more innovative and extend the traditional occupational therapy role in mental health. The Pitsmoor service has demonstrated that people with severe, enduring mental illness can be helped to live a more satisfying life through occupational therapy intervention at the primary care level, without having to access secondary mental health services. The Pennywell project showed the contribution that occupational therapy can make in promoting good mental health, in partnership with community organisations, through designing activity programmes for different age groups.

Occupational therapy has been slow to move to develop mental health interventions in primary care but these schemes demonstrate that there is a variety of ways of doing this and that the profession has a significant role to play.

REFERENCES

Birchwood M, Smith J et al 1990 The social functioning scale: the development and validation of a new scale of social adjustment for use in family intervention programmes with schizophrenic patients. British Journal of Psychiatry 157: 853–859

Blom Cooper L 1989 Occupational therapy: an emerging profession in health care. Duckworth, London

Department of Health 1996 Building bridges: a guide to arrangements for inter-agency working for the care and protection of severely mentally ill people. Department of Health, London

Freeman H 1994 Schizophrenia and city residence. British Journal of Psychiatry 164 (supplement 23): 39–50

Gauntlett N, Ford R, Muijent M 1996 Teamwork, models of outreach in an urban multi-cultural setting. Sainsbury Centre for Mental Health, London

Hopkins H L 1988 An historical perspective on occupational therapy. In: Hopkins H L, Smith H D Willard and Spackman's Occupational therapy, 7th edn. Lippincott, Philadelphia

Lancashire S 1994 Modified version of Krawiecka, Goldberg, Vaughn 1977 KGV symptom scale (Available from THORN, School of Nursing, Coupland 3 Building, University of Manchester, Oxford Road, M13 9PL)

Law M et al 1996 The person–environment occupation model: a transactive approach to occupational performance. Canadian Journal of Occupational Therapy 63(1): 9–23

Ruggeri M, DallAgnola R, Agostini C, Bisofi G 1994 Acceptability, sensitivity and content validity of the VECS and VSSS in measuring expectations and satisfaction in psychiatric patients and their relatives. Social Psychiatry and Psychiatric Epidemiology 29: 265–276

Sainsbury Centre 1998 Keys to engagement. Sainsbury Centre for Mental Health, London

Spreadbury P, Cook S 1996 Measuring the outcomes of individualised care: the binary individualised outcome measure. Nottingham City Hospital NHS Trust OT Department, Nottingham

Wilcock A A 1998 An occupational perspective of health. Slack, New Jersey

Wing J, Curtis R, Beevor A 1994 Health of the nation outcome scales. Royal College of Psychiatrists, College Research Unit, London

Zubin J, Spring B 1977 Vulnerability – a new view of schizophrenia. Journal of Abnormal Psychology 86: 103–126

26

Working in a transcultural context

Saroj Gujral

INTRODUCTION

Forty years ago the term 'transcultural psychiatry' began to come into use. It was a topic of discussion at the World Federation of Occupational Therapists' Congress in 1979.

Intercultural interactions are a normal part of occupational therapy practice. Some see such interactions as exciting challenges, others see them as a problem to overcome. An understanding of the nature of these interactions and the issues involved is vital to the development of strategies to make such interactions satisfying and productive for both the occupational therapist and the client.

The purpose of this chapter is to provide occupational therapists with the knowledge of how to recognise the need for interactive strategies. These have changed, from trial and error and a focus on assimilation, to the recognition that cultural diversity enhances society. This chapter describes what culture means and how it affects ethnic minorities and immigrants. The incidence and presentation of psychiatric illness in immigrants is reviewed and factors influencing treatment are examined. A section on occupational therapy with transcultural clients considers aspects of provision of a good occupational therapy service, including treatment planning, implementation and outcome. Recommendations are made concerning the responsibilities of students and occupational therapists and how their perceptions and roles affect occupational therapy for transcultural mental health clients.

Culture

Culture is a concept that varies according to the context in which it is being used. For the purposes of this chapter, it may be regarded as comprising traditional beliefs and social practices that lead to accepted rules for social interaction within a particular locality or social group. Culture evolves continually in response to external influences such as changes in population structure, the media and ideological influences. Specific information about the beliefs of the culture can be passed on from one generation to another.

According to Krefting & Krefting (1991) culture has been identified as one of the least developed aspects of occupational therapy knowledge. It is for this reason that many schools are now designing and offering courses in multiculturalism (Peters 1992). However, many people think of culture in terms of race and ethnicity. Hinojosa & Kramer (1994) wrote that traditions, beliefs, values and patterns of behaviour must be included in the study of culture so that therapy can be personalised.

Cultural competence

Cultural competence has been defined by Dillard and colleagues (1992) as having an awareness of, sensitivity to and knowledge of the meaning of the culture. Added to this must be an appreciation of the historical and geographical background of that culture in order to realise how deeply rooted many of the beliefs and traditions of the host country are, both culturally and religiously.

Chan (1990) described the elements of cross-cultural competence as including:

- awareness of one's own cultural background and values
- knowledge of information specific to each culture
- the ability to interact with others successfully.

For occupational therapists, cross-cultural competence is more easily developed in learning situations which require active engagement of students and occupational therapists along with integration of prior knowledge, current research and personal experiences.

Cultural factors have potentially far-reaching effects on the provision of care, including selection and interpretation of assessment instruments, interpersonal communication, intervention and outcome expectations. This is particularly true because of the occupational therapist's emphasis on independent function and the client's ability to perform daily life activities in the context of his roles and responsibilities.

Culture shapes perceptions, explanations and experiences of illness which in turn influence help-seeking patterns and responses to treatment (Kleinman 1978, 1980; Harwood 1981).

THE MULTICULTURAL SOCIETY

Several benefits of a multicultural society outweigh any disadvantages. Shared knowledge of a rich variety of experiences and resources from several cultures can benefit the entire community. For example, the variety of restaurants and supermarkets offering different styles of food, the art and music enjoyed and appreciated by different communities and sharing the understanding and knowledge of religious practices such as meditation and yoga can all be enriching.

Cultural differences may enrich society, but they may also create divisions within it. Differences may be evident in dress, personal habits, religious beliefs, values and attitudes. Some differences can be discovered only on closer acquaintance, once mutual trust has been established.

This section looks at how some of these factors may create situations of conflict or lead to difficulties in settling in the host country.

Adapting to a new country

Any obstacles to socialisation must be overcome in becoming resocialised to another culture. Briefly, as the child grows and develops, he learns the social rules of the society in which he lives. The adult has thus absorbed, and usually conforms to, a vast number of rules and complex sociocultural patterns of behaviour.

Someone moving to another culture has to compare the new behaviour patterns required with his previous experience and decide within himself the degree to which he wishes to modify his behaviour to become resocialised and, therefore, more acceptable to the host community. This may be a subconscious or a deliberate decision to adapt.

Beliefs, values and customs are also transmitted from generation to generation. These act as a filter through which individuals interpret daily events. It can be painful to relinquish religious practices interwoven with the social network.

Assuming that the individual wishes to change, he may do so at three different levels:

1. adjustment, where there is no change in values but behaviour is modified to enable harmonious relationships
2. adaptation, to modify his attitudes in line with those of the host culture
3. integration into the social networks, becoming more like the native population. This implies a degree of change on both sides, but to a greater extent on the part of the immigrant.

ASSIMILATION

Assimilation is a process of socialisation, or the merging of the social networks of two ethnic groups. When a person has mastered the social processes and achieved acculturation (see below), he has reached the stage at which he is accepted as an individual by the host society. He then has to become assimilated at a deeper level in order to be fully integrated. Someone who might be regarded as a 'nice chap' but is not accepted as a town councillor or a potential son-in-law is not fully integrated.

The higher the level of assimilation reached, the more alike the native and the immigrant become. For the second-generation immigrant, who is socialised from birth into the host culture, the differences may be negligible. He may expe-

rience some clashes between parental behaviours and those which he learns at school but still be able to cope with this.

Acculturation

Acculturation signifies the adoption by one ethnic group of the cultural traits of another. It is a part of assimilation.

The culture shock experienced by new immigrants is stressful and the constant endeavour to do the correct thing and not cause offence can be very tiring. Learning new skills in adulthood is not an easy process, and learning to cope in an unfamiliar culture may cause loss of confidence and identity.

Separate groupings may occur in the effort to preserve cultural identity.

Family break-up may be an additional stress. The desire to assimilate is facilitated by a wish to settle in the host country. This may have a negative effect if the pressure to succeed is too great.

Refugees may have been exposed to torture and brutality, imprisonment or fear of being caught. These experiences may scar the person for life and make adjustment to an alternative culture especially threatening.

Factors affecting assimilation

Some of the main factors affecting the extent to which assimilation occurs are the following:

- Cultural distance between immigrant and host community. This includes the history, culture and ideology of the host country.
- Previous contact with the host country prior to immigration.
- Lack of familiar cues, heightening the feeling of separateness.
- Ability to learn new social skills; if individuals are not willing to admit the existence of gaps in knowledge of everyday behaviour in the host country, then small points, like using a knife and fork or operating an electric gadget, can lead to a feeling of incompetence that reduces self-confidence.

- Availability of models to demonstrate new skills.
- Adjustment from rural to urban life can cause stress in some cases.
- Different appearance, such as skin colour and dress.
- Standard of living; this may be different between the host and original countries.
- Language barrier and difficulty communicating.
- The length of time for which an established group has lived in the community. Existing cultural links and named contacts ease the transition.
- Racism and prejudice, although often denied, cause the most obvious difficulties.
- Unavailability of familiar items, such as foodstuffs or clothes, or being unable to enjoy festivals, may contribute to a sense of loss.

IMMIGRATION

Immigration means to enter a foreign country as a permanent resident. The immigrant is leaving his country of birth to establish a home and life in a new country. Broadly, migrants can be divided into two groups: voluntary and involuntary.

Voluntary immigration

People may voluntarily decide to emigrate for the purposes of study, for better job prospects, because of business or industrial interests, for an improved quality of life, for missionary work, or for social reasons such as marriage.

As modern travel makes international movement easier, more people are staying for short periods in other countries for career purposes, or on vacation. Occupational therapists are also highly mobile professionals and may experience working in several different countries, especially in the early years of their career.

Involuntary immigration

Involuntary departure from one's homeland is usually the result of a natural disaster, or a serious politically based disturbance such as war or religious persecution. Even when a move in these circumstances is premeditated it cannot be regarded as voluntary.

Often, refugees will have the additional stress of a hasty departure, possibly having had to leave family and friends without knowing what has happened to them. Refugees or those in exile (long-term absence from country of origin) may find that their families have become split up, with members living in countries that are thousands of miles apart.

Resettlement via transit camps brings its own traumas which can leave lifelong psychological scars. The impact of such events could even be experienced by the second generation.

Second-generation immigrants

It must be noted that many apparent immigrants have been born in the host country. It is upsetting for people to be asked where they have come from when they have spent all their lives in the UK and therefore feel British. As second-generation citizens, their expectations and experiences are different from those of their parents. Why should their rights and entitlements be different from those of any other British citizen?

The culture of their parents may lead to children having an identity split between home and the wider society. The clash that may ensue between the cultures of the different generations can create considerable stress. Kolvin & Nicol (1979) have described some of the psychiatric problems affecting the children of immigrants.

An Asian girl, whose parents expect her to remain at home after school, may resent not being able to join her friends at the disco. She may also get into trouble if she speaks to male fellow pupils at the bus stop. Many such teenagers can accept family life, watching Indian videos, and gain a sense of cultural identity from participating in worship at the local temple. Other young people may see this as a continuous source of conflict causing them to develop a rebellious personality. The stability of the teenager's sense of identity often depends on being able to merge with the peer group.

Social integration. Second-generation immigrants may experience different difficulties from those of their parents, leading to intergenerational conflict. To be a member of a minority group, or to live in a ghetto, can cause problems. It can be difficult to follow religious practices or some customs, for example following the rules of purdah. Maintaining an extended family structure with close kinship may be difficult as the British system of the nuclear family is so different. Male and female roles in the family can be different and may be in conflict with previous conventions.

ILLNESS AND IMMIGRANTS

Living in a foreign country, or any unfamiliar society, may be an alienating experience but this is, of course, not always the case. Many people adapt over time and enjoy the variety of experiences and opportunities available without having any feeling of being set apart.

Others, however, feel that they do not fit in and this can aggravate existing problems. Depression may result, or hostility and anger towards the host community may be expressed both verbally and physically. Frank psychiatric symptoms may emerge but these may be difficult to detect if the psychiatric staff involved represent the alien group in the eyes of the client.

TRANSCULTURAL PSYCHIATRY

Are there real differences in presentation rates between races and, if so, why? Is transcultural psychiatry a valid concept?

Incidence of illness

Cochrane (1977), in a study of mental illness among immigrants admitted to hospitals in England and Wales, identified relatively high admission rates for particular diagnoses among different ethnic groups. Irish and Scots immigrants had the highest admission rate, compared to the native-born population of England and Wales, with high levels of alcohol- and drug-related disorders. All immigrant groups had higher rates of admission for schizophrenia, due, perhaps, to differences in age structure between the groups.

The high incidence of admissions may be either a cause or an effect of migration. For example, social drift may be a consequence of schizophrenia, with people moving to seek a solution to their problems. On the other hand, the level of stress that results from immigration may precipitate psychiatric problems. Sometimes there is an acute reaction to immigration but, in other instances, years may elapse before psychiatric conditions manifest themselves. More research is needed on the following questions. How many hidden cases are there? Are patients known to their general practitioner or do they receive support from their own ethnic group? Is there considerable under-representation of certain groups among those who do get admitted? Does presentation affect diagnosis and are diagnoses accurate? Are there language or cultural blocks which prevent take-up of National Health Service resources, or does the absence of alternative support actually precipitate admission? The person's attitude towards illness is often reflected in his help-seeking behaviour.

Help-seeking behaviour

Each community has its own informal rules about how a sick person seeks help and from whom. Much care may be provided by lay people without any recourse to professional help; alternatively, a sick person may be encouraged to seek medical help fairly rapidly. The family may influence the decision, or other people in respected positions, such as teachers or priests, may suggest seeking help. Help-seeking behaviour will also be governed by past experience and the ways in which the individual has learned to obtain help for an illness. It will also depend upon the level of social support available to the individual. If there is a family network and tried and tested family remedies, solutions may be sought through the advice of older or respected members rather than from the NHS. People may accept illness as being the will of God, and outside their control. This apparently passive reaction may be puzzling to hospital staff when the problem is one that is easily dealt with. Some immigrants believe solely in the medical model, expecting medication to cure all and absolving themselves from any active role in their rehabilitation.

The sick person may not believe that Western medicine has the answer to a particular problem. Help may be sought from a practitioner of alternative medicine, such as a herbalist or faith healer. This may be for language and communication as well as cultural reasons. Knowledge of what medicine can provide is also relevant, as is an understanding of the nature of the illness itself. Fear of having a serious illness can often be a deterrent to seeking help, as is fear of stigma and shame on the family.

Loss of face

This is a concept that can only be partially understood by Western cultures. Status and standing in the community may be of paramount importance to an immigrant and loss of face is devastating. Suicide is sometimes seen as the only option. Any slur or stigma, such as mental illness, extends to the family and, for this reason, many immigrants try to mask quite severe problems and may seem superficially uncooperative. Sensitive handling of the situation may overcome this.

Somatisation

Probably the most well-documented example of how presentation of symptoms may vary from one culture to another is that of somatisation. Instead of the agitated, perhaps tearful, client who voices feelings of unhappiness, delusions of worthlessness or guilt, the doctor may be confronted by a person with a headache or sore stomach, for which no physical cause can be identified. Rather than pressing the individual, it may be possible to treat him for depression in the knowledge that this is a recognised presentation in people who have no language or concepts with which to describe it, other than physical symptoms.

Conceptual differences

A common language does not necessarily mean common conceptual patterns or symbolism and at this level communication becomes far more complex. For example, colours may have different meanings. Red is an auspicious colour for the Chinese and in Indian cultures white signifies mourning. Most people in the UK use an umbrella to give protection from rain but someone from a warmer part of the world may think of it as a sunshade.

On a social basis, family relationships may be understood differently. Instead of the clearly defined relationships linked to the nuclear family, somebody from West Africa may talk about having many mothers, meaning his aunts and cousins. The extended family draws different distinctions. Conceptual differences become integrated into value systems so that understanding and communication of illness behaviour may vary from group to group. A man who declares that his wife is ill because she will not cook his meals will not find much sympathy for his attitude in some Western households.

Perceptual differences

These are complex. People growing up in rural or urban surroundings will learn to perceive their environment in different ways. The high-rise blocks of Hong Kong provide different sensory input from the villages of Bangladesh. There may even be different interpretations of 'round' and 'straight'; people who have been reared in a village with circular houses and an absence of straight-sided buildings will have a different sense of perspective (Gregory 1972).

When conceptual differences are involved, incidents may be interpreted completely differently and this may be relevant in psychiatric practice. A hearing from a spiritual healer, or seeing evidence that the evil eye has been cast upon one, may be readily understood by someone from West Africa. In the UK, to have a second sight or communication with spirits may be regarded as a family gift. Neither of these is the same as hallucinating but both may be interpreted as such. Careful questioning is necessary to identify beliefs and the normality of the person's experience within the context of family values, even if it is at variance with that of the local community.

Obtaining information

There may be problems in gaining sufficient material upon which to base diagnosis and assessment. Information is often contained within the family and rules of medical confidentiality do little to alter this. The social stigma of psychiatric illness may be seen as so damaging that help is not sought when it is required. The psychiatric team may therefore lack information that may be crucial to the diagnosis and management of the client. The occupational therapist can obtain information by observing behaviour and so contribute to the diagnostic formulation and management of the client. There may be a reluctance on the part of a group to provide details about cultural norms. Fear of ridicule, resentment about prying, or a feeling of intrusion, together with doubts as to how the information may be used, can all be problematic if mutual trust is not established.

Factors influencing treatment

Environmental factors

Clients present with problems which are partly shaped by the environments in which they live. These physical and social environments slowly evolve into the culture of the client and affect his health and well-being. Some of these environmental factors may well be beyond his control but still affect his performance, attitudes, values, traditions, beliefs and behaviour. Occupational therapists assess a client in relation to the environment in which he lives. The goals agreed between the therapist and the client take into account environmental factors, some of which are mentioned below.

Occupational therapists need to prepare themselves with the skills which their clients need or expect them to have, hence, the occupational therapist's role and the service are shaped accordingly. Refugees, people who have fled from a culture of war and other asylum seekers may carry major psychological scars which affect their mental health. Therapists need to acquire slightly different skills to meet the needs of totally different cultures and environments.

Social influences

In colder countries, social interaction tends to be restricted due to the weather which encourages people to stay indoors, thus reducing their opportunities to meet people. The level of interaction and support within communities can impact on an individual's health and well-being and, therefore, affect the occupational therapist's role.

Family dynamics can hinder or facilitate the achievement of occupational therapy aims. Good family support, focused in the right direction, is always helpful.

There are few day centres, clubs, sheltered housing and nursing homes which are appropriate for people from ethnic minorities, and this restricts social interaction and the achievement of occupational therapy aims. The more people are isolated, the more likely they are to develop mental health problems.

Expectations

A client may regard a cure through Western medicine as being impossible or, in contrast, a total cure may be expected from medication. Doctors and other members of the treatment team may find themselves being expected to provide an instant solution, often when little information is being volunteered by the client. For the psychiatric practitioner this raises particular difficulties when the client is not willing to accept responsibility for his own progress.

The family

The family unit is given priority over individualism. People in Asian cultures are expected to work hard to keep the family unit together, which can be a source of stress in an environment where practicalities do not facilitate this.

Family structures may not consist of a nuclear family of husband, wife and two children but be an extended kinship system in the context of which all decisions are made. Having the family participating in the decision-making process may not be compatible with the team's goals of independence for the individual, even if there is no clash of opinions. It can be frustrating for the medical team to have to wait while relations overseas are consulted.

Occupational therapists need to recognise who is the decision maker in the family. Decisions can sometimes be made under the umbrella of culture which are not in the best interest of the client. It might be difficult for a Western therapist to decide how much respect should be given to the culture and where to draw the line. Occupational therapists need to take into account the client's interests in the context of his culture and, if appropriate, adjust the goals of treatment to keep an appropriate balance under the circumstances.

Children may not be able to speak freely with parents as they face the dilemma of which of the two cultures to follow. All children are expected to respect their parents and not to talk back. In most Asian cultures there is a strong emphasis on teaching children from an early age to respect teachers and parents.

Older people are well respected in the clan or families. The oldest member in the family is usually given an important place when families gather, served first, greeted first while in a group and used as a source of experienced advice for the younger generation(s). Grandparents take a lot of interest in their grandchildren, enriching their thinking by narrating stories, teaching culture and history. Usually parents in the later years of life live with sons, not with daughters.

Psychiatric illness can greatly affect the marriage prospects of a relative in the family, with the consequence that the disabled person may be hidden. It also poses a problem for social integration.

Men's and women's roles

These may be closely linked to religious and family customs, often with distinct division in sexual roles. A woman who has always maintained pur-

dah may accompany her husband to Britain when he comes to study. Without her female relations her social network is nonexistent, and how can she establish contacts in her new environment? She may not even be allowed to go to the shops alone. A Muslim woman might want to continue purdah, and may keep herself fully covered in the hospital and refuse to be seen by a male therapist. If she is forced to see a male therapist her inhibitions may hinder treatment.

Women may find the freedom of their Western counterparts quite alien or, in some cases, despicable. Caring for children may prove problematic and, if they are of school age, their experiences in the classroom may be totally alien to their parents.

The occupational therapist must remember that topics such as assertiveness training for women may be quite unsuitable. It is not appropriate to impose ideas of liberated behaviour on women who belong to male-dominated cultures. If it has to be done it should be to a small degree and very selectively. Equally, the gender difference between the Western female therapist and the male client from a male dominated society can cause problems (Box 26.1). The client may find it difficult to accept and follow advice from a woman therapist.

Religion

For many people, religion may have a far greater significance in day-to-day life than that to which

---

Box 26.1 Case example 1

Mr Leonidou from Greece was given a driving assessment. He demonstrated some lack of insight and it was agreed that therapeutic intervention might improve this. When this was suggested, Mr Leonidou became very loud and verbally aggressive. The occupational therapist's assessment of the situation was 'the Greek male is a dominant-type character and would not accept constructive criticism from a woman'.

The multidisciplinary team discussed whether an Asian man would have responded in the same way. Such expressive behaviour seems much less surprising and less gender-related when viewed with an awareness of culturally generated differences.

people in the West have become generally accustomed. Respect should be accorded to religious practices, such as specific times for prayer, dietary and cleanliness rules and the need to have significant objects to hand. For example, it may be standard practice to cease work for prayer. Preferred foods may not be available and required dietary items unobtainable. This will cause distress, the extent of which may not be fully understood.

Some rituals which are part of daily life activities need to be taken into account while planning treatment, for example, saying prayers four to six times a day, specific foods being prohibited and some rituals and foods being prohibited at specific times of the day (Box 26.2). Prayer rooms/places should be hygienically clean and away from an unhygienic environment, for example a toilet. The client might expect to take a shower or wash two or three times a day. Shoes may not be allowed inside the house, in the kitchen or in the prayer room. While doing a home visit the occupational therapist should check with the client/carer for the routine to be followed.

When the client is under treatment it is helpful to encourage the observance of religious festivals, which can prove more therapeutic than newly created activities, although it should be done within practicable limits. Most religious festivities around the world follow similar themes, for example, thanksgiving, charity, closeness of family and friends, goodwill exchange, good food, cleanliness, morality, fun, enjoyment, relaxation and remembering God.

Box 26.2   Case example 2

Mrs Jones refused to drink coffee and tea in the ward. The nurse labelled her paranoid, based on the explanation Mr Jones provided. Mrs Jones was treated for this symptom until a specialist nurse, who had more awareness of the differing beliefs within the Christian church, discovered that Mrs Jones belonged to the Seventh Day Adventists who prohibit tea and coffee drinking. When the specialist nurse identified this cultural belief, an alternative drink of milk and herbs was immediately provided.

Political and legislative influences

The practice of occupational therapy is influenced by what is essential, important or desirable. It may be essential to provide a certain level of service because there is an expectation that the therapist will act within the law of the particular country. The political and legislative framework of the government's policies affects how the occupational therapist approaches goal setting with the client which, in turn, affects the occupational therapist's role. Treatment planning and implementation are done within given resources, therefore, what is important or desirable must be balanced against those resources.

Cultural aspects of the client are an important part of the assessment process and may even be considered essential in order to achieve a satisfactory outcome. It is hoped that, in a state managed health care system such as that in the UK, cultural aspects can be incorporated effectively into assessment and intervention.

The open market health care system has an impact on people's expectations which shape their attitudes and values. This subsequently modifies their help-seeking behaviour and responses to intervention and, thus, affects the occupational therapist's role.

Economic influences

The level of industry and the economic development of the country of origin has an impact on what the client values and what he would consider to be sufficient service provision. The client may be happy with an ordinary old chair with a cut-out hole and a bucket to use as a commode or, alternatively, he may be unhappy with even the provision of a sophisticated chemical commode.

The values of the client are also shaped partly by the economic status of the country or the province in which he lives, and partly by his own economic status.

Technical influences

The level of technical advancement of the country in which the client is living will determine whether a sophisticated computer training section can be provided or a less complex training centre is sufficient.

The carer's role

The carer's role can be harder for immigrants. The expectations from family members are high, and it is not easy to fulfil the carer's role in a foreign land, especially when the disability is permanent. If expectations are not met it can lead to frustration on the part of the carer at not being able to do what he wishes to do for his relatives.

The reasons for not being able to fulfil the role of carer may include:

- being away from the home country and not having support from the family network
- not being used to coping with a cold climate; not being able to go out easily because of cold weather, with transport difficulties adding to the problem
- being unaware of the rights of carers and the help available to them, and continuing to struggle alone for a long time
- a slow build-up of stress when there is not enough respite; racial discrimination; lack of festivals; lack of a social or support network.

Additional stress factors should be identified if carers are living with the family; for example, high levels of expressed emotions and high dependency and adoption of sick roles are more prevalent among clients from Eastern cultures.

Bereavement

Occupational therapists may have an important role in helping patients through mourning, and in giving extra support to grieving individuals who also experience mental health problems. Those who have not coped well before their loss are in danger of becoming depressed again.

The bereavement process in most Eastern cultures and religions is quite different from Western culture (see Box 26.3). It adds to the stress level of clients, at such a time, when they have to conform to a great extent to the host culture. For example, in most Eastern communities

mourning is conducted for several days with several rituals being performed. Relatives and friends visit quite a lot and create opportunities for the mourner to talk about the loss as much as is practically possible. There is a series of prayer sessions with special themes conducted by relatives, and friends come to stay with the mourners and take responsibility for food, accommodation, the funeral and immediate financial arrangements. There are special mourning songs, sung in groups and by individuals, with beating of chest or head in rhythmic movements, and outbursts of crying.

All the above-mentioned activities provide the mourners with an outlet for grief. The mourning process in Eastern culture is extremely therapeutic, and especially so for a client with psychiatric problems. As far as is possible, clients should be encouraged to go through the full process and rituals of mourning according to their culture. Staff and other associated people should be encouraged to facilitate the process followed by the client's cultural value system.

A few lines of sympathy in letter form are appreciated rather than a card. It can be offensive to send a card. Things are kept simple. People are not expected to be very smartly dressed at funerals but to wear very simple and plain clothing. Very smartly dressed people at the funeral can cause offence.

Resettlement into the community

Hospitalisation carries a social stigma, so there should be preparation for settling back into the community, in conjunction with the carers or agencies involved. They should be prepared to receive the client.

Box 26.3 Case example 3

A woman from Zaire received information that her father had been killed. Her grief reaction appeared hysterical, with loud crying, which is a normal reaction in her culture. However, she was diagnosed as a psychiatric case, until she was seen by a doctor who understood the accepted norm and offered bereavement counselling.

When a patient is resettled into the community, the emphasis on independence is often so strong that attention towards cultural needs can often be forgotten (Box 26.4). It is important to consider the cultural background, role in the family and role in the community. For example in some cultures women do not go out to work, so teaching them work skills may be inappropriate.

When accommodation is obtained for people from ethnic minorities, if possible a place should be found where their needs are catered for. It may be more appropriate for a person with particular cultural needs to go to a smaller place, such as a flat, group home or care home, rather than larger accommodation such as a hostel. Placing the client with a smaller group will enable the providers to pay individual attention to that client.

When introducing such clients to community resources, the occupational therapist must be aware of cultural needs and use appropriate facilities. It may be essential that the client is introduced to a community network that deals with ethnic needs. Some ethnic minority organisations provide excellent residential and community support facilities and these should be explored. However, it is also important not to assume that the ethnic minority client will want to live exclusively with others of the same minority group.

Racist attitudes

Psychiatric staff, who regard themselves as sensitive to clients' needs and behaviour, will resent any suggestion of racist attitudes. Nevertheless, the problem still does arise.

Box 26.4 Case example 4

An adolescent Chinese boy was not well received by the family after he had learned how to cook in hospital, as cooking was seen as a female role. The boy went back into a depression. It may not be appropriate to teach skills to someone who is not likely to use them after discharge.

Most staff in hospital or community settings would reject any racist label but, because of their attitudes, lack of knowledge and assumptions about other cultures, they may harbour subconscious prejudices which affect the way they relate to different cultural groups, even though there is no conscious intent to be racist.

When circumstances are such that the individual seeks psychiatric help, he may encounter racism within the hospital setting. Racial stereotyping may affect choice of treatment as well as aggravating difficulties that may have led to the stresses which caused the client's admission in the first place. Limited experience may result in limited resources but may also lead to standardised responses. There may be greater use of electroconvulsive therapy (ECT), or attribution of a particular diagnosis more often than with clients from the dominant culture. Such generalisations are obviously detrimental to client care.

Outright racism may occur, sometimes within the client group and sometimes between the client and staff. White clients may resist treatment from black or coloured staff. The reverse is unlikely. Covert prejudice is more difficult to deal with. Mimicking can be stopped but more subtle action may be less obvious.

Disregard for values and behavioural norms may not be seen as racism, but failure to provide the correct diet or to respect religious customs is both distressing and offensive to the individual.

In some parts of the country the person may be the only visibly different member of the client group and this situation requires close monitoring to avoid scapegoating. Racial hostility, in addition to the stress of hospital admission, should be quickly countered and can, if circumstances are right, be put to educational use in breaking down existing barriers. Burke (1986) describes this issue in greater detail. Research by MIND (Rogers & Faulkner 1989) has shown that poorer housing conditions and discrimination in the education system contribute to the aetiology of mental illness. Lack of understanding and sensitivity on the part of the police add to

Box 26.5 Case example 5

Late one night, police doing a spot check questioned Mr X, an Afro-Caribbean young man, as to why he was walking late at night. Mr X replied that he was going home. The police constable cross-examined him and during the course of the conversation asked the question, 'Do you believe in God?' Mr X replied, 'Yes, He directs my life.' That led to further conversation. Mr X, being a devout Christian, took the opportunity to state his beliefs about God. As a result Mr X was taken to see a psychiatrist who happened to be white and did not hold the same beliefs about religion. Ultimately the man was diagnosed as having a psychiatric disorder and was admitted to hospital.

Mr X's statement was wrongly interpreted because most people do not talk in that way about God. Some communities are more open about expressing their religious views; others prefer to remain reserved.

harassment and, for some people, unnecessary admission to hospital (Box 26.5) (Rogers & Faulkner 1989). Police forces are currently working to recruit liaison officers whose remit includes dealing with the sensitive issues of culture and mental health.

OCCUPATIONAL THERAPY WITH TRANSCULTURAL CLIENTS

The ability to achieve health is acknowledged to be influenced by our circumstances, our beliefs, our culture and our social, economic and political environment (Dyck 1989).

The development of culturally sensitive practices must be based on a greater understanding than we currently have of the complex interrelations between cultures, the environment and people's experiences of health and illness. Particular attention must be given to how culture is conceptualised in research and how research findings are used to guide practice. Differences between the practitioner and the client in values, beliefs and ways of doing things, complicated by language difficulties, provide considerable challenges to all those engaged in the therapeutic process.

A successful occupational therapy intervention is predicated on the active involvement of the client in the therapeutic process. It is important to recognise that the cultural interpretations of the occupational therapist will directly affect how the problems are defined, how goals are set and how meaningful activity is defined and chosen. The ideas, beliefs and practices of our profession provide only one way of viewing health problems and disability. Occupational therapists need to know what the disease or injury means to the client for interventions to be consistent with the client's everyday life experiences. The primary focus should be on the differences in values and beliefs of occupational therapist and client and how these may impinge on the ways in which goals are set and activities chosen (see e.g. Cromwell 1987).

COMMUNICATION

In order to understand the everyday life circumstances of clients which will affect the therapeutic process, it is necessary to have effective communication within the health care encounter. This may be inhibited by the differing communication styles of occupational therapist and client. Lack of differentiation between words, and nuances in language, particularly in emotional descriptions, may create blocks to communication. Literal translations may be highly misleading.

The occupational therapist should use straightforward language, avoid colloquial phrases and ensure that the instructions are understood by the client. With a little imagination, much can be conveyed by sign language. The occupational therapist, by using a few words of the client's language, may help improve rapport.

In addition to verbal communication, literacy and numeracy must be considered. In our form-filling, welfare state, written communication is virtually essential, and not being able to read bus and street signs or food packaging is frustrating for the client. In areas where there are large ethnic minority populations, the occupational therapist should endeavour to get written translations of important forms. Some councils now provide funding and expertise for this task.

If the client wishes to speak in his own language to anyone, in the presence of others, that should not be considered offensive. Speaking his native language can help the client to express himself in a better way; in particular it can help to establish a common bond which leads to a good rapport while interacting with the occupational therapist or other people.

In order to understand the everyday life circumstances of our clients which will affect the therapeutic process, effective communication in the health care encounter is necessary. All practical and social problems must be interpreted according to the requirements of particular nationalities. For further information, the local Community Relations Council, ethnic organisations and colleagues of the same ethnic background as clients can be consulted, and further literature can be sought out and studied.

ASSESSMENT

It is essential to assess clients' skills in the context of their own culture. Assessment of the level of integration in all aspects of the client's life should be carried out. It is important to find out how much the client is already integrated into the host community, how much he would like to be and how much is forced upon him. It is important to know in what areas the client would prefer to keep his own culture and identity. In the 1990s there has been increasing emphasis on providing a needs-led service in which the client's wishes are paramount.

Regular assessment of client's needs should also focus on cultural aspects. Though most standard assessments ignore this, some cultural factors should be included. Special assessment forms should be devised, or conventional assessment forms should incorporate specific cultural aspects, based on the following:

- activities of daily living – domestic and personal care
- leisure
- work (where relevant)
- interpersonal relationships
- linguistic/communication ability, verbal and non-verbal

- religion/beliefs
- diet
- norms in household management
- length of residence in this country
- contacts within the local community
- awareness of legislation linked with the client's environment
- support available/carers/dependants
- family values
- marital or sexual situation
- social skills
- ethnic network beyond immediate family
- attitudes to and acceptance of new culture
- bereavement
- level of integration
- financial situation
- political status
- fluency/command of language/whether mother tongue is spoken and understood
- acceptance of new way of life/other cultural norms
- pride in own ethnic origin
- integration and assimilation into the host country's culture
- reasons for leaving country of origin
- role expectations
- desire for assimilation.

TREATMENT PLANNING

Client-centred practice seeks an active engagement on the part of the client in defining problems and in setting goals. There must be continuing development in understanding how culture shapes conceptions of, and responses to, illness and disability.

Models for the practice of occupational therapy, such as the model of human occupation (Kielhofner 1985), urge us to include culture as an integral component of the clinical reasoning process, as we consider complex interactions between the individual and the environment.

Understanding and examination of the problem of culture in clinical practice has focused on a number of topics, and some issues have been found to be fundamental. These include:

- sensitivity to a particular culture and beliefs and the possible discordance of values between client and occupational therapist (Hume 1984, Blakeney 1987, Kanemoto 1987, Swaski 1987)
- problems of intercultural communication and the choice of appropriate activities and programmes (Levine 1984, Lightfoot 1985, Morse 1987, Robinson 1987)
- cultural differences in learning styles and special problems relating to intervention with specific community problems
- evaluation of the utility of current occupational therapy models in addressing cultural issues in practice (Levine 1984, Tebbutt & Wade 1985, Iannone 1987, Wieringa & McColl 1987).

While findings from various studies are useful to practitioners in increasing awareness of alternative views and lifestyles, which may clash with Western rehabilitation procedures, other work suggests that it is important that occupational therapists should also develop awareness of their own values and beliefs. This awareness needs to include consideration of the cultural biases of occupational therapy frames of reference and their practice, which match the broader social attitudes of society. In particular, any tendency towards stereotyping is decried, for, if we are to meet the needs of clients in the context of their own lives, the uniqueness of each client must be recognised. An uncritical focus on cultural characteristics may lead practitioners to explain the practical difficulties they encounter in treatment planning primarily in terms of the different values and beliefs of their clients, so detracting from the importance of the overall circumstances of an immigrant client's life.

A developing understanding of the complexity of culture and its relationship to the environment is needed, if the holistic approach framing occupational therapy practice is to address fully the health problems of immigrants. Rather than understanding the culture as a social characteristic or property of an individual, it is necessary to recognise that ideas, beliefs and practices are changeable and that the form they take has a close relationship to the everyday context of people's lives.

The socioeconomic circumstances of many immigrants' lives have not been widely considered in studies focusing on cultural characteristics; therefore generalisations about a group's ideas, beliefs and customary practices must be treated with caution when planning treatment.

Awareness of the everyday routines of the client's life, housing conditions, work, family and neighbourhood relationships, must be an integral part of the clinical reasoning process. It may be beyond our ability to change the socioeconomic conditions framing our clients' lives, but we should acknowledge how they impinge on everyday decisions, including those concerning adaptation to disability. This will affect how we name client problems and define goals. Furthermore, they indicate the importance of follow-up care whenever this is possible.

The occupational therapist should consider the links with mental health problems for those who have lost confidence and self-esteem and have withdrawn from society. How do such difficulties relate to psychiatric illness? Can they be aetiological factors or do they mask signs and symptoms? It is important that hospital staff, including occupational therapists, are aware of transcultural variations in the presentation of illness. The onus must be on the occupational therapist to learn about and recognise the needs of the client, whether it is to be sensitive to the fact that some languages have no words to describe certain models, or to be aware that depressive symptoms can be totally somatised. Textbooks can provide background theory but, as the occupational therapist is concerned with clients' functional abilities, the main focus should be on this aspect of behaviour. However, it is necessary to understand clients' attitudes towards illness before beginning to plan treatment programmes.

TREATMENT IMPLEMENTATION

Media and techniques should be selected according to the needs of the client. For an ethnic minority client, the objective of teaching or sharing knowledge with other clients or staff, for example teaching Indian cooking, sharing yoga or meditation or modelling a pot linked with a traditional Chinese model, can be extremely therapeutic.

Teaching and learning techniques should be adapted according to the intellect, learning ability and cultural background of the client; for example baking is a familiar activity for many people and is often used to raise self-esteem and confidence. However, for an Asian lady, who is not used to baking cakes, the activity can be counterproductive. A more therapeutic approach would be for her to cook something familiar. In the later stages of treatment she may even be able to demonstrate this to other clients, enhancing the therapeutic effect.

Warm-ups and other sessions of games should also be of a nature that clients can understand. Using a rhyme or a song which is unfamiliar is not therapeutic.

Activities of daily living

Activities of daily living vary from one client to another and depend on which country the client has come from and how much he has adapted to the ways of the host country. These activities are changeable according to the weather, diet, clothing, household management, religion and personal care. They are also linked with culture, value systems and customs.

Weather

In most hot countries clients may not have experienced indoor life. Village or urban life has been focused upon the street, and the social isolation consequent on being behind doors is in itself a problem. It is a strain to feel perpetually cold, and grey days are depressing. Additional heating and clothing can be a burden. Educating the client about the cost of heating and alternative ways of staying warm may form part of the treatment process.

Diet

Clients might wish to continue the same diet as in their country of origin but the ingredients may not be available. People migrating from hot countries have different dietary habits and requirements. Their religious beliefs might not allow certain foods to be consumed. For example, Hindus do not eat beef, Muslims and Jews do not eat pork. This should be taken into account when planning a cookery session. Some diets could be restricted at certain times of the day, night, week or month. Hindu and Muslim communities have strict regimes of fasting in a routine and disciplined way.

Clothing

Occupational therapists may need to teach or give practice in dressing, for example putting on a sari. It might be therapeutic to ask the client to demonstrate how to put on a sari, either to the occupational therapist or another client. Sensitivity to clothing should be observed.

Household management

In many Asian countries, people can employ home helps and often relatives are helpful. Having to manage all the household affairs in Western countries can be stressful. The operation of household appliances may need explanation, and the occupational therapist should patiently help the client to learn.

Day-to-day cooking of Asian recipes is often very laborious and complicated so short cuts can be advised if needed. If relevant, clients could be asked to teach some recipes to staff.

It might take clients some time to get used to the British habit of a weekly shopping trip when they are used to buying fresh food from a local stall on a daily basis.

The role of gender in home management is important. In Asian culture most males will not do housework and some females may not do household shopping. Young boys in the family may not give a hand with household chores whereas girls will be expected to help.

Personal care

There is a very strong emphasis on hygiene, not just on cleanliness. Shoes may be taken off before entering the kitchen or even the house. A daily bath is considered essential; merely washing instead of having a bath is not acceptable, and a shower is preferred to a bath. Cleaning after going to the toilet may be with water rather than tissues. A suitable water container with an appropriate spout should be provided for this purpose. The left hand is used for ablution and the right hand for eating.

Grooming, hair care or make-up should be according to the client's value system. Some communities and religions do not wear make-up. If a Sikh client senses that his turban and hair care is seen as a problem, this will give a lot of stress to him and his family.

Groupwork

A drama or music session may prove therapeutic for one client and frustrating for another and therefore the selection of the type of subject and group should be careful. It may be helpful to group together two or three patients of similar background for greater success. The occupational therapist should always remain sensitive to the culture of the group and should be able to gain their confidence. Problems may be so personal that they cannot all be dealt with in a group. It may be unacceptable to a client to reveal his personal problems. Accepting the group as a norm can take time. Clients should not feel left out in a group and there should be a feeling of togetherness. If a person cannot relate their beliefs and values with the group, it is difficult for the group to become cohesive.

Drama

Drama could mean very little to an ethnic client if the content is not congruent with the emotions, history or value system of the client, or sometimes is not even understood. For example, in most ethnic communities the mother-in-law normally lives with the son and daughter-in-law, as compared to the Western world where the mother-in-law lives with the daughter and son-in-law. The client may find that some experiences he has had are opposite to what is expressed in the drama session.

If it is appropriate, a group from the same community can be formed, which has some advantages. Physical contact may not be acceptable so the occupational therapist should ask the client about this first. If a shy young girl is hesitant to hold the hands of a male client, the occupational therapist should respect her feelings.

Music

It may be difficult for a client from an ethnic culture to enjoy a music session with an unfamiliar style of music or one in which he is not interested. It is unlikely that such music would prove effective. The occupational therapist might need to do some research into the music which interests the client. Carers, ethnic staff or local organisations may be able to help.

Craftwork

The selection of craftwork should be linked with the client's background knowledge, his interest and ability to learn a new craft or practise one learned previously. What is a leisure activity for one may be work for others. Whether the task is culturally acceptable should be considered.

- *Yoga, meditation and relaxation techniques.* These might be easier to implement, especially when a client has either experience or knowledge of them. In such cases the effectiveness of therapeutic intervention is much greater.
- *Clay modelling.* An Asian girl might make an Indian pot in spite of being shown and taught an English-style pot. The reason may be that what she learned in her childhood is easier for her to reproduce. A child from an Indian Punjabi family may make a clay chapati instead of a cake, as cakes are not as popular in Asian countries as they are in the Western world.

Social skills

Social norms are different in different cultures. There are no universally accepted norms for social behaviours and skills. Therefore, when training people in social skills it is important to consider the ethnic and cultural background of the person.

Social isolation or withdrawal, a classic symptom in conditions like schizophrenia, can cause additional problems in integrating the client into the community. When the stigma of mental illness is unacceptable in his community, the withdrawal of a person with schizophrenia may be even more marked. In this case it is important to work with the family as well as the client.

Communication is an important area which can easily be overlooked with an ethnic group of clients. When working with people with an ethnic minority background, a detailed assessment of their language problems – to differentiate the communication problem caused by the illness – will assist in training them. For example, in a person suffering from depression the communication problem may be due either to the depression or to a language problem.

Non-verbal communication should also be taken into account. The greeting rituals of other cultures can be enigmatic, and gestures may have totally different meanings from one culture to another. Mastery of non-verbal social conventions is a prerequisite to effective interpersonal contact (Morris 1977).

Eye contact with senior or older people is not always a regular practice among certain ethnic groups. Young girls may be shy and speak in a low tone of voice and this could be misunderstood. Assertiveness must also be looked at in the context of the cultural background. What is considered to be assertive behaviour in some cultures can be seen as aggressive or undesirable behaviour in another. For example, saying 'no' is used in some cultures more often than in other cultures. Special training for social skills may be needed to identify areas of faulty communication based on a misunderstanding of non-verbal cues. A simple example is that nodding the head means 'no' to a Greek.

Reminiscence therapy

This therapy should be linked with the client's past experiences. English songs of the early 1940s played for an Asian lady may not be therapeutic if she was living in an Indian village at that time and had never heard the songs before.

To make reminiscence therapy effective, the occupational therapist will need to make an effort to find material which is relevant to the past experiences of the client. Many shops and libraries stock video and audio tapes which could be used to provide effective reminiscence therapy. Most ethnic clients have access to their own newspapers. Community voluntary organisations may also help provide appropriate material.

OUTCOME EVALUATION

It is essential to evaluate outcomes within a cultural context. When an elderly Asian patient returns home to her family to be dependent on them, this may be considered a successful outcome by her family who see the situation as enabling them to fulfil their role of caring for and respecting the elderly. In Western culture this degree of dependence may be unacceptable. The therapist must judge whether or not unrealistic pressure is being put on the family.

Differences in values, beliefs and ways of doing things between practitioner and client, complicated by language difficulties, provide considerable challenges to all those engaged in the therapeutic process. These are not isolated problems; the individual concerns of a variety of health professionals over, for example, nonadherence or early termination of treatment, are part of a pattern reflected in research literature, including high rates of ineffective treatment and under-utilisation of services (Health and Welfare Canada 1986a, b).

Occupational therapists need to know whether a client is able to follow recommendations within the particular configuration of family roles and relationships, location of services and local job opportunities, and how the information provided is evaluated and used when the client has left the simulated situation and structure provided in the clinical setting.

Findings in the health care literature suggest that where there is incongruence between evaluation and explanation of a disorder and expectations of treatment on the part of the client and practitioner, there are likely to be lower levels of client satisfaction and adherence to treatment regimes (Kleinman 1978, Health and Welfare Canada 1986b, Jenkins 1988).

The treatment planning stage should incorporate cultural aspects which will be reflected in the outcome stage, and monitoring of cultural issues should be introduced in all mental health services.

OCCUPATIONAL THERAPISTS AND MULTICULTURALISM

Attitudes of occupational therapists

Occupational therapists should consider their own professional responsibilities for educating themselves and examining their own attitudes.

The occupational therapist should have a deep respect for and innate sensitivity to clients, their families and the very process of therapy itself. Mosey (1981) described several personal characteristics thought to be commonly shared by masters of the art of practice. These include the belief in the dignity and rights of the individual within the context of family and culture, respect for the client's needs and values, empathy, and involvement in one's own professional growth and development. The tendency of health care professionals to label disabled clients from some ethnic groups as malingerers or poorly motivated can fail to unmask the particular difficulties of individual clients if they have poor language skills, a low level of education, and differences in cultural values, beliefs and norms. Failing to consider the life circumstances surrounding a client's ill-health or disability may lead to both inappropriate intervention and misinterpretation of its effectiveness (Tebbutt & Wade 1985, Wieringa & McColl 1987).

The covert framework, which many occupational therapists do not realise they use in practice, is that which stems from personal experience. This may be formed from the therapist's nationality, gender, religion and socioeco-

nomic stratum, but it also includes family background, education, including professional training, the media to which she has been exposed and the people with whom she has mixed.

If culture is reduced to merely race and ethnicity, then an occupational therapist's perception of a client may relate to his ethnic group rather than to him as an individual, and it will probably be biased. Occupational therapists have, therefore, to examine their own values and beliefs before they can explore those of others (Hinojosa & Kramer 1992). While working in India, S. E. Ryan felt he was constantly challenged to examine his own values, beliefs and patterns of behaviour (Ryan & Tuli 1994).

If occupational therapists are to offer culturally sensitive therapy, they must be able to understand clients in the context of their physical and social environments and in a social, economic and historical perspective. This ability implies knowledge about different cultures, as well as learning at a personal level regarding one's own beliefs and values and those of others. The latter development occurs through interaction between individuals from different backgrounds.

The expectations of the occupational therapist and client should match, therefore there should be joint planning of treatment goals.

Student training

Students have usually had limited exposure to individuals from different backgrounds. They should be prepared for sociocultural diversity in treatment. Students can learn at a personal, empathic level through reflective practice and interaction with individuals from different backgrounds. Sociocultural diversity in treatment can be effective in helping students to discover the pervasive effect of culture on occupational therapy intervention, while avoiding an ethnocentric approach.

Students can learn in a cognitive manner, but more importantly, they can learn at first-hand that many of their perceptions, fears and biases related to people of other cultural and socioeconomic backgrounds are based on a lack of knowledge or incorrect information. The more one knows, the more one finds out how much one does not know. This insight, coupled with the experience of exploring a new and perhaps rather uncomfortable social environment, should make the students more sensitive to their clients' needs and more confident in approaching new challenges in their practice as occupational therapists.

The educational content of student training should relate to sociocultural factors and their effect on practice (American Occupational Therapy Association 1991) so that students are able to collaborate with families and other professionals.

Occupational therapy education should address demography, the exploration of students' own cultural backgrounds and broad issues related to occupational therapy intervention. These should include:

- cultural influences
- access and willingness to use health care services
- assessment in occupational therapy
- communication
- joint goal setting with clients
- help-seeking behaviour
- care giving.

The training should take a lifespan perspective, exploring the influence of culture on the performance of daily activities, work, play and leisure in childhood and adolescence, adulthood and old age. It should address the needs of culturally diverse populations as defined by ethnicity, gender, disability, cultural background, socioeconomic status and lifestyle aspects.

The multidisciplinary team

It is important to remember that the occupational therapist is not only concerned with clients but that team relationships are important, and overseas colleagues also may face difficulties in adjusting to local practices. For example, friendly hints on ward procedures can lead to more effective working relationships.

Colleagues from overseas often need extra support from their managers and peers. There can be instances when managers should have a particularly understanding attitude to facilitate adjustment and improve competence in occupational therapists who have immigrated.

Colleagues from overseas are affected by being away from their own culture and by not being able to keep their religious social conventions; for example, the Muslim doctor who finds the long hours of summer daylight difficult during Ramadan or the occupational therapy student whose father expects her to be home in the evenings rather than participating in the clients' disco.

During ward rounds, highlighting or having open discussion about cultural aspects of clients' treatment helps improve awareness and understanding of other team members.

SUMMARY

It is clear that occupational therapists need to be conscientious, sensitive, willing and interested in their interaction with clients. Successful interaction leads to correct assessment, and then an acceptable solution can be found to meet treatment goals. Recognition of culture as an issue helps therapists to develop strategies that lead to satisfying and successful interaction.

Occupational therapists should not view the complex issue of culture simplistically. The latter leads to simplistic assessments and plans, and the outcome of the interaction can be anger and frustration on the part of both the client and the therapist.

Occupational therapists who are successful in their intercultural interactions recognise culture, in its complexity, as a potentially critical factor in their clients' adaptations to life changes and they communicate this awareness and concern, which reinforces one of the basic tenets of occupational therapy, that is, its holistic perspective.

In Western societies there is a long tradition of the separation of mind, body and society, of treating them as separate entities, when in fact they are merely strands in the same fabric and no single strand is, or reflects, the whole. The same applies to cultures in multicultural societies: no single culture, whatever the magnitude of its impact, reflects the whole.

Clients have a right to keep their culture and identity and these should be respected by the occupational therapist.

REFERENCES

American Occupational Therapy Association 1991 Essentials and guidelines for an accredited educational program for the occupational therapist. American Journal of Occupational Therapy 45: 1077–1084

Blakeney A B 1987 Appalachian values: implications for occupational therapists. Occupational Therapy in Health Care 4: 57–72

Burke A 1986 Racism, prejudice and mental illness. In: Cox J (ed) Transcultural psychiatry. Croom Helm, London

Chan S Q 1990 Early intervention with culturally diverse families of infants and toddlers with disabilities. Infants and Young Children 3: 78–87

Cochrane R 1977 Mental illness in immigrants to England and Wales: an analysis of hospital admissions. Social Psychiatry 12: 5

Cromwell F S (ed) 1987 Sociocultural implications in treatment planning in occupational therapy. Occupational Therapy in Health Care 4: 1

Dillard M, Andonian L, Flores O, Macrae A, Shakir M 1992 Culturally competent occupational therapy in a diversely populated mental health setting. American Journal of Occupational Therapy 46: 721–726

Dyck I 1989 The immigrant client: issues in developing culturally sensitive practice. Canadian Journal of Occupational Therapy 556(5): 248–255

Gregory R L 1972 Eye and brain, the psychology of seeing, 2nd edn. Weidenfeld and Nicholson, London

Harwood A 1981 Ethnicity and medical care. Harvard University Press, Cambridge, Massachusetts

Health and Welfare Canada 1986a Achieving health for all: a framework for health promotion. Department of National Health and Welfare, Ottawa

Health and Welfare Canada 1986b Review of the literature on migrant mental health. Department of National Health and Welfare, Ottawa

Hinojosa J, Kramer P 1994 Defining multiculturalism for occupational therapy. World Federation of Occupational Therapists 11th International Congress, vol 3, 1301–1303

Hume CA 1984 Transcultural aspects of psychiatric rehabilitation. British Journal of Occupational Therapy 47(12): 373–375

Iannone M 1987 Cross cultural investigation of occupational role. Occupational Therapy in Health Care 4: 93–101

Jenkins J H 1988 Conceptions of schizophrenia as a problem of nerves: a cross-cultural comparison of Mexican-Americans and Anglo-Americans. Social Science and Medicine 26: 1233–1244

Kanemoto J S 1987 Cultural implications in treatment of Japanese American patients. Occupational Therapy in Health Care 4: 115–125

Kielhofner G (ed) 1985 A model of human occupation: theory and application. Williams and Wilkins, Baltimore

Kleinman A 1978 Concepts and a model for the comparison of medical systems as cultural systems. Social Science and Medicine 12: 85–93

Kleinman A 1980 Patients and healers in the context of culture. University of California Press, Los Angeles

Kolvin I, Nichol A R 1979 Child psychiatry. In: Granville-Grossman K (ed) Recent advances in clinical psychiatry. Churchill Livingstone, Edinburgh, vol 3

Krefting L, Krefting D 1991 Cultural influences on performance. In: Christiansen C, Baum C (eds) Occupational therapy: overcoming human performance deficits. Slack, New Jersey

Levine R E 1984 The cultural aspects of home care delivery. Occupational Therapy in Health Care 4: 3–16

Lightfoot S 1985 Culture shock in the health context. Australian Occupational Therapy Journal 32: 118–121

Morris D 1977 Manwatching: a field guide to human behaviour. Cape, London

Morse A 1987 A cultural intervention model for developmentally disabled adults: an expanded role for occupational therapy. Occupational Therapy in Health Care 4: 103–114

Mosey A C 1981 Occupational therapy: configuration of a profession. Raven, New York

Peters C 1992 Developing a course in international occupational therapy. Education Special Interest Section, Newsletter 2(4). American Association of Occupational Therapists

Robinson J 1987 Patient compliance in occupational therapy home health programs: sociocultural considerations. Occupational Therapy in Health Care 4: 127–137

Rogers A, Faulkner A 1989 A place of safety. Mind Research, Croydon, Surrey

Ryan S E, Tuli U 1994 Professional and cultural issues: rehabilitation in India. Amar Jyoti Charitable Trust, New Delhi

Swaski K A 1987 Ethnic/racial considerations in occupational therapy: a survey of attitudes. Occupational Therapy in Health Care 4: 37–48

Tebbutt M, Wade B 1985 Frames of reference in the care of migrant patients. Australian Occupational Therapy Journal 32: 91–109

Wieringa N, McColl M 1987 Implications of the model of human occupation for intervention with native Canadians. Occupational Therapy in Health Care 4: 73–91

27

Forensic psychiatry

Alison Rogowski

INTRODUCTION

'Forensic' means 'pertaining to, or connected with, or used in courts of law' (Faulk 1994). Forensic psychiatry describes the specialist area of psychiatry that deals with individuals whose mental illness has brought them into contact with the law or is likely to do so. Forensic psychiatry is practised in special hospitals, regional secure units (RSUs) and prisons. In addition, it is practised within interim units and locked or 'intensive care' wards. The Fallen Report (1999) notes increasing involvement of occupational therapists following up in-patients in the community.

The mentally disordered person who is difficult to care for, formerly cared for in locked wards in local hospitals, is now more often found in special hospitals, regional secure units, prisons, young offenders' institutions or on the streets, often passing from one institution of social control to another. This has happened largely as a result of legislation during the late 1950s, including the Mental Health Act 1959. This period introduced the open door policy and community care. The advent of the use of major tranquillisers played a part in unlocking the doors of previously locked wards. The impact of these changes was felt in the prison medical service, in the special hospitals, in the inception of regional secure units and in the community. As early as 1961, a Ministry of Health report warned of the dangers of dispensing with security precautions in local hospitals. Hospitals without well considered security plans made applications to transfer in-patients to special hospitals more often than those with such plans.

The courts, and parts of the mental health service, have experienced difficulties in finding beds in local psychiatric hospitals for patients with complex mental health needs in conjunction with offending behaviour. Local hospitals are not able to provide an adequate service for those mentally disordered individuals who require care under conditions of some supervision and control but are not sufficiently dangerous to be placed in prisons, special hospitals or regional secure units.

The Glancy Report (DHSS 1974) suggested that in the early 1970s there were 13 000 patients in local hospitals who required some degree of security and whom hospitals wished to transfer to more secure hospitals. At that time, the security provided by local hospitals was neither planned nor therapeutic, simply involving locked doors, the use of seclusion and physical restraint.

Where hospitals have maintained locked wards, they have often not been a part of a well considered security plan but have been caused by staff shortages. It is cheaper and administratively more convenient to lock a door to contain potentially disruptive or absconding patients than to increase staffing levels. Inadequate security in local hospitals has been widely accepted by successive governments as being a problem. So too has the solution: the development of regional secure units.

It would appear that the new millennium will present development opportunities for occupational therapists working in special hospitals, regional secure units and prisons. This chapter will describe the history and background of these three areas in order to explore the different settings in which occupational therapists work as an increasingly vital part of the multidisciplinary team. Aspects of occupational therapy in the forensic psychiatry setting will then be discussed, including working collaboratively with the multidisciplinary team. The characteristics of the patient groups with whom occupational therapists work and the role of the occupational therapist will be examined. Finally, issues of risk assessment are addressed.

THE SETTINGS

SPECIAL HOSPITALS

The three special hospitals in England are Broadmoor Hospital in Berkshire, Rampton Hospital in Nottinghamshire, and Ashworth Hospital in Merseyside which consists of Moss Side Hospital and Park Lane Hospital combined. Carstairs Hospital in Lanarkshire is the equivalent to a special hospital in Scotland and Dundrum Hospital in Dublin serves as a special hospital in Eire. These hospitals provide treatment for psychiatric patients who need to receive care in conditions of maximum security because of their potential dangerousness. The term 'maximum security' has been defined as not less security than that required for the most dangerous category A prisoners (HMSO 1968). The first special hospitals in England were originally administered by the Home Office but all came within the National Health Service (NHS) at its inception in 1948.

The Mental Health Act 1959 made it possible to transfer any psychiatric patient detained on a civil section from an ordinary psychiatric hospital to any special hospital on the grounds of dangerousness. This arrangement thus allowed non-offender patients to be transferred to a special hospital. In reality, there are now very few such patients, especially in the light of the new contracting agreements (Mee, personal communication, 1995).

Since 1989, the special hospitals have been managed by the Special Hospitals Service Authority (SHSA). The SHSA has been directly accountable to the Secretary of State for Health and funded separately from other National Health Service secure psychiatric facilities through a central allocation from the Department of Health. The SHSA has implemented a major programme of change in the special hospitals service. It focused principally on improving the level and quality of patient care, bringing the special hospitals more closely into line with the wider NHS and forging links with the NHS and other, related services.

Organisation of high security psychiatric services

In 1995, a statement was issued by the Department of Health regarding future changes in the management and funding of the services provided by Ashworth, Broadmoor and Rampton Special Hospitals. These new arrangements have aimed to integrate the special hospitals more closely with other mainstream NHS mental health services. This will help to reduce the isolation of special hospitals and will remove financial and organisational barriers which have impeded the movement of patients through services in relation to their clinical and security needs. These changes will ultimately facilitate the development of services for patients who need longer-term care at lower levels of security than are currently offered by the special hospital service.

The government is making the legislative changes necessary to allow the high security hospitals to be managed by NHS Trusts. This will promote better integration of high secure services into the wider NHS and extend the range of clinical provision available to those who need mental health care within a secure setting (Broadmoor Hospital communication, 1999).

Security and treatment in special hospitals

As places of maximum security, special hospitals aim to prevent patients from absconding. Thus, physical security includes a perimeter wall or fence, surveillance cameras and routines of locking doors and checking on patient movements which are rigorously adhered to. Within these restrictions, the hospitals endeavour to incorporate all contemporary mental health assessment, treatment and management techniques and procedures. The hospitals are staffed by psychiatrists, nurses, psychologists, social workers, technical instructors (previously called occupations officers) and, more recently, occupational therapists and creative therapists. Because of the historical link with the Home Office, many nurses previously belonged to the Prison Officers' Association, however, membership of other unions, including the Royal College of Nursing and Unison, is currently growing. There is a higher staff-to-patient ratio than at other psychiatric hospitals and there now exists a wide range of therapies, including work related and educational opportunities for in-patients. Occupational therapy students have had successful field-work placements at the special hospitals in recent years (Hirst 1998).

The level of increased expenditure in the special hospitals over the past few years has been remarkable. The three hospitals in England have benefited from a substantial increase in health spending at a time when the NHS has been facing retrenchment and cuts in services. Despite a fall in the number of special hospital patients (from 2028 in 1979 to 1569 by the end of 1984), during the same period the Department of Health and Social Security (DHSS) sanctioned a rapid increase in expenditure, from £15 million to over £40 million. The number of patients stood at just over 1500 in 1995 (NHS Executive 1995). Rampton now holds approximately 450 (Rampton Hospital Authority 1999) and Broadmoor's Chief Executive was quoted as saying that 'even with the highest quality and lowest or fairly competitive prices, I feel this hospital will not have 480 beds in 5 years time.' The Reed Report (DoH and Home Office 1992) recommended that the special hospitals should have between 200 and 250 beds. Much positive change has had to be assimilated by secure hospital staff.

The interests of security and those of treatment sometimes conflict, and reduced security may be a consequence of increased treatment and rehabilitation programmes. It has been suggested that special hospitals should provide flexible security so that patients who need more intensive rehabilitation should be able to have more freedom and greater opportunity for leave or parole for specific purposes, for example shopping, visits or leave with family. Special hospitals are implementing this by introducing systems of parole where some patients have opportunities for greater freedom within the hospital grounds, leave of absence and escorted shopping trips. However, patients rarely have the opportunity to handle money and generally choose their clothes from mail order catalogues.

Patterns of admission

The special hospital system is no longer organised on a national basis with no formal catchment areas. Each special hospital now serves a defined regional catchment area, taking into account a patient's former place of residence. Visiting by friends and family has thus been made slightly easier. For example, from April 1996, Broadmoor Hospital Authority has formed part of the south-east region, covering health authorities in Kent, Surrey, Sussex, Hampshire, the Isle of Wight, Berkshire, Buckinghamshire, Oxfordshire and Northamptonshire.

All special hospitals may admit patients classified under any category of mental disorder but, for historical reasons, each has developed differently. Broadmoor and Park Lane (now Ashworth) used to admit primarily mentally ill and personality disordered patients while both Rampton and Moss Side (now Ashworth) took a significant number of patients with learning disabilities. Rampton now treats patients with a mental illness or personality disorder, mostly from the northern and eastern side of England. In addition it has sole responsibility for providing maximum security services for people with a learning disability for the whole of England and Wales (Rampton Hospital Authority 1999).

Moss Side has, in the past, taken children as young as 11 and 12 years old. Admission to a high security psychiatric hospital can be extremely detrimental to a young person. At Moss Side, young people were removed from family or parent figures, losing most of their contact with other children. They were, at times, subject to seclusion, physical restraint and high doses of drugs, and they suffered the lifelong stigma of having been detained in a special hospital. As a matter of policy, it is wrong to place any child or young person in a special hospital and it has been suggested that only patients over the age of 18 should be eligible for admission (Faulk 1994). By 1985, no patients remained who were below the age of 16.

REGIONAL SECURE UNITS
Provision of regional secure units

The change in mental hospitals from closed, secure institutions to open conditions, which occurred from the 1950s onwards, brought with it an awareness that a small group of patients would not be provided for under the new arrangements. A recommendation in 1961 by the Working Party on Secure Hospitals that regional secure units be provided for these patients met with very little response.

The idea of regional secure units (RSUs) was reintroduced in 1974, in the interim report of the Committee on Mentally Abnormal Offenders, chaired by Lord Butler (Home Office and DHSS 1975). It proposed the urgent provision of secure units in each regional health authority. It was estimated that 2000 beds would be needed nationally. The committee urged the government to finance these units by allocating funds directly from central government. The revised report of the working party on security in NHS psychiatric hospitals, chaired by Dr Glancy (DHSS 1974), was published at about the same time as the interim Butler report. It also recommended the development of RSUs but proposed 1000 beds instead of 2000. RSUs would fill the 'yawning gap' between maximum security and open psychiatric wards to enable further assessment, rehabilitation and risk management to continue while being a smaller adjustment for patients assessed as being able to move towards life in the community after several years inside. It was some 19 years after the DHSS first decided that there was an urgent need for regional secure unit provision that England's first and, until 1983, only regional secure unit, providing 30 of the 60 beds originally planned, opened in the grounds of St Luke's Hospital, Middlesbrough.

RSUs are separate, specially designed units with the exclusive purpose of caring for potentially difficult or dangerous patients. Four kinds of provision have been proposed and developed:

1. large secure units which are purpose-built and take patients from the entire region
2. low secure units, providing a longer time-scale for in-patients still requiring some security

3. smaller units, closely associated with local hospitals, to which they are attached, and with the facility to exchange patients and staff between the unit and the hospital
4. a capability for secure provision in each psychiatric hospital.

These units vary in size from about 30 to 100 beds. Their primary purpose, in each regional health authority, is the assessment and treatment of those patients who are too difficult or dangerous for the open psychiatric hospitals but not in need of the maximum security a special hospital would provide.

Regional secure unit patients

A White Paper on mental illness (DHSS 1975a) made a positive statement about the kind of patient that should be admitted to an RSU: 'Patients who are continuously behaviourally disturbed or who are persistently violent or who are considered a danger to the public, albeit not an immediate one'. The units are intended to admit most types of patient: offenders and non-offenders, male and female, in-patients, outpatients, patients being assessed for the courts, adults and adolescents (not below 18 years). There is a small amount of provision for adolescents needing secure care, for example the Gardner Unit, Manchester. Due to the much larger ratio of male to female patients and the management difficulties of mixed wards, the needs of women are being reassessed in order to deliver care and treatment more sensitively in conditions of medium security.

RSUs are not intended for individuals with severe learning disabilities. There has been little planning for people with learning disabilities placed in secure provision such as special hospitals until the development in recent years of medium secure facilities.

Treatment and security in regional secure units

RSUs usually aim to keep patients for as short a period as possible (the remit is a maximum of

between 18 months and 2 years) and to have a high turnover of patients, although this is not always the case. In reality, the stay may be a period up to 5 years. RSUs provide medium security. They have the capacity to prevent patients absconding but to a lesser degree than the maximum security special hospitals.

At the same time, RSUs run treatment programmes which include leave outside the unit as the patient progresses. When first admitted, the majority of patients have no leave. As time goes by, and depending on the assessed mental state and behaviour of the individual patient, progress may be made to ground leave. Initially a patient may have ground leave, escorted by two members of staff, who have a hand-controlled radio linked to the staff at the unit (if this is thought necessary, depending on the individual). Then the escort consists of two staff without radio, then one member of staff, then unescorted in the grounds for shorter then longer periods. If the patient's behaviour remains appropriate, as observed on the wards, in therapeutic groups, in individual work and on leave, the patient will then have escorted community leave followed by unescorted freedom of movement into the community. This will build up gradually over time with a carefully planned structure, for example leave for specific purposes, including activities the patient is interested in, such as voluntary work, swimming or shopping for clothes, and will involve longer periods and overnight leave.

RSUs aim to provide a good range of therapeutic facilities within their boundaries. They are highly staffed to provide greater therapeutic efficacy and greater security to reflect the complex needs of the patient group. A conflict or tension can be felt by staff between the functions of therapy and security. The patients will almost invariably be detained under the Mental Health Act 1983 and the majority will have been through, or will go through, the courts.

Patterns of admission

In terms of the total number of patients admitted to psychiatric hospitals in each region, RSUs admit only a small percentage. This number consists of those patients whose management may be causing considerable anxiety or difficulty who have been referred from open psychiatric hospitals. Some individuals will be admitted from the community where their behaviour has caused concern. Others are admitted from prison. Individuals may have been ill at the time of the offence or become ill in the remand or convicted prison setting. Some patients will be admitted from special hospitals, having undergone rigorous assessment from the special hospital setting and from the receiving RSU setting.

PRISONS

Types of prison

The penal system is divided into two types of facilities: those for prisoners on remand (awaiting trial) and those for convicted offenders. The system is currently segregated into male and female prisons. There are prisons for adults over 21 years and young offenders' settings for individuals aged between 17 and 21 years.

While on remand, the prisoner has several rights which are lost if he is subsequently convicted. For example, inmates may wear their own clothes and visitors are permitted at frequent intervals. If convicted, however, the imprisoned offender is placed in an institution with security appropriate to the individual. This will vary from category A prisons to category D prisons. Category A presents conditions of highest security, for example housing terrorists. Category D prisons are open prisons which often house people serving a life sentence. Prison clothes must be worn, for example, trousers and a striped shirt. Visitors are restricted and prison rules apply, governing discipline and management.

Prison inmates

Inmates requiring psychiatric intervention are a diverse group. Their characteristics often include: poor work records, failed relationships, impoverished social and interpersonal skills, lack of structure in their lives, and lack of satisfy-

ing roles and habits. They are often materially impoverished, have little or no family and may have come into prison as a result of poor adjustment to life within the community.

It is worth remembering that the vast majority of inmates will be released. This has implications for the future. There is the need to consider whether and how an individual will have changed. Will he have had the opportunity for reflection, self-analysis, growth and change, or will he emerge angry and embittered against society, ready to reoffend in the vulnerable weeks after release?

Health care for prisoners

The total health care of prisoners is the responsibility of the Prison Medical Service. This service consists of some 100 doctors employed by the Home Office to work full time in the penal system. They are complemented by a similar number of practitioners employed to work on a sessional basis within the prisons.

The prison medical officer is based in the prison health care centre. This consists of either a new building or a converted wing of the prison. This provides some, but not all, of the facilities of a hospital. Its purpose is to care for the physically and mentally ill until they recover or can be transferred to NHS hospital care under section. However, some mentally ill individuals do not meet the criteria of the Mental Health Act 1983 for admission to an NHS hospital. These people will remain in the prison health care centre or on the wings.

These health care centres are not recognised as hospitals within the Mental Health Act 1983. Prison doctors are therefore currently unable to treat any patient against his will except in certain emergencies. Floridly psychotic patients may have to remain untreated for many months unless they are willing to cooperate with treatment or their condition deteriorates to the extent that treatment becomes imperative. This situation is far from ideal and is in need of review.

If a convicted prisoner becomes mentally disturbed then this will be brought to the attention of the prison doctor who, depending on the degree of disturbance, may arrange transfer to the prison health care centre for further observation. If a serious mental disturbance is diagnosed, requiring treatment in a psychiatric hospital, the prison doctor will make a recommendation that the prisoner be transferred to an NHS hospital. In practice, prisons often find considerable difficulty in obtaining a bed in an NHS hospital. The difficulty is centred around the anxiety of psychiatric hospitals regarding the possible danger posed by the inmate. Other, very real, concerns that hospitals face in accepting mentally disordered prisoners are: low numbers of staff, the difficulties staff are likely to encounter in terms of treatment and management of such patients, and the inability of hospitals to prevent absconding.

Prisoners who become mentally ill will sometimes be transferred to a regional secure unit following assessment of need. This may be to provide a comprehensive multidisciplinary team assessment and review of medication of an individual who has become depressed, suicidal or psychotic. Individuals may go back to serve their remaining sentence in prison after this or, if on remand, may be transferred to the RSU until their earliest date of release (EDR) following recommendations by their responsible medical officer (RMO) and a court diversion.

Many inmates with mental disorder are treated in prison by the prison medical officer or by visiting psychiatrists employed on a sessional basis. Minor disorders can be treated in the local prison hospital but there are also specialised prisons and wings which concentrate on treating particular disorders. For example, Grendon prison has a therapeutic community treatment programme for psychopathic disorders as well as a wing for psychotic offenders. C wing in Parkhurst prison runs a programme for inmates with severe personality problems and Feltham Youth Custody Centre specialises in the care of psychiatrically disordered young adults.

Due to new government initiatives recommending that the standard of health care for prisoners should be made similar to that in the NHS in general, another opportunity is presented for focus on the value of occupational therapy input in prison.

OCCUPATIONAL THERAPY AND FORENSIC PSYCHIATRY

Working with the multidisciplinary team

The Department of Health and Social Security (1975a) strongly encouraged the adoption of a multidisciplinary approach in regional secure units, prior to their inception. The skills necessary for the treatment and resocialisation of mentally disordered offenders who require a degree of security require a multifaceted approach of psychiatric nursing, medicine, psychology and occupational therapy.

Creative therapies, including art, music and drama therapy, are sometimes available, as well as adult education. Physiotherapy is included in some secure units. Social work interventions are provided from admission and, in conjunction with medical and community psychiatric nurse follow-up, after discharge. Occupational therapy has begun to be seen as an important area of follow-up from some RSUs. Lloyd (1995a) has commented on the tensions and conflict that can arise regarding roles and role overlap in this setting. It is important to be clear about core skills and interdisciplinary work and to build strong collaborative relationships within the multidisciplinary team in order that the patient may gain maximum benefit from a variety of perspectives on his assessment and treatment.

This is also the case within the special hospitals. Existing technical staff, who have worked at the hospitals for years, may feel threatened by the employment of occupational therapists, particularly as they see some similarities in the work they undertake. Some technical instructors are beginning to appreciate the differences in the skills that occupational therapists bring to the work. However, some have taken the option to undertake in-service training as occupational therapists and some occupational therapists have deliberately highlighted the difference in approach by undertaking different interventions.

Work in prisons may involve a clash of culture and philosophies for occupational therapists who come from a therapeutic background and some (but not all) prison officers who come from a security/punishment philosophy.

Treatment approaches

All the traditional approaches used in other areas of mental health are used in forensic psychiatry. Thus, the medical model and behavioural, developmental, psychodynamic and cognitive approaches are used in special hospitals and RSUs. In prison hospital settings, the medical model (Box 27.1) is in use. While the behavioural approach could be relevant, there would be practical difficulties in using behavioural techniques, given the environment. The psychodynamic approach is also used, for example via individual psychotherapy interventions. This approach is used more comprehensively in some prisons than others. Grendon prison, for example, is established on psychodynamic lines. Other prisons may use this approach to a greater or lesser degree, dependent on the number of psychologists, counsellors and psychotherapists employed.

Apart from these traditional approaches, examples of appropriate occupational therapy models underpinning practice include:

- adaptation through occupation (Reed & Sanderson 1983)
- the model of human occupation (Kielhofner & Burke 1980)
- activities therapy (Mosey 1973, 1978)
- sensory integration (Ayres 1968)
- cognitive disability (Allen 1982, 1985)
- occupational behaviour (Reilly 1974)
- activities health (Cynkin & Robinson 1990).

Lloyd (1995b) has argued that the model of human occupation provides useful theoretical underpinning to the work of forensic occupational therapists. Assessments based on this model may prove valuable, for example the Occupational Case Analysis Interview and Rating Scale (OCAIRS) (Kaplan & Kielhofner 1989) and the interest check-list (Matsutsuyu 1969, Kielhofner & Neville 1983).

OCAIRS is being replaced by new assessments, including the Occupational Performance History Interview II (OPHI II) and the Assessment of Communication and Interaction Skills (ACIS) which can be used, for example, as an integral part of the assessment of a practical session for a small number of inmates, such as a cooking group or art and craft activity group. It is also possible to respond to the needs of the individual with a genuinely eclectic approach, using several models to treat individuals in a specific setting (Creek 1990). This means having a well grounded knowledge of the theory base of each model and

---

Box 27.1   The medical model

Occupational therapists need to have an awareness of these diagnoses and knowledge regarding how these impact on function. As a result of this, coping mechanisms can be taught.

Functional psychosis and neurosis

The functional psychoses are classified by the tenth revision of the International Classification of Diseases (ICD10) (WHO 1992) into:

- schizophrenic disorders
- affective psychoses
- paranoid states
- other non-organic psychoses (which are largely attributed to recent life stresses)

Organic brain disorders

- dementia

- delirium (confusional state)
- epilepsy and its associated psychiatric conditions
- organic personality syndromes
- organic psychosis
  — organic delusional syndrome
  — organic hallucinations
  — organic affective syndrome
- substance-induced organic disorders
- amnesic syndrome

Psychopathic disorders

Clinical features of a psychopathic disorder:

- antisocial personality or personality disorder with predominantly sociopathic or asocial manifestations
- borderline personality
- explosive personality
- sexual sadism and paedophilia

a thorough understanding of how each model could be applied, as well as having undertaken a critical analysis of which models will be helpful in any given clinical setting.

All these occupational therapy models would be relevant in the prison health care setting for the needs of individuals but will need careful thought regarding the influence of the security restrictions and the often high turnover of patients in prison hospital settings (Rogowski & Fowler 1995a).

THE ROLE OF THE OCCUPATIONAL THERAPIST

OCCUPATIONAL THERAPY IN SPECIAL HOSPITALS

The first special hospital to employ an occupational therapist in the UK was the state hospital at Carstairs, Scotland, in 1991. Before then it had employed occupations officers (now technical instructors) whose role it was to occupy patients throughout the day in various different activity areas. These areas tended to concentrate on specific vocational activities, such as book-binding. While these areas provided the opportunity to learn certain skills and fostered work habits, the input was in the style of diversional or industrial therapy rather than having an occupational therapy approach.

In recent years, occupational therapists have been recruited as managers and clinicians within special hospital settings in order to provide a theoretical framework and to implement occupational therapy practice using a critical mass of occupational therapists to influence change. The skills of occupational therapists are acknowledged as a necessary and important aspect of the habilitation and rehabilitation of the mentally disordered offender. This is because of occupational therapy's focus on: assessment, individual goal setting in collaboration with the individual, functional and daily living, quality of life, and preparation for possible return to the community. The occupational therapist also highlights temporal adaptation (or the use of time) and the health giving balance of activities of self-care, rest, productivity and leisure.

The latter is a vital part of the rehabilitation of the mentally disordered offender. In an age of high unemployment, with the double stigma of being mentally ill and an offender, it is unlikely that more than a few individuals will gain paid employment. These few are usually well motivated, with social and life skills and a previous positive work history. The development of skills to use leisure time constructively is imperative to increase quality of life and prevent relapse and recidivism.

The danger of institutionalisation

There is a very real danger of institutionalisation in special hospitals. The high security environment and high staff-to-patient ratio may contribute to institutional dependence. The prospect of institutionalisation may be heightened where there is a high proportion of long-term chronic patients.

Over 50% of the residents of special hospitals have been detained in a special hospital for over 5 years and 5% have been detained for 20 years or more (Faulk 1994). However, every year Rampton Hospital discharges about 80 patients. Sixty percent of these transfer to other NHS health care services and about 40% go back to prison (Rampton Hospital Authority 1999). Once a person enters a special hospital, the effects on his life are profound and, arguably, worse than admission to a prison or to any other institution. Patients are detained for psychiatric assessment and intervention. If a patient admitted from prison recovers, he will be returned to prison to serve the rest of his sentence unless it is felt by the team to be detrimental to his mental health. Individuals who have committed similar crimes are sometimes detained for varying lengths of time. The stigma is enormous and continuing and they may receive treatment against their will. However, individuals have the same access to mental health tribunals as patients in open psychiatric hospitals.

Before the 1980s it would have been difficult to find many ex-special hospital patients who claimed that their time at a special hospital was a therapeutic or useful experience (Cohen 1981). This situation is changing, following the recognition that individual patients' needs must be addressed, as highlighted in various reports on the special hospitals in recent years.

Rehabilitation

The majority of patients will be rehabilitated, that is, prepared for their return to less secure conditions and, eventually, to open mental health settings or other settings within the community, such as landlady accommodation or a staffed hostel. Rehabilitation is the process of enabling a patient to develop or retain competence to live in the community. Rehabilitation (from the Latin root *habilis*, meaning to invest again with dignity) is the greatest single challenge to staff in the special hospital system. The concept of rehabilitation requires mental health professionals to make an assessment of how a patient will react under increasingly less secure and less controlled conditions. There is a whole variety of tasks, activities and relationships which the patient must have the opportunity of coming to terms with if he is to be discharged or transferred as a more integrated, confident person. These range from practical skills such as shopping, budgeting and making everyday decisions to how to relate to friends, family, the opposite sex and other people in the community.

Given the previous catchment areas of special hospitals, rehabilitation has been difficult to achieve. An individual may have been detained hundreds of miles from the community where he will live when he is discharged and could easily lose contact with those people who might have been the most important in helping him to rebuild his life. This situation has improved somewhat as the special hospitals now have circumscribed catchment areas. Social workers do their utmost to ensure contact with families and friends, where it is appropriate and beneficial to all parties concerned.

Because special hospitals must be secure enough to contain the most determined absconders and the most dangerous people, it is only possible to give patients a certain amount of freedom and autonomy. The environment of the special hospitals is necessarily restrictive for the patient.

This regime may not ultimately best protect the public because there is relatively little opportunity to assess how patients will react to more autonomy and freedom or, for example, how a patient might react to alcohol or to relationships with the opposite sex. The multidisciplinary team can have little idea about how someone will behave outside the restrictive confines of the special hospital. This means that a highly controlled psychopath may seem reasonably safe inside a special hospital but may be dangerous or may relapse when transferred to the open conditions of a local hospital or discharged into the community with little or no supervision or after-care. Currently, risk assessments are undertaken to assist clinical teams to make these decisions and rehabilitation trips are being undertaken more frequently into the community as part of treatment.

In addition, awareness of the need for community care has been highlighted. Section 117 of the Mental Health Act 1983 and the Care Programme Approach (CPA), originating from the National Health Service and Community Care Act (1990), both address follow-up care for discharged inpatients.

Changes in approach and attitude to rehabilitation

Prior to the setting up of the Special Hospitals Service Authority (SHSA) in 1989, there had been a distrust within special hospitals of the concept of rehabilitation which was referred to by almost every report dealing with them. For example, the NHS Hospital Advisory Service report on Broadmoor (DHSS 1975b) stated, 'it is a fact that Broadmoor staff in general view rehabilitation with some suspicion. They equate it with certain policies which are welcome in an open hospital but which are incompatible with Broadmoor.' The report concluded that there is 'no evidence of a coordinated rehabilitation policy for the hospital'. The Elliott (1973) and Boynton reports (DHSS 1980) on Rampton came to very similar conclusions. Hamilton (1985) also showed concern:

'Criticisms made by the Elliott Report on Rampton in 1973 and the Hospital Advisory Service on Broadmoor in 1975 on the lack of effective rehabilitation policies are to a large extent unanswered.' The Trent Regional Health Authority (DHSS 1982) and the Rampton Review Board (DHSS 1980) also expressed reservations about the priority given to rehabilitation at Rampton.

However, following the inception of the SHSA, one of its first priorities was to appoint a director of rehabilitation in each of the special hospitals in order to bring about a much needed focus on rehabilitation. Since then, there have been significant changes in the approach to rehabilitation including the introduction of a range of specialist therapies, in particular occupational therapy.

OCCUPATIONAL THERAPY IN REGIONAL SECURE UNITS

It is worth asking the question, is forensic mental health really a specialism or another area of mental health work where the same skills, expertise and knowledge are used?

Occupational therapists have worked in RSUs since their inception. The role of occupational therapists in a forensic setting is essentially the same as their role in any other mental health setting. Thus, the occupational therapy process involves assessment, collaborative goal setting, group and individual intervention and evaluation. The only differences are the special awareness and consideration required regarding issues of security in relationship to therapy and concerning some very specific interventions for example, with sex offender groups. Risk assessment is an important issue but this has been an increasingly important area in mental health generally. The role of the occupational therapist in regional secure units is illustrated by the following case study of a psychotic patient admitted to an RSU.

Case example

Mental state

On admission to the RSU Alan was acutely psychotic, displaying inappropriate responses to conversation, laughing, smiling and talking to himself. His speech was aggressive and the content was delusional. He experienced flight of ideas and evidenced paranoid thinking. He felt persecuted. He thought the television was broadcasting programmes about him and lacked insight into his illness, taking little responsibility for his actions.

He remained orientated in time, place and person at all times and was aware of his environment. He was aware of people and events in the unit. His mood and behaviour were unstable and changeable and he was uncooperative, verbally abusive and disorganised within the structure of the unit.

Physical state

He had not taken care of his appearance and had few clothes. Overall, his appearance was one of neglect. His personal hygiene was poor and needed prompting and supervision. A dental appointment was noted as necessary at a late stage in admission. His diet was also poor and he tended to eat very little. He was unwilling to eat with the others in the dining room.

Alan had difficulty in sleeping and was prescribed medication. His routine was upside-down, being up in the night, agitated and restless, and sleeping during the day.

Medication and physical tests

Alan suffered with low blood pressure, thought to be caused by chlorpromazine. This was changed to thioridazine and his blood pressure was monitored with no further incidents or adverse reactions. Routine blood tests were taken, with some persuasion from staff, and came within the normal range. A routine urine test proved normal and physical examination showed no abnormalities.

Social situation

Alan was admitted from prison where little contact had been made with his family. He had a long previous psychiatric history and, in recent years, dealings with the police. He had had many problems with short-lived relationships, lack of ability to hold down a job and a generally chaotic lifestyle with an inability to retain stability in these areas for any length of time. In addition, he had problems with substance misuse.

Management

This presented a few problems for the team. Alan smoked heavily and would often smoke lying in bed, in spite of requests not to do so, thus presenting a fire risk. He also wrote on the walls of the dining room. Following disturbed behaviour he spent a 2-week period in the intensive care area (ICA) until he was more able to concentrate and able to take care of ward property. The medication regime was monitored for its effect.

Occupational therapy assessment and intervention

Following thorough reading of the occupational therapy notes from previous admissions, and discussions with the occupational therapist from the prison Alan was admitted from, the occupational therapist met with Alan to start the initial assessment process. As a result of assessment, a very low-key occupational therapy programme was implemented in order to: continue to form a rapport with his named occupational therapist, begin to structure Alan's time, have opportunities for continued assessment, gather data through observation and encourage engagement in a therapeutic programme. Alan was unable to participate in deciding upon his occupational therapy programme of groups in collaboration with his named occupational therapist in the initial stages of admission, due to his mental state. Initial assessment and treatment included 15-minute periods with his named occupational therapist in the intensive care area. This low-key programme was aimed at improving his concentration and providing a routine and structure to the days, in an attempt to meet his needs and match his abilities at this time.

Alan was encouraged to pursue his interests which included using an exercise bicycle, writing, drawing and other art work, and going for walks, initially in the enclosed garden area until he obtained leave. Self-care and daily living skills also required assessment and intervention, working mainly on a one-to-one level in conjunction with nursing colleagues.

As Alan's mental state improved, the occupational therapist was able to use structured methods of data gathering via specific occupational therapy assessments based on the model of human occupation (Kielhofner 1995) and use this information to review Alan's programme, now in collaboration with Alan. He was able to take a more active part in group activities, including sports in the gym area.

Alan's programme became more balanced, incorporating both group and individual work. Group interventions now included: an activity group, woodwork, a current affairs and discussion group, a music group, a social group, a drug and alcohol group, a support group and others. The occupational therapists were aware that Alan enjoyed creative work and, after discussion with him, referred him to the art therapist. Individual work, at this stage, involved completion of a domestic assessment followed by a course of domestic training to meet identified needs, including budgeting.

Emphasis on social interaction skills became more appropriate at a later stage in treatment and Alan began to take part in more groups whose purpose was the exploration and development of these skills, including social skills, assertiveness and self-awareness. Alan's emotional life also needed to be addressed. He engaged in a course of closed psychodrama groups. Individual work concentrated on a specific agreed number of anger management sessions at this time.

Evaluation

Since admission there had been a noticeable improvement in Alan's mental state. He settled into a routine and there remained no evidence of psychotic thinking except very occasional references to the television.

Alan began to take an active interest in self-care and to manage daily living skills, the ward routine and his therapeutic programme with only minimal prompting. He benefited from the security and stability in the unit which met his basic needs, made him feel safe and supported and also enabled him to develop considerably. He made constructive use of his time and his interactions with staff and patients became more appropriate. His medication also proved beneficial. However, he had to take medication to counteract the side-effects of medication. In the past he had been given follow-up support on many occasions by community psychiatric nurses and social workers and had failed to cooperate, leading to frequent admissions and, over the past 5 years, criminal offences, usually as a result of the need to obtain illegal substances to misuse.

Looking through his extensive past psychiatric history, there was evidence that he suffered from recurring psychotic episodes. It was unrealistic to think that Alan would be able to live independently in the community without follow-up support and medication.

At this stage, Alan became involved in one-to-one patient education regarding his illness with the ward doctor, followed up by a group run by medical staff, occupational therapists and nurses in which the emphasis was on recognising symptoms as a common problem, obtaining self-knowledge and taking responsibility for recognising signs of illness in order to prevent relapse. He was also given guidance regarding the importance of activity, structured use of time and coping strategies in the prevention of future break-down. Alan was transferred from the acute to the rehabilitation ward after about 11 months. His leave status was reviewed as the treatment process progressed, increasing to full unescorted community leave to engage in specific interests, including sport in local community centres. He continued to participate in a full occupational therapy programme of groups that met the goals he had highlighted with the occupational therapist following the use of Occupational Performance History Assessment (OPHI II) and the Self-Assessment of Occupational Functioning (SAOF) (Baron &

Curtis 1990). As discharge drew nearer, the emphasis shifted to encouraging independent living and working together to analyse Alan's balance of occupations, habits and roles. To facilitate this, the Role Checklist was used (Oakley et al 1986). To enable ongoing support regarding substance misuse prior to discharge. Alan started attending Narcotics Anonymous (NA) meetings, a self-help group that became an ongoing source of strength and hope.

The occupational therapist continued to liaise with the multidisciplinary team in order to ensure that all team members were aware of the aims of occupational therapy intervention and the treatment plan in order to support the team working together to the same ends.

Alan was subsequently transferred to an open rehabilitation ward, under Section 37 of the Mental Health Act 1983, with full community leave. Later he moved to a group home. Support from the community psychiatric nurse, occupational therapist, social worker and responsible medical officer was maintained, with a facility available for self-referral for admission to hospital if necessary. He then remained under this section of the Mental Health Act for approximately 2 years, with one readmission.

OCCUPATIONAL THERAPY IN PRISONS

About half of the prison population at any one time is in need of mental health support. Given a population of 4700 in the 160 prisons in Great Britain this is a significant number (Oliveck 1993). In the light of the Reed Report (DoH and Home Office 1992), purposeful activity has been highlighted as an important part of a prisoner's sentence. It has been acknowledged that occupational therapists are trained in this area and could be usefully employed in prison health care settings. However, there has been no overall strategy to implement occupational therapy in prison hospital wings nationwide (James & Rogowski 1994). This situation is expected to change, given the recent government focus on quality of care in prisons when compared with mainstream health care services.

There have been several pilot schemes to provide occupational therapy in prison health care settings, for example in Birmingham and Bristol (Rogowski & Fowler 1995b). The number of prisons that contract occupational therapists to work as part of the wider mental health service is growing and includes Brixton, Crumlin Road (Belfast) and Maghaberry (Moira). A service is also provided in Manchester. These examples still demonstrate a piecemeal approach of individual initiatives but, encouragingly, a study day for occupational therapists working in prisons, held at the College of Occupational Therapists in 1998, was attended by 20 therapists.

The client group is diverse (some of the index offences for which prisoners will have been convicted are shown in Box 27.2). Prisoners are either remanded or sentenced. Most have no wish to be in prison although some seem to prefer the structure that prison offers to the uncertainty of the length of time spent in a regional secure unit. Some individuals seem to like the

---

Box 27.2 Index offences

Index offences or crimes are often referred to and it is important for the occupational therapist to be aware of these. The following headings cover the most common offences.
Offences against property include two types:
- acquisitive offences (e.g. burglary)
- destructive offences (e.g. arson)

  Offences against the person: the most common are:
- homicide
Unlawful homicide includes:
— murder
— manslaughter
— infanticide
- death of infants

Assault
This group of offences includes:
— wounding
— assaults, divided into: grievous bodily harm; actual bodily harm; common assault; assaulting a policeman
- driving offences
- sexual offences include:
— rape
— indecent assault on a male, female or child
— indecent exposure
- armed robbery
- non-accidental injury to children

---

security that being locked in prison appears to provide them. Prisoners are an unstable population who may be transferred to other prisons at any time. This means that the occupational therapist may only have access to treating them for a short time. Although there are exceptions to this, providing opportunities to develop therapeutic relationships does take time, therefore, a lot of the work will be in sowing seeds for the future.

Applying occupational therapy

The prerequisites for an occupational therapist working in prison are: having some knowledge of the prison system, gaining the confidence of prison officers and communicating the role of the occupational therapist to others. A high tolerance of frustration and a sense of humour are necessary. Firm professional boundaries are required between staff and inmates. A good management and supervision structure is essential in order to recruit and retain staff and ensure consistent standards. Strong links with colleagues from outside or, preferably, based at the local regional secure unit are all important, as is awareness of the limitations of what can be achieved.

The occupational therapy assessment skills that are necessary in the prison setting are of needs, function, dysfunction and potential, followed by the intervention skills needed to address these. Rehabilitation can include life skills training and practice of work, domestic, interpersonal, social and leisure activities in order to increase coping strategies for everyday life when released. Other important interventions include enhancing self-expression and encouraging the application of adaptive behaviour to everyday life. Creative media may be used to facilitate self-awareness and awareness of others. It may also be beneficial to address communication skills.

Farnworth and colleagues (1986) described the work of occupational therapists at a psychiatric unit within a high security prison in Australia. Issues of working with the multidisciplinary team and the difficulties that occupational therapists faced were addressed. These included previous failures which had reduced morale, the prisoners' limited repertoire of coping skills, the fact that the prisoners were a diverse group, and the limitations of the prison environment. The occupational therapy programme consisted of daily activity, recreation, self-development, social interaction, life skills, education and communication skills using video feed-back. Sport and music were also used and were found to be beneficial because they did not need a wide range of verbal skills. Relaxation training and insight-orientated groups were also used successfully.

Challenges for occupational therapists working in prison

Occupational therapy interventions will often need to be short term. Some of the staff working in prison health care settings may be untrained in mental health issues and sometimes lack experience of multidisciplinary work within the prison environment. Staff may feel threatened initially by the presence of other workers (for example the occupational therapist) who may then have a low status in addition to having to work in what is a challenging but can also be an unattractive setting. Resources and facilities for treatment may be poor. However, the skills, perseverance and creativity of occupational therapy staff can usually overcome these potential difficulties, leading to positive and productive relationships with staff and therapeutic gains for prison inmates.

An occupational therapy service in prison could:

- address occupational deprivation (Whiteford 1997, Molineaux & Whiteford 1999 and Whiteford 2000)
- provide treatment opportunities equivalent to those that could be found in an NHS hospital for mentally disordered offenders
- turn doing time into using time (Tumin 1993)
- equip offenders with skills which they lacked before offending
- reverse the negative effects of life in prison
- contribute to a more positive culture.

THE OCCUPATIONAL THERAPIST'S ROLE WITH PEOPLE WITH PERSONALITY DISORDER

The Department of Health and the Home Office are currently reviewing how treatment/care will be organised for the extreme end of this patient group, that is, those with severe personality disorder. It could be argued that occupational therapists have a central role to play in work with this client group, utilising the whole range of skills that an occupational therapist would use in mental health work in relation to assessed need.

RISK ASSESSMENT

Risk assessment has become increasingly important in the light of recent events which have received much publicity at a national level, for example the case of Christopher Clunis (HMSO 1994) and the death of the occupational therapist Georgina Robinson (Blom-Cooper et al 1995). A definition of dangerousness has not been agreed (Faulk 1988, 1994). Dangerousness has been defined by Scott (1977) as 'an unpredictable and untreatable tendency to inflict or risk serious, irreversible injury or destruction or to induce others to do so'. Others have disagreed with the words 'unpredictable and untreatable' (Tidmarsh 1982). The Butler Committee (Home Office and DHSS 1975) described dangerousness as having 'a propensity to cause serious physical injury or lasting psychological harm'.

Risk factors

A number of authors (Scott 1977, Steadman 1983, Gunn 1990, Prins 1991) have identified factors which predispose to and precipitate dangerous behaviour. These include:

- Personality factors: poor impulse control together with a wish for instant gratification; quick temper coupled with the aggressive expression of anger; resorting to violence easily as a coping mechanism or habit
- Social factors: including a deprived upbringing and environment; experience of

abuse, which may have included verbal, physical and/or sexual abuse in the formative years; lack of positive attention or neglect

- Lack of family contact and support; lack of worthwhile activities, employment, recreation and education; thwarted ambition
- Cognitive impairment and brain damage
- Conflict and/or provocation
- Stressful life events combined with poor coping strategies
- Alteration in mental state; disinhibition with alcohol, drugs or other substances; the presence of onlookers
- The presence of both weapons and victim.

Occupational therapists working within the forensic psychiatric setting have an important part to play in the assessment, management and treatment of dangerousness. Little is known about the prevalence of violence or other dangerous behaviour within the setting of the occupational therapy department or towards occupational therapy staff. A study examining 'whether inactivity was an important precipitator of patient violence and if so whether engagement in purposeful activity could be used as a means of reducing violence' (Wheatley 1993) clearly demonstrated the importance of engaging in purposeful activity. In addition, evidence from research conducted at Fromeside RSU by psychologists indicated that occupational therapists are very rarely the focus of patient violence when compared with nursing staff (Torpy & Hall 1993).

Prior to assessment and engagement in a therapeutic programme, it is important to consider a number of factors. The occupational therapist should have a complete knowledge of the individual's personal, psychiatric and criminal history in order, for example, to be aware of possible transference to staff. It is crucial to be aware of current factors surrounding the mental state of an individual patient. In addition, the following questions need to be considered:

- Have the main precipitating factors been removed or managed, for example alcohol and/or drugs, disturbed mental state and immediate stress factors such as a difficult relationship with a parent or partner?

- Are there new possible precipitants, such as anger at detention, the presence of other patients or the pressure of court appearances or tribunals?
- Does the patient feel held, supported and nurtured or restricted and persecuted?
- Has the patient insight or does he not consider himself ill and therefore resent being detained?
- Will the context in which the patient is seen have similarities to the context of the original offences?
- Are there possible grounds for transference to the therapist or other group members, including age, gender, race, cultural background or personality type?
- Has the patient been very isolated, for example with a diagnosis of schizophrenia in prison? Will he therefore find the presence of others on a busy admission ward disturbing and difficult?
- Does the therapist feel safe with the patient?
- Prior to engaging the patient in purposeful activity, has careful thought been given to realistic goals/objectives in collaboration with the patient, taking into account instant gratification, age-appropriateness, purposefulness and attractiveness of activities?
- Are there objects/equipment which could be used as weapons?
- What limits/boundaries is it appropriate to set?
- Is the therapist aware of the use of self as a therapeutic tool, for example, using humour or positively reframing negative comments towards the individual made by other patients?

The above list is daunting and no question can be answered to complete satisfaction. What is important is that these areas are considered before therapy begins so that risks can be taken with maximum information.

Managing risk

Even in the best managed unit, potentially dangerous situations will arise. The following guidelines are given with regard to the management of such situations:

- Be aware of situations/factors that could be confrontational.
- Use disturbance alarms.
- Be careful in one-to-one situations, especially when out in the community with no staff support.
- Be aware of where you are in the room, for example, by an exit.
- Be aware of the depth at which the conversation is pitched. It may be less appropriate to converse at a deep level while alone in the community, when strong emotions may be aroused in the patient and the boundaries provided by the unit are not present.
- Use a calm tone of voice and body language, for example minimal arm, head and body movements. Eye contact should be steady but not over-intense.
- Weigh up individual situations; sometimes it may be better to keep some distance between yourself and a patient. At other times it is helpful to get closer and perhaps make appropriate physical contact.

Additional points to consider when working in a group are as follows:

- Be aware of how much attention you are giving each group member and do not include too many patients in the group.
- If another member of staff is not available to act as an escort, consider running the session with fewer patients who are also well known to the therapist and appear very stable, or run the session on the ward instead of the department, or cancel the group. (The last option is obviously a last resort but, if necessary, individual work can be commenced in place of the group intervention.)
- Keep a balance between having patients that the therapist knows well and introducing new patients to the session.
- Be aware of conflict, for example because of negative transference from a specific patient to a specific staff member or between two patients. Decisions must be made regarding whether the patients come to different groups or the group runs with both present or with an extra member

of staff, being aware of where the patients will be sitting.

- Have a minimum amount of dangerous equipment available. In a therapeutic session such as woodwork, tools can be shadow-boarded and must be checked before and after the session, also during the session if a patient wishes to return to the ward. It may be useful to use a tick-box list for checking tools which is objective, auditable and not too time-consuming.
- Management of incidents will involve other members of the multidisciplinary team. This may include the use of time out or control and restraint procedures, that is humane techniques that can be taught to and used by a minimum of three members of staff to restrain the individual, avoiding injury to patient(s) and staff. Medication is sometimes used as required by the situation. Seclusion may be used, but this is a last resort. These interventions are used if verbal or other management of the situation has not proved successful (James & Rogowski 1994).

Long-term strategies

The occupational therapist has a major role to play in reducing an individual's dangerousness in the long term. This is achieved through various therapeutic interventions to enable patients to develop new coping strategies and ways of interacting which decrease the need for immediate gratification. The occupational therapist will need to address anger management, impulse control and provocation in individual and group settings, in appropriate ways. The individual's immediate coping strategies, skills, roles and habits will also benefit from occupational therapy assessment and interventions. The latter include assessment and training in daily living skills, home management, budgeting and money management (including dealing with the Department of Social Security). Specific educational approaches include substance misuse groups which enable the patient to reevaluate misuse of alcohol, drugs or glue.

It is important to improve the patient's ability to gain support from others so that, if required, an individual can verbalise the need for this, rather than acting out in negative and attention-seeking ways. Interpersonal skills will be addressed, together with increasing self-awareness and awareness of others. Social skills and assertiveness may also provide appropriate areas for intervention. Occupational therapists will also involve patients in a variety of activities, including opportunities for education, employment and satisfying use of leisure time. The occupational therapist can help the patient to find an appropriate balance between the activities of self-care, rest, productivity and leisure (Rogowski 1995).

When planning discharge, Prins (1991) recommended that a number of questions should be asked, as follows:

1. Have the past precipitants and stresses been addressed and/or removed or is there further work that needs to be done?
2. What is the patient's current capacity for dealing with provocation?
3. Does the patient now possess a range of strategies for dealing with conflict or is he brittle with a limited range of strategies?
4. What is the patient's current level of self-esteem and self-confidence?
5. Was the patient's behaviour person-specific and is rage still being harboured?
6. Has the patient come to terms with what he did? Does he understand why and how the index offence happened? Does he express remorse?
7. How does the patient react when he does not get what he is asking for/seeking, both immediately or not at all? Is the individual currently pursuing instant gratification or is he able to, for example, save up for something he wants to buy or wait during the time it takes to organise and access opportunities for further education, work or voluntary work options?
8. Lastly, it is crucial to ask what the patient's current attitude is to, and involvement with, disinhibiting substances such as alcohol, glue and drugs.

These questions can be best answered following a combination of assessment, intervention and rigorous observation, during individual and group treatment activities on the ward, in the department and in community settings.

Reduction of dangerousness is an important part of the activity of all those working in the forensic setting and has important implications for work within the clinical setting as well for decisions regarding discharge and aftercare (James & Rogowski 1994).

SUMMARY

The settings for occupational therapy in forensic psychiatry were described at the start of this chapter. Treatment approaches in occupational therapy and working in the multidisciplinary team in this area were then explored.

The role of occupational therapists in special hospitals, regional secure units and prisons was discussed. This was followed by a consideration of risk assessment.

REFERENCES

Allen C K 1982 Independence through activity: the practice of occupational therapy (psychiatry). American Journal of Occupational Therapy 36: 731

Allen C K 1985 Occupational therapy for psychiatric diseases: measurement and management of cognitive disabilities. Little Brown, Boston

Ayres J 1968 Sensory integrative processes and neuropsychological learning disability in learning disorders. Special Child Publication, Seattle, vol 3

Baron K, Curtis C 1990 A manual for use with self-assessment of occupational functioning. Unpublished manuscript. Department of Occupational Therapy, University of Illinois

Blom-Cooper L, Hally H, Murphy E 1995 The falling shadow: one patient's mental health care, 1978–1993. Duckworth, London

Cohen D 1981 Broadmoor. Psychology News Press, London

Creek J (ed) 1990 Occupational therapy and mental health: principles, skills and practice. Churchill Livingstone, Edinburgh

Cynkin S, Robinson A M 1990 Occupational therapy and activities health: towards health through activities. Little Brown, Boston

Department of Health and Home Office 1992 Review of health and social services for mentally disordered offenders and others requiring similar services. (Reed Report) HMSO, London

Department of Health and Social Security 1974 Revised report of the working party on security in National Health Service hospitals. (Glancy Report) (Unpublished)

Department of Health and Social Security 1975a White Paper on mental illness. HMSO, London

Department of Health and Social Security 1975b NHS Hospital Advisory Service report on Broadmoor. HMSO, London

Department of Health and Social Security 1980 Report of the review of Rampton Hospital. HMSO, London

Department of Health and Social Security 1982 The Trent RHA review of Rampton Hospital. HMSO, London

Elliott J 1973 Report on Rampton. HMSO, London

Farnworth L, Morgan S, Fernando B 1986 Prison-based occupational therapy. Australian Journal of Occupational Therapy 34(2): 40–46

Faulk M 1988 Basic forensic psychiatry. Blackwell Scientific, Oxford

Faulk M 1994 Basic forensic psychiatry, 2nd edn. Blackwell Scientific, Oxford

Gunn J 1990 Clinical approaches to the assessment of risks. In: Carson D (ed) Risk taking in mental disorder. SLE Publications, Chichester

Hamilton J R 1985 The special hospitals. In: Gostin L (ed) Secure provision. Tavistock, London

Hirst M 1998 OT student's big challenge. Therapy Weekly

HMSO 1968 Second report session, 1967–68. The special hospitals and the state hospital. HMSO, London

HMSO 1994 Report of the inquiry into the care and treatment of Christopher Clunis. HMSO, London

Home Office and Department of Health and Social Security 1974 Interim report of the committee on mentally abnormal offenders. (interim Butler Report) HMSO, London

Home Office and Department of Health and Social Security 1975 Report of the committee on mentally abnormal offenders. (Butler Committee) HMSO, London

James A, Rogowski A 1994 Working with dangerous patients in occupational therapy. Therapy Weekly (April)

Kaplan K, Kielhofner G 1989 The occupational therapy case analysis interview and rating scale. Slack, Thorofare, New Jersey

Kielhofner G 1995 A model of human occupation: theory and application, 2nd edn. Williams and Wilkins, Baltimore

Kielhofner G, Burke J P 1980 A model of human occupation, part 1. Conceptual framework and content. American Journal of Occupational Therapy 34(9): 572–581

Kielhofner G, Neville A 1983 The modified interest checklist. Unpublished manuscript. University of Illinois, Chicago

Lloyd C 1995a Forensic psychiatry for health professionals. Chapman and Hall, London

Lloyd C 1995b Trends in forensic psychiatry. British Journal of Occupational Therapy 58(5): 209–213

Matsutsuyu J 1969 The interest checklist. American Journal of Occupational Therapy (23): 323–328

Mee J 1995 Personal communication.

Mental Health Act 1959. HMSO, London

Mental Health Act 1983. HMSO, London

Molineaux M, Whiteford G 1999 Prisons: from occupational deprivation to occupational enrichment. Journal of Occupational Science 6(3): 124–130

Mosey A C 1973 Activities therapy. Raven Press, New York

Mosey A C 1978 Behavioural models in occupational therapy. The 7th International Congress of the World Federation of Occupational Therapists, Jerusalem

National Health Service and Community Care Act 1990. HMSO, London

NHS Executive 1995 High security psychiatric services: changes in funding and organisation. Department of Health, London

Oakley F, Kielhofner G, Barris R, Reichler R K 1986 The role checklist: development and empirical assessment of reliability. Occupational Therapy Journal of Research 6: 157–170

Oliveck M 1993 Report of the College of Occupational Therapists' conference on the rehabilitation of mentally disordered offenders. Therapy Weekly (28 Jan 1993)

Prins H 1991 Dangerous people or dangerous situations? Some further thoughts. Medicine, Science and the Law 31(1): 225–237

Rampton Hospital Authority 1999 Annual report.

Reed K L, Sanderson S R 1983 Concepts of occupational therapy, 2nd edn. Williams and Wilkins, Baltimore

Reilly M (ed) 1974 Play as exploratory learning. Sage, Beverley Hills, California

Rogowski A M 1995 College of Occupational Therapists 19th annual conference, 12–14 July 1995, Edinburgh. British Journal of Occupational Therapy 58(8): 356–357

Rogowski A M, Fowler M C 1995a College of Occupational Therapists 19th annual conference, 12–14 July 1995, Edinburgh. British Journal of Occupational Therapy 58(8): 357

Rogowski A M, Fowler M C 1995b OT goes to prison for one year. Occupational Therapy News 5: 12

Scott P D 1977 Assessing dangerousness in criminals. British Journal of Psychiatry 131: 127–142

Steadman H J 1983 Predicting dangerousness among the mentally ill. International Journal of Law and Psychiatry 6: 381–390

Tidmarsh D 1982 Implications from research studies. In: Hamilton J R, Freeman H (eds) Dangerousness: psychiatric assessment and management. Gaskell for the Royal College of Psychiatrists, London

Torpy D, Hall M 1993 Violent incidents in a medium secure unit. British Journal of Psychiatry 4(3): 517–544

Tumin S 1993 H M Chief Inspector of Prisons' report: doing time or using time. HMSO, London

Wheatley E 1993 Inactivity as a precipitator of patient violence towards staff in a forensic psychiatry unit. (Unpublished study)

Whiteford G 1997 Occupational deprivation and incarceration. Journal of Occupational Science; Australia 4(3): 126–130

Whiteford G 2000 Occupational deprivation: global challenge in the new millennium. British Journal of Occupational Therapy 63(5): 192–204

World Health Organization 1992. The ICD-10 classification of mental and behavioural disorder: clinical descriptions and diagnostic guidelines. WHO, Geneva

FURTHER READING

Bluglass R 1992 The special hospitals. British Medical Journal 305(8): 323–324

Broadly Speaking 1996 Issues 51, 52, 53

Chiswick D 1994 High security for mentally disordered people. British Medical Journal 309(8): 423–424

College of Occupational Therapists 1993 Challenges in the rehabilitation of mentally disordered offenders. COT, London

College of Occupational Therapists 1993 The role of occupational therapy in the rehabilitation of the mentally disordered offenders. COT, London

College of Occupational Therapists 1998 Forensic psychiatry. OT Current Awareness Bulletin

Crawford M 1991 Broadmoor: protects society and treats. Therapy Weekly (30 May 1991), p. 5

Department of Health 1992 Health of the nation. HMSO, London

Department of Health 1992 Report of the committee of enquiry into complaints about Ashworth Hospital. HMSO, London, vols 1 and 2

Department of Health 1994 Report of the working group on high security and related psychiatric provision. Department of Health, London

Eaton L 1993 Top security hospitals. Health Service Journal (12 Aug 1993)

Flood B 1993 Implications for occupational therapy services following the Reed Report. British Journal of Occupational Therapy 56(8): 293–294

Gunn J, Taylor P J 1993 Forensic psychiatry: clinical, legal and ethical issues. Butterworth Heinemann, Oxford

Holt J, Hayward H, Mulligan M 1994 The variety of roles of occupational therapists within the three special hospitals. World Federation of Occupational Therapists 11th World Congress, London

Lloyd C 1983 Forensic psychiatry and occupational therapy. British Journal of Occupational Therapy 53(12): 348–350

Lloyd C 1987 The role of occupational therapy in the treatment of the forensic psychiatric patient. Australian Journal of Occupational Therapy 334(11): 20–25

Lloyd C, Guerra F 1988 A vocational rehabilitation programme in forensic psychiatry. British Journal of Occupational Therapy 51(4): 123–126

McConnachie K 2000 The way forward: developing the existing role of OT within the prison service: a therapists' perspective. Final year thesis, Brunel University

Nelson A M, Taylor P, Hawkins B et al 1995 Special Hospitals Service Authority review. SHSA, London

Oliveck M 1993a Care for mentally ill, not prison. Therapy Weekly (28 Jan 1993)

Oliveck M 1993b Cornerstone of rehabilitation is integration. Therapy Weekly (4 Feb 1993)

Report of the review of Rampton Hospital 1980 Boynton report on Rampton. HMSO, London

Shallah D 1993 Can forensic psychiatric services be quality and consumer driven? Journal for Nurses and Other Professionals in Forensic Psychiatry 3: 4–7

Stein E, Brown J D 1991 Group therapy in a forensic setting. Canadian Journal of Psychiatry 12: 18–22

Taki 1990 Nothing to declare: prison memoirs. Viking, London

Therapy Weekly 1993a New report urges better therapy for offenders. Therapy Weekly (7 Jan 1993)

Therapy Weekly 1993b Occupational therapists have key to help offenders. Therapy Weekly (2 Dec 1993)

Whiteford G 2000 Occupational deprivation: global challenge in the new millennium. British Journal of Occupational Therapy 63(5): 192–204

ACKNOWLEDGEMENTS

Michelle Walsh, OT from Broadmoor Hospital who gave advice and kept me updated regarding the exciting developments in the Special Hospitals.

Dr Adrian James, Consultant from Leander Unit, for permission to use information from jointly written and researched papers.

Eileen Pollard and Maggie Moloney for their IT skills.

My Mum and Dad, extended family and friends for their love, interest and support.

Particular thanks go to Robert, Isobel, Matt, Tom and Simon, Liz, Charlie and Elizabeth, Nathan and Mike, Alison and Roger, Helen, Andrew, Henry and Margaret.

Finally, thanks to my husband, Mark, to whom I dedicate this chapter.

28

Substance misuse

John Chacksfield
Jenny Lancaster

INTRODUCTION

This chapter is about an issue that occupational therapists will find themselves facing with an increasing range of client groups in both mental and physical health settings. It is intended as a starting point for occupational therapists interested in the specialism of substance misuse as well as those who work in other areas of mental health and are likely to encounter substance use alongside psychiatric disorder.

The term 'substance use' generally means the ingestion of alcohol or other chemical substances that have the potential to be addictive. 'Substance misuse' refers to any ingestion of alcohol or drugs that is illegal, causes harm to the consumer or other people, or damages society. 'Substance dependence' is a specific diagnostic term describing what is commonly termed 'addiction'.

History and culture

The use of addictive substances has been intertwined with human occupation for a considerable proportion of mankind's history. For example, according to Nunn (1996), archaeological evidence exists for the use of alcohol in Ancient Egypt from as early as 6000 BC. Cannabis and other plant-derived drugs were in use from about 2600 BC, and were employed to heal, to reduce tension and to alter consciousness. A number of famous historical figures, including Alexander the Great, Stalin and Hitler, have been addicted to various substances. Modern examples abound among the glamour of Hollywood and the international music industry. Recently, a well known footballer, Tony Adams, has declared himself an alcoholic (Adams 1998).

Culture mediates views of drugs in terms of how dangerous they are, how legal they should be and how good or bad they are. For example, the Christian, moralist, Temperance movement in 19th-century Britain set out to reduce alcohol consumption (Berridge 1993). At the end of the 19th century, cocaine was highly popular and recommended by doctors such as Sigmund Freud and Sir Clifford Albutt. At the same time, Albutt (cited in Gossop 1993) held a different view of another drug, popular today, as illustrated in a quote from his medical textbook: 'The sufferer is tremulous and loses his self-command, he is subject to fits of agitation and depression. He loses colour and has a haggard appearance. As with other such agents, a renewed dose of the poison gives temporary relief, but at the cost of future misery.' The drug described was coffee.

Many cultures use and have used drugs in social ritual or religious ceremony, to enhance skill in war and for pleasure. In some, the cultivation of drug crops, though often illegal, is a major industry that offers considerable employment opportunities and contributes to the national economy (Henman 1985). Drug profits have been known to drive political movements, such as the suggested use of heroin trafficking by the People's Republic of China to fund Communist Party activities (Musto 1993).

Alcohol has long been considered to be the dominant drug of European culture, whereas in the Americas plant-based drugs unknown in Europe, such as nicotine and cocaine, were widely used for centuries before alcohol was popularised with the coming of immigrants from Europe (Gossop 1993).

Substance misuse from the 18th to the early 20th century was primarily seen as a sin. The drunk and the 'opium sot' were seen as morally degraded. The turn of the 20th century saw this attitude change towards a much more disease-oriented concept that offered a cure. In the 1960s

came the idea of *dependence* as a concept that acknowledged psychological reliance on a drug and, in the 1970s, this was developed into the modern *dependence syndrome*. More recently, social models of substance misuse have been developed that take into account wider cultural, economic and psychological factors.

What this chapter is about

This chapter discusses the nature and extent of substance misuse in the UK. It offers an occupational perspective on why people take drugs and considers the types of problems that the individual drug user may experience. The treatment process is outlined and the role of the occupational therapist highlighted. Three models of intervention are described: the Twelve Steps, the Stages of Change and Relapse Prevention. The chapter finishes with an account of some of the occupational therapy intervention strategies available for problem drug and alcohol users.

SUBSTANCE MISUSE: A GREAT AND GROWING ISSUE

Currently, in the UK, substances misused are generally categorised as either legal or illegal, are subject to restrictions according to age or cultural acceptability, and are either natural plant extracts or manufactured.

Substance misuse, if frequent, is known to lead to problems of a physical, psychological or social nature. Extensive regular use can lead to dependence and to severe dependence, with a range of associated negative consequences (Royal College of Psychiatrists 1987). Most of the results of problem use of substances or dependence on them can be observed in the patterns of human occupation exhibited by the user and their impact on the user's quality of life. Some of these effects are described later in the chapter.

As a result of the growing problems relating to substance misuse, the British government has recently given the issue of drug misuse considerable attention. Recent key documents have outlined their concerns and strategies (HMSO 1995, SO 1998, Institute for the Study of Drug Dependence 1999). In 1997, the first UK anti-drugs coordinator was appointed.

The policy paper *Tackling Drugs to Build a Better Britain* (SO 1998) acknowledged that 'Drug problems do not occur in isolation. They are often tied in with other social problems, for example, poor housing, rough sleeping and school exclusions'. The government has set up the Social Exclusion Unit to address these related social problems. The programme of action outlined in this paper contains two key strategies:

1. to support problem drug misusers in reviewing and changing their behaviour towards more positive lifestyles, linking up where appropriate with accommodation, education and employment services
2. to provide an integrated, effective and efficient response to people with drugs and mental health problems.

It is clear that both substance misuse and dependence are on the increase worldwide, are becoming increasingly widespread among younger people and are to be seen among the mentally ill and physically disabled populations as both causes and consequences of their illness.

The impact of alcohol misuse on society can be illustrated by two statistics (DoH 1999):

- In 1996, 27% of men and 14% of women aged 16 and over were drinking more than the recommended amount (21 units and 14 units respectively). Drinking at these levels among men has remained stable at around 27% since 1986; that of women has risen from 10% to 14% in the same period.
- It is estimated that the annual prevalence rate of alcohol dependence in private households is 75 per 1000 population among men aged 16–64 years and 21 per 1000 population among women in the same age group.

The huge cost to communities caused by illegal drug use gives the issue a high profile in politics and in the media, as the examples below illustrate (Institute for the Study of Drug Dependence 1999):

- the general costs to the criminal justice system of drug-related crime are, at a very conservative estimate, at least £1 billion every year (preliminary results from Drugs Comprehensive Spending Review)
- 32% of the adult population have used an illegal drug at some time in their life but 80% of this group do not continue to use regularly
- the highest prevalence of drug use is found among the unemployed, with 40% reporting drug use within the last year.

Of particular concern are the increase in heroin use among younger people, the 'crack epidemic' and the generation of new 'designer drugs' (such as Ice). These substances are very pure and often act very quickly on the brain, making them far more addictive and far more dangerous in terms of long-lasting effects. Ice, or methamphetamine, is known to induce long-term psychotic effects. Crack is a crystalline form of cocaine that is highly addictive.

Where alcohol and drugs are used by people with mental health diagnoses, they can severely exacerbate symptoms and disrupt treatment. They are associated with disrupted lifestyles, suicide (Duke et al 1994) and violent behaviour (Swanson et al 1990).

What are drugs and other substances?

Drugs and other substances are usually grouped according to psychotropic action or legality.

Drug action

The action of drugs on the human brain determines whether they are considered an opiate, a stimulant, a depressant, a hallucinogen or a minor tranquilliser. Some drugs, such as cannabis, nicotine and volatile inhalants, do not conform to any of these classifications.

It should be noted that drug action and effect can be influenced by: the route of administration, for example smoking, drinking or injecting, personality characteristics of the user, cultural expectations, and the immediate setting and expectations. Taking a drug together with another drug, or taking drugs when mentally ill, can also influence drug action and effect.

Alcohol and drugs act on specific centres of the brain. For example, opiates (e.g. heroin) act on the opiate receptor in areas of the brain such as the limbic system, specifically the nucleus accumbens and the ventral tegmentum (Stellar & Rice 1989). Changing the state of these receptors by using drugs results in pleasurable experiences.

Many drugs are thought to act on the dopamine system. Dopamine is a chemical messenger which plays an important role in the brain's reward centre. It is released when we do pleasurable things, from eating good food to having sex. Drugs such as cocaine and heroin cause a massive surge of dopamine to be released, and this extra dopamine leads to the sensation of pleasure. Over time, repeated drug use can lead to dopamine receptor sites in the brain being reduced or shut down. Therefore, the drug user finds less effect from using a drug, which leads to an increase in the amount used. The other significant effect is that the drug user is likely to experience a decreased ability to feel pleasure or satisfaction in activities of daily life. This can lead to further drug use or thrill seeking activities.

Alcohol has a variety of complex actions but is generally a nervous system depressant. The reason alcohol appears to produce euphoria is that it depresses frontal cortex functioning resulting in loss of inhibition.

Legality

Alcohol is legal for use by people over the age of 18. Nicotine can be used from age 16. Pharmaceutical drugs generally depend on a doctor's prescription (governed by Sections 12–17 of the Misuse of Drugs Act 1979). The legality of other drugs is determined in the UK by the Misuse of Drugs Act (HMSO 1979). This classifies drugs as Class A, Class B or Class C. Each class carries particular penalties for use and supply of the drug.

Table 28.1 illustrates some of the most common substances in terms of legal classification and psychoactivity.

Measurement

Alcohol is measured in units of 10 mg. One unit of alcohol can be found in a single measure of spirits, a glass of wine or a half pint of ordinary strength beer.

Table 28.1 Drugs and substances according to psychoactive quality and legality

	Drug name	Method of consumption	Legal class/status
Stimulants ('uppers')	Nicotine	Smoking in cigarette, cigar, pipe	Legal if aged 16+
	Caffeine	Mixed with hot water	Legal
	Cocaine	Heated and inhaled or smoked	Illegal: Class A
	Crack cocaine	Smoked	Illegal: Class A
	Amphetamines	Tablets or injected	Illegal: Class A
Depressants ('downers')	Alcohol	Oral ingestion via carrier substance	Legal if aged 18+
	Benzodiazepines	Tablet form, oral or injection	Legal if prescribed
Opiates	Heroin	Injected or smoked by heating and inhalation ('chasing the dragon')	Illegal: Class A
Hallucinogenics	Lysergic acid diethylamide (LSD or 'acid')	Manufactured as 'tabs', small squares of paper which are placed on the tongue	Illegal: Class A
	Psilocybin ('magic mushrooms')	Infusion (tea) or smoked after drying	Illegal: Class A if prepared for use, e.g. by drying
	MDMA ('ecstasy')	Tablet form	Illegal: Class A
Other	Cannabis	Resin, dried leaves or flowers	Illegal: Class B

Drugs are also measured in terms of amount purchased or mode of delivery. Heroin, cocaine and cannabis (resin or leaf forms) are generally measured by weight, although for non-cannabis drugs in powder form, the purity of what is purchased is variable according to what the powder has been mixed (or cut) with. LSD and Ecstasy are sold in units or 'tabs'.

Why do people use substances?

People are known to use substances for many and varied reasons (Edwards 1987, Gossop 1993). Alcohol, for example, is widely used as a social lubricant, to reduce tension, to intoxicate as a way of coping with bad feelings or as a sedative. Drugs such as cannabis are used to remove the symptoms of glaucoma, to relax, bring pleasure, alter consciousness or as part of initiation into a social group. Glue sniffing is often commenced as a result of peer pressure or as a consequence of problems in the home (Royal College of Psychiatrists 1987). Heroin use is described as offering a warm, dreamy 'cocoon' and, for many compulsive users, it serves as antidote to emotional pain and the stress of a life lacking in meaning (Tyler 1995).

Reasons for substance use: an occupational perspective

Substance use is often closely tied to human occupational behaviour. It could be said that the most common reasons for the use of substances lie in their ability to either enhance or disrupt human occupation. Some of the reasons for substance use can be categorised under the headings listed below. These reasons can be found applied to almost all substances, including alcohol, nicotine, caffeine and tranquillisers as well as illegal drugs. It is important to note that each individual drug user will have his own very specific reasons and the following list is unlikely to be exhaustive:

Enabling occupation

- by reducing tension
- by removing inhibition

- by stimulating mental alertness
- by imitating others' drug use.

Avoiding occupation

- through intoxication
- through stimulus-seeking via drug use
- through escape into drug culture
- through denial of responsibility by drug use.

As a coping mechanism

- to cope with anxiety
- to relieve or avoid facing pain
- to mask distress
- to increase confidence, peer acceptance
- as self-medication for mental health problems.

To alter perception

- in order to develop wider understanding of life
- for desired spiritual attainment
- as part of religious ritual
- to assist creativity
- because drug-induced perception is considered more pleasant than normality.

To develop meaning in life

- through the ritual of drug-taking behaviour
- through the routine of drug obtaining or dealing activities
- through the excitement of avoiding legal services
- through interacting and sharing a culture with associates in a drug-using network.

To enhance occupation

- by celebrating positive events
- by enhancing good feelings
- by removing negative emotional states.

Applying some of these ideas, using the Human Open System (Kielhofner 1985, 1995), a possible model of their interaction can be constructed (Fig. 28.1).

When does drug use go wrong?

In general, it is likely that most people can regulate their use of alcohol, caffeine and some other drugs

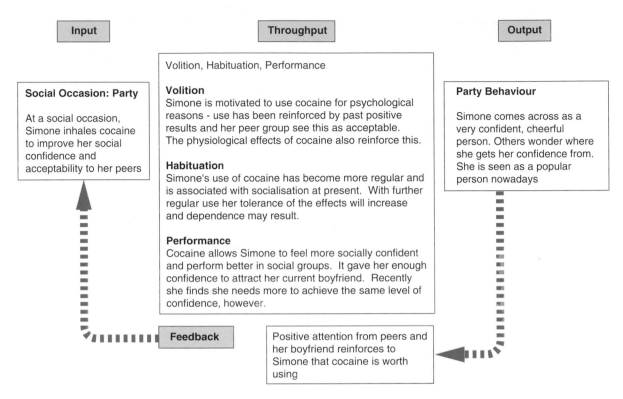

Figure 28.1 Drug use and the Human Open System: an example (all names are fictitious).

without this use leading to damage to themselves, others or their occupational behaviour patterns. However, the use of alcohol and other drugs can and does lead to a considerable range of physical, psychological and social problems.

User surveys reported by the Department of Health (1996) suggest that drug use cannot be tackled in isolation. It is often associated with factors such as unemployment, family break-up and crime. Failure to address the wider life context issues can slow down or reverse progress in treatment of the drug problem itself.

Research has shown that substance users have higher rates of psychiatric disorder than the general population (DoH 1996). Either the disorder may be induced by drug ingestion or drugs can be used to self-medicate the symptoms.

Other studies show that drugs and crime are interlinked (Forshaw & Strang 1993). An American study revealed that violent behaviour is approximately three times more likely in people who both use drugs and have a mental disorder than those who do not suffer either (Swanson et al 1990).

Drugs have been associated with homelessness, sexual abuse and prison populations.

Problems and dependence

Two issues represented in the academic literature on substances are problems and dependence. These are illustrated in Figure 28.2.

The quadrants in Figure 28.2 do not represent distinct categories but each axis lies on a continuum (Drummond 1992):

Sector A: those who experience problems related to non-dependent use (e.g. often young people)
Sector B: a group who experience both dependence and problems (typical in the clinical setting)
Sector C: a group in the population who take a substance but experience neither significant dependence nor problems

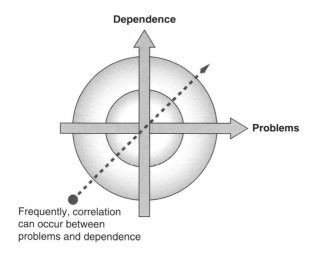

Frequently, correlation
can occur between
problems and dependence

Figure 28.2 Diagram to show how problems and
dependence coexist (after Edwards et al 1977).

Sector D: those who are significantly dependent
but do not experience problems.

Research by Drummond (1990) suggested that
people who are more dependent on alcohol
experience more problems, but that certain problems are more closely related to dependence than
others. Also, dependence can lead to abnormal
drinking patterns. Where alcohol problems may
be subject to sociodemographic effects, dependence is more likely to exist independently of most
sociodemographic variables. Dependence and
problems can be seen as coexisting and interrelated but not as separate entities (Drummond
1992, Gossop 1994).

Problems

Alcohol or drug problems can be said to occur
when their use severely disrupts a person's normal lifestyle balance or physical state.

Consumption of more than 50 units of alcohol
per week for men and over 35 units weekly for
women is likely to cause problems (Gossop
1994a).

Patterns of drug use can cause problems, such
as binge use of a particular drug, or drug use as
the only way to cope with difficulties.

Physical problems can range from malnutrition to heart problems and lung, liver and gastric

disease. Psychological problems can range from
memory loss to neurological damage, chronic
psychotic symptoms and dementia. National figures show that drug and alcohol users die
younger that those who are non-users.

Dependence

Dependence on substances is diagnosed using
the dependence syndrome (WHO 1981). This
consists of a list of seven problems, three of
which at least have to be present in a greater or
lesser degree to indicate dependence:

1. Subjective awareness of compulsion to use a
   drug or drugs
2. A desire to stop using the drug in the face of
   continued use
3. A stereotyped drug-taking habit, that is, a
   narrowing of the repertoire of drug-taking
   behaviour
4. Experience of withdrawal symptoms
   (evidence of neurodaptation/tolerance)
5. Use in order to relieve withdrawal symptoms
6. Primacy of drug use over other activities in
   life (salience)
7. Rapid reinstatement of dependence after a
   period of abstinence.

The dependence syndrome is the most widely
used method of diagnosing substance dependence. It consists of both physical and psychological aspects and aims to emphasise the
importance of psychological dependence on a
substance as well as physical symptomatology.
Edwards & Gross (1976, Edwards 1987), who
developed the dependence syndrome concept,
emphasised the need to take a clinical picture in
its social and environmental context and to tailor
the picture to the individual.

Dependence on alcohol is generally identified
either through interview or by using questionnaires such as the Severity of Alcohol
Dependence Questionnaire (SADQ) (Stockwell et
al 1979). The SADQ is the instrument recommended by the World Health Organization
(Anderson 1990).

Other concepts of dependence include the
addictive personality concept, which suggests

that addiction is a form of personality disorder, or that people dependent on a drug are predisposed towards this because of their personality characteristics. The validity of this view has been largely dismissed on the research evidence (Gossop 1994a). Another approach to understanding drug dependence is the conditioning approach, first developed by Wickler (1948). This idea suggests that drug-related behaviours occur because they become paired with the reinforcing effect of the feelings a drug produces. Other conditioning models exist, as do social models and the basic biomedical approach.

DRUG AND ALCOHOL TREATMENT IN CONTEXT

Drug and alcohol treatment services are operated by both the National Health Service and the private and charitable sectors. Treatment settings include hospital and community locations, and treatment can commence in either. Most frequently, new episodes of treatment will begin via a general practitioner referral, the police or court, another NHS service or self-referral. Often, referrals will come from employers or employee assistance programmes. Specific services exist for the treatment of addicted health professionals.

Once referred, the client will then either leave treatment of his own volition or engage in a process of treatment and support.

TRIGGERS TO TREATMENT ENTRY

Entry into treatment is usually triggered by a crisis. For example: a family seek help from their general practitioner as they can no longer tolerate their son or daughter's growing drug habit; a young person is caught breaking into houses to fund a growing crack cocaine habit; a patient is admitted to hospital because his liver is failing as a consequence of his drinking; a City of London businesswoman is taken to a private clinic by her partner out of concern for the amount of whisky she drinks at work; a vulnerable, homeless person with schizophrenia has been sexually assaulted when incapacitated on tranquillisers; or a prostitute seeks help at her latest attendance to a needle exchange in a Manchester treatment facility.

Referral

Referral generally starts with an assessment. With alcohol use, if the person is intoxicated at the time of referral then a detoxification period will be given. Heroin users are often stabilised on prescribed methadone. During this time the client will be monitored for withdrawal symptoms. He may also be breathalised or have urine and/or blood tests to monitor the alcohol or drug content. After the client becomes sufficiently coherent, the professional receiving him will carry out a verbal assessment.

ASSESSMENT APPROACHES
Screening assessment

Assessments are initially adisciplinary. The person at the first point of contact may be a nurse, a doctor or a duty drug worker of any profession. The goal of the assessment, in addition to establishing physical risk issues, is to discover the primary issues surrounding the client's substance use, his motivation to change his habit and how long and how severe the habit is.

A number of screening assessments can be used. The widely used CAGE questionnaire (Box 28.1; Mayfield et al 1974) or the S-MAST (Pokorny et al 1972) provide fast, rough guides to the extent of drinking problems. For drug use there are the Severity of Dependence Scale (Gossop et al 1992), which is designed to be generic to a range of drugs. It is essential to monitor withdrawal (Edwards 1987) and assessments are often used to assist this, such as the Short Opiate Withdrawal Scale (Gossop 1990) or the Selective Severity Assessment (SSA; Gross et al 1973).

An interview is used to decide the next course of action, which is usually to refer to an inpatient setting, outpatient department or community for a detoxification period.

Box 28.1 The CAGE questionnaire

1. Have you ever felt you ought to *C*UT DOWN on your drinking?
2. Have people *A*NNOYED you by criticising your drinking?
3. Have you ever felt bad or *G*UILTY about your drinking?
4. Have you ever had a drink first thing in the morning to steady your nerves or get rid of a hangover? (*E*YE-OPENER)

Two or more affirmative replies are said to identify the problem drinker. Research has supported this assertion.

Multidisciplinary assessment

During the detoxification period, a multidisciplinary team will usually carry out further assessments. These can include:

- structured questionnaires
- interviews
- observation
- self-assessment and contracts
- physiological assessments (for example, blood analysis, ECG)
- neurological assessments (for example, EEG, CAT or MRI scan).

Interview techniques

Interviews add to the assessment. These can follow a standard mental health interview approach but should also include questions about the client's substance use. These can include:

- number of different drugs used
- amount used
- a typical day of use
- history of use, including first drug use occasion and changes in use over time.

Structured assessments

Multidisciplinary, structured questionnaires aim to investigate the severity of dependence, the range and complexity of problems associated with substance use and motivation to engage in treatment or change substance use behaviour.

Other issues may include measurement of specific symptoms, such as anxiety, and rehabilitation potential, using occupational therapy assessments.

Occupational therapy assessment

Occupational therapy investigates three domains (American Occupational Therapy Association 1994):

1. *Performance areas*: categories of human daily activity, such as activities of daily living, leisure, self-maintenance and work/productivity. Substance use affects each of these areas in different ways.

Occupational therapists are concerned that substance misuse and dependence disrupt the balance of work, self-care and leisure (Lindsay 1983, Busuttil 1989, Nicol 1989, Rotert 1990, Chacksfield 1994, Morgan 1994). Recent quantitative research by occupational therapists such as Mann & Talty (1990), Scaffa (1991), Stoffel et al (1992) and Chacksfield & Lindsay (1999) has highlighted poor use of leisure by alcohol dependent clients as a key problem area.

2. *Performance components*: fundamental human abilities that are required for successful engagement in performance areas include sensorimotor, cognitive, psychosocial and psychological components. Drug action can create both short- and long-term effects on performance components.

Occupational therapy research has suggested that low motivation and low self-esteem are significant in substance misusers (Viik et al 1990, Stoffell et al 1992).

3. *Performance contexts*: environmental factors and situations that influence the client's engagement in performance areas. These are significant in substance-using clients due to the way environmental cues can impact and trigger substance use, called 'environmental press' by Kielhofner (1995).

This idea has been supported by a growing body of research into cue exposure (Drummond et al 1995). Cue exposure concerns environmental cues or stimuli that trigger addictive behaviour in individuals. A client returning to the same lifestyle on discharge is likely to relapse to substance use and will need work on coping strategies to counteract environmental effects.

Occupational therapy assessment tools

Occupational therapists will wish to supplement the standard initial interview with open questioning to obtain information about how substance use is impacting on the client's occupational performance areas, components and contexts.

Some occupational therapists may wish to use the Occupational Performance History Interview (Kielhofner et al 1998) as a structure for initial interview into which a substance use perspective can be integrated. However, this instrument can be time-consuming.

Some appropriate tools include:

- Occupational Self Assessment (OSA)
- Rosenberg Self-Esteem Inventory
- Self-Efficacy Scale
- Volitional Questionnaire
- Coping Responses Inventory (CRI)
- Interest Checklist
- Role Checklist
- Assessment of Motor and Process Skills (AMPS)
- Internal/external locus of control scale.

Use of these instruments will be limited by the time available, that is, the length of admission. It is recommended that occupational therapists identify which areas are most important during the initial interview and apply relevant questionnaires accordingly. For example, the AMPS assessment (which requires the assessor to be trained) will be relevant for those clients with obvious neurological problems.

INTERVENTION

Intervention is a complex process in the field of substance misuse due to the complex needs presented by clients, therefore, a multidisciplinary, multi-modal, multi-agency approach works best (Edwards 1987, DoH 1996). Some principles of intervention include:

- tailoring treatment to the individual client
- fostering a relationship between the client and the treatment institution
- setting achievable goals for intervention
- involving the family or carers
- emphasising empowerment of the client in overcoming substance problems or dependence.

Treatment strategies tend to aim towards the following goals:

1. detoxification
2. re-balancing external and internal problems not directly related to substance use
3. reducing external and internal problems that are related to drug use
4. reducing harmful or hazardous behaviour associated with the use of drugs (for example, sharing dirty needles)
5. developing the internal resources (self-esteem, motivation, knowledge) to address the drug problem or dependence
6. establishing a safe, controlled pattern of drug use that is not harmful or dependent
7. establishing abstinence from the problem drug (or drugs)
8. establishing abstinence from all drugs
9. establishing an independent lifestyle.

These goals are not mutually exclusive and can be carried out in combination. For instance, many physical problems, such as muscle atrophy or memory loss, may continue to require treatment during many of the other stages.

Occupational therapists contribute to the intervention programme by enhancing occupational performance via activity based and other, related, interventions.

Treatment approaches

Detoxification

Detoxification is carried out using a drug similar to the substance of misuse. This is done to minimise the harmful or uncomfortable effects of withdrawal.

Treating physical problems

Physical problems are often extensive if a person has misused drugs for a long time and if they have maintained poor levels of nutrition (Royal College of Psychiatrists 1987). Neurological damage is a major issue, and includes memory loss and dementia. Physical problems can initiate contact with health services.

In addition, there has been a spread of fatal diseases such as human immunodeficiency virus (HIV) and hepatitis C in the drug-using community far greater than the incidence in the general population. A key intervention approach here is harm reduction. This focuses on safer drug use, healthier behaviours, safer sexual behaviour and education about the risk of spreading HIV, acquired immune deficiency syndrome (AIDS) and hepatitis C.

Outreach services attempt to reduce harm in populations that are outside the treatment services, such as prostitutes or the street homeless. Some of this work includes needle exchanges, where drug users can reduce harm to health by obtaining and exchanging injection equipment, obtaining contraceptives and receiving education.

Occupational therapists can be involved in outreach drug work, and goals will be to support harm reduction and to increase positive self-maintenance through educational and milieu approaches. Milieu approaches offer informal, passive environments in which a drug user has the opportunity to ask about advice or treatment should they want to engage in it. This can then lead to further treatment. Occupational therapy task-based activities, such as art groups, can be valuable in encouraging informal contact in these settings.

Substitute prescribing

Some opiate users require prescription of a substitute drug, methadone. This aims to stop the user experiencing unpleasant withdrawal symptoms but does not provide a 'high'. The rationale behind substitute prescribing is that the drug user no longer has to inject street heroin with its associated health risks, or be involved in illegal activities in order to fund a habit. Long-term prescription of methadone, or methadone maintenance, aims to allow users to stabilise their drug use and therefore their lives and, combined with psychological and social support, enables users to make positive lifestyle changes. It it usually only considered after a user has tried to detoxify and failed, and requires close monitoring to ensure that the client ceases illicit drug use.

MODELS OF INTERVENTION

The main treatment models currently fashionable in the treatment of substance misuse include: the 'Twelve Steps', or Minnesota model, made popular by the Alcoholics Anonymous movement (1955; see Box 28.2), and the Stages of Change model, or Model of Change (Prochaska & DiClemente 1982, 1986)

Box 28.2 The Twelve Steps of Alcoholics Anonymous

1. We admitted we were powerless over alcohol – that our lives had become unmanageable.
2. Came to believe that a Power greater than ourselves could restore us to sanity.
3. Made a decision to turn over our will and our lives to the care of God as we understood him.
4. Made a searching and fearless moral inventory of ourselves.
5. Admitted to God, to ourselves, and to another human being the exact nature of our wrongs.
6. We were entirely ready to have God remove all these defects of character.
7. Humbly asked Him to remove our shortcomings.
8. Made a list of all the persons we had harmed, and became willing to make amends to them all.
9. Made direct amends to such people wherever possible, except when to do so would injure them or others.
10. Continued to take a personal inventory, and when we were wrong promptly admitted it.
11. Sought through prayer and meditation to improve our conscious contact with God as we understood Him, praying only for knowledge of His will for us and the power to carry it out.
12. Having had a spiritual awakening as a result of these steps, we tried to carry this message to alcoholics, and to practise these principles in all our affairs.

(see Fig. 28.3). These are often augmented by brief therapies, such as:

- Motivational Milieu Therapy (Van Bilsen & Van Emst 1986, Van Bilsen 1988)
- Solution Focused Therapy (Berg & Miller 1992)
- Cue Exposure Therapy (Dawe & Powell 1995).

The Twelve Steps

Alcoholics Anonymous (AA) and its associate Narcotics Anonymous (NA) offer an extensive international support network for substance users and their families. Meetings of these organisations occur at various times during the day and are supplemented with Step Meetings, for those serious about abstinence, and individual support from a sponsor. The sponsor is a person who has been successful in his abstinence for a significant length of time and who has worked his way through the Twelve Steps (Box 28.2). As it is so comprehensive, this approach is widely advocated and some research evidence exists to show it works for about 26% of members (Bebbington 1976).

Criticism has been made of the requirement that those who attend have to adhere to the idea that dependence is a disease and that people attending have to constantly remind themselves that they are alcoholic, even when they have been abstinent for many years. Additionally, criticism is directed at the idea that a higher power is responsible for an AA or NA member's abstinence, suggesting that this removes the responsibility for sobriety from the individual.

The Stages of Change

When working with clients with any addictive behaviour (or any client working towards behaviour change), the Stages of Change model is a useful tool for guiding the selection of treatment goals and interventions (Fig. 28.3). Therapeutic intervention can be targeted to help clients progress through the stages of change.

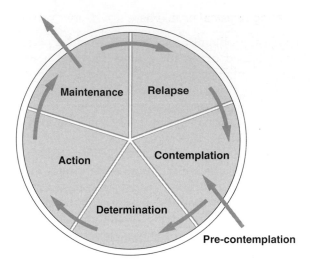

Figure 28.3   A model of change (adapted by Jenny Lancaster from Prochaska & DiClemente 1982, 1986).

Prochaska and DiClemente (1982, 1986) first developed this model with smokers, who they found reported movement through different stages of change as they attempted to give up. These same stages have since been observed in all other addictive disorders (Gossop 1994b).

This is a transtheoretical approach, therefore it can be used across a variety of approaches, including occupational therapy.

It reflects the reality that it is normal for an individual to go round the process several times before achieving lasting behaviour change. Most of us can relate to attempting behaviour changes ourselves, for example, dieting, starting regular exercise or stopping smoking, where we have not succeeded in maintaining the change at the first attempt. In fact, Prochaska and DiClemente's initial research was with smokers who went round the cycle between three and seven times before finally giving up for good.

Therefore, addiction can be viewed as a chronic, relapsing condition in which relapses are viewed as normal events that can be learned from rather than seen a failure.

The central concept of this model is that behaviour change takes place through the following discrete stages:

- *Pre-contemplation*. These are people who do not recognise that they have a problem, therefore they are outside the 'wheel of change'. 'Pre-contemplators' rarely present for treatment. However, when they do it is in order to assuage the concerns of others.
- *Contemplation*. In this stage, the person recognises that his behaviour is problematic and considers doing something about it. This change is characterised by ambivalence. Unless this ambivalence is resolved the person could remain in this stage indefinitely.
- *Determination*. This is the period in which ambivalence is resolved and the person decides to change.
- *Action*. The person attempts to change the problem behaviour, for example stop drinking, with or without outside help.
- *Maintenance*. If the person is successful in achieving this behaviour change, their next goal is to maintain or sustain the change.

Due to the circular nature of this model, it follows that a person may slip back a stage or exit the cycle into pre-contemplation at any time.

By using this model the therapist can establish which stage the client is at and use this to select the most appropriate treatment. For example, a client in the maintenance phase may benefit from learning stress management or assertive skills. This would boost self-confidence and reduce the risk of relapse. However, these strategies would probably be wasted on someone in the pre-contemplation phase.

In addition to assisting in treatment matching, this model is helpful for both client and therapist in helping to set realistic and achievable goals, that is, to move to the next stage in the cycle rather than try to stop the behaviour immediately. Also, it is a more optimistic approach in that relapse is viewed as a normal part of the process of achieving long-term behaviour change rather than as failure.

Occupational therapy input is most effective when the client has reached the maintenance phase. The occupational therapist can help the client to develop coping skills, such as anxiety management and assertiveness, and satisfying occupations in day-to-day life which are important in preventing relapse into drug or alcohol use.

Relapse Prevention

Based on the Model of Change, Relapse Prevention (RP; Marlatt & Gordon 1985) has become one of the most widely used intervention approaches in the field of addiction. Marlatt (Marlatt & Gordon 1985) suggested that RP is a self-management programme that is designed to enhance the maintenance phase of the process of change.

The RP approach uses cognitive behavioural strategies to help clients who are trying to stop or reduce drug use to learn how to anticipate and cope with situations and problems that might lead to a relapse. The model focuses on the notions of high-risk situations and coping strategies available to the individual.

Research has shown that people who are aware of potential relapse situations and use specific strategies can effectively reduce their risk of relapse (Litman 1986, Kirby et al 1995). Boredom and negative mood states are most likely to precipitate a relapse. Second comes social pressure and being offered, or talking about, drugs. Other risk factors beyond these include alcohol use, interpersonal violence and environmental cues.

Environmental cues or triggers to relapse are important factors in prognosis, therefore these are given high significance in relapse prevention. Initial stages of relapse prevention focus on enabling the client to develop good awareness of internal and external triggers to craving. Methods used include diary keeping, where clients regularly chart substance use and the antecedent and consequent feelings, activity and location of use. Clients are encouraged to identify possible relapse triggers unique to themselves and work on these with the therapist. The therapist, either in a group setting or individually, can help the client to analyse these situations. The client will also be taught how to analyse situations for himself.

Structured problem-solving techniques are used as well as role-play or rehearsal of relapse situations.

Specific cognitive techniques used to assist the client in preventing relapse include:

Seemingly Irrelevant Decisions (SIDs). This works on how to identify and prevent covert planning that may lead to relapse, such as 'happening' to go into the local pub to buy cigarettes and eventually obtaining alcohol.

Urge Surfing. This is a technique for coping with craving. When craving is experienced, the client must allow the feeling to 'wash over' and beyond him. Coping strategies, such as relaxation methods, distraction, biofeedback or other approaches, may assist this technique.

Relapse prevention is an approach that fits well with occupational therapy in particular because it focuses on lifestyle and real situations that cause relapse. Here, occupational performance areas, components and contexts are critical to treatment success.

Developing psychological performance components, such as self-esteem and volition, for example, can help an individual cope with environmental triggers to relapse, also called environmental press (Kielhofner 1985).

OCCUPATIONAL THERAPY AND SUBSTANCE MISUSE

The earliest papers describing occupational therapy with alcoholics highlight areas for concern that are close to those identified by modern occupational therapists after research and the experience of time. For example, a Canadian occupational therapist, Hossack, writing in 1952, highlighted reduction in former interests and activites as well as social connections, difficulty concentrating, tension and family problems. She suggested that the alcoholic 'must look to a more fully rounded life with a balance of activity.' Doniger, in 1953, suggested unpredictability, elusiveness, relationships, leisure and motivation as areas for concern.

The issues raised by these two pioneers of occupational therapy in the field of addiction remain key throughout much of the subsequent occupational therapy literature.

Occupational therapy can have a significant impact in preparing a client for change and in changing from substance misuse to a more controlled or abstinent life. For many clients with substance misuse problems, prior to treatment their lives have centred around their drug/alcohol use. After becoming engaged in treatment clients can be left feeling a vacuum in their day-to-day lives which leaves them de-skilled, vulnerable and bored. Occupational therapy can help clients to develop skills and coping strategies, as well as a more satisfying, balanced lifestyle.

Some of the general issues occupational therapy can address are divided under the three occupational performance area headings of work, self-care and leisure. Intervention is usually via individual work and groupwork. It can involve both task-oriented and person-centred activities aimed at developing performance components in a range of contexts, for example learning to cope with anxiety without alcohol or saying 'no' if offered drugs. Group contexts and community locations can provide the chance for try-outs of performance components. Individual work can focus on enhancing very specific components through counselling and/or role-play.

Leisure

Leisure is one of the key problem areas for alcohol and substance misuse clients. This is principally because leisure activities and contexts are where alcohol and drugs are most commonly used. Negative mood states, such as boredom, and social pressure are the two most common factors in relapse.

Whether taken alone or with other people, leisure is a major part of most drug users' lifestyle and most will know few or no other leisure activities apart from those that involve substance use.

The goals of occupational therapy will focus on learning how to use leisure time and how to counteract negative mood states. During treatment, new or forgotten leisure activities can be tried out. Sport and fitness related activities will raise self-esteem and confidence and counteract negative affect. Discovering or rediscovering leisure can help develop motivation to change and move clients round the process of change, in conjunction with other therapies.

Groupwork can be used to explore leisure seeking and leisure replacement techniques and self-motivation. As part of a relapse prevention programme, rehearsal and role-play around leisure-based relapse situations can be useful. This can be linked to cue exposure therapy programmes, where role-play is carried out in the environment where substances may have been used or obtained.

Leisure intervention may form an important part of family therapy, where family oriented leisure has been involved with or affected by substance use. In the authors' clinical experience, activities that help enable a substance user engage in adaptive interactions with family members are often highly successful. This is especially so where the client enjoys and can remember the activity and where it stimulates both client and relative. Examples include practising magic tricks (described by Chacksfield & Darnley 1995), cooking group meals, learning day trip locations, swimming, playing racket sports, bowling and visiting theatres, cinema or art galleries. Activities that individuals can take up as a hobby and talk about with the family are effective. The impact of substance misuse on family is often highly significant.

Box 28.3 Case vignette (based on a true case in a London alcohol unit)

Brian was a 32-year-old alcoholic man who had a history of verbal and sometimes physical violence towards his two young children. He valued his role as a father but felt he did not know what to talk to his children about. Occupational therapy involved attendance to six weekly group sessions on magic tricks. After the third week his children visited him and he showed them one of the coin tricks he had learned. They were delighted and spent an hour talking to him about it and trying to learn what he could do. He took magic up as a hobby and obtained the admiration of family and friends for his abilities. He remained sober for over a year.

Work/productivity

Work and productivity in substance misuse cover two distinct areas of discussion:

1. drug use during everyday, legal employment
2. drug use or dealing following similar patterns to paid work and providing similar rewards and meaning to life.

Work-based substance use

Where substances are used during a job, this use can be very subtle and often either linked to peer pressure or coping with work pressure. Substance use can be considered a part of work when the entertainment of business clients is part of the working day.

Substances are often hidden at work and used covertly. Initial experiences of high achievement reinforce this pattern of substance use, however, errors of judgement usually ensue and crises occur. Jobs are often affected negatively or lost altogether once substance misuse patterns become established.

Other non-paid work, such as housekeeping and voluntary work, will exhibit similar features to the above.

Occupational therapy goals focus on helping a client cope with work without using the drug. In addition, intervention aims to develop resistance to relapse triggers in work settings. Work may involve liaison with an employer to develop graded re-entry into work and to identify coping strategies and support strategies for both employer and employee. People who, owing to their substance use, have lost work or have been unable to hold down a job may need to start with low-pressure, voluntary work until they have developed the confidence, tolerance and skills to enter full-time employment.

Substance-based productivity

Where maintaining a drug habit becomes work, an individual's effort can be directed to obtaining a regular supply of the substance, selling the substance or engaging in regular criminal activity in order to fund the drug habit.

These three types of behaviour can follow patterns and display characteristics that are very similar to legal employment. A certain amount of a product will have to be obtained during the day. Where dealing is involved, this product will have to be sold to obtain money to either buy more or maintain a regular supply of drugs. In order to achieve this, and avoid arrest by the authorities or violence from peers, a considerable repertoire of specialised dealing, trading and bargaining habits can be developed. Alcoholics often describe a daily routine of waking, drinking, obtaining money, going to purchase alcohol and drinking it. When withdrawal occurs, more alcohol is purchased. This pattern can be as regular as the routines in a 9-to-5 office job.

Occupational therapy can focus on identifying habit maintaining skills and transferring these to non drug-related activities, such as voluntary work or sheltered work. Clients can be encouraged to enrol in training to develop business skills or apprenticeship-type work where a gradual skill transfer can occur. This type of intervention should ideally occur in conjunction with appropriate support. Alcoholics Anonymous and Narcotics Anonymous offer opportunities for members to engage in voluntary work to help run the organisation. This can work well, as support from peers with experience of abstinence is available.

Self-maintenance

Self-maintenance activities tend to decrease the more substances are used. The need and compulsion to use a drug eventually supersedes any awareness of nutrition, health, cleanliness, safety or responsibility for finances.

Drug users, once abstinent or stabilised in treatment, often feel particularly de-skilled to cope with day-to-day household activities such as budgeting or basic time management.

Evaluation of outcomes

Outcome measurement is possible through a wide range of occupational therapy-specific and other questionnaires or assessment tools. Some of these are described in the assessment section (above). Most of those described are used as pre and post measures of blocks of intervention. Others can be used on a sessional basis, such as the Hospital Anxiety and Depression Scale. The Canadian Occupational Performance Measure (COPM) can be administered at any time during treatment and is effective as a measure of client perception of performance and satisfaction. As an outcome measure it should be administered at the start and end of treatment and at regular intervals if indicated.

SUMMARY

This chapter has focused on the range of issues presented by people who misuse substances and the intervention strategies open to them.

It is clear that there is considerable scope for occupational therapists to contribute to substance misuse treatment. Substance misuse occurs at the very centre of human occupation, in work, leisure and self-care, and it gradually takes over as the most central driver of occupational behaviour, changing and damaging performance components as it progresses.

Occupational therapy approaches work well with the key clinical approaches already developed in the field of addiction. Furthermore, occupational therapists can learn and enhance practice through their work with the subtle and complex issues that clients in this field present.

Further research is recommended in this area, as is further education, especially as substance use exists within all areas of mental health practice and is more likely to increase than decrease in everyday practice.

REFERENCES

Adams T 1998 Addicted: his open and inspiring autobiography. Collins Willow, London

Alcoholics Anonymous 1930 The big book. Alcoholics Anonymous, London

American Occupational Therapy Association 1994 Uniform terminology for occupational therapy, 3rd edn. American Journal of Occupational Therapy 48(11): 1047–1054

Anderson P 1990 Management of drinking problems. WHO Regional Publications, European Series, No. 32. WHO, Geneva

Bandura A 1977 Self-efficacy: towards a unifying theory of behavioural change. Psychological Review 84: 191–215

Bebbington P E 1976 The efficacy of Alcoholics Anonymous: the elusiveness of hard data. British Journal of Psychiatry 128: 572–580

Berg I K, Miller S D 1992 Working with the problem drinker: a solution-focused approach. W W Norton, New York

Busuttil J 1989 Setting up an occupational therapy programme for drug addicts. British Journal of Occupational Therapy 52(12): 476–479

Chacksfield J D 1994 Occupational therapy: the whole in one treatment for alcohol dependent clients. In: World Federation of Occupational Therapists, 11th International Congress. Congress Summaries 3: 995–997

Chacksfield J D, Lindsay S J E 1999 The reduction of leisure in alcohol addiction. Paper presented at College of Occupational Therapists Conference, 1999

Dawe S, Powell J H 1995 Cue exposure treatment in opiate and cocaine dependence. In: Drummond D C, Tiffany S T, Glautier S, Remington B (eds) Addictive behaviour: cue exposure theory and practice. Wiley, Chichester

Department of Health 1996 The task force to review services for drug misusers: report of an independent review of drug treatment services in England. Department of Health (H87/001/04/96/0032 1 P 5k April 96 (01)), Wetherby

Department of Health 1999 Statistics on alcohol: 1976 onwards. Department of Health Statistical Bulletin 1999 (24)

Doniger J 1953 An activity program with alcoholics. American Journal of Occupational Therapy 7(3): 110–112, 135

Drummond D C 1990 The relationship between alcohol dependence and alcohol-related problems in a clinical population. British Journal of Addiction 85: 357–366

Drummond D C 1992 Problems and dependence: chalk and cheese or bread and butter? In: Lader M, Edwards G, Drummond C (eds) The nature of alcohol and drug related problems. Oxford University Press, Oxford, pp. 61–82

Drummond D C et al 1995 Cue exposure. Wiley, New York

Duke P J, Pantelis C, Barnes T R E 1994 South Westminster schizophrenia survey. British Journal of Psychiatry 164: 630–636

Edwards G 1987 The treatment of drinking problems. Blackwell Scientific, Oxford

Edwards G, Gross M M 1976 Alcohol dependence: provisional description of a clinical syndrome. British Medical Journal 1: 1058–1061

Forshaw D M, Strang J 1993 Drug, aggression and violence. In: Taylor P J (ed) Violence in society. Royal College of Physicians, London

Gossop M 1990 The development of the short opiate withdrawal scale (SOWS). Addictive Behaviours 15: 487–490

Gossop M 1993 Living with drugs, 3rd edn. Ashgate, Aldershot

Gossop M 1994a Drug and alcohol problems: investigation. In: Lindsay S J E, Powell G E (eds) The handbook of clinical adult psychology, 2nd edn. Routledge, London

Gossop M 1994b Drug and alcohol problems: treatment. In: Lindsay S J E, Powell G E (eds) The handbook of clinical adult psychology, 2nd edn. Routledge, London

Gross M M, Lewis E, Nagarjan M 1973 An improved quantitative system for assessing the acute alcoholic psychoses and related states (TSA and SSA). In: Gross M M (ed) Alcohol intoxication and withdrawal: experimental studies: Plenum, New York, pp. 365–376

Henman A 1985 Cocaine futures. In: Henman A, Lewis R, Malyon T Big deal: the politics of the illicit drugs business. Pluto Press, London

HMSO 1979 Misuse of Drugs Act. London

HMSO 1995 Tackling drugs together: a strategy for England. HMSO, London

Hossack J R 1952 Clinical trial of occupational therapy in the treatment of alcohol addiction. American Journal of Occupational Therapy 6(6): 265–282

Institute for the Study of Drug Dependence (ISDD) 1999 Drug situation in the UK – trends and update. Available online at *http://www.isdd.org.uk/*

Kielhofner G 1985 A model of human occupation. Williams and Wilkins, Baltimore

Kielhofner G 1995 A model of human occupation: theory and application, 2nd edn. Williams and Wilkins, Baltimore

Lindsay W P 1983 The role of the occupational therapist in the treatment of alcoholism. American Journal of Occupational Therapy 37(1): 36–40

Litman G 1980 Relapse in alcoholism. In: Edwards G, Grant M (eds) Alcoholism treatment in transition. Croom Helm, London

Mann W C, Talty P 1990 Leisure activity profile: measuring use of leisure time by persons with alcoholism. Occupational Therapy and Mental Health 10(4): 31–41

Marlatt G A, Gordon J R 1985 Relapse prevention. Guilford, New York

Mayfield D et al 1974 The CAGE questionnaire: validation of a new alcoholism screening instrument. American Journal of Psychiatry 131: 1121–1123

Morgan C A 1994 Illicit drug use: primary prevention. British Journal of Occupational Therapy 57(1): 2–4

Musto D F 1993 The rise and fall of epidemics: learning from history. In: Edwards G, Strang J, Jaffe J (eds) Drugs, alcohol and tobacco: making the science and policy connections. Oxford Medical Publications, Oxford

Nicol M 1989 Substance misuse – who cares? British Journal of Occupational Therapy 52(1): 18–20

Nunn J F 1996 Ancient Egyptian medicine. British Museum Press, London

Pokorny A D et al 1972 The brief MAST: a shortened version of the Michigan Alcoholism Screening Test. American Journal of Psychiatry 129: 342–345

Prochaska J O, DiClemente C C 1982 Transtheoretical therapy: towards a more integrative model of change. Psychotherapy Theory, Research and Practice 19: 276–278

Prochaska J O, DiClemente C C 1986 Towards a comprehensive model of change. In: Miller R J, Heather N (eds) Treating addictive behaviours: processes of change. Plenum, London

Rosenberg J 1965 Society and adolescent self image. Princeton University Press, Princeton

Rotert D A 1989 Occupational therapy in alcoholism. Occupational Medicine: State of the Art Reviews 4(2): 327–337

Rotert D 1990 Occupational therapy and alcoholism. Journal of Occupational Medicine

Royal College of Psychiatrists 1987 Drug scenes: a report on drugs and drug dependence by the Royal College of Psychiatrists. Gaskell, London

Scaffa M E 1991 Alcoholism: an occupational behaviour perspective. Occupational Therapy in Mental Health 11(2/3): 99–111

SO 1998 Tackling drugs to build a better Britain. Stationary Office, London

Stellar J R, Rice M B 1987 Pharmacological basis of intracranial self-stimulation reward. In: Royal College of Psychiatrists Drug scenes: a report on drugs and drug dependence by the Royal College of Psychiatrists. Gaskell, London

Stockwell T, Hodgson R, Edwards G, Taylor C, Rankin H 1979 The development of a questionnaire to measure severity of alcohol dependence. British Journal of Addiction 74: 79–87

Stoffel V C, Cusatis M, Seitz L, Jones N 1992 Self-esteem and leisure patterns of persons in a residential chemical dependency treatment program. Occupational Therapy in Health Care 8(2/3): 69–85

Sutherland G, Edwards G, Taylor C et al 1992 The measurement of opiate dependence. British Journal of Addiction 81: 485–494

Swanson J W, Holzer C E, Ganju V K, Tsutomo Jono R 1990 Violence and psychiatric disorder in the community: evidence from the epidemiological catchment area surveys. Hospital and Community Psychiatry 41(7): 761–770

Tyler S 1998 Street drugs. Hodder and Stoughton, London

Van Bilsen H 1988 Motivating drug users to change. In: Bennett G (ed) New directions in the treatment of drug abuse. Routledge, London

Van Bilsen H, Van Emst 1986 Heroin addiction and motivational milieu therapy. International Journal of the Addictions 21: 707–713

Wickler A 1948 Recent progress in research on the neurophysiologic basis of morphine addiction. American Journal of Psychiatry 105: 329–338

USEFUL ADDRESSES AND INFORMATION

Association of Occupational Therapists in Mental Health, Substance Misuse Representative,
120 Wilton Road, London SW1V 1JZ
Tel: 020 7 233 8322 Fax: 020 7 233 7779
E-mail: *profbriefings@msn.com*
Web *http://www.profbriefings.co.uk/assoc/aotmh.htm*

Drugscope, Waterbridge House, 32–36 Loman Street, London SE1 0EE
Tel: 0207 928 1211 Fax: 0207 928 1771
Web *http://www.drugscope.org.uk/*

Drugscope (formerly ISDD and SCODA) provides information on drugs and drug misuse. It maintains an extensive library and a consultancy and research service on information provision in the drugs field.

Alcohol Concern, Waterbridge House,
32–36 Loman Street, London SE1 0EE

Tel: 0207 928 7377 Fax: 0207 928 4644
Web: *http://www.alcoholconcern.org.uk/*

Alcohol Concern is a national alcohol misuse agency. It provides a range of publications, and has a library, bookshop and information unit. Membership is open to individuals or organisations.

Alcoholics Anonymous (AA), London Region Telephone Service, 1st Floor, 11 Radcliffe Gardens, London SW10 9BG Tel: 0207 352 3001

Narcotics Anonymous (NA), 202 City Road, London EC1V 2PH Tel: 0207 730 0009 (Helpline) Tel: 0207 251 4007 (Office) Fax: 0207 251 4006 Web *http://www.ukna.org/*

National drugs helpline 0800 776600

Drinkline 0800 917 8282

29

Loss and grief

Clephane A. Hume

INTRODUCTION

Loss encroaches on all aspects of life, and is an important topic and highly relevant in the field of mental health. Indeed, all clients will have experienced a sense of loss by virtue of their inability to cope with the demands of life and consequent referral for help.

Paradoxically, the prevalence of AIDS and recent incidences of wars and disasters have increased public awareness about some of the issues related to loss. Despite this universality of experience, and the increasing amount of literature about bereavement, it is still an area about which many people are reticent. Social taboos and stigmas persist, adding to the painful feelings of the individual concerned.

In the context of illness, losses might include alteration in roles and reduction in cognitive or physical abilities, choices, self-esteem and hope. Some people will be additionally distressed by loss of faith.

Unacknowledged loss, or feelings which are ignored, may lead to mental health problems in the future and the occupational therapist therefore requires an understanding of some of the issues facing clients.

Much documented work about the impact of loss on health relates to terminal illness, bereavement and unemployment. The aim of this chapter is not simply to repeat material which already exists about the theory of loss but rather to consider the nature of loss, people's reactions, and factors which may influence mental health and well-being.

Case examples of loss consequent on ill health and bereavement are included and consideration is given to how such losses may add to existing feelings of loss for patients and relatives.

In some instances, the intensity of the grief reaction may necessitate specialist intervention, and sources of help are included.

TYPES OF LOSS

In considering the nature of loss, it is helpful to identify some of the most common contexts in which loss may be experienced. Bereavement and redundancy are obvious examples, illness less so. The recurrence of schizophrenia or depression after a symptom-free period can be a real blow.

Social pressures and expectations may also contribute to feelings of loss. In a success-oriented society, those who do not come first may lose everything. Being second does not secure the job.

Sometimes the loss may be felt retrospectively or reflect a gap in the person's life – a living loss. For example, Morley (1996) wrote movingly about her feelings of loss in relation to not being a parent.

In practical day-to-day terms, loss may occur as the result of many situations which cause changes in relationships. Table 29.1 is not a hierarchy of the gravity or severity of any loss, since

each individual's experience is entirely personal. Clients will have their own examples.

These contexts can be summarised in the functional perspective outlined by Mitchell & Anderson (1983), who divided loss into 6 types:

1. *Material*: loss of possessions, for example, through theft
2. *Relationship*: an unavoidable aspect of human life
3. *Intrapsychic*: loss of self-image because of a change in circumstances, for example, on completion of a task or as a result of failure
4. *Functional loss*: loss of autonomy
5. *Role loss*: retirement, acquiring a new level of responsibility, becoming a patient
6. *Systemic loss*: loss of function within an existing system, for example, a child leaves home or one family member's retirement impacts on the function of the entire family.

Of these, types 3, 4 and 5 obviously have particular significance in relation to loss of health of the individual. The other categories may also occur as sources of stress and are therefore of relevance to the occupational therapist.

Marris (1974) wrote of the 'crisis of discontinuity': 'If we believe that the meaning of life can only be defined in the particular experience of each individual, we cannot at the same time treat that experience as indifferent . . . . Change implies loss, and . . . losses must be grieved for, unless life is meaningless anyway.'

Table 29.1 Contexts of loss

Cause of the loss	Nature of the loss/person who is lost
Bereavement	Spouse, parents, siblings, friends
Miscarriage, stillbirth	Expectations of parenthood
Death of a pet	
Unemployment/redundancy	
Divorce	Also affects children and grandparents
Breakdown of a relationship/friendship	
Remarriage	From the child's perspective, loss of previous relationship with a parent
Ill health	Enduring or recurrent illness, sudden accident
Loss of familiar environment	Move to another town, to long-term care
Failure	Not getting a job or passing exams, etc.
Empty nest syndrome/retirement	
Loss of relationships through neglect	The busy parent/spouse who has little time for the family
Loss of opportunities	Childlessness
Loss of valued objects	Loss of precious mementos, due to breakage or theft

Characteristics of loss

Features of the presenting situation merit consideration since these undoubtedly affect the characteristics of the loss experience. Using as an example a teenage girl who sustains a spinal cord injury, the loss may be:

- *Avoidable or unavoidable*? This is debatable. Her mother says: 'if only I had prepared a meal for her before I went out she wouldn't have had to go the chip shop and that car wouldn't have knocked her down . . .'.
- *Temporary or permanent*? She will never be able to walk again.
- *Actual or imagined*? This example is a fact. It has happened.
- *Anticipated or unanticipated*? This injury was not expected. The sudden onset of a CVA will likewise be unexpected. Insidious conditions or terminal illness may give the individual time to anticipate further loss.
- *Static or deteriorating condition*? Unlike a degenerative, progressive illness, once the period of rehabilitation is complete, this girl should be relatively healthy and able to lead an active, albeit altered, life.

Timescale

As reactions to loss necessarily vary according to the individual situation, so does the timescale during which the intensity of feelings may be experienced. It may reasonably be expected that sad and painful feelings will diminish with time, as usually happens in bereavement, but it would be wrong to assume that they will completely disappear. Grief may persist for a long time and the following personal anecdote may be helpful:

My collar hides a scar. The surgeon did an impressively neat job and the line is not nearly as visible as it used to be, so that a lot of people don't notice it. However, I know that it is there and I shall always be aware of it. Sometimes it twinges.

Loss may be experienced in terms of the following timescales:

- *Immediate*. The immediate feelings of loss in response to trauma or diagnosis which, in the case of an accident, may be mingled with relief that the person is still alive.
- *Anticipatory*. The response to an expected loss, when the person begins the grieving process in advance of the actual loss, for example following diagnosis of terminal illness or dementia in a loved one.
- *Episodic*. Feelings experienced from time to time, particularly in relation to lack of achievement of normal milestones – the parents of the young man who, but for his head injury, would have been graduating with his peer group.
- *Future*. The parents of this young man are now unlikely to be grandparents.
- *Anniversaries*. It was on this date, 5 years ago, that 'X' was diagnosed/'Y' died.

It is documented by hospital chaplains in the field of general medicine that within the bereavement process there is generally a 2-year average period of adjustment, and it could be speculated that this would be comparable in the context of illness (Ainsworth et al 1982). However, opinions vary. My own experience has indicated that, for some people, loss is an enduring feature of disability, a view described by Monteith (1987, p. 10) in respect of inability to participate in normal, childhood activities.

In contrast, Whalley Hammell (1997), writing in the field of spinal cord injury, found reduction in expression of loss after a period of time similar to that described in relation to bereavement. She suggested that, for some people, the experience of physical disability enhances quality of life. Unexpected opportunities may result, such as for the girl accidentally blinded in a bomb attack who was subsequently invited to the USA to play the piano for the president.

It should be noted that apparently small losses may add to the cumulative experience of grief and provide the last straw which leads to seeking help or medical intervention. Breaking a mug given by a deceased person may trigger a reaction far in excess of what might have been expected by the onlooker.

The implications of multiple bereavements are obvious, but any experience of loss may contribute to mental health problems or act as a precipitating factor in the onset of illness. Illness itself may give rise to further experiences of loss and these secondary experiences are worthy of attention.

REACTIONS TO EXPERIENCES OF LOSS: THE GRIEF PROCESS

Theories of loss have been well documented by authors working in different contexts, who describe similar patterns of functional and psychological reactions. Bowlby (1985, p. 85) observed children who were separated from their parents and described stages in separation anxiety. He described an initial phase of protest, followed by withdrawal and regression when the loved person has gone. Thirdly, he noted a stage of restructuring when new attachments are formed.

Theories of loss in relation to bereavement have been developed by doctors and counsellors, Kubler Ross (1970), Parkes (1986) and Worden (1991) among others. Briefly, these theories describe common features and pathways towards the resolution of grief:

- Denial – disbelief and numbness
- Anger – usually directed towards God, or the person for going away
- Depression – the pain of reality and realisation of the permanence of the situation
- Acceptance – gradual accommodation to the situation.

Bereaved people will often express feelings of guilt: 'If only I had . . .'.

These stages have been extended in relation to terminal illness by Kubler Ross (1975) and can be translated into experience of loss consequent on disability:

- Denial – 'When I get home everything will be alright.'
- Anger – 'What have I done to deserve this? Am I being punished?'
- Bargaining – 'If I become a better sort of person . . . maybe things will work out.'

- Depression – 'I'm no good to anyone like this.'
- Acceptance – 'Being able to get out again makes me feel I can still be of some use'.

A parallel concept is that of stages of loss, grief, depression and sorrow, encompassing earlier, intermediate and later reactions (Livneh and Antonak 1997).

People will not follow these stages neatly – they may move rapidly between different aspects of the grief process.

Mitchell & Anderson (1983) described 'shapes of grief'. Initially, there is searching for the lost object, immoderation and disorderliness of behaviour, as the person seeks to make sense of the chaos around him. They described the pattern of grief as spiral, not linear, with distortion of time. They noted that grief is self-oriented and suggested that grieving never wholly ends.

The realisation of loss and grief may occur suddenly. The woman who returned home having purchased bananas, which she did not eat but which were a favourite food for her mother who had recently died, stated that this was when it really hit her that her mother had gone for ever. Isolated events may trigger feelings of loss at any time, possibly producing unexpected flash back reactions which demonstrate the fickle and enduring nature of the experience.

Grief may also be regarded as a crisis of coping. Caplan (1969), who pioneered the development of crisis theory in community psychiatry, noted that a person who faces either a threat of loss or an actual loss, which he does not have an existing repertoire of skills to cope with, experiences a crisis which has to be resolved in order to return to a state of equilibrium. Subsequent crises rekindle the feelings associated with earlier losses.

The usual experience and process of grieving as a reaction to loss may be summarised as: disbelief, acknowledgement of the reality of the situation, experience of pain and grief and rebuilding over a period of time unique to the individual. There can be no predicted time by which the process will be complete.

FACTORS TO CONSIDER IN REACTIONS TO LOSS

Previous work in relation to psychiatric rehabilitation (Hume & Pullen 1994) identified that how someone copes with a physical disability depends on a variety of factors which can also apply to mental illness:

- the nature of the onset of the disability/illness
- the nature of the disability/illness itself
- what the disability/illness means for that person
- the reaction of others to the disability/illness.

A not dissimilar perspective was taken by Livneh & Antonak (1997), who proposed four classes of variables which must be considered in relation to outcomes of psychosocial adaptation:

1. those associated with the disability itself
2. those associated with sociodemographic characteristics of the individual
3. those associated with personality attributes of the individual
4. those associated with characteristics of the physical and social (external) environment.

From this they devised a model of psychosocial adaptation to chronic illness and disability (CID). This incorporates functional performance, quality of life and medical status as indicators of level of adaptation.

Those with curious and intellectual minds, especially in the medical and allied professions, may ask particularly searching questions about the nature of their experience of loss. In addition, responses will depend upon the age of onset and therefore the stage of life the person has reached and his general social circumstances: 'If this had happened when I was younger, I don't know what I would have done . . .'.

The physical and social environment may, or may not, be readily adaptable. Friends and family may be flexible in their outlook and the person will have variable individual personal resources with which to cope with what has happened (Hume & Pullen 1994). Many people will be living on their own, and when it comes to public transport and other resources there is a

world of difference between being alone in a rural area and in the city.

Particular circumstances necessarily have an impact on reactions, for example the families of siblings diagnosed with the same life-threatening illness, such as cystic fibrosis, face the prospect of multiple bereavements. A family where the prospect of redundancy threatens will be more susceptible to the extra strain imposed by the worry of having a sick family member.

Previous experience also will influence the person's response, as in the lady who was, not unnaturally, upset when her husband sustained a spinal injury. Reassurance as to the relatively positive outcome was of no avail and it transpired that the lady's brother had died following a similar injury. This, however, had been several years earlier, before the availability of antibiotic medication. Understanding advances in medicine helped to reduce the lady's distress.

The cumulative effect of multiple losses should also be remembered. Talking of his wife's final admission after years of treatment for cancer, one man said, 'The dog died just 2 days before she went back into the hospice.' This left him completely alone.

RISK FACTORS AND PROBLEM REACTIONS

Grief is a *normal* reaction to loss; however, there are certain factors which can be recognised as putting the person at greater risk of developing problem reactions to loss.

Mitchell & Anderson (1983) described some impediments to grieving. These include intolerance to pain, in the sense that the individual does not allow himself to feel it. This may be linked to a need to maintain control, and therefore acceptability, according to cultural and family influences, or to lack of external encouragement, such as lack of privacy or supportive listeners. The expression of distress may also be hindered by intellectualising or masked by the use of sedatives, medicalising a normal response.

Some people may employ coping tactics, such as the use of humour or keeping busy as a distraction or avoidance technique. Such behaviour may create more difficulties for the observer than for the individual who may be cocooned in a state of denial or preoccupied with maintaining a fragile front.

Further risk factors include traumatic death, other recent losses and problems arising due to the nature of the relationship, for example, the parent/child relationship in which there are tensions or a marriage in which the couple are totally enmeshed with each other. Those relieved of a burden of care may feel guilty for feeling thankful, whereas post traumatic grief may give rise to feelings of guilt in those who have survived the accident. Shared grief may lead to bonding experiences in which onlookers find themselves excluded. A few people may fling themselves into a new lifestyle with no apparent regrets – the merry widow syndrome. This is usually hard for the onlooker to tolerate but it remains a possibility that the individual may be in denial.

While these reactions have their origins in the context of bereavement, they are also valid for the person struggling to come to terms with loss of health. Bright (1996), a music therapist and grief counsellor, stressed the need for the person to grieve over disability and not to be overwhelmed by therapeutic optimism.

THE CONSEQUENCES OF LOSS

BEREAVEMENT

It should be remembered that grief, individual or shared, however it is expressed, cannot be avoided and needs to find expression within a supportive environment. Grieving may be a lonely experience and the world can be very critical of people who have not recovered after a period of time. People must be allowed to grieve at their own pace.

Worden (1991) suggested four tasks to be undertaken in bereavement:

1. accept the reality of the loss
2. experience pain and grief
3. adjust to a new environment
4. withdraw emotional energy and reinvest it in other relationships.

For the therapist, this means providing a supportive environment for the expression of painful feelings. People may feel a lack of support from others (real or perceived), so listening is of paramount importance. Careful attention to the person's use of language can identify those at risk. 'I wish I could see *the* light at the end of the tunnel' does not mean the same as 'I wish I could see *a* light at the end of the tunnel.'

Gomez (1987) outlined a problem solving process very similar to that of a treatment planning cycle, in which the person is encouraged to identify areas of difficulty. Possible alternatives are then considered and a course of action planned. Re-evaluation of the situation leads to any other problems being identified.

Restructuring of life might include the acquisition of practical skills and building social networks. Support and encouragement in doing things alone should lead to increasing confidence and self-esteem for the individual adjusting to a new status.

Guidelines for working with people who grieve

What the person seeks, above all, is someone who has time to listen in a non-judgemental way, someone who will accept the painful feelings and the anger which need to be expressed. Worries about upsetting the person or saying the wrong thing are natural, but tears need to be shed and it is preferable for this to happen in a supportive environment. Some people will want a hand to hold or a touch on the shoulder and this must be sensitively gauged. Non tactile people can usually make their feelings obvious!

Start where the person is and let him take the lead. Give him time to talk and be gentle in encouraging self-disclosure. Use the deceased person's name and ask questions which demonstrate an interest in knowing what the person was like. The reality of the loss has to be acknowledged, both in the present and in what the future will now mean.

Asking what the grieving person does not miss may help to promote expression of anger or negative thoughts, which may be concealed as being unacceptable when other people are focusing on the positive attributes of the deceased person.

It may be necessary to cover the same ground more than once, and it is important to realise that once the initial period of numbness and shock is passed, when society thinks the person is back to normal again, feelings of grief become more painful.

Never be tempted to compare your own experience of grief with the person and say, 'I know how you feel.' You don't. Although your experiences may help you to understand, the person's sense of loss is unique to him.

In summary, be there for the person. Stay there. People suffer more when others avoid them than they do from supportive attempts to help.

Disability/loss of health

It is necessary to consider the consequences of loss in practical terms. What effect has the loss had on the individual's life? The following examples are by no means comprehensive but are a starting point for understanding and, therefore, for intervention.

Israel (1981, p. 88) described painful reactions to loss of health:

When a person is confronted with the fact of his powerlessness in the face of ill-health . . . he undergoes different phases of response. Childish incredulity . . . when the reality of the new situation has been fully grasped, the sufferer tries to wriggle out of it by devious routes . . . Recourse to alternative therapies including spiritual healing . . . Return to progressive enfeeblement and despair grounded in reality. Final realisation that the process is irreversible. One can go on but there is no turning back . . . Moment of truth . . . Period of revolt.

A serious or fatal diagnosis is usually delivered in a supportive context, and present-day routine counselling for the newly diagnosed eliminates the referrals for psychiatric help which were not uncommon in previous decades. Realisation that the diagnosis means long-term dependence upon medication may provoke a grief reaction or a form of Russian roulette in which erratic compliance becomes problematic.

Psychological/emotional

The emotional suffering caused by loss in all its forms, but especially loss of control over one's life, isolation, abandonment and inability to carry out normal roles, always merits consideration. Difficulties related to sexual expression may not readily be talked about and loss of friends, just when most needed, is painful.

Inability to work or to maintain the same level of occupation may create feelings of worthlessness and alter social status. Reduced financial status means material constraints. It can feel that nothing will ever be the same again.

Cognitive

Processing information, organising thoughts and making decisions may all take extra time and energy and detract from other activities. Perplexity and anxiety may result. For example, a man with schizophrenia said 'I can listen to the content of the conversation or determine whether or not the other person is friendly, but not do both at the same time.'

The problems of deteriorating memory are more easily understood but are painful for those who experience them.

Physical

Problems may be visible or invisible, affecting movement, mobility, and function and therefore impacting on level of independence. A CVA patient commented that 'I know it's obvious, but it's not having two hands to do things . . .'.

Loss of sensory function, for example sight or hearing, may also create profound feelings of grief, as in, 'I'll never be able to see what my grandchildren look like.'

Spiritual

The spiritual dimension of treatment is receiving more attention from the medical professions than previously. From being a neglected area, it is verging on being a fashionable topic (Hume 1999). In the context of psychotic illness, people may become confused by religious ideology or make statements such as 'I've lost God'.

In the secular world, spirituality is acknowledged as having a wider meaning than organised religion, so that the individual's beliefs about health care, thoughts about the meaning of life and personal values will be recognised as having an influence on his spiritual needs.

Social

Alteration in interpersonal relationships and social activities must be considered, both on account of the individual's feelings and because these experiences will be shared by relatives and friends. Withdrawn, unpredictable or antisocial behaviour can seriously curtail social contacts, while role reversal can give rise to difficulties in relationships. Leisure activities or holidays may be impossible.

Carers

Those closest to the individual have their own experience of loss, such as the living death of Alzheimer's disease. 'He's not the person he used to be.' 'I've become his carer, not his wife.' Such feelings may be particularly difficult where the problems are not immediately obvious to others, for example in a relationship confused by delusional ideation.

It is also necessary to remember the future which may not now happen, the hopes and ambitions for the family that cannot be realised due to the limitations imposed by disability or financial constraints (Hume 1994, Bright 1996).

Loss and the elderly

Footballing grannies and jet-setting pensioners notwithstanding, old age can be a time of loss. This is multifactorial – memory, physical health, stamina, cognitive ability. Friends may die before you or become lost through dementia. For those unable to live at home, loss of symbols, objects, possessions and, perhaps, a pet, exacerbate feelings of incompetence at relinquishing independence.

The special needs of those growing old in an alien culture, who may never return to their roots, should be acknowledged (see Ch. 26).

Loss comes in many guises but can be summarised as meaning loss of control over one's life, loss of roles and loss of choices, any of which give rise to feelings of isolation and abandonment and to loss of self-esteem.

It is obvious that support and respite for carers are important.

CASE EXAMPLES

Joan's husband died unexpectedly following minor surgery. Surrounded by a supportive family and friends, she was able to express her feelings and to pick up the threads of life again, without any medical intervention.

Freda had threatened to pour boiling oil over her daughters in order to purify them. In later years they expressed their feelings of terror and sense of loss of their mother as 'a real mother' rather than someone strange and frightening.

Sarah was an elderly lady with a long history of mild arthritis which would not have been a problem to most people. Her considerable gifts as a pianist were much enjoyed by those round about her. She, however, experienced lifelong grief because her physical illness had deprived her of her career as a professional violinist. This led to bouts of depression and withdrawal and repeated hospital admissions for psychiatric intervention.

Paul contracted encephalitis at the age of 17. This left him with a limited field of vision in his right eye, some arm movement and the ability to move three fingers, both in his dominant hand. His parents and siblings cared for him devotedly but his girlfriend's visits diminished and eventually she stopped coming to see him. Likewise, his hopes for going to university and his ambitions for having a family faded.

David had spent many years in hospital and sometimes reminisced about the early days in the hospital. Seeing him wandering about outside my office one wet morning, I called to him to come in before he got soaked. 'I like to feel the rain,' he replied. 'The nurses would never take us out when it was raining.' This was an aspect of institutionalisation I had never considered.

Jim had a very responsible job in banking. On his retirement, he became seriously depressed, believing that he was no longer of any use. Reassurance from his friends that they would welcome his company on the golf course had little effect. Fortunately, a course of antidepressant medication was effective and his wife was able to persuade him to go to America to visit his grandchildren. On his return, he took up voluntary work and began to enjoy life again.

SOURCES OF HELP

There will be occasions when the therapist needs to refer someone for more specialised help. This is not an admission of failure on the part of the therapist but rather a mature professional judgement.

Various self-help groups may provide support for those experiencing loss in relation to a specific diagnosis, perhaps from fellow sufferers who can also offer practical advice on coping strategies. These groups are too numerous to list but may be contacted through local libraries, voluntary organisations, information officers or resource workers.

There are also specialist organisations to which people may be referred for bereavement counselling in relation to specific circumstances. The best known is Cruse, the bereavement care organisation. There are also groups such as SOBS (Survivors of Bereavement by Suicide), SANDS (Stillbirth and Neonatal Death Association), Compassionate Friends (death of a child) and the Miscarriage Association.

Care for the therapist

Working with people expressing loss can be distressing and may awaken memories of loss experienced by the therapist. Identification with clients may to some extent be helpful in creating empathy, but it may also tempt thoughts of self-disclosure. While this is useful in some instances, too much equates to stealing the person's problem and may be embarrassing to the client. It may also create loss of confidence as the person has doubts about the ability of the therapist, who has apparently not dealt successfully with her own problems, to help.

If the therapist finds herself personally distressed and unable to respond to loss situations in others, it would be wise to discuss things with a supervisor. It is only the stony-hearted who remain unmoved by the pain of others, but overwhelming reactions are counterproductive to therapy. Avoidance of the situation means unresolved problems for the client.

A FINAL CAVEAT

The reaction of the individual may not be consistent with what the loss implies to others. The treatment team congratulated themselves on curing Jimmy's hallucinations. After 30 years of companionable voices, Jimmy reported feeling lonely and did not perceive the change as totally beneficial.

Reality, which might mean a confirmed diagnosis, however bleak that may be, can be easier to cope with than uncertainty, for it gives a clear starting point for action.

SUMMARY

Loss encompasses many aspects of everyday life. This chapter has reviewed the context and characteristics of a variety of situations and outlined common grief reactions.

Examples of reactions to bereavement and loss of health have been described.

REFERENCES

Ainsworth Smith I, Speck P 1982 Letting go: caring for the dying and bereaved. SPCK, London

Bright R 1996 Grief and powerlessness. Jessica Kingsley, London

Bowlby J 1985 Attachment and loss, vol 3. Loss: sadness and depression. Penguin, London

Caplan G 1969 An approach to community mental health. Tavistock, London

Gomez J 1987 Liaison psychiatry. Croom Helm, London

Hume C 1994 Working with terminally ill people and their relatives. Therapy 20(50): 6

Hume C 1999 Spirituality: a part of total care? British Journal of Occupational Therapy 62(8): 367–370

Hume C, Pullen I (eds) 1994 Rehabilitation for mental health problems. Churchill Livingstone, Edinburgh

Hume C, Stuckey N 1994 Physical handicap. In: Hume C, Pullen I (eds) Rehabilitation for mental health problems. Churchill Livingstone, Edinburgh

Israel M 1981 The pain that heals. Hodder and Stoughton

Kubler Ross E 1970 On death and dying. Tavistock, London

Kubler Ross E 1975 Death, the final stage of growth. Prentice Hall, New Jersey

Livneh H, Antonak R 1997 Psychosocial adaptation to chronic illness and disability. Aspen, Maryland

Marris P 1974 Loss and change. Routledge and Kegan Paul, London

Mitchell K, Anderson H 1983 All our losses, all our griefs. Westminster Press, London

Monteith G 1987 Disability, faith and acceptance. St Andrew Press, Edinburgh

Morley B 1996 Grieving for what has never been. Contact, the Interdisciplinary Journal of Pastoral Studies 120

Parkes C M 1986 Bereavement: studies of grief in adult life, 2nd edn. Penguin, London

Whalley Hammell K 1997 Spinal cord injury: quality of life; occupational therapy: is there a connection? British Journal of Occupational Therapy 58(4): 151–157

Worden J 1991 Grief counselling and grief therapy: a handbook for the mental health practitioner, 2nd edn. Routledge, London

Organisation and management

30

Management

Lynne Barr

INTRODUCTION

This chapter will try to clarify what is meant by 'management' and address its application and importance to the profession of occupational therapy. Various models and structures of management will be introduced because the environments in which occupational therapists are employed are increasingly more diverse. An understanding of different models is therefore more relevant than knowledge of historical structures in the traditional institutions, such as the National Health Service.

This chapter will also differentiate between the key issues of management and leadership, as the terms are frequently confused. This is also an important issue to clarify for the practitioner therapist who may have concerns about her role versus the management structure and responsibilities within the working environment.

There are many popular preconceptions about management. Most of them are negative, especially in respect of management in the public sector. The practising therapist needs to understand concepts, styles and models of management in order to enhance her therapeutic role and gain advantage for her patient/client group appropriately by responding to, or creating, the management opportunities that arise.

WHAT IS MANAGEMENT?

An early management theorist, Mary Parker Follet (cited in Steers et al 1985) said that 'management is the art of getting things done through people'. This statement implies that more or better things can be achieved through working with others than by an individual working alone. However, those efforts need to be coordinated so that all the effort is directed towards a common goal. Hence, the role of the manager emerged.

Steers and colleagues (1985) updated this concept to one which occupational therapists will recognise more readily: 'Management is the process of planning, organising, directing and controlling the activities of employees in combination with other organisational resources to accomplish stated organisational goals.' This concept will be used to demonstrate the specific aspects of management that apply to professions in the modern health and social care agencies.

The role of the occupational therapy manager is not only that of coordinating the efforts of others but also of generating a sense of direction and energy that is compatible with the aims of the organisation. In addition to meeting the organisational goals, the manager of a profession such as occupational therapy also usually has a role as an advisor, which may be explicit in the job description or implicit in how the organisation functions. This advisory role may require the manager to deal with diverse professional issues and to advocate for the client groups that they represent.

The key functions of a manager can be discussed within the four domains referred to above (Steers et al 1985):

1. planning
2. organising
3. directing
4. controlling.

Planning

Planning is often referred to in one of two ways, strategic or operational.

Strategic or long-term planning

Strategic planning in modern management terms usually involves a 3–5 year plan. Planning for a longer period ahead becomes too vague as the influencing factors are more unknown and difficult to predict.

The strategic plan influences the annual planning cycle. The external environment, that is, political and financial influences, have a major impact upon the vision of the strategic plan. The national government agenda has both a direct impact and indirect influence on occupational therapy by such means as its central funding policy, national priorities such as the public health targets (DoH 1997), and social policy decisions, for example the NHS Plan (DoH 2000), affecting some of the client groups with whom occupational therapists work. It is important that the strategic plan for occupational therapy recognises the impact of the external environment and uses appropriately the opportunities that exist. A successful manager will anticipate and prepare occupational therapy staff and other senior colleagues for the future with this framework in mind. The current development of primary care groups and primary care trusts in the UK is a fundamental change that the profession needs to be responding to. This will include the need to forecast the workforce requirements that will enable therapists to respond to the new demands and new expectations of them.

Operational planning

This is the planning and scheduling of workloads within the resources available. To some extent, every occupational therapist is a manager when planning her own schedule with that of junior colleagues or students and balancing what is required with whom and what is available. The manager frequently needs to address these issues across a whole service, ensuring that the urgent and important work is done and that preparation and investment in the longer-term needs are not ignored. This balancing act also needs to take into account the workload and complexity of the work, together with the development needs of staff.

Operational planning is frequently done uniprofessionally on a weekly or monthly basis and reviewed as and when necessary or discussed with other professional colleagues in regular meetings.

Organising

Organisational skills are required on a day-to-day basis. The operational manager needs to be able to respond to the daily demands and fluctuations of the service. The manager who knows the service and staff well is able to handle several situations at once, keep calm in stressful situations and consistently deliver what is required. This manager will respond to situations in a way that supports the longer-term strategy of the service wherever possible. She will communicate openly with all concerned, so that staff respond positively to the changes required. Changes may be temporary or permanent and opportunities can arise from such events, if handled well. An example of this would be if a colleague in the multidisciplinary team was unable to fulfil his normal role due to sickness or other absence. In this instance, the occupational therapist could contribute to the programme in an enhanced way by rescheduling her day and/or the programme. This could be an opportunity to demonstrate to the multidisciplinary team and the patient how the occupational therapy aspect of the programme could be enhanced on a regular basis through this act of helpfulness in a problem situation. This would be a particularly proactive gesture if it is part of the strategic direction of the service. The alternative, but less proactive, way would be to just rearrange that aspect of the programme to a time when the other member of staff is available.

Directing

Directing is activity that enables managers to gain the participation of the workforce. It is necessary to understand the dynamics of workgroups, key individuals and how they respond to situations. There are different cultures within workplaces and professions and it is important to recognise the impact of these issues and how to handle each situation. Textbook solutions do not exist in the workplace and a good manager will exhibit leadership skills in order to resolve or, better still, to prevent the occurrence of problems that disrupt work or dishearten the staff unnecessarily.

Directing involves setting and being able to implement the objectives of the organisation, involving staff in negotiating the direction and the specific objectives, and keeping the impetus to achieve them in the timescale proposed.

Occupational therapists are familiar with group dynamics with their client groups but frequently do not apply their understanding to their workplace behaviour or relationships with colleagues. Once the value of this knowledge is recognised, the transference into management ability is relatively straightforward.

Controlling

The term 'controlling' implies a rigid and constraining force in order to achieve the desired outcome of the service. This is not the case in management terms. Controlling arises out of the availability, knowledge and interpretation of the data that are required by the manager to enable her to manage. Managers must now have skills in information technology (IT), budgets and audit. Information is the means by which managers gain tangible evidence to explain service activities carried out by the staff over a period of time. The information, or management reports, as they are frequently referred to, assist in communication with other management colleagues and help managers to understand how the occupational therapy service is perceived by others. The types of reports that are usually generated are detailed in Table 30.1. The emphasis, however, will vary according to the project or employing organisation. Each organisation has to demonstrate its effectiveness and value for money and, in the case of public sector organisations, there are specific information reports engendered from the information required by, for example, the Department of Health.

Data must be interpreted by managers who understand the service they manage. Data should be used with caution and conclusions

Table 30.1 Types of management report

Report	Description/purpose	Frequency
Annual report	Summary of achievements and resources available within the year	Annual
Financial statements	Summary statements on expenditure and income Predictions of the annual expenditure based on past performance Explicit over or underspend statement on the annual budget	Monthly
Activity	Number of patients/clients received treatment Sub-section: • by speciality/doctor or referrer • by therapist • by location of treatment • by time spent in treatment • by time spent on other duties Ratio of new referrals to treatments Number of non attenders Number waiting for treatment Length of waiting times for appointment	Monthly
Staffing	Staff employed/leavers/hours worked Sickness/absence rates	Monthly
Audit reports (internal and external)	Relevant to quality initiatives: • Investors in People award • evaluation of training • clinical governance • recruitment factors such as vacancy times, responses and number of applicants, turnover of staff by grade	Quarterly or annual

should not be drawn without analysis of the situation. Data are best used over time, to identify trends and issues of concern or progress. Timely feedback to the staff, who frequently spend an inordinate amount of time completing data input sheets, is important so that they see the impact of their contribution to the service as a whole.

It is worth noting that modern computer systems still have difficulty in representing the therapeutic professions. However, while data collection is costly in terms of staff resources and financial capital, the profession does need to continue in the quest for improvement in this field if services are to be able to produce the required results in the future.

MANAGEMENT ROLES

There are other models of management that will become familiar to therapists as they progress in their career. These are based on management roles rather than tasks. Henry Mintzberg (1973) described a model, based on his research of the 1970s, in which he examined how different managers at all levels spent their time. Mintzberg's model was a pragmatic approach to defining management activities which can assist the therapist to understand that the role of management is an integrated whole. It is more than a series of tasks, which the first, functional approach to management would lead us to believe.

From this research emerged the following constellation of roles (Lessen 1990):

• decisional roles
• informational roles
• interpersonal roles.

Decisional role

This can be subdivided into four types of role. Each is involved with decision making from a different angle or context:

1. *Entrepreneur.* The proactive decision maker, initiator of change

2. *Disturbance handler*. Instant decision maker, responding to situations beyond his control
3. *Resource allocator*. Pre-planned decisions about resource management
4. *Negotiator*. Decision making in the context of negotiations involves both pre-planned and improvised responses, depending on the circumstances.

Informational role

Mintzberg (1973) considered that the communication and receipt of information is the central issue for the manager. This includes both informal and formal aspects of communication. These informational roles are of three types:

1. *Monitor*. Seeking information to be used to the best advantage, such as the management reports referred to in Table 30.1. This information can be gained from formal or informal sources.
2. *Disseminator*. Distributing information that would not be otherwise available to those senior and junior to her. This information would usually be passed on by personal contact.
3. *Spokesperson*. Taking formal responsibility for communicating information up and down the organisation, or even outside the organisation. This is a key role that frequently reflects the function of the organisation and the individual style of the manager.

Interpersonal role

Interpersonal relationships help to keep the service running smoothly at all times. The interpersonal role has three facets:

1. *Liaison*. The liaison person deals with people outside the immediate span of control. Success depends upon the interpersonal skills of the individual rather than decision-making skills.
2. *Figurehead*. This role is that of a formal representative at important functions.
3. *Leader*. The leadership role is by far the most important and involves projecting values and

creating a sense of direction, empathising with others according to their needs and inspiring or motivating.

Leadership issues will be dealt with more thoroughly later in this chapter.

MANAGEMENT STRUCTURES

Management structures are a formal framework of accountability and responsibility within an organisation. The framework will indicate the levels and type of management required to fulfil the goals of the organisation. These are outlined briefly below.

Levels of management

Levels of management are frequently referred to as tiers, as shown in Table 30.2.

While the manager has a complex role that involves many dimensions and numerous tasks, the tier of management will determine the major skills required for the fulfilment of the job. That is to say, the first line manager will direct and monitor the day-to-day issues, making sure that tasks are completed as well as possible, and bringing problems to the attention of

Table 30.2   Management tiers

Tier	Skills
Senior management	Conceptual and coordinating skills Sense of vision and direction Negotiating and planning Awareness of trends and influences
Middle management	Frequently uni-professional Organisational and personnel/staff management skills Attention to detail and monitoring of information Able to respond quickly to changes and demands
First line management	Team leaders Specialised/limited scope of responsibility Knowledge and skills primarily related to specialist field Day-to-day responsibilities for the service

the middle manager. The senior manager will be more involved in longer-term issues that will affect the workforce, such as planning staffing and recruitment levels. The senior manager needs to be able to rely on the middle and first line managers to organise and carry out the jobs that are required. Essentially, the senior manager needs to be in contact with the other tiers of management in order to be able to plan effectively so that the expectations on the staff are realistic and services are planned where and how they are needed. This interrelationship is paramount to the success of any management structure. Each tier is as important as the others, and the communication between them needs to be open and honest and supportive.

It is important to recognise that each manager, while at a recognised level of management within the service, will be a part of another, often wider management structure across the organisation. Therefore, the relationships and skills will need to be adaptable for the complex nature of this position. For example, the most senior manager of occupational therapy could be at the top of the career structure within the professional structure, but would be considered as a middle or first line manager within the management structure of the organisation as a whole (Figure 30.1).

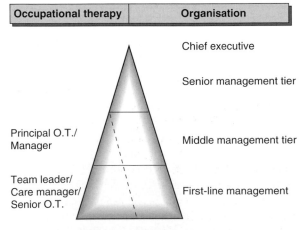

Figure 30.1 The position of the occupational therapy manager.

Organisational structures

The lines of communication and number of tiers in an organisation will reflect the management style and structure. There are wide variations in the style and manner of communication depending upon the culture and historical patterns of behaviour within each organisation. These may be based on the type of work and responsibilities of the organisation, or on the type and level of technical skills and knowledge base and working patterns of the workforce. Whatever the format of the organisation, it is essential not to underestimate the impact that this will have on the responses of the workforce, particularly during periods of change. Occupational therapists will experience this in particular when relating to colleagues working in other organisations, such as historical differences between the health and social services departments. Different management structures will affect the scope of influence and/or responsibility of the managers of the service. Most organisations operate in a hierarchical structure within themselves. The structure resembles a family tree and the number of branches between the chief executive or management board and the manager demonstrates the lines of communication and, therefore, the level of authority of the manager within the organisation.

Structure can group different aspects of the organisation according to:

- division of work
- span of control and responsibility
- the nature of the work, that is, level of formality required
- preferred number of levels of management.

Familiar groupings include:

- *Functional*. Such as specialist areas, usually in small organisations.
- *General*. Full span of control over the whole process for particular population or client groups, such as a disability resource team.
- *Divisional*. These structures become efficient in dealing with their own area but largely operate as autonomous entities within the organisation. Duplication of resources can

occur, for example within clinical divisions in a hospital setting.

- *Geographical*. These structures allow the service to be as close to the action as possible. This can be seen in community based services, for example in community mental health teams.
- *Matrix*. These are mixed structures that attempt to be flexible and responsive to complex, changing environments. These are more common in the current public service arena as integrated approaches are being sought to resolve some of the increasing and chronic health and social care needs of the clients that occupational therapists work with. This structure works well between different organisations which may well have their own internal structures more akin to the above.

The occupational therapy manager

The manager of an occupational therapy service may or may not be an experienced occupational therapist. If she is an occupational therapist, she may be regarded as a skilled technical/professional manager. She will be required to be a practising therapist with modern skills in a particular field that is relevant to the employing organisation. More frequently now, occupational therapists are managed by general managers or managers from other professional groups, particularly in community settings where the team structure is truly multiprofessional. This may also be a feature for occupational therapists working in a partnership situation where the matrix management structure exists between the organisations involved. In this instance there should be a lead occupational therapist recognised by the organisation, who would advise both individual therapists and the organisation on the professional issues that arise. This role can include professional supervision of individual therapists (Fig. 30.2).

The important additional elements required if the manager of the service is not an occupational therapist are communication skills. It is vital that

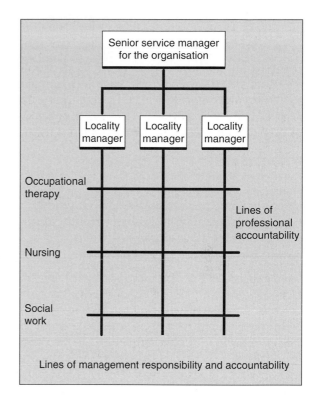

Figure 30.2   Matrix organisational structure.

the manager listens well to staff about the service and its requirements but, equally essentially, that the occupational therapists themselves learn to articulate their needs, aspirations and achievements in a manner that is heard by their manager.

The role of the occupational therapy manager is diverse as the actual tasks of the manager will vary according to the organisation that he is working for. The profession needs to produce and support the development of eloquent and competent managers. Indeed, for the increasing number of occupational therapists who are now working in private practice, or for independent agencies, management tasks become even more important in respect of responsibilities and the need to address professional clinical frameworks required by the clinical governance agenda. The role of manager needs self-discipline and organisation. However, this can be more readily achieved and maintained if some leadership qualities and attitudes are present.

LEADERSHIP

This part of the chapter attempts to demonstrate the differences between leadership and management and the importance of leadership to the profession of occupational therapy as a whole and to each individual occupational therapist.

Leadership is a complex activity of social interaction involving:

- processes of influence
- people who are both leaders and followers
- the commitment of individuals to common goals and the enhancement of group cohesiveness (Saddler 1999).

Management is concerned with the achievement of plans through tasks and processes, whereas leadership is about aligning people and gaining their commitment to the vision and direction of the service. Individuals in organisations can rarely be successful on their own, they must influence, lead and coordinate efforts to achieve their goals. The success of leadership rests on the ability to influence different groups in the organisation.

Leaders are people in a position of influence either by their status, which can be as a specialist or expert, or their particular personal qualities, popularity or sense of judgement. Therefore, leaders are not always managers, although some managers are leaders. Some of the best known managers have become famous because of their leadership qualities. This explains why management and leadership can become confused.

Leadership in occupational therapy

Occupational therapists of any grade can find themselves in a position of influence and leadership, possibly much more frequently than some of their other working colleagues, because of the relatively low numbers of staff in each working situation. There will regularly be only one occupational therapist in a rehabilitation team compared, for example, with physiotherapists or nurses; that individual occupational therapist will, therefore, have a significant personal and professional influence on whatever contribution she makes to that team. In that instance the individual is required to be a role model for the profession, even at a relatively junior grade. Some people are natural leaders in some situations, for example the person who can organise a successful social evening for a staff group, or the person who gathers people around her in order to resolve issues successfully.

Personal leaders are consistent in their values and commitment and people respond willingly to them. 'Personal leadership is not an event, it is an ongoing process of clarifying (your) vision, values and aligning yourself with timeless principles' (Covey 1996).

Leadership is consistent with the ethos and values of occupational therapy and therefore is compatible with the role of the committed and inspired occupational therapist. It is important, when trying to understand the dimensions of leadership, to recognise and understand the sub-sets of motivation, essential tools of the occupational therapist:

- goal setting and ownership
- energy and agreed action plan
- intrinsic reward system

The occupational therapist will link the three sub-sets to the needs and rehabilitation goals of the patient or client, whereas the organisational leader will use the same skills with individual staff or colleagues. By linking goals, energy and rewards (often intrinsic), the effective leader can use the valuable skill of motivation to empower people to perform effectively.

In work based teams, motivation and rewards for the individual need to be compatible with the ethos and objectives of the team and the organisation or project. The occupational therapist or manager working in an interagency or multidisciplinary team needs to be able to recognise the leadership role and the challenges that arise. She should be able to respond constructively to, and operate within, the dynamics and motivational factors that affect the team. However, team cultures need proactive development. An effective team is much more than a group getting on well, and it requires leadership to recognise the team's requirements and strengths. A successful leader will encourage and value openness and reflexivity which, in turn, will allow the team to challenge, learn and grow together to increase their effectiveness as a whole.

Leadership traits and behaviours

The elements of leadership can be observed as attitudes and behaviours, succinctly described by Sundstrom et al (1990, cited in Leadership Effectiveness Analysis TM 1998) as 'Management is doing things right . . . leadership is doing the right thing'. These behaviours or traits are easily recognisable but often difficult to describe, particularly in an objective manner in the work situation (see Box 30.1). The list in Box 30.1 is taken from the Leadership Effectiveness Analysis TM

Box 30.1 Leadership traits and behaviours (reproduced with permission from the Leadership Research Group)

Leadership trait	Behaviour demonstrated
Creating a vision	
Traditional	Studying problems in the light of past practice, to ensure predictability and reduce risk
Innovative	Feeling comfortable in fast changing environments; being willing to take risks and to consider new approaches
Technical	Acquiring and maintaining in depth knowledge in a particular field, using the expert knowledge to draw conclusions
Self	Recognising the need for independent decision making
Strategic	Taking a long range, broad based approach to problem solving, thinking ahead and planning
Developing followers	
Persuasiveness	Building commitment by convincing others, winning others over to the point of view
Outgoing	A capacity to quickly establish easy relationships, a friendly and informal manner
Excitement	Operating with a good deal of energy and expression, keeping others involved and enthusiastic
Restraint	Maintaining a low key interpersonal demeanour by working to control emotional expression
Implementing the vision	
Structuring	Developing and utilising guidelines, an organised approach
Tactical	Emphasising production of results, practical strategies
Communication	Clear expression of what is expected and needed, maintaining flow of information
Delegation	Enlisting the talents of others by giving important jobs to others and autonomy to do it
Following through	
Control	Setting deadlines for actions and ensuring progression to completion
Feedback	Letting people know in a straightforward manner how well they are performing against the expectations
Achieving results	
Management focus	Seeking to exert influence over others
Dominant	Pushing to achieve results
Production	A strong orientation towards achievement, with high expectations of self and others
Team playing	
Cooperation	Accommodating the needs of others in order to assist with the achievement of their objectives
Consensual	Collecting and valuing the contributions of others in decision-making processes
Authority	Showing loyalty and respecting the opinions of people in authority
Empathy	Demonstrating an active concern for the needs of others through relationships

(1998). This leadership model is employed to clarify the terminology that is used to identify the spectrum of behaviours we recognise in our leaders and some of our managers. All the behaviours will be desirable in particular situations, but each individual role or management position will require the predominance of a particular range of traits or behaviours.

A good leader will be able to select and use the above skills and behaviours appropriately to the best effect in the situation in which she finds herself. The skill of the leader is in being able to adapt herself, to know when to use some traits and hold back on others. She will use these skills alongside her clinical or technical skills and make decisions with a balance of judgement, positive acknowledgement and a proactive stance.

The leadership contribution to management is often referred to as the 'soft' issues and management as the 'hard' issues. All occupational therapists will be familiar with this concept as many of the areas with which we are clinically involved rely not just on the application of technical knowledge but also on the inclusion of the less tangible, emotional and relationship issues that affect the client's ability to cope and function.

The leadership element of management is now a requirement of the modern day manager. However, it can be a beneficial and highly effective trait in all grades of staff, such as a coordinator of a graduate therapist group, a lead therapist in research or a health and safety representative. Individual therapists could find themselves in specific projects, clinical audits or trail-blazing ventures, where the approach that they take could have a minimal impact or could make a radical difference. Most occupational therapists want to make a difference. The behaviours of leadership portray skills and qualities that would help them to do just that, whether they have the title of manager or not.

SUMMARY

It is essential that the management of occupational therapists is in competent hands. It may be that the manager of the team within which the individual works is not an occupational therapist. Whilst this may not be the preferred model of management it is not necessarily a problem as long as the professions within the team are well respected and represented at senior levels through a professional lead person. The structure of the organisation and fairness of the manager will determine if this can be achieved successfully. Management tasks can well be achieved by a sensitive and empathetic manager with good leadership skills. The career path into management from practising therapist is not a popular one and it may be beneficial in some areas for the skills of the practitioner to be retained, rather than be diluted to an inefficient level. However, the profession does need occupational therapists to be leaders. The long-term future of the profession, in its many and diverse roles and functions, needs individuals to 'do the right thing', whatever their status and place of work.

Occupational therapists frequently work with client groups who are under-represented in the structure of our society – they frequently need us to be advocates on their behalf, to lead the cause and represent their needs. The role of the modern manager is changing. Additional qualities are required in order to be able to achieve, with and through others, what needs to be done. The role of the manager could become more popular within the profession when the importance of the leadership element is recognised and the confidence of practitioners can be reflected in their achievements as leaders.

REFERENCES

Clutterbuck D 1998 How teams learn. Training Officer 34(7): 198–200

Covey S 1992 Seven habits of highly effective people: restoring the character ethic. Simon Schuster, London

Covey S 1994 Covey Leadership Centre Inc. 10/94 AE6S7HB.

Department of Health 2000 NHS plan. HMSO, London

Department of Health 1997 Our healthier nation. HMSO, London

Department of Health 1998 The new NHS. HMSO, London

Leadership Effectiveness Analysis™ 1998 Management Research Group GabHm, Munchen

Lessen R 1990 Global management principles. Prentice Hall, Hertfordshire

Mintzberg H 1973 The nature of managerial work. Harper Row, New York

Saddler P 1999 Leadership in tomorrows company. Centre for Tomorrows Company, London

Steers R M, Ungson G R, Mowday R T 1985 Managing effective organisations. Boston Publishing, Kent

31

Budgeting

Lynne Barr

INTRODUCTION

Every occupational therapist operates within a service framework and within control systems, whether as an individual therapist in private practice or as a member of a therapy team within a larger organisation. The framework for an individual therapist will be that of her own business plan and the scope of her own skills and service, while that of the team therapist will be the main purpose of the organisation and the role of the occupational therapist within it. The role and requirements of a social services department, for example, will determine the structures and systems that impact on all of its services, including those of the occupational therapy team.

There are at least three types of control systems for every organisation (Hussey 1994):

1. Budget and financial controls
2. Operational and production controls: clinical standards, clinical governance and legislation in respect of patient/client care
3. Employee related controls: employment law, health and safety at work, grievance and disciplinary procedures, trade union activity and state registration (or minimum standards of competence).

This chapter will examine the budget and financial controls that affect the occupational therapy services.

BUDGET CONTROL WITH MANAGEMENT

As with the management of occupational therapy, there is no one model that applies to the service as a whole. The diversity of management models and structures throughout the profession will be reflected in the financial and budgetary control systems that are in place. On the whole, the structure of an organisation will determine the level of budgetary devolution and accountability of each manager. The flatter the management structure, the more the devolution of responsibility for the service and the budget.

The Chartered Institute for Management Accountants (Hussey 1994) defined a budget as: 'a quantitative statement, for a defined period in time, which may include planned revenues, expenses, assets and liabilities and cash flows. A budget provides a focus for the organisation, aids the co-ordination of activities and facilitates control.' The concept of budget management in occupational therapy is not always grasped willingly and there are potential problems in maintaining the service when attention focuses on the budget. The language of financial management provides another cognitive and emotional barrier to the new occupational therapy manager. It is another area where the importance of clear communication is essential in order to promote understanding from both the financial advisor's perspective and the occupational therapy manager's perspective.

Apprehension about managing budgets is also reinforced by lack of experience at junior grade level or senior clinician level. It is essential that training is undertaken by the new manager, in particular, training for non financial managers, which will help to clarify the terms and legislative requirements.

The financial statement should be seen as an information tool to assist the manager in the achievement of her goals. Every organisation has to operate within defined and frequently limited resources, even if the organisation operates on a profit-making basis. The shareholders of the company would complain if the company's resources were being inefficiently managed. Public sector organisations, however, have to operate within other additional constraints. These will be explained later in the chapter.

BUDGETS IN PLANNING

Budgets are a useful planning and control tool (see Ch. 30, 'Control', p. 543). They are a financial statement of future expenditure and income (revenue) that helps a manager to plan the best use of her resources. Resources can be people or machinery, equipment, basic materials or utilities, such as communication systems, heating or lighting. Budgets allow the manager to quantify whether there are adequate resources, and to plan accordingly.

Budgets are normally set, within given constraints, by first or middle line managers who are familiar with the operational elements of the service, and approved by the senior managers. Once budgets are set they are only modified under extreme circumstances. It is for this reason that it is important, when establishing a new service, to take into account the full costs of the service so that financial problems do not occur at a later date. Larger organisations, particularly those in the public sector, have a historical protocol for modelling the resourcing of services. It is important both to know the protocol and to use it and, in turn, know its limitations so that any planning or predictions will be realistic and the services not overstretched.

It is equally important to recognise that the protocols for different organisations will vary and if submitting bids for new developments it is vital that the relevant protocol is followed.

Budgets serve several purposes. They:

- aid communication between managers about their commitment to the priorities of the organisation
- require a periodic review of the service objectives because of the fixed timescale related to the objectives
- contribute to the measurement of effectiveness of the use of resources
- clarify the scope and range of responsibility of the manager.

Budgets are usually set annually, with monthly statement reports. The financial year, or fiscal year as it is referred to, can be established to suit the organisation. Public sector organisations in the UK usually mirror the tax year, which runs from April to March the following year.

The budget-setting process will follow the annual planning cycle of the organisation, so that corporate and individual service objectives can inform the budget setting exercise (Fig. 31.1).

Six-months' notice is usually given of any major changes to patterns of service, so there should not be any sudden changes in the budgetary position that cannot be accommodated in that time. Annual budget setting cycles, however, are not conducive to strategic long-term planning or the development of the types of service that occupational therapists are usually involved

in. There has been a move in more recent health and social care policies, such as *The New NHS* (DoH 1997), to extend the contractual cycle to 3 years wherever possible. This should achieve more stability in services that need to have year-on-year investment in order to make some impact for the client or population groups they are intended to help. Long term service agreements will be commissioned by primary care groups/trusts, where they are being set up to address this very problem.

FINANCIAL PARADIGMS

There are four main financial paradigms that occupational therapy managers may encounter within their department's financial structure.

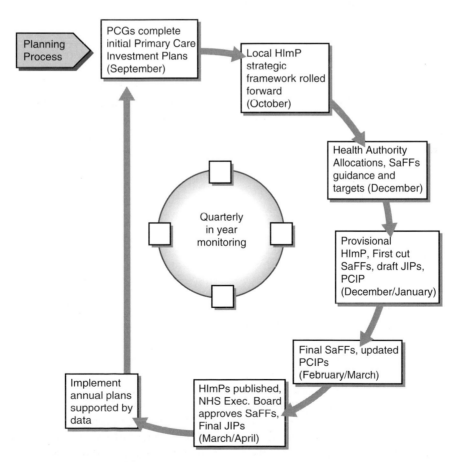

Figure 31.1 The NHS planning cycle (DoH 1999a).

The occupational therapy budget may well be constructed from one or more of the following:

- the bid system
- financial planning system
- planning programme budget system
- zero based budget system.

They are all subject to 'best practice' guidelines produced by the NHS Audit Commission, the National Audit Office and the professional accounting bodies (Wilson 1998).

The bid system

This is an incremental budget. Each department prepares its own estimates of future plans and requirements. These are aggregated and compared to the resources available. The total of the proposed bids inevitably exceeds resources, so the bids are cut to balance the resources.

The disadvantages of this system are:

- it is often difficult to respond to the frequently tight time constraints for submitting the bids, therefore bids are ill prepared
- the system is open to manipulation by internal politics and produces winners and losers
- long-term planning is restricted by the year-on-year allocation process
- arbitrary cuts to match bids to resources give negative feedback to the bidders, so overbidding occurs
- there is little review of base expenditure, only of the increases or cuts necessary
- bids need to be monitored closely to ensure that they address corporate or local/national policies.

Financial planning

This financial model follows the guidance from central government and tends to address the medium term issues on a year on year basis. It operates as follows:

Base line expenditure plus inflation
Minus a reduction due to efficiency savings
Plus growth for committed targets set
Plus new money for new developments.

This results in a disjointed incrementalism to service budgets but is typical of the funding of hospital based occupational therapy services over the years.

The system works well when there is a stable environment and no major changes are required. The disadvantages are:

- the baseline budget is not consolidated so the starting point for each year is the same rather than recognising that the service is evolving over time
- this system leads to an individual departmental approach and reduces the scope for achieving shared or corporate objectives, such as team developments.

Planning programme budget system (PPBS)

This is referred to as a rational system, as it relates to established objectives and outcomes, but it is difficult to implement because of the detail required.

The process is based on the planning and analysis of costs budgeted for and actual costs, by each area of activity. Alternative means of achieving the objectives are analysed by asking the question 'What ought to be done?' and then considering the impact of the alternatives on other services. This is a very complicated task and difficult to prepare and assimilate. It does, however, promote and enable major changes in the way services are delivered, therefore, in the current climate of shifting resources from secondary, hospital based care to primary and community care, it has a very useful role. This system is particularly advantageous across a range of services for specific client groups, such as rehabilitation services, and can be combined with outcome and target driven objectives, or health priorities, such as those proposed in the health strategy *Our Healthier Nation* (DoH 1998).

Zero based budgeting

This starts the budget-setting process with a clean sheet. This is a radical approach not commonly applied to existing services unless a major change is forecast. The budget is built up by examining possible service levels or packages of care and establishing what can be achieved within the resources available. In this system, nothing from the past is automatically rolled over or brought forward. This does not work well as an annual routine because of the need for some stability in services. It works well when applied as a result of a major policy change, in selected areas (Wilson 1998).

In order to be able to manage a budget it is essential to know how the organisation that is funding the service receives its own income. This will vary and, in the case of private practitioners operating as sole agents, it will be self-evident. For the purpose of this chapter a brief outline of the funding of public sector organisations is included.

THE ECONOMIC ENVIRONMENT

Public sector organisations include central and local government offices and public corporations. They exist to provide services on a 'not for profit' basis and funded by income raised from public taxes (84.5%), national insurance (11.3%) prescription charges and other sources. The size and efficiency of the organisation is measured by the public expenditure level, rather than the profit made, as would be the case in an independent agency or by an individual operating on a private basis.

The UK has what is known as a mixed economy and public sector organisations operate in that external environment. However, the funding of the public sector is that of a planned economy in which budget negotiations take place annually. This is mainly because the level of taxation is fixed and the amount of money available can largely be predicted, given the set of social and economic circumstances that the country is experiencing at the time.

FUNDING THE NATIONAL HEALTH SERVICE

In the UK, the National Health Service has existed since 1948 with the sole aim to provide a national service and to overcome the imbalances of better hospital services in the wealthier areas and worse health in the less advantaged areas. To achieve this, district health authorities were allocated funding with which to deliver health services.

Since 1991, the funding process has required health authorities to specify the type of health service that is required within their area and to contract formally with providers to deliver to that contract. This agreement was intended to improve the quality of the service and to enable a service to be provided to deal with specific priorities. In the main, contracts reflected the historical pattern of service except that some quality and activity targets could be incrementally increased, thus achieving more within the financial constraints imposed. This created a business market environment that resulted in a competitive culture being promoted. Services that require a coordinated inter-agency approach, such as occupational therapy, suffered during this period.

The latest approach, the allocation of budgets against national and local priorities, focused through Joint Investment Plans and Partnership Grants, is largely supportive of the type of investment in which occupational therapy services are involved. Client groups are well represented, such as mental health groups, older people and those requiring rehabilitation and recuperation (Fig. 31.2). However, occupational therapy needs to be integrated into a truly cohesive plan rather than be an isolated series of interventions. This means that the occupational therapy manager must work closely with other professional colleagues in order to take the advantage of the opportunities that are available through this planning programme budget system.

New services or service developments are most likely to be resourced in this way. Health authorities and primary care groups/trusts are required to perform their functions within their total funds (DoH 1977, 1986, 1999b). They will now do this through Health Improvement Programmes (HImP) by:

- identifying national and local priorities, according to national priorities guidance

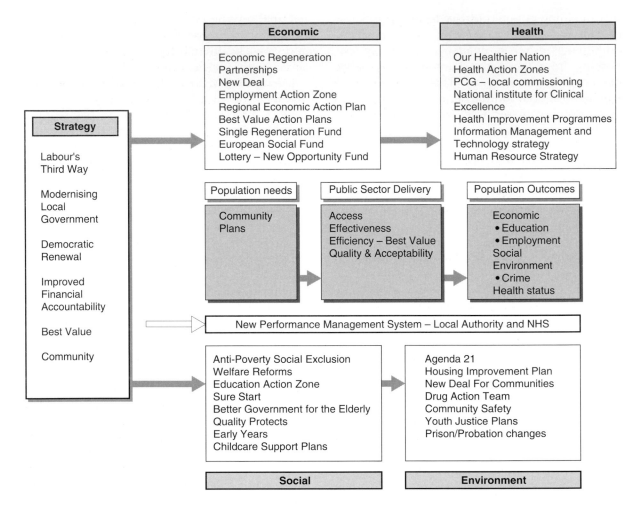

Figure 31.2 Overview of strategic planning framework (Brown 1999).

- confirming the resources available
- monitoring commissioned services against national targets and objectives for the NHS – (DoH 1998, 1999a).

This is achieved through the planning process outlined in Figure 31.1.

The Health Improvement Programme is underpinned by the Service and Financial Framework (SaFF) which sets out the levels of NHS service activity and financial investment required to achieve the targets and the Primary Care Investment Plans (PCIPs). Improvements in health care will only be delivered by the performance of all local partners including the

newly established primary care groups, in some areas primary care trusts, in partnership with local authorities and other local agencies. Joint Investment Plans (JIPs) focus on the development of services at the interface of health and social care. Funding is allocated to jointly commissioned ventures for specific client groups and targeted over a 3-year period to reshape services to address the needs identified. The executive boards of primary care groups include representation from the local authorities, the public, general practitioners and nursing.

The occupational therapy manager needs to understand this fundamental shift in how the National Health Service is funded in order to be able to recognise and address health priority targets for her locality. It is also important to be able to influence the primary care groups/trusts as it is they who approve and support new developments for their locality. As there is very little new money around, it is important to recognise that the historical pattern of services may not be how the local PCG wants it to be, and it may be necessary to reconfigure and shift services and resources to where they are required. The needs of the local population and client groups must be paramount. If the therapy manager is involved and able to influence the strategic planning, shifts in services, although disruptive and needing careful handling of staffing issues, can often be achieved to the benefit of clients. In turn, staff could also benefit and the frustrations of their working environment could be reduced as investment in new priorities improves the effectiveness of the service they can deliver. This effect is increased if services are shifted by client needs, thus including the full range of services for the client group and promoting improved team working.

The fixed budget system, as applied through health authorities and primary care groups/trusts, allows for close monitoring of activity and performance against the budget. This principle applies all the way through the system and includes the occupational therapy service. The means by which monitoring is carried out will become increasingly sophisticated and relevant to occupational therapy services. Outcome measures or targets that we use to reflect the effectiveness of our contribution need to address the needs of the commissioners as well as the clinical effectiveness framework within which we work (NICE 1998).

SETTING THE BUDGET

Despite the above planning mechanism for service developments, the main public sector bodies are essentially constrained by central government's control of funding. Change can only be achieved by rethinking existing services. The costing exercise for the National Health Service is carried out on an activity-based costing and budgeting basis. The activity base is becoming increasingly target orientated, with financial penalties for default. Targets are largely influenced by the political agenda of the day.

Close monitoring of the budgetary situation reflects activity towards the targets and is used as an indicator throughout the year. Although it is possible to modify and influence activity as a result of analysis of the budget versus activity, there are only limited options available for action because of the political nature of the situation.

Unfortunately, the production of alternative measures of effectiveness is very complex and problematic, not just for occupational therapy, so the use of the cost-based activity model is liable to be maintained for some time to come.

The total amount of resources for the coming year is often uncertain, but there is a baseline budget that can be set relating to the fixed costs, especially those where there is an ongoing commitment, either through employment contracts or lease arrangements of the premises. In occupational therapy services, the baseline budget is usually largely related to the costs of staffing. Within each financial year, allowances need to take into account recruitment factors, the impact of inflation and rising costs, the influence of competition from other organisations, the need for support, such as travel arrangements, cover for staff absences, stationery, methods of communication and more.

This baseline budget setting exercise produces the allocation from which the core service is provided. It relates most closely to the financial planning model.

It is vital that the budget should be predicted as accurately as possible, as it will significantly affect the level of service which can be provided throughout the next year. Prediction is, however, not an exact science and the manager can only predict on the information that is available. The historical pattern of services can demonstrate trends over time, but will not identify details.

Some of the management reports identified in Table 30.1 (p. 549) in Chapter 30, will help to inform the manager about changing trends in the service and where resources need to be directed.

THE OCCUPATIONAL THERAPY BUDGET

The occupational therapy budget is usually set once a year, several months ahead of the end of the financial year, that is, January, basing costs on the fixed costs of the service, projected forward to the end of the financial year.

The occupational therapy budget can contain three elements.

1. *Pay costs*. These are related to the costs incurred by the employment and payment of staff.
2. *Non-pay costs*. These are related to the expenses incurred from running the service, such as materials used, stationery, training costs and travel.
3. *Income*. These accounts are established to monitor credits received by the department, usually in respect of services provided additional to the core or central services, income derived from providing training or income from the sale of goods.

Financial statements about the cash flow, month-on-month, are received monthly. These statements reflect the income and expenditure of the service for that specific month, and are used to predict the financial situation at the end of the year.

A responsible attitude must be taken to managing the budget, if only to avoid the penalties of not doing so. The amount of overspend or debt incurred at the end of the financial year will usually be carried forward into the next financial year, so that a deficit is incurred by those services who do not manage their service within the constraints of the organisation. The problem, therefore, is only moved on to the following year. As it is rare that there is any windfall of extra funding for the next year, and there are frequently additional constraints, it becomes more difficult to redress the balance as times moves on.

PAY COSTS

Predictions for the resourcing of a service need to identify the costs of relevantly skilled staff, for the length of time required, as frequently as they are required. Staff will be employed under contract with the organisation or subcontracted to the service.

People who work in the public sector or major organisations will have well established terms and conditions of employment, some of which will relate to the amount of remuneration (salary) that they will receive. There are scales of payment to which grades and responsibilities will have been designated. The employee's own contract of employment will clearly state the remuneration that she will receive. However, these salary figures do not appear on the budget statement because there are additional costs incurred by the organisation which will be included in the financial statement. These additional costs include the employer's national insurance fund contribution and the superannuation fund, if applicable. These 'on costs', as they are referred to, are approximately 12% of the salary the individual receives.

There are now various pay structures in operation, even within the National Health Service, so the actual remuneration will vary from place to place.

Annual increments and pay bonuses or incentives need to be predicted as accurately as possible. In the case of the public sector, it is commonplace in recent years for annual pay rises not to be fully funded by the budget allocation from central governments, in which case additional costs need to borne by the services themselves. This is done to try to increase efficiencies in the service and to avoid the excess that occurs through the implementation of the bid system, where managers try to over-bid in order to achieve additional funding.

There is no additional funding to pay for staff absences due to sickness, study or maternity/paternity leave. Local arrangements may apply to recoup some costs related to maternity leave, depending on the length of time this will apply and it is always worthwhile investigating every individual situation. In general terms, all extra staff time has to be met from the base budget already established.

The financial statement, usually received monthly, can resemble the example given in Figure 31.3.

NON-PAY BUDGET

The content of the non-pay budget will be very specific to the type of service and to the organisation within which it operates. For example, the non-pay budget of a local authority social services department could be hundreds of thousands or even a million pounds or more, where as the non-pay budget of an occupational therapy service in a small hospital or general practice could be only a thousand or so, being based upon travel costs to client homes for the whole year. Increasingly, as management of services is being devolved to the point of service delivery, the specific costs of a service are being defined. This could include stationery costs, telephone, photocopying, electricity and heating as well as typical transport and uniform costs. An example is given in Figure 31.4.

INCOME

The recent history of changes in how the NHS and, indeed, social services departments have been funded, through contractual arrangements, shows the promotion of a more businesslike environment. In the NHS, it has become a reasonable option to contract with external organisations in exchange for payment for services. This enables occupational therapy services, and others, to generate income in order to redress some of the shortfall in their budgets. While this needs to be carried out conservatively, in order not to stretch staffing levels beyond their capacity, market forces can prevail.

An example of this is the increased use of occupational therapy services by solicitors to provide independent assessment of a client's function following injury or illness in order to make a suitable claim against the responsible party.

BUDGET MANAGEMENT

Understanding how the budget management system operates enables the manager to maintain control. All expenditure goes through the accounts ledger and is charged to the appropriate account by a system of accounting codes. The coding of expenditure is therefore important if the correct budget is to be charged with the correct amount of expenditure.

Cost Centre = 1234   *Occupational Therapy*

Date: 12 February 2000
Period: January 2000

Staff expenditure	MPE budget	MPE actual	Annual budget	Current month	Variance month
Senior manager	1.00	1.00	28 500	2500	125
O.T. grade 11	1.00	1.00	24 600	2150	100
O.T. grade 10	5.60	6.55	157 206	12 025	(1075)
O.T. grade 9	4.53	4.00	72 570	6748	(894)
O.T. grade 8	6.75	5.00	116 346	5610	(1963)
Tech inst. 5	0.00	1.00	0	0	0
O.T. asst. 4	1.00	1.00	12 500	1500	458
O.T. asst. 3	5.50	6.50	55 000	5416	573

The figures in parentheses indicate an underspend. The variance for the month is an indicator. Predictions for the year end will be forecast by the variances and how much under or over the budget will be, depending on how long the variances occur. Variances may occur because the budget setting exercise was not done well. In the case of this example, by the month of January the forecast should be quite clear and there would be another column indicating the forecast situation for the end of the financial year.

Figure 31.3   Therapy budget statement: pay.

Cost centre = 1234   Occupational therapy

Date: 12 Feb 2000
Period: January 2000

Non-staff expenditure	Annual budget	Monthly budget	Actual	Variance
Therapy mats and equipment	2000	166	250	84
Provisions	300	50	25	(25)
Printing and stationary	1000	84	150	66
Lease car	2000	166	800	634
Uniforms	0	0	120	120

Some non-staff expenditure may not be funded although there are accounts open, such as uniforms in this example. In this instance, the total figure for non-staff expenditure will be the one that is taken into account. However, in the case demonstrated above, the whole of the non-staff expenditure can be predicted to be in a grossly overspent situation by the end of the financial year unless some additional action is taken. The monthly budget totals £465. The monthly expenditure is £1345, therefore the overspend would be 12 × the difference between the two, that is £880 × 12 = £10,560. However, this may have been an unusual month and a forecast based on one month could be grossly inaccurate. The trend over the whole year needs to be taken into account.

Figure 31.4   Non-pay budget statement.

Centralised coding system

This type of system tends only to operate in very small organisations where there are few sections or types of expenditure. This system requires that all orders and invoices are passed on to the finance department who allocate a code to each item of expenditure and then process them for payment. This means that the finance department determines exactly which budget holder is charged so that the budget holder is not able to manage her budget adequately.

Source coding

Source coding usually applies in larger organisations and reflects the devolution of management responsibilities. Each budget holder is responsible for a series of budget accounts, each one of which has a code number allocated to it, rather like a bank account code number. Every invoice or request for payment has to be aligned to an appropriate budget account code within the remit of the budget holder. There are usually a very restricted number of signatories, that is, authorised people to sign for each account. Each one will have a financial limit up to which she can authorise, such as £ 1000 or £ 5000 per order. This system allows for full management control

while reflecting the flexibility of the day-to-day requirements of the service.

Income is similarly assigned to budget accounts via the code system, so that income can be directed to balance out the expenditure. For example, if a member of staff is contracted out to provide a service to an external agency, the income can be coded against the employee's salary and the money directed into the correct account to balance the expenditure incurred.

Financial control

The manager's contract of employment and service objectives usually require that she works within the financial framework of the organisation and the constraints that this imposes on the service. The best use of resources must be made and efficient budget control is part of the monitoring system in place to achieve this. There are strict instructions to ensure that honest brokerage of the funds is maintained. This means that all movements of money have to be accounted for, either through the balance of costs from payment for staff salaries or payment for goods and services through invoices.

The language of budget management is not explained fully here, but it is useful for the occupational therapist to be aware of the following, frequently used terms:

Virement

This is the system that allows the transfer of money from one financial account to another. Normally, the transfer of money is not allowed. However, particularly with the advent of contracts and internal service agreements between different parts of a large organisation, it is now an accepted means of paying one department for a service that has been given to another. It is also sometimes possible to vire money from one account to another, in special circumstances, to offset unpredicted costs.

Audit

Auditors oversee the financial management of the service. The main function of audit is to:

- prevent and check against fraud
- check that standing financial instructions are being followed
- check that the organisation's procedures are robust
- ensure that value for money is being achieved
- ensure that public money is being used appropriately.

There are two main audit departments usually in contact with the occupational therapy departments, the financial audit department and the NHS Audit Commission.

Financial audit department. The financial audit department will be in contact at least once a year to examine the accounting system for items for resale and for the sale of any goods produced by the department. This requires that all items are counted if still in stock, or accounted for and appropriately charged for if sold. This task, known as the stock take, needs to be carried out at the end of each financial year, as close to 31 March as possible.

NHS Audit Commission. The other audit department that occupational therapists may encounter is the NHS Audit Commission. The NHS Audit Commission reports to Parliament on the economy and efficiency of services. It usually carries out the audits by visiting departments at prearranged times but at relatively short notice. Frequently, the same services across the country will be audited for a 6- or 12-month period. This allows the Commission to benchmark the audited services and gain an overview of the situation at that time, across the country. This type of audit will happen only very infrequently for the same services.

SUMMARY

The concept that this chapter hoped to convey is one of budget and financial management as an information tool for the occupational therapy manager. Skills and a sense of purpose are fundamental to the successful use of the tool, as with any other. Once the monthly financial statement becomes a useful source of information for the manager it holds few areas for concern. The information it conveys includes level of activity, who is doing what and how much it is costing to do it. The statement should only reflect what the manager already knows about the service and, if there are any surprises, they are quickly investigated with the help of the financial advisor.

The relevance of strategic planning mechanisms and financial models is included to aid the manager in recognising opportunities that exist for the development of client-focused services. It is only by relating services to these strategic objectives and submitting bids through these routes that service developments will be recognised. These are more likely to be achieved if they are submitted through shared approaches with our colleagues. However, whatever the planning mechanism, the financial models that apply should be recognised and utilised to resource adequately the service developments required.

REFERENCES

Brown H 1999 Personal communication. Planning Directorate, Tees Health Authority, Teesside

Department of Health 1977 National Health Service Act. DoH, London

Department of Health 1986 National Health Service Act (amended). DoH, London

Department of Health 1997 The new NHS, modern, dependable. DoH, London

Department of Health 1998 Our healthier nation. DoH, London

Department of Health 1999a Planning for health and health care. HSC1999/244. DoH, London

Department of Health 1999b Health Act. DoH, London

Hussey J 1994 Understanding business and finance. DP Publications, DoH, London

NICE (National Institute for Clinical Excellence) 1998 A first class service. HSC113/98. DoH, London

Wilson J 1998 Financial management for the public services. Open University Press, Philadelphia

32

Fieldwork education

Sheena E. E. Blair   Jean McLean

INTRODUCTION

What is fieldwork education?

When graduating occupational therapists are asked what the most memorable and important aspects of their education were, the chances are high that they will identify fieldwork education. This form of learning is potent and long lasting, with many people finding that it provides the main reason for wanting to enter a particular field of occupational therapy. Fieldwork education has also been the focus of important additions to the literature since the last edition of this book, notably Alsop & Ryan (1996) and Ilott & Murray (1999). Similarly, journals of occupational therapy from all parts of the world frequently publish research concerned with student attitudes or reactions to particular aspects of working in psychiatry (Gilbert & Strong 1997) Thus, it would appear that this is an area of growing academic interest whether related to specific aspects such as clinical reasoning where the differences between experts and novices is studied (Robertson 1996) or concerned with broader issues of professional socialisation.

Fieldwork education refers to the totality of opportunities offered to students within an educational experience to synthesise theory and practice, reflect upon experience and undergo assessment related to that area. Students are required to undertake placements in a range of areas which reflect current practice in occupational therapy. Placements are of varying duration and are usually interspersed with academic studies in order to maximise opportunities to integrate theory and practice. Fieldwork is a vital component of the educational process whereby students can reflect upon knowledge, gain therapeutic skills and form attitudes which are fundamental to professional judgement. The minimum period of fieldwork practice suggested by the World Federation of Occupational Therapists is 1000 hours and it is usually organised in an incremental manner with gradually increased expectations as the course progresses. In many occupational therapy education programmes, fieldwork constitutes approximately one third of the total course time.

Since the second edition of this book, further changes have occurred in health and social policy which have had a direct influence on fieldwork education, leading to a greater variety of placement opportunities, work with more acutely ill people within the community and the ramifications of greater client and carer control. It is also possible to detect a shift towards greater autonomy over the nature of learning and the setting of individual learning goals by the student within the fieldwork experience.

The change of terminology from clinical education to fieldwork education, as noted by Alsop & Ryan (1996), reflects the move from placements in predominantly medical venues to a host of possibilities within local authorities, voluntary agencies and other community settings.

Many changes have also occurred within the curricula of occupational therapy courses. Most undergraduate courses are offered at honours degree level and, within institutes of higher education, there has been a switch to modularity. This offers greater choice for students and more flexibility in modes of study. Throughout these educational changes, the emphasis on both the importance of fieldwork education and the necessity for it to be integrated within the curriculum has been enduring.

Non-traditional fieldwork opportunities in housing associations, high street chemists, prisons, residential care, nurseries and different community venues are increasing. This may mean that, although the core skills of occupational therapy are being practised, supervising personnel are not occupational therapists. Overall, fieldwork supervision is likely to be carried out by an occupational therapist but, particularly in the later stages of the course, students may at times be supervised by other professional personnel.

The field of mental health offers a diversity of experience which is challenging for the learner. The current changes within mental health services, which often lead to a very rapid turnover of clients and to working with more acutely ill clients within the community, can be bewildering for the novice. There may still be perceived disparities between what was learned in the educational institution, in terms of how and where clients are treated, and the reality of fieldwork.

Within this complexity there is a necessity for students to feel comfortable with their professional identity and to have opportunities to reflect upon the theory–practice continuum. This requires corresponding attention to the educational needs of fieldwork educators, ensuring that there are frequent opportunities for continued professional development in this area.

This chapter will examine features which are of particular relevance to fieldwork education in the field of mental health. In particular, features of the educational process in this area, common difficulties, student support and assessment of competence will be covered. The basic philosophy underlying the chapter is that there is an interdependent relationship between theory and practice and that collaboration and dialogue should be the key features of fieldwork education.

The context of fieldwork education

Occupational therapy in mental health was the focus of a project, under the auspices of the College of Occupational Therapists, to develop a position paper which would reveal a direction for research, education and practice (Craik et al 1998). This paper, published in 1998, revealed that 'good fieldwork placements' are valued by practitioners and highlighted the importance of an educational experience which emphasises occupation as the key concept, value and principle for undergraduate programmes of study. The position paper provided a useful focus for educational planners in terms of curriculum design and research.

The work also revealed how the relationship between the professions and society has changed fundamentally, with a demand for accountability, and greater partnership and clinical governance. Inter-agency cooperation is a feature of community care, often with complex logistical and financial ramifications. The aim of restructuring health and social services is to achieve greater efficiency and cost-effectiveness and more involvement of the users of services.

All these changes have resulted in a very steep learning curve for students on fieldwork placements who require to develop rapidly the skills necessary to cope with the swift turnover of clients and the changing ethos.

The venues for fieldwork education are also changing. More traditional hospital and community settings are still being used for early blocks of fieldwork experience. Towards the final stages of the course of study, however, it is also possible that students will be increasingly involved in a variety of non-traditional placement experiences, many of which will be electives organised by the student.

Fish et al (1992) investigated the supervision of pre-service practice and raised a number of theoretical issues which have a bearing on how students learn. Central to the discussion were theoretical arguments about what constitutes professional knowledge. The curriculum content of most occupational therapy courses reveals an awareness of the need to broaden the scope of knowledge. There is a noticeable departure from a concentration on medical and condition-specific knowledge towards the study of human occupation, social policy, management, health related social science and discipline specific theories.

The intellectual challenges facing the student necessitate a theoretical approach completely different from the simplistic application of a theory to practice model or, as Schon (1987) described it, the 'technical rational' model.

Alternatives to this model, examined by Fish and colleagues (1992), include:

- the critical self-appraisal approach which is the precursor to performance appraisal
- a problem solving approach which suggests that the placement allows refinement of skills within a supervised situation
- the reflective practitioner approach which is the favoured model in that it is more comprehensive in terms of values, skills and knowledge and promotes 'professional artistry'.

This last approach seems to be the basis for the work of Cohn (1989) who, from an American context, offered practical suggestions for how fieldwork education can provide the scaffolding for clinical reasoning. She felt strongly that the analysis and interpretation of dynamic situations is highly complex and that the supervisor has an obligation to provide situations in which this intellectual process can be nurtured.

An important element in discussing the context of fieldwork experience is accreditation of clinicians and their sites. Openshaw & Goble (1991) explained that the 'process of accreditation aims to provide a mechanism for developing effective clinical placements by providing empirically defined standards'. They went on to explore the essential supervisory practices from which standards and practice guidelines could be designed. Accreditation originated in Canada where a national system exists and is monitored by the Canadian Association of Occupational Therapists. The College of Occupational Therapists (1994) have produced guidelines concerning the accreditation of fieldwork educators and those accredited assume the responsibility for the standards of fieldwork education.

It is imperative that close working relationships are forged between educational establishments and fieldwork educators and that the educational institution takes responsibility for providing learning opportunities and support for therapists who offer fieldwork education.

FEATURES OF FIELDWORK EDUCATION RELATED TO COMMUNICATION

Fieldwork education most closely resembles what Bryne & Long (1973) called the 'attachment relationship', in which the novice is placed with an experienced practitioner. Within this situation, the novice is able to witness the direct application of specific knowledge and skills and the processes by which clinical judgements are reached and decisions made. The attachment relationship offers the possibility of mutual exploration of the student's and supervisor's respective roles. Rogers (1986) included this exploration of roles in her concept of mentorship. Wallis (1977) also considered the negotiation of roles in the course of a learning experience as intrinsic to and necessary for learning.

The quality of experiential learning that occurs depends upon many factors, including the motivation of the learner, the teaching skill of the clinician and the strength of the supervisor–student relationship. Ultimately, the dream of education is to free, not control, and to nurture the desire to learn for life. Ekstein & Wallerstein (1972) urged that the natural scepticism of the student be used to fuel curiosity rather than be interpreted as doubt and criticism by the supervisor.

Fieldwork educators' styles of teaching

Styles vary widely and depend on a variety of factors which include:

- the personal and professional confidence of the fieldwork educator
- the fieldwork educator's preferred teaching style
- the supervision culture in a department, attitudes to students in particular and to placements in general
- the level a student is at
- the ability of the student.

While different styles of teaching and learning occur between educators, a general rule is that, as the course of study progresses, greater control is taken by the student to determine the nature and type of learning required. Alsop & Ryan (1996) outlined several models of supervision which are relevant to fieldwork education:

- The apprenticeship model relates to training and mastery of skills and tends to encourage students to reproduce supervisors' behaviours without necessarily knowing what the basis for these is, so that rote performance is seen rather than performance based on understanding from a sound theoretical base.
- Growth models are influenced by personal development psychology and focus on the student's personal experience, self-awareness and affective responses. The belief is that an increase in self-awareness is a useful underpinning for therapeutic practice.
- Educational models focus on the interplay between student learning, educational aims and learning outcomes.

A more extensive overview of models and roles was offered by the interdisciplinary group of McLeod and colleagues (1997). They subdivided models of clinical education into:

- descriptive models which explain the perceived components of this type of education, including personnel involved, the content and associated key concepts
- integration models which attempt to reveal the close relationship between academic and clinical subject matter
- developmental models which acknowledge the individual needs of students and how meaning is constructed from each experience. They also perceive different learning needs at different times and how they can be accommodated by fieldwork educators
- interactive process models which involve study of the exchanges between the educator and student. They usually involve explanation of learning cycles within the supervisory process, permitting analysis of where problems or issues arise
- collaborative models which refer to the merging of the roles and responsibilities of

student and educator and where greater partnership in learning is the norm.

More recently, Higgs & Edwards (1999) offered a new model of the interactional professional which represents the transactional nature of practice. It highlights the requirement for the emerging health professional to recognise the broader remit of social responsibility and to work within the local and global context to advance practice. Such an array of potential models for fieldwork education is valuable considering the breadth of experience offered to students. Models act as tools of analysis and communication about the learning/teaching process. Nevertheless, certain commonalities are evident and relate to the drive towards lifelong learning and help students work within ever-changing philosophies and practice.

THE STUDENT/FIELDWORK EDUCATOR RELATIONSHIP

Occupational therapy practice within the field of mental health carries intrinsic pressure that makes it necessary for staff to give each other support and encouragement. Support is also vital for students, especially those with no prior experience in mental health. Initial exposure to this area of work can, for many, be anxiety provoking. Throughout a placement fieldwork educators have a major responsibility to create a safe learning environment for students in which 'permission' is given to make mistakes and to learn and develop from them.

The student and fieldwork educator must work together to:

- define individualised aims for the placement
- agree areas for, and levels of, responsibility
- clarify expectations
- identify feedback strategies and timing.

For the relationship to be effective, communication between the student and the fieldwork educator must be good at all times and each participant in the partnership should be alert to both verbal and non-verbal interactions and cues and to any potential variations in interpretation of these. The relationship frequently progresses from educator to mentor as the student's experience and confidence grows.

Mentorship was described by Rogers (1986) as a teaching model that has significant advantages. It is a nurturing process that encourages the professional growth of the student. The mentor is actively involved in and accepts responsibility for guiding student development. Within this model the locus of control is shared between the student and the supervisor.

Historically, students have tended to work with supervisors on a one-to-one basis; however, there has been a recent emergence of shared supervision models. Tiberius & Gaiptman (1985), Ladyshewsky & Healy (1990) and Jung et al (1994) advocated approaches which involve supervisors being responsible for two or more students at one time. The major advantages are that opportunities exist for collaborative learning between the students involved and the fostering of interactive problem solving and team-building skills.

A key issue in effective fieldwork education is the recognition of each student as an individual with both professional and personal needs and aspirations. The educator must be flexible in approach and be willing to negotiate the nature of supervision suitable for each student. Students in turn should be encouraged to participate actively in defining the nature of the supervisory relationship, to specify learning goals and the level of supervision required. The latter should, in normal circumstances, diminish as the placement progresses.

Effective supervision

There is a need for the fieldwork educator to examine personal preferences and prejudices and to attempt some self-understanding prior to assuming a supervisory role. It is easy to state that an atmosphere of openness should exist, where queries and criticisms are heard nonjudgementally, but it must be acknowledged that raw nerves are touched, insecurities stirred and defensiveness aroused when teaching, planning or practice is questioned. Recognising this is vital in order to prevent didactic or over-critical evaluation of students.

Entwistle (1983), from an educational research perspective, suggested that teachers will often adopt methods of teaching that reflect their own preferences in learning. In fieldwork education, students sometimes comment that if they emulate their supervisor's style and practice they are given more positive feedback. Clearly, teaching style will affect attainment and therefore, since not all students are the same, a repertoire of teaching behaviour is necessary to give the best opportunity for learning to the greatest number of students.

Methods vary from very structured programmes to ones that allow freedom to develop the student's own ideas and clinical approach. Teachers whose approach is considered enabling by students are those who:

- are realistic about the student's level of study
- acknowledge individual learning styles
- accept responsibility for helping to integrate theoretical and research based knowledge with fieldwork
- appreciate that students learn best by doing
- permit enquiry, criticism and challenge without defensiveness
- offer remedial action for difficulties experienced
- share knowledge
- offer guidance for future practice.

Within the short time span of a fieldwork placement, the most likely role model for the student is the supervisor. Over the 3 or more years of an occupational therapy programme, a variety of role models will be presented to the student and the most comfortable or credible behaviours will be adopted.

The American medical educator Irby (1978) described the need for clinical teachers to demonstrate high professional standards. Characteristics that attract imitation are:

- personal and professional confidence
- a capacity for self-criticism

- acceptance of responsibility
- recognition of personal limitations
- respect for others.

Students in the early stages of a fieldwork placement feel it safer to replicate directly the therapeutic approach of their supervisor. This is noted particularly in speciality areas such as group psychotherapy, centres for the treatment of alcohol and drug abuse or forensic work. As experience grows, personal style emerges. This pattern of initial compliance, leading to identification with the place or person and, finally, to internalisation of meaningful characteristics was outlined by the psychotherapist Kelman (1963) in terms of growth of therapeutic confidence and professionalism.

THE RELATIONSHIP BETWEEN UNIVERSITY AND FIELDWORK PLACEMENT

Supervised fieldwork experience is an essential part of the educational programme, providing opportunities to synthesise theory with practice as well as to learn new skills and information. A close relationship between the educational institution and fieldwork placement is imperative to ensure a shared frame of reference for teaching and learning. This relationship can be established by:

- regular meetings between fieldwork educators and university staff
- lecturers' visits to placements
- mutual exchange of techniques or information and shared teaching resources
- reciprocal teaching arrangements involving university staff in in-service training and fieldwork staff in course work
- mutual involvement in fieldwork educators' courses
- joint development of teaching aids, such as videos, tape/slide presentations or static teaching displays
- involvement of fieldwork staff in course planning
- regular updates for fieldwork staff on course changes, development, etc.

- workshops for and with fieldwork educators on both supervision and practice.

Overlap between classroom and fieldwork situations

Within a period of fieldwork education it is possible to identify how a student learns and makes sense of occupational therapy. The setting may emphasise 'doing' but this does not inevitably lead to understanding of the philosophical and theoretical bases or frame of reference that underpin practice. It is the joint responsibility of university and clinician to ensure that integration of knowledge, development of skills and growth of constructive attitudes to occupational therapy in mental health are taking place. Fieldwork education offers a reality of involvement for the student that is both frightening and exciting. It has been stated that modelling is a useful teaching behaviour. Learners rapidly sense a 'Do as I say and not as I do' approach. When such discrepancies occur, the supervisor's credibility suffers and the student's sense of professional identity is threatened.

The gap between the ideal situation that is often taught in universities and the clinical reality is illustrated by Box 32.1. Treatment planning is a core skill of occupational therapy; however, much confusion may occur in the student's mind over where and when this takes place.

A transfer of focus occurs for students in fieldwork practice. In university they are the central focus, while in the fieldwork area there is a shared focus of attention between patient care, management and countless other duties. This necessary juggling of priorities often causes anxiety and a feeling of dependency in the student, and can create a dilemma for the supervisor. The student may be concerned about not receiving sufficient attention, obtaining sparse feedback on performance and feeling that experiences are not tailored to her individual needs. The need for a mediator arises frequently, and this may be the head of department, the designated lecturer or another university lecturer who acts as an objective evaluator. This contact with university is vital in maintaining the student's academic and personal link with the educational base. Visits from university staff usually occur following the midway report. This is also a time for reviewing the objectives and expectations of the placement.

COMMON PROBLEMS FOR OCCUPATIONAL THERAPY STUDENTS

Working in the field of mental health is a daunting prospect to some, in that it demands a personal investment. Although this could be said of all areas in which occupational therapists are deployed, the therapeutic use of self is deemed to be an essential ingredient within this field. Each area within mental health has inherent features that can complicate learning. These have to be allowed for in compiling learning objectives and in the assessment of performance. Problems that

---

Box 32.1   Case example 1

Anna was a friendly and adaptable student who found the weekly timetable on an acute psychiatric admission ward both stimulating and well-balanced, in that it catered for a variety of emotional, interpersonal and practical needs. However, at her midway report it was considered by her supervisor that Anna could not analyse or articulate individual treatment aims within the programme of group activities.

In discussion with the visiting university lecturer, Anna explained that, despite her having an awareness of individual needs and aims, at no time had she witnessed other staff or her supervisor formally record or definitely state clear goals within the programme for each individual client, apart from changes in medication. It appeared to the visiting lecturer that the specifics of planning and judgement were not clearly outlined either in the course of daily events or in supervisory teaching sessions. Hence, Anna was confused about the insistence by the university on specific analysis and sound treatment planning when she considered that what was occurring in the unit was proving therapeutic and useful without it. In turn, the supervisor considered that individual treatment planning was carried out continually 'in her head' but that there was insufficient time to record it formally.

Consequently, the problem for Anna's learning was that she was being criticised for lacking a skill that everyone agreed in theory was important but that could not be observed in practice.

may arise for the student include personal problems, professional role confusion and lack of clinical skills.

PERSONAL PROBLEMS
Overidentification

An anxious student may identify strongly with the fieldwork educator in the hope that, by adopting the same style, she may achieve the same success. The danger of this behaviour is that individuality is lost and a personal style is not developed. Unconsciously or not, such imitation may be fostered by the supervisor and a frequently heard comment from students is that 'she only wants me to be like her'. There is a danger too that students may learn practice by rote and copy the actions of the fieldwork educator without understanding the theoretical concepts which underpin these. Learners have to maintain their integrity and learn, with support, to value their own judgement.

Overidentification with clients can occur in practically every area, for example with problems such as eating disorders, depression, anxiety and interpersonal difficulties. This shows in many ways, such as intense sympathy with the client, desire to solve problems personally, wanting to become a valued and sought after carer, staying late at work or intervening passionately on the client's behalf. These may all be indicators that objectivity is being affected by personal needs. This is not to be confused with commitment, enthusiasm and individual styles of caring; the danger signals are shown when the student gives an excessive amount of time to one client for a variety of personal reasons. This needs discussion, either with a personal tutor, fieldwork educator or some other objective person.

High levels of anxiety

Occupational therapy is a profession dependent upon doing and the acquisition of skill but this may be rendered impossible by anxiety. Fear has a paralysing effect and can inhibit learning

(Anderson & Graham 1980). Within occupational therapy in mental health, certain areas of performance are likely to create anxiety, such as verbal reporting, leading groups, or any situation where the student is heard by other health professionals. A progressive desensitisation has to occur by rehearsing the event and building upon small gains.

Students may also feel anxious about their initial experience of work in mental health. Many students have little experience of mental health prior to commencing their professional education, and negative media representations of mental health issues can generate considerable anxieties for them. Careful preparation in the university setting, an empathetic fieldwork educator and honesty on the part of the student should all help to allay these anxieties.

Certain client conditions, such as behavioural disturbance and aggressive behaviour, require special training procedures and considerable support from more experienced staff. Students should be alerted, in the early stages of the placement, to how they should obtain assistance in situations with which they do not have the skills or knowledge to deal.

Feelings of therapeutic frustration

These may be caused by a number of factors, not least by rapid turnover of clients. Consequently, students may feel that their involvement consists solely of assessment and emergency intervention rather than longer-term therapeutic intervention. Frustration may also occur with those clients who appear to change very little during the allotted weeks of fieldwork practice. Such frustrations may be experienced with longer-term clients but are also encountered in interventions within acute and community care settings. Here, policies relating to rapid discharge from hospital, patient choice and staffing levels may serve to frustrate the student in carrying through a desired intervention. Opportunities for personal experience of tasks, such as problem solving, or for seeing change in clients over time may be restricted, thus leading to reduced opportunity for students to gain insights into the potential of occupational therapy.

The task of providing opportunities for students to understand current situations in the context of past events, to envisage what long-term interventions may be utilised, and to explore possible or probable outcomes lies with the fieldwork educator. Lack of this vision may leave students feeling that their interventions are futile and do not lead to change.

Frustration may also be felt by students who consider that they cannot emulate the skills of qualified staff. They may feel therapeutically naive and afraid of doing or saying something wrong. Fieldwork educators have a role in encouraging students to explore what they have encountered in the past, both in theory and practice, and to consider its application within that particular placement at that time.

There may be additional frustrations associated with closed groups or one-to-one work with clients where the service user does not feel comfortable to have another person involved. This can cause additional difficulties in relation to the student gaining sufficient real life experience to feel confident in utilising techniques and approaches that they only know from a theoretical perspective.

Personal experience

For all students, fieldwork is an intensely personal experience. It is important that fieldwork educators remember this and take into account the individual student's starting point in relation to experience in mental health. A student's first experience in mental health has many issues to deal with which subsequent ones will not have. The individual and her experience, knowledge, fears and aspirations should all be taken into account in planning learning experiences. It is also important that at all times students should be judged in relation to the agreed aims for the placement.

PROBLEMS WITH PROFESSIONAL ROLE

Professional identity

The professional identity of the occupational therapy student is formed to a significant extent through identification with her fieldwork educator. When occupational therapists are seen to be integrated, at ease and accepted within the multidisciplinary team the student gains confidence in her professional role. Alsop & Ryan (1996) pointed out that much time is spent discussing core occupational therapy skills but argued that a more useful way of thinking is to focus on the 'core approach' which is employed by occupational therapists, focusing on the client's unique world. Such an approach may help to minimise insecurity about role blurring which occurs in some settings. Increasingly, students are working in settings where the occupational therapist has been employed under another title and a focus on core approach would help to enhance development of professional identity. Similarly, Higgs & Hunt (1999) advocated the adoption of what they described as an interactional professional approach to health care education, in which there is recognition of both core and generic skills and how exploration of these might be utilised to best effect in dealing with service users.

Students need encouragement to drop their professional defensiveness and learn from other professionals. In order to help them do this, the fieldwork educator has to be prepared to acknowledge the potential difficulties of role blurring, provide learning situations that study collaborative working with other disciplines, and show the student how she can contribute professional expertise.

Team relationships

Occupational therapists frequently describe their role as 'integral' to the multidisciplinary team. Students are confused by this assertion if they do not observe the occupational therapist to be such an important member of the team. Sometimes, they are caught between what the fieldwork educator wishes could take place and the actual reality.

Teams come in many shapes and forms and it is difficult for the newcomer to find a niche. It is unrealistic to expect a student on placement for a few weeks to take an active part in the team unless the climate and ethos of the unit is to welcome and use newcomers' impressions. The ideal in mental health is for a multidisciplinary or a transdisciplinary team (Alsop & Ryan 1996). In the former, all members work together and each contributes specific profession-related skills. In the transdisciplinary team, all of the members work in similar ways and their role is much more generic. Students need to be alerted to the type of team they are working in so that they can begin to understand roles and responsibilities within it.

Common difficulties for students include:

- unrealistically high expectations of the cohesiveness and effectiveness of the team – the student hopes for an ideal harmonious entity that values opinions from all sources
- disappointment when time in team meetings is taken up with, for example, discussion of pharmacological management, with less attention paid to social and interpersonal issues
- professional boundary problems and uncertainty about whether they can contribute to the management of clients in areas traditionally outwith the occupational therapist's role.

The fieldwork educator needs to impart the attitudes and values of an integrative approach. Philosophies of teamwork are best taught within fieldwork education where the constraints can be witnessed alongside the strengths.

Coping with an eclectic approach in mental health

Appreciating an eclectic approach should not represent a major conceptual shift for occupational therapy students. The profession traditionally encompasses flexibility of thought, application and process, which are inherent qualities of eclecticism. Work in the community increasingly demonstrates that a variety of approaches and treatment techniques can be used to meet client needs. Selection of the method of treatment that offers the greatest promise for alleviating problems and symptoms

as quickly as possible is the core skill of an eclectic approach.

In the very short time of the fieldwork placement, problems may exist in learning how to choose from many possibilities without becoming bewildered. Students will have learned the major models and approaches to treatment and can usually identify corresponding techniques. However, personal ideological preferences may exist to favour the psychodynamic, behavioural or humanistic approach. The fieldwork educator's task is to increase therapeutic and conceptual flexibility.

Active supervision is needed to help the student cope with the experience. This can include suggesting reading assignments, allowing ample time for reflection, discussing the alternatives and setting specific learning objectives.

PROBLEMS WITH SKILLS

Limited interpersonal skills

There will be students who, by personality and preference, are more suited to working in other areas of health and social services than in mental health. Psychiatry demands high levels of interpersonal skills and the use of self is often thought of as the primary therapeutic factor. Certainly, it is necessary for any therapist to engage the motivation and participation of the client and this is partly engineered through the therapist–client relationship.

Within the study of occupational therapy, time is spent in the curriculum on social skills, interactional skills or interpersonal skills training. Despite this training, the reality of the event in fieldwork practice is often far removed from the role play in the classroom. Fieldwork practice provides opportunities for direct observation, practice of and feedback on a variety of interpersonal skills.

Learning objectives can be graded to allow progression from one-to-one encounters to small groups and ultimately to large groups. In this way, the student is able to develop increased self-awareness and security in interpersonal skills.

Interactional skills can be subdivided into listening skills, interviewing skills, counselling and group leadership skills. Students may be competent in one area but not in another. For example, they may demonstrate competent listening skills but lack group skills.

It would be a mistake to equate interpersonal effectiveness only with a vivacious outgoing personality. The steady reflective style of the gentler personality can be equally successful.

Problems in group situations

As Priestly & McQuire (1983) stated, it is not unusual for experienced professionals to disclaim any interest in working with groups. Groups may be experienced as frightening, unpredictable and possibly damaging, therefore the newcomer understandably wishes to remain an onlooker.

In order to make the group experience less overwhelming, the model of treatment or approach must be first identified: is it geared to uncovering unconscious material, to supporting the client through a crisis or to self-help? The occupational therapy student faces a confusing array of approaches, techniques and milieus and the confidence to contribute can only follow identification of culture and observation of process.

Modelling plays an important part in learning how to work in groups, with cues taken from more experienced staff on what to say, how to phrase it and when to interject. Instruction, practice and feedback can be given on preparing for a group, introducing a session, facilitating interaction and ending a session. Difficulties arising with any one of these skills do not automatically imply that the student is unable to work in groups.

Confidence grows with success, allowing the student to attempt more complex interactions. Supervisors must hold a realistic view of what skills can be acquired in a short time and be accurate in diagnosis of areas of weakness, otherwise groupwork and a large section of psychiatry is 'written off' as not being within the individual's capabilities.

STUDENT COUNSELLING IN THE FIELDWORK SETTING

Sometimes a problem may arise that requires particular assistance from either university staff or clinical staff. Such problems may include:

- difficulties with integration of constructive criticism
- student–educator communication conflict
- finding it hard to bear the intense emotion of some psychiatric disorders
- feeling overwhelmed by role blurring, failure to grasp the rationale of occupational therapy in psychiatry, or anxiety engendered when people appear not to improve
- lack of interpersonal skill highlighted by the length of 'settling-in time', inter-staff difficulties or poor group skills
- fear of failure, leading to compliance and superficial understanding.

Counselling in the fieldwork practice arena is chiefly concerned with listening, exploring possibilities and mutually setting goals. Two types of counselling may be used with students on placement:

1. academic counselling, concerning problems with meaning and transfer of knowledge or difficulties in achieving clinical competency
2. personal counselling, concerning relationships or personal conflicts.

These are interlinked and combine to affect development.

Time and expertise put a boundary on the amount of counselling possible, therefore it is always wise to involve the student's personal tutor or university fieldwork coordinator. It is usually more useful if the student can take this initiative herself. Difficulties experienced in one placement may affect performance in the next, so it is imperative to maintain a consistent support system. The ultimate aim of all counselling is to enable the person to generate solutions for herself. It is also vital that staff involved with the student recognise the limits of their interactions with students and that, if necessary, when issues are outwith their own remit and abilities, they refer students to a trained counsellor.

STUDENT DEVELOPMENT

McAllister et al (1997) suggested that fieldwork experience allows the development of knowledge and skills in a real-life setting and that this enhances the integration of theory and practice, the development of skills and the reorganisation of knowledge to enable the student successfully to make safe decisions, solve problems and plan in the work context. The following are some of the factors that can contribute to student development within fieldwork studies.

ESTABLISHING A LEARNING CLIMATE

Setting a learning climate is a feature of all educational environments. The antennae of students are alert from the first few moments in a placement to the expectations, ethos and affective nature of the place. During the orientation period, familiarisation with people, places and timetables is taking place on one level, while attitudes towards learning are more subtly communicated on another.

If the student perceives that active learning is the norm in a placement, she will be influenced by it. This includes:

- the enthusiasm, for the student's learning, of the fieldwork educator and other staff
- the provision of books, journals and learning aids
- access to library facilities
- freedom of access to a variety of resource materials, such as tape slides, directed reading material, learning packages, photographs and learning cassettes
- overt statements by the fieldwork educator that it is all right not to know and to make mistakes and that the placement is a learning opportunity.

These provisions encourage development of knowledge and skills and offer opportunities for students to focus on the areas of theory with most relevant application to the placement setting. Numerous audio-visual aids which enrich learning are commercially available and can be used in tutorials, seminars and lectures. A balanced tutorial system, including interdisciplinary teaching, is effective in enriching the learning experience.

Fostering attitudes of enquiry

Encouraging a desire in the student to learn is the joint remit of clinical and academic staff. If a curriculum encourages intellectual curiosity, the student can rehearse presenting sound arguments. This ability to argue a theoretical point precedes problem solving with 'real' problems and gives confidence to apply theoretical knowledge. The teaching behaviour of the supervisor can keep alive a wish to investigate. Irby (1978) described five positive aspects of the clinical teacher that foster the growth of the learner:

1. being accessible
2. observing, giving feedback on and evaluating student performance
3. guiding students, providing practice opportunities and developing skill in problem solving
4. giving case-specific comments
5. offering professional support and encouragement.

Value of peer group support

Whenever several students are on placement together a healthy cross-fertilisation of ideas can occur. Small group teaching can be useful, particularly for dealing with difficult moral or ethical problems or for understanding the feelings of students working in psychiatry. In the case of students who are finding difficulties in coping with aspects of their studies, McAllister et al (1997) advocated the use of Schulman's (1984) mutual aid model. This involves students sharing their problems and fears as well as their ideas for solutions to their perceived difficulties. Tutorials are the most likely places for students to meet, to identify and discuss issues common to the practice of occupational therapy. A number of teaching methods can be used on these occasions, including brainstorming sessions, buzz groups, workshops, seminars and case presentations.

The value of peer support is very clearly highlighted in the collaborative or 2:1 model of supervision. This is where more than one student at a time is assigned to one fieldwork educator. In this situation there are many more opportunities for collaborative learning and the student's reliance on the fieldwork educator, especially for more trivial matters, is generally reduced. Ladyshewsky (1995) suggested that this type of supervision is best suited to placements which are located in the later stages of the course.

Care must be taken in collaborative models of supervision to ensure that students have opportunities to present evidence of their own work so that judgements about performance are made on the basis of work carried out by the individual and that one student does not become overshadowed by another. It is also important that competition between students is discouraged since this is counterproductive to the establishment of an effective, collaborative learning climate.

Multidisciplinary learning

Occupational therapy in mental health cannot exist in isolation but requires input from other disciplines. Such interaction gives the student opportunities to learn sensitivity to the roles of others. This educational function of the multidisciplinary team is well recognised within the health service. Boufford (1978) believed that any health professional education must prepare the student to:

- be aware of the resources that other health professionals can provide for a client, and
- co-ordinate their care of the client with that of other involved professionals.

He said that the basic goals of the team are clear communication, goal setting, role negotiation and decision making. Defensiveness about professional boundaries can be lessened if education about the team is included in fieldwork studies.

PLANNING

Prior to the start of a placement, planning is essential to consider how students will meet the placement aims and learning outcomes which are defined by the academic institutions, supervisor and/or student. The method selected should help to guide the student towards successfully meeting the aims without necessarily channelling all students along the same route. This allows for individual variations in learning styles and recognises that each student has a unique knowledge and experience base. As in other aspects of fieldwork, the degree of fieldwork educator control can vary from student to student.

Some fieldwork educators and students prefer working within a well defined framework, with clear, written, weekly objectives identified prior to and/or during the placement. Others prefer the use of a more flexible system where the overall aims and direction of learning are reviewed on a regular basis. Another alternative is the use of learning contracts within which students have the major responsibility for defining the aims and the process involved in achieving these. Learning contracts need to be reviewed on a very regular basis throughout the placement and to be seen as both flexible and evolving.

There are similarities in all methods of planning for fieldwork, the crucial elements are that both student and fieldwork educator:

- are conversant with the structure and content of the academic elements of the course
- are aware of the student's prior learning
- know what must be achieved
- clearly understand all aims, objectives and learning outcomes
- are agreed on the process of achieving placement aims

- know how and when the student will be assessed
- know the level at which aims are to be achieved
- are flexible in how and when placement aims are achieved.

Aims, objectives and learning outcomes

Aims

Aims are general statements of intent which provide guidelines for action. They must be realistic and relevant to the stage of learning. For example, on a first placement an aim could be:

- to conduct an interview under supervision and record the information.

Objectives

Objectives are more specific statements of intent and describe what the student will be expected to do and to achieve during the learning process. They focus on the steps involved in successful completion of the aims. Using the aim previously mentioned, the objectives during a 5-week placement could be:

Weeks 1/2

- The student will observe the fieldwork educator carrying out interviews.
- The student will revise theory relating to interviewing and communication.
- The student will make notes on the process of at least two interviews, and discuss these with the fieldwork educator.
- The student will make notes on the information obtained at interview, taking account of both verbal and non-verbal communication, and compare these with the information obtained by the fieldwork educator.
- The fieldwork educator will give the student feedback on both observations and written work.

Week 3

- The student will observe the supervisor carrying out at least two interviews and record the information from them in a format agreed with the fieldwork educator.
- The student will compile a reflective diary of the process of preparing to undertake interviews under supervision.

Weeks 4/5

- The student will carry out interviews under supervision and make notes on the processes involved.
- The student will make notes on and record information obtained at interview.
- The supervisor will give feedback on the student's interview technique, observations and written documentation.
- The student will complete a reflective diary about the interview completed and use this information in supervision.

Objectives can offer structure to both student and fieldwork educator; however, there must be room for flexibility in the achievement of them due to variations between students and to circumstances outwith the control of both students and supervisors.

Learning outcomes

Learning outcomes relate to what the student will have achieved and/or be able to do by the end of the learning process. For example, by the end of the placement the student will be able to:

- conduct interviews with clients under supervision
- collect information at interview in a logical and appropriate manner
- record information obtained at interview logically, accurately and precisely
- relate and understand theory and practice of interviewing
- reflect on personal performance in preparing for, carrying out and reviewing interview sessions.

In some instances, students and fieldwork educators work more effectively by deciding on plans of action from week to week. This usually involves the supervisor organising the first week and, at the end of it and in all subsequent weeks, reviewing with the student what has been achieved and planning objectives for the following week. This approach allows for greater student involvement in negotiating how placement aims will be achieved. This method is often more suited to those students in the later stages of training who are more aware of their own learning needs and styles.

Learning contracts

A further development in increasing student involvement in planning is the use of learning contracts which are said to have many advantages (Solomon 1992, Donaldson 1992, Martenson & Schwab 1993, Stephenson & Laycock 1993, Anderson et al 1996). Knowles (1990) described them as a 'potent tool' in the field of adult learning.

Learning contracts involve the student in negotiating with the supervisor, prior to the placement, the aims and the processes involved. There are several major strands to the learning contract:

- *Placement aims.* Identify major areas which the student will focus on during the placement.
- *Learning goals.* Identify the stages involved in achieving the aims.
- *Process/resources.* Expand on how the learning goals will be achieved and quantify time required from others and resources required such as library facilities and travel time.
- *Intended learning outcome.* This relates to what the student anticipates will be achieved during or by the end of the placement.
- *Proposal for assessment.* This indicates how the student will demonstrate that the placement aims have been achieved.

The major advantages of learning contracts are that they place the locus of control for learning with the student and involve the student in negotiation of the learning process so that she is an active participant rather than a passive recipient. Used effectively they also encourage reflective learning.

It is not necessarily appropriate for students to define all placement aims, but they can at least be involved in setting personal goals and in defining the processes involved in the achievement of aims defined by others.

There can be disadvantages to using learning contracts, not least of which is the variations between students' aspirations and effort. This can be controlled by careful monitoring by both university based and fieldwork staff. In this way students can be guided to set aims at a level which is appropriate for their stage of education. Students often need assistance in recognising their ability to shape their own learning while at the same time meeting curriculum needs in a professional course.

REFLECTIVE LEARNING IN FIELDWORK EDUCATION

Much has been written about the topic of reflection in professional work and education (Schon 1987, Cross 1993, Alsop & Ryan 1996). The process of reflection is an integral part of any learning experience as, without this, opportunities for continuing development will be lost. Students usually require assistance to develop a reflective learning style and need to be encouraged to reflect before, during and after an event. Many universities now advocate the use of reflective diaries. Through using these students can commit to paper their thoughts about carrying out a particular task as well as list theories to be reviewed and planning to be done before the task is carried out. This helps the student to recognise, ahead of time, any areas which need to be discussed, prepared or dealt with. Students can also be encouraged to reflect as they carry out a task, although it can be difficult to do and reflect at the same time. It is also vital for students to review what they have done following completion of a task and to reflect on what they will have to accomplish before carrying out another, similar task. Using a reflective style of learning forms the foundations for effective clinical reasoning; it takes time, effort and commitment on the part of the student and the establishment of a supportive culture on the part of the fieldwork educator.

The use of reflective diaries can also be invaluable in helping a students to prepare for supervision sessions. The full content of the diary need not be exposed to the fieldwork educator but it can be used to highlight main points for discussion and development. This approach encourages an interactive supervisory model and gives the student more control over personal learning.

FEEDBACK

Feedback is a crucial element in all learning and accurate information about performance is vital for the learner. In the context of fieldwork education, feedback should provide students with information not only about performance but also about how to change that performance to improve it in the future.

Fieldwork educators can experience many dilemmas in relation to giving feedback; this is especially so when a student is performing poorly. For many reasons, which have been thoroughly explored by Ilott & Murray (1999), fieldwork educators find it very difficult to give negative feedback, indicating a weak performance. Fieldwork educators may feel that the student needs more time to settle and to become accustomed to the area of work, especially in fieldwork settings unfamiliar for the student. If, in the early stages of the placement, student performance is weak, fieldwork educators may be reluctant to state this openly for fear of compromising the student's confidence. Fieldwork educators may avoid taking action until it is too late and then feel unable to assign a fail grade even when it is the most realistic one. This situation need not occur if fieldwork educators consider carefully not only what feedback is given but also how it is presented. Hawkins & Shohet (1989) identified that there are several facets of good feedback, namely that it is clear, owned, regular, balanced and specific. They suggested that educators must:

- be clear about the message they want to give
- recognise ownership of feedback and phrase it in such away that it reflects their perceptions of a situation, for example, 'I had

some difficulty in understanding why you did that' rather than 'You did that wrong'
- give regular feedback and not keep it all for one time
- try to balance the feedback over time
- be specific about what is being said, rather just stating that everything is fine.

We all have our own information-processing systems, whereby we assimilate non-verbal cues and sift verbal communication before incorporating what is acceptable into our own frame of reference. The quality of communication and the student's interpretation of the feedback determine its effectiveness. Effective feedback requires effective listening before effective communication is possible! Non-specific comments about performance are as unhelpful as no feedback. Learners need coaching, acknowledgement of their strengths and remedies to overcome learning blocks. Judicious pacing is required to maintain readiness for accepting comments on personal development or skill; the individual's threshold for accepting praise and criticism needs to be shrewdly gauged. It is a complex task for the supervisor to match the amount of feedback she gives with the threshold of acceptance in the learner. Pacing is the greatest skill in feedback, ensuring that the wish to try again is continually encouraged.

However, it must be acknowledged that both parties have needs within this relationship. The supervisor needs:

- feedback on teaching style
- frank evaluation of the placement by the student
- scope to apply individual style and not be compared with other supervisors
- confidence to relinquish authority and allow the student to develop skills
- continued opportunities to develop clinical teaching strategies, for example regular short courses or other forms of study.

The student needs:

- coaching on a regular basis
- regular and planned supervision sessions
- scope to express individuality and not be compared to other students

- opportunities to practice clinical skills
- clarification of the purpose of fieldwork education
- opportunity to reflect on all aspects of performance and practice.

ASSESSING COMPETENCE

The purpose of assessment

Every educational process requires assessment: the profession must be satisfied that competency is assured, the fieldwork educator must decide whether or not objectives have been met and the student needs feedback on performance. Fieldwork education combines ongoing formative assessment designed for the benefit of the learner with regular formal summative grading designed to identify the level of competence. For each placement there will be specific requirements which must be met in order for the student to be assigned a pass grade.

Assessing competence to practice is a very difficult task. In itself, competence can be defined as an ability to do a task, however, when this is combined with practice, problems in clarity of what is being assessed begin to arise. Practice in occupational therapy is very complex and multifaceted and some aspects are difficult to define and, consequently, difficult to assess. Indeed, Burrows (1989) pointed out that it is often easier to identify incompetent behaviour than it is to recognise competent practice.

Bond & Spurritt (1999) suggested that there are three main challenges of assessment, namely:

1. to be clear about why the assessment is being carried out
2. to match process and desired outcome
3. to make assessment a positive experience for all involved in it.

All too often people make assumptions about assessment but it is important for all fieldwork educators to be very clear about what and how they are assessing and to convey this clearly to the student.

ASSESSMENT STRATEGIES

Assessment formats

Student report forms cover the essential elements of competence and provide a permanent record of performance. Most forms include a section for students to evaluate the learning experience, which provides a more complete account of the placement.

Although there are many ways to design a fieldwork assessment form, some common features exist. The form is usually subdivided into salient professional characteristics, for example:

- professional development
- interpersonal relationships
- communication
- assessment
- practice of occupational therapy
- treatment planning
- organisation and management.

Each of these sections is further analysed for core skills and aptitudes that the student should attain at different stages of the course. Additionally, a method of differentiation may be required to indicate to the student the extent of success or failure.

Most fieldwork educators would agree that the most vital formative assessment procedure occurs in the section where the clinician writes comments in support of the assessment decision. It is important to ensure that the nature of the assessment form reflects the desired personal and professional changes throughout the period of education.

Finally, in any process of assessment, opportunities must be offered to the student to reflect upon the fieldwork experience and suggest to the clinician what the most and the least helpful aspects of the placement were. Again, the design of such a form will vary according to the stage the student is at but it usually includes the following areas:

- level of supervision
- quality of feedback
- special features of the placement
- assessment procedures
- links between university and academic work
- any recommendations or changes.

The report form is given to fieldwork educators along with an accompanying guide for completion. Each fieldwork educator is reminded of the main emphasis of the university work immediately preceding the placement and the aims of the assessment.

Student–supervisor evaluation

A report form that judges the performance of the student without an accompanying report from the consumer is incomplete. An honest exchange of views between teacher and student is the most potent way of giving feedback to the fieldwork educator. It can be difficult for the student to write a report on her placement but such a report gives practice in realistic reporting.

It can be just as painful for educators to accept that they may, for example, be seen as authoritarian and difficult as it is for the student to accept negative appraisals. A period of fieldwork practice is just that for all concerned. We are all learning, practising and changing in this context.

Review of the learning experience

At the end of a placement it is wise for the supervisor and student to review the experience together. This has many advantages, including:

- giving the student time to wind down and put the experience into perspective
- highlighting areas of the placement that require rethinking by the supervisor
- offering the supervisor feedback on the learning environment and whether it is conducive to growth.

The review is a reflective process that can be conducted by questionnaire, interview or group activity. One method is to brainstorm with a group of students, writing words, comments and thoughts about the placement on a blackboard until the surface is covered. Following this, the words are ranked into potentially positive or potentially negative phenomena. This offers a profile of the placement as seen through the eyes of each group. Over a year this can show if students have been overloaded, if they are happy with the facilities, if more help is needed to make sense of theory and a host of other important information.

SUMMARY

This chapter has sought to highlight the specific characteristics of teaching in the clinical setting. It particularly stresses:

- the context and features of fieldwork education
- the importance of the supervisor–student relationship and the need to achieve a constructive working alliance
- the variety of supervision styles that a student may experience
- the relationship between the university and the fieldwork placement
- common difficulties encountered by students while on mental health placements
- student autonomy in learning
- ways in which a learning climate can be encouraged that allows all concerned to grow and develop skills.

The need for a better understanding of fieldwork education is recognised by all health professionals. This is especially so in occupational therapy when over 1000 hours is devoted to such studies. The following list suggests areas for further research:

- validity studies of existing fieldwork assessment procedures
- evaluation of the process of acquiring fieldwork competence
- application of recent research on students' learning styles in the fieldwork setting and investigation of the implications for fieldwork education
- exploration of alternative methods of supervision in fieldwork locations
- the use of learning contacts and reflective diaries to promote autonomy of student learning in fieldwork education.

REFERENCES

Alsop A, Ryan S 1996 Making the most of fieldwork education: a practical approach. Chapman and Hall, London

Anderson J, Graham A 1980 A problem in medical education: is there an information overload? Medical Education 14 (1): 4–7

Anderson G, Bond D, Sampson J 1996 Learning contracts: a practical guide. Kogan Page, London

Bond H, Spurrit D 1999 Learning practical skills. In: Higgs J, Edwards H (eds) Educating beginning practitioners: challenges for health professional education. Butterworth Heinemann, Oxford

Bryne P S, Long B E L 1973 Learning to care. Churchill Livingstone, Edinburgh

Burows E 1989 Clinical practice: an approach to the assessment of clinical competencies. British Journal of Occupational Therapy 52(6): 222–226

Cohn E S 1989 Fieldwork education: shaping and foundation for clinical reasoning. American Journal of Occupational Therapy 43(4): 240–244

College of Occupational Therapists 1994 Recommended requirements for the accreditation of fieldwork educators. College of Occupational Therapists, London

Cross V 1993 Introducing physiotherapy students to the idea of reflective practice. Medical Teacher 15(4): 293–307

Donaldson I 1992 The use of learning contracts in the clinical area. Nurse Education Today 12: 431–436

Ekstein R E, Wallerstein R S 1972 The teaching and learning of psychotherapy. International Universities Press, New York

Entwistle N 1983 Styles of learning and teaching. Wiley, London

Fish D, Twinn S, Purr B 1992 How to enable learning through professional practice. West London Institute of Higher Education, London

Gilbert J, Strong J 1997 Australian occupational therapy students: attitudes towards and knowledge about psychiatry. British Journal of Occupational Therapy 60 (1): 12–16

Hawkins P, Shohet 1989 Supervision in the helping professions. Open University Press, Milton Keynes

Higgs J, Edwards H (eds) 1999 Educating beginning practitioners: challenges for professional education. Butterworth Heinemann, Oxford

Higgs J, Hunt A 1999 Rethinking the beginner practitioner: introducing the interactional professional. In: Higgs J, Edwards H (eds) Educating beginning practitioners: challenges for health professional education. Butterworth Heinemann, Oxford

Ilott I, Murray R 1999 Success and failure in professional education: assessing the evidence. Whurr Publishers, London

Irby D M 1978 Clinical faculty development. In: Ford C W (ed) Clinical education for the allied health professions. Mosby, St Louis

Jung B, Martin A, Graden L, Awrey J 1994 Fieldwork education: a sharing supervision model. Canadian Journal of Occupational Therapy 61(1): 12–19

Kelman H C 1963 The role of the group in the induction of therapeutic change. International Journal of Group Psychotherapy 13(4): 399–432

Knowles M S 1990 The adult learner: a neglected species. Gulf Publishing, Houston, Texas

Ladyshewsky R 1995 Enhancing service productivity in acute settings using a collaborative clinical education model. Physical Therapy 75(6): 502–510

Ladyshewsky R, Healey E 1990 The 2:1 teaching model in clinical education. University of Toronto, Toronto

McAllister L, Lincoln M, McLeod S, Maloney D 1997 Facilitating learning in clinical settings. Stanley Thornes, Cheltenham

McLeod S, Romanini J, Cohn E S, Higgs J 1997 Models and roles in clinical education. In: McAllister L, Lincoln M, McLeod S, Maloney D Facilitating learning in clinical settings. Stanley Thornes, Cheltenham

Martenson D, Schwab P 1993 Learning by mutual commitment: broadening the concept of learning contracts. Medical Teacher 15(1): 11–15

Openshaw S, Goble R 1991 Development of a method for setting standards of clinical experience. British Journal of Occupational Therapy 54(1): 16–18

Openshaw S, Goble R 1992 Setting standards and developing practice guidelines: accreditation of clinical experience. British Journal of Occupational Therapy 55(8): 305–309

Priestley P, McQuire J 1983 Learning to help. Tavistock, London

Robertson L 1996 Clinical reasoning. Part 2: Novice/expert differences. British Journal of Occupational Therapy 59(5): 212–216

Rogers J C 1986 Mentoring for career achievement and advancement. American Journal of Occupational Therapy 40(2): 79–82

Schon D 1987 Educating the reflective practitioner. Jossey-Bass, San Francisco

Schulman L 1984 The skills of helping individuals and groups. E Peacock, Illinois

Solomon P 1992 Learning contracts in clinical education: evaluation by clinical supervisors. Medical Teacher 14(2/3): 205–210

Stephenson J, Laycock M 1993 Using learning contracts in higher education. Kogan Page, London

Tiberius R, Gaiptman B 1985 The supervisor – student ratio: 1:1 versus 1:2. Canadian Journal of Occupational Therapy 52(4): 179–183

Wallis M 1977 Aspects of management. British Journal of Occupational Therapy 40(11): 273–276

Glossaries

GLOSSARY OF OCCUPATIONAL THERAPY TERMS

Ability: a measure of the level of competence with which a skill is performed.

Action: the exertion of motivation into mental and physical effort, resulting in the creation of a tangible or intangible end product.

Activity: an activity is performed by an individual for a specific purpose on a particular occasion.

Activity analysis: involves breaking down an activity into sequences of component tasks and identifying the skills required to perform these tasks.

Activity synthesis: the process of combining different elements of activity and environment into an activity suitable for assessment or therapeutic intervention.

Adaptation: the process by which the individual adjusts to changes in his environment in a way that enables him to continue to function adequately.

Adaptive skill: a learned pattern of behaviour that assists the individual to function adequately within his environment.

Approach: ways and means of putting theory into practice.

Client-centred therapy: a method of intervention in which the client is helped to become aware of his own potential and of ways in which he can work towards realising it.

Cognition: faculty of knowing, understanding, perceiving and conceiving.

Competence: the ability to perform skills to a level that allows satisfactory performance of life roles.

Creative act: the final result of an individual's creative response and creative participation (de Witt P A 1992 Creative ability – a model for psychiatric occupational therapy. In: Crouch R B (ed) Occupational therapy in psychiatric and mental health. Lifecare Group, Johannesburg, pp 1–2).

Creative capacity: the creative potential which an individual has (de Witt 1992).

Creative participation: the process of being actively involved in all activities concerned with living (de Witt 1992).

Creative response: the positive attitude which an individual displays towards any opportunity which is offered (de Witt 1992).

Dysfunction: inability to maintain the self within the environment at a satisfactory standard because of lack of skills necessary for coping with the current situation.

Environment: the human and non-human surroundings of the individual, including objects, people, events, cultural influences, social norms and expectations.

Frame of reference: a system of theories, serving to orient or give particular meaning to a set of circumstances, which provides a coherent conceptual basis for therapeutic intervention.

Function: possession of the skills necessary for successful participation in the range of roles expected of the individual.

Health: the ability to function adequately in a balanced variety of roles, and achieve a sense of satisfaction from them.

Human development: the gradual evolution of the individual through a series of predictable stages to full growth.

Humanism: a system of beliefs and a theoretical approach that is concerned with what it means to become fully human.

Identity: sense of self; knowledge of one's own individuality.

Intrinsic motivation: an innate drive to use one's capacity for action.

Model: a simplified representation of the structure and content of a phenomenon or system that describes or explains the complex relationships between concepts within the system and integrates elements of theory and practice.

Motivation: the force that causes people to act.

Occupation: occupation defines and organises a sphere of action over a period of time and is perceived by the individual as part of his social identity.

Occupational behaviour: active engagement in occupation; 'the entire developmental continuum of work and play' (Reilly M 1969 The educational process. American Journal of Occupational Therapy 23(4): 299–307).

Occupational choice: a developmental process, extending over many years, through which people make the series of choices that lead to decisions about major occupations.

Occupational form: the sociocultural and physical characteristics of an occupation that exist independent of the person engaging in the occupation.

Occupational genesis: 'the evolving adaptive process in which humans engage in purposeful activities that are meaningful to their lives as their world and their experiences change' (Breines 1995).

Occupational performance: the actions of the individual elicited and guided by the occupational form.

Occupational role: the main social position held by an individual and the tasks performed in that position, for example, student, worker or volunteer.

Occupational science: 'an academic discipline, the purpose of which is to generate knowledge about the form, function, and the meaning of human occupation' (Zemke & Clark 1996).

Occupational therapy: the restoration or maintenance of optimal functional independence and life satisfaction through the analysis and use of selected occupations that enable the individual to develop the adaptive skills required to support his life roles.

Occupational therapy practice: the actions taken by the therapist to serve the need of the client for development of optimum function and independence.

Occupational therapy process: the series of steps by which professional philosophy, theory and content are translated into practice.

Personal causation: the individual's capacity to initiate action with the intent to affect the environment.

Philosophical assumptions: basic suppositions about the nature of living beings, the nature of the universe and the relationships between them, upon which we build our knowledge.

Play: a variety of occupations that constitute a pleasurable way of passing time and are also the medium through which a wide range of skills can be learned and rehearsed.

Potential: innate aptitude which is capable of development.

Process: a sequence of actions ordered for a particular purpose to achieve a result.

Professional philosophy: shared beliefs, assumptions and values that provide the profession with its sense of identity and exert control over theory and practice.

Quality: degree or standard of excellence; characteristic trait or attribute.

Quality assurance: a method of ensuring that a service consistently achieves client satisfaction.

Role: the set of expectations placed on an individual in a particular social context that become part of his identity and influence his behaviour. Each person plays a large number of roles, such as worker, parent, friend.

Self-care: occupation that enables the individual to survive and that promotes and maintains health, including mental health.

Skill: a performance component which evolves with practice.

Synthesis: combining separate elements together into an integrated whole.

Task: a constituent part of an activity.

Task analysis: identification of the tasks that are performed in sequence to make up an activity.

Therapeutic medium: any activity which is used to develop competence in skills that the individual can use to sustain a satisfactory range of life roles.

Value: internal guidelines for assessing worth, desirability or utility, which allow the individual to set priorities for action.

Volition: the ability to choose between alternative actions; exercise of the will. Or the inner condition of the organism that initiates or directs its behaviour towards a goal (Coleman 1969, in de Witt 1992).

Work: any productive activity, whether paid or unpaid, that contributes to the maintenance or advancement of society as well as the individual. The work in which an individual spends most time usually becomes both an occupation and a major social role.

GLOSSARY OF ETHICAL TERMS

Autonomy: literally, to be a law unto oneself (Greek *autos* = self, and *nomos* = law), but while 'being a law unto oneself' usually has derogatory connotations of lawlessness, it was introduced by Kant to emphasise that the responsible moral agent must internalise and make the moral law their own, and not merely act from some duty imposed on them by authority (heteronomy).

Beliefs: beliefs comprise the sub-set of attitudes for which we personally make truth claims and which we should therefore be prepared to defend – by producing sound reasons or evidence.

Code of conduct: a systematic collection of rules or regulations relating to official conduct which serves as the basis for the discipline of misconduct or fraud, etc.

Code of ethics: a general statement of fundamental principles, values and standards for behaviour, not necessarily having the force of disciplinary rules.

Common good: the public interest as defined by any moral community and serving as a focus for individual and collective action (cf acting *pro bono publico*).

Confidentiality: a duty of care (especially important in the consulting professions) not to disclose information that may be damaging to the interests of a client, whether or not the client has asked for the information to be kept secret.

Deontological ethics: (Greek *deon* = duty) a general approach to ethics, in which priority is given to fundamental principles and rules, rights and duties as defining what actions are unconditionally right or wrong.

Ethic: 'An ethic' refers to the 'belief-and-value system' of any moral community, or to the formal code of practice of a corporate body, or profession.

Ethics: In general, ethics (Greek *ethos*), means the spirit of a community. It refers to the formal cooperative endeavour of a moral community to define its values, the necessary conditions, practical requirements, and protective rules which will ensure its well-being and the flourishing of its members.

Mores: (Latin *mores* = manners or fashion): this term refers to the traditions or social customs that define one's social comportment or acceptable ways of relating to others, including rules of dress, manners, sexual conventions, court ceremonial and professional courtesies.

Norm/normative: (Latin *norma* = carpenter's square) a standard or scale by which we check, compare, or measure things, or assess people's performance and the consistency of their actions. A norm or standard allows degrees of comparison to be made (e.g. 'bad', 'worse', 'worst', or 'good', 'better', 'best') on a continuum where terms like 'good' and 'bad' mark the limits of the scale at either end.

Philosophy: philosophy is not just another science, but the activity of seeking to understand the fundamental presuppositions common to all sciences. It is reflective knowledge of knowledge, for example the critical consideration of the theoretical foundations of ethics as such.

Principle (moral): (Latin *principium* = a beginning or starting point) a statement of a basic and universal moral truth, or general moral requirement that serves as the starting point for further moral reasoning, and from which various duties and rights may be derived.

Rights: justified legal or moral entitlements which may be based on particular agreements (such as promises, bets, oaths, vows, covenants or contracts) or claimed universal entitlements of human beings as human beings (such as the rights embodied in the UNO *Universal Declaration of Human Rights*).

Rule: a statement of what can, should or ought to be done (or not done). A rule is a prescription which seeks to regulate or governs what we do. Rules define our duties, and are based on some source of 'legislative' authority (e.g. parents, church, school, government).

Teleological ethics: (Greek *telos* = end or goal) theories which focus on the goals or consequences of an action, to define whether actions are morally justifiable, rather than focusing on ethical principles or the means adopted to achieve the end. Teleological eudaimonism (cf Aristotle) argues that all human action aims towards some end and the tendency to seek our own happiness.

Utilitarianism: the theory, advocated in particular by Bentham and Mill, that the guiding principle for all conduct should be to achieve the greatest happiness for the greatest number, and that the criterion of the rightness or wrongness of an action is whether it is useful in furthering this goal (utility principle).

Values: while beliefs do not necessarily commit us to action, values do, for we stake our lives and our decisions on our choice of values as our chosen means to attain both our short- and long-term life goals. Values are based on beliefs, and may encourage us to change some inherited attitudes or cultivate others.

Index

swimming as therapy 220
systemic loss 530

T

task analysis 124, 125–128
teaching techniques 286–291
    attitude of therapist 286–287
    emotional skills 289–290
    learning environment 287
    methods 287–290
    styles of 568–569
team work *see* multidisciplinary team
technical influences
    transcultural psychiatry and 479
teleological theories 197
temporal adaptation 38
terminology, learning disability
    417–418
tests for older people, standardised
    384
theories of occupation 35–42
    balance 37–38
    behaviour 41
    biological sciences 42–43
    choice 41, 89
    classification 36–37
    definitions 35–36, 46
    developmental therapy 43–44
    framework for 47–48
    function of 36
    genesis 38–39
    physical medicine 44
    psychology 45
    psychiatry 45
    roles 39–40, 89
    sociology 45
therapeutic relationships 327
therapist
    core skills 74–75
    experience and skill 134
    interpersonal skills of 75–76
    personality 134
    reflective practice 134
    relationship with client 135
    staff availability 135
thought disorders 337
tic disorders 403
time sampling 107
timescale of loss and grief
    531–532
toys and play materials

constructive/latency/post-oedipal
    310
display and storage of 307
motor/anal/pre-oedipal 308–309
representational/phallic/oedipal
    309–310
sand and water 307
sensory/tactile/oral/narcissistic 308
types of 307–310
training, staff 13
    in rehabilitation setting 365–366
transcultural context, working in
    471–490
    assessment 483
    attitudes of occupational therapists
        488
    communication 482–483
    culture 472
    cultural competence 472
    multidisciplinary team 489
    outcome evaluation 487–488
    psychiatry *see* psychiatry,
        transcultural
    student training 488–489
    treatment implementation 484–487
    treatment planning 483–484
    see also multicultural society
treatment 80–81
    clients' right to 201–202
treatment implementation 129–137
    key elements of intervention 132–136
    motivation 129–132
treatment media for learning disability
    426–427
treatment planning 119–138
    activity adaptation 124–125,
        128–129
    activity analysis 125
    data analysis 120–121
    goal setting 121–124
    process 120
    task analysis 125–8
triangulation 62
Tuke, William 5
Twelve Steps Model 521, 522

U

urge surfing 524
USA, development of profession in
    7–8
Utilitarianism 197

V

validation 115–116
validation therapy 387
values 231
    assessment of 102–103
    related to goods 194
videotape records 142–143
virement 563
virtue ethics 197
volunteers to help old people 389

W

walking as therapy 221
ward in the community
    359–360
weather, effect of, on immigrants
    485
Wechsler Adult Intelligence Scale –
    Revised 229
well-being, factors promoting
    21–22
women's health promotion
    group 468
work 37
    rehabilitation 364–365
work activities in community
    care 450
work-based substance use 525
work programmes
    for learning disability 429
World Federation of Occupational
    Therapists 13

Y

Yoga as therapy 220–221
young people
    mental health 468–469

Z

zero-based budgeting 556–557